Springer Wien New York

Marc G. Jeschke, Lars-Peter Kamolz,
Folke Sjöberg, Steven E. Wolf *(editors)*

# Handbook of Burns

## Acute Burn Care

## Volume 1

SpringerWienNewYork

**Marc G. Jeschke, M.D., Ph.D.**
Sunnybrook Health Sciences Centre, Department of Surgery, Division of Plastic Surgery, University of Toronto, Sunnybrook Research Institute, Toronto, ON, Canada

**Lars-Peter Kamolz, M.D., M.Sc.**
Plastische, Aesthetische und Rekonstruktive Chirurgie, Landesklinikum Wiener Neustadt, Wiener Neustadt, Austria

**Folke Sjöberg, M.D., Ph.D.**
Department of Hand and Plastic Surgery and Intensive Care, Linköping University Hospital, and Department of Clinical and Experimental Medicine, Linköping University, Linköping, Sweden

**Steven E. Wolf, M.D.**
Brooke Army Medical Center, Fort Sam Houston, TX, USA

© 2012 Springer-Verlag/Wien
Printed in Austria

SpringerWienNewYork is part of
Springer Science+Business Media
springer.at

Typesetting: Jung Crossmedia Publishing GmbH, 35633 Lahnau, Germany
Printing: Holzhausen Druck GmbH, 1140 Wien, Austria

Printed on acid-free and chlorine-free bleached paper
SPIN: 12679065

With 95 (partly coloured) figures

Library of Congress Control Number:  2011943771

ISBN 978-3-7091-0347-0 SpringerWienNewYork

# Preface

Severe burn injuries are maybe not the most common injuries occurring on a daily basis however, it is estimated that within North America approximately 300,000–500,000 patients are hospitalized annually due to a burn related injury and that worldwide approximately 500,000–1,000,000 people die due to a burn related injury. Once a burn injury has occurred it is one of the most severe forms of any injury, inducing a complex cascade of various responses including inflammatory, hypermetabolic, immune, as well as infectious responses. These responses interact with each other and are extremely complex and difficult to treat. Specialized centers, protocolized treatment, multi-centre trials and close collaborations improved morbidity and mortality after severe burn injury over the last two decades. However, a vast morbidity and mortality post burn still occurs and represent one of the major problems in burn treatment.

One of the major characteristics of burn injury that has been evolving over the last 5 years is that a burn injury is not treated and healed once the wounds are healed. This used to be a landmark that no longer exists. Various studies have indicated that a burn injury and its pathphysiologic sequelae persist for at least 5-10 years, and not only in terms of scarring, infection, metabolism and the various other responses. Therefore this leads to the importance of the current two volumes of these burn books. It has been speculated and hypothesized that early intervention and alleviation of these detrimental responses benefit in terms of clinical outcomes, therefore the individual book chapters focus on the treatment and complexity of each of these responses to improve outcomes. The up to date chapters provide evidence based medicine and current state of the art treatments for any practitioner dealing with acute burn wounds, chronic burn wounds, and all other types of burn wounds. The second volume will then delineate the importance for long term treatment as it describes the reconstructive and alternative approaches of long term treatments post burn. Therefore the design of the two volume book was now to focus on early treatment as well as later treatment. This is unique and therefore will hopefully improve the outcome of burn patients by guiding various kinds of burn practitioners from nursing, physicians, occupational therapy, physical therapy, pharmacy and so forth. The focus of each chapter is not only to give an overview but also to focus current best treatments and to make it easy for each reader to easily access the treatment options and knowledge.

We hope that these books will raise as much enthusiasm as it has for the contributors of these books.

*Marc Jeschke, MD PhD FACS FRCSC*

# Contents

# List of contributers

**Gerard J. Abood, M.D.**
Stritch School of Medicine;
The Robert J. Freeark Professor Department of
Surgery
Burn and Shock Trauma Institute
Burn Center
Loyola University Medical Center
Maywood, IL, USA

**Benjamin Amis, M.D.**
Department of Orthopaedic Surgery
University of Washington
Seattle, WA, USA

**Harald Andel M.D., Ph.D., M.Sc.**
Department of Anaesthesie and General
Intensive Care
Medical University of Vienna
Vienna, Austria

**Anna Arno, M.D.**
Burn unit and Plastic Surgery Department
Vall d'Hebron University Hospital
Autonomous University of Barcelona
Barcelona, Spain

Ross Tilley Burn Centre
Sunnybrook Health Sciences Centre
Department of Surgery
Division of Plastic Surgery
University of Toronto
Toronto, ON, Canada

**Brett D. Arnoldo, M.D.**
UT Southwestern Medical Center
Dallas, TX, USA

**Joan Pere Barret, M.D.**
Val D'Hebron Hospital
Barcelona, Spain

**Mette M. Berger, M.D.**
Adult ICU and Burn Unit
University Hospital (CHUV)
Lausanne, Switzerland

**Ludwik K. Branski, M.D., M.M.S**
Department of Plastic, Hand and Reconstructive
Surgery
Hannover Medical School
Hannover, Germany

**David A. Brown, M.D.**
University of Washington
Department of Surgery
WA, USA

**Pavel Brychta, M.D., Ph.D.**
European Burns Association (EBA), President
Department of Burns and Reconstructive Surgery
University Hospital Brno
Czech Republic

**Kathryn L. Butler, M.D.**
Shriners Hospital for Children
Massachusetts General Hospital
Harvard Medical School
Boston, MA, USA

**Leopoldo C. Cancio, M.D., FACS**
USAISR
Ft. Sam Houston
TX, USA

**Roberto Cartotto M.D., FRCS(C)**
Ross Tilley Burn Centre at Sunnybrook
Health Sciences Centre
Department of Surgery
University of Toronto
Toronto, ON, Canada

**Amalia Cochran, M.D., FACS**
Burn-Trauma Center
University of Utah Health Center
Salt Lake City, UT, USA

**Manuel Dibildox, M.D.**
Ross Tilley Burn Centre
Sunnybrook Health Sciences Centre
Department of Surgery
Division of Plastic Surgery
University of Toronto
Toronto, ON, Canada

**DI(FH) Johannes Dirnberger**
Research Unit for Medical-Informatics
RISC Software GmbH
Johannes Kepler University Linz
Upper Austrian Research GmbH
Hagenberg, Austria

**Peter Dziewulski, M.D., Ph.D., FFICM FRCS
FRCS (Plast)**
St. Andrews Centre for Plastic Surgery and Burns
Chelmsford, Essex, UK

**Richard L. Gamelli, M.D., F.A.C.S.**
Stritch School of Medicine
The Robert J. Freeark Professor Department
of Surgery
Burn and Shock Trauma Institute
Burn Center
Loyola University Medical Center
Maywood, IL, USA

**Gerd G. Gauglitz, M.D.**
Department of Dermatology and Allergy
Ludwig Maximilians University
Munich, Germany

**Günter Germann, M.D., Ph.D.**
ETHIANUM, Clinic for Plastic,
Aesthetic & Preventive Medicine at Heidelberg
University Hospital
Heidelberg, Germany

**Nicole S. Gibran, M.D.**
Director, UW Burn Center
Professor, Department of Surgery
Harborview Medical Center,
Seattle, WA, USA

**Michael Giretzlehner, M.D.**
Research Unit for Medical-Informatics
RISC Software GmbH
Johannes Kepler University Linz
Upper Austrian Research GmbH
Hagenberg, Austria

**Richard Girtler, M.D.**
Abteilung für Anästhesie und Intensivmedizin
am Wilhelminenspital der Stadt Wien
Vienna, Austria

**Caran Graves, M.D.**
Burn-Trauma Center
University of Utah Health Center
Salt Lake City, UT, USA

**Burkhard Gustorff, M.D., Ph.D.**
Abteilung für Anästhesie und Intensivmedizin
am Wilhelminenspital der Stadt Wien
Vienna, Austria

**Herbert L. Haller, M.D.**
UKH Linz der AUVA
Linz, Austria

**Bernd Hartmann, M.D.**
Zentrum für Schwerbrandverletzte mit
Plastischer Chirurgie
Unfallkrankenhaus Berlin
Berlin, Germany

**John L. Hunt, M.D.**
UT Southwestern Medical Center
Dallas, TX, USA

**Mary Jako, M.D.**
Ross Tilley Burn Centre
Sunnybrook Health Sciences Centre
Department of Surgery
Division of Plastic Surgery
University of Toronto
Toronto, ON, Canada

**Marc G. Jeschke, M.D., Ph.D., FACS, FRCSC**
Ross Tilley Burn Centre
Sunnybrook Health Sciences Centre
Department of Surgery
Division of Plastic Surgery
University of Toronto
Toronto, ON, Canada

**Kunaal Jindal, M.D.**
Ross Tilley Burn Centre
Sunnybrook Health Sciences Centre
Department of Surgery
Division of Plastic Surgery
University of Toronto
Toronto, ON, Canada

**Lars-Peter Kamolz, M.D., Ph.D., M.Sc.**
Section of Plastic, Aesthetic and
Reconstructive Surgery
Department of Surgery
Landesklinikum Wiener Neustadt
Wiener Neustadt, Austria
Division of Plastic and Reconstructive Surgery
Department of Surgery
Medical University of Vienna
Vienna, Austria

**Maike Keck, M.D.**
Division of Plastic and Reconstructive Surgery
Department of Surgery
Medical University of Vienna
Vienna, Austria

**Matthew B. Klein, M.D., MS, FACS**
David and Nancy Auth-Washington
Research Foundation
Endowed Chair for Restorative Burn Surgery
Division of Plastic Surgery
University of Washington
Seattle, WA, USA

**Judy Knighton, M.D.**
Ross Tilley Burn Centre
Sunnybrook Health Sciences Centre
Department of Surgery
Division of Plastic Surgery
University of Toronto
Toronto, ON, Canada

**Leila Kolios, M.D.**
Clinic for Hand-, Plastic & Reconstructive Surgery
– Burn Center –
Clinic for Plastic and Hand Surgery at Heidelberg
University Hospital
BG Trauma Center Ludwigshafen
Ludwigshafen, Germany

**Paul Kraincuk, M.D.**
Universitätsklinik für Anästhesie
Allgemeine Intensivmedizin und Schmerztherapie
Vienna, Austria

**David B. Lumenta, M.D.**
Division of Plastic and Reconstructive Surgery
Department of Surgery
Medical University of Vienna
Vienna, Austria

**Jonathan B. Lundy, M.D.**
US Army Institute of Surgical Research
Fort Sam Houston
TX, USA

**Alexis McQuitty, M.D.**
Shriners Hospital for Children
Department of Anesthesiology
UTMB
Galveston, TX, USA

**Christian Ottomann, M.D.**
Plastische Chirurgie und Handchirurgie
Intensiveinheit für Schwerbrandverletzte
Universitätsklinikum Schleswig Holstein
Campus Lübeck, Germany

**DI Robert Owen, MSc.**
Research Unit for Medical-Informatics
RISC Software GmbH
Johannes Kepler University Linz
Upper Austrian Research GmbH
Hagenberg, Austria

**Tina L. Palmieri, M.D.**
University of California Davis Regional Medical Center
Shriners Hospital for Children Northern California
USA

**Michael D. Peck, M.D., Sc.D., FACS**
Arizona Burn Center
Maricopa Medical Center
Phoenix, AZ, USA

**Tam N. Pham, M.D.**
University of Washington Burn Center
Harborview Medical Center
Seattle, WA, USA

**Gary F. Purdue, M.D.**
UT Southwestern Medical Center
Dallas, TX, USA

**Jeffrey R. Saffle, M.D.**
Burn-Trauma Center
University of Utah Health Center
Salt Lake City, UT

**Shahriar Shahrokhi, M.D., FRCSC FACS**
Ross Tilley Burn Centre
Sunnybrook Health Sciences Centre
Department of Surgery
Division of Plastic Surgery
University of Toronto
Toronto, Canada

**Robert L. Sheridan, M.D.**
Shriners Hospital for Children
Massachusetts General Hospital
Harvard Medical School
Boston, MA, USA

**Edward Sherwood, M.D.**
Shriners Hospital for Children
Department of Anesthesiology
UTMB
Galveston, TX, USA

**David A. Sieber, M.D.**
Stritch School of Medicine
The Robert J. Freeark Professor Department of Surgery
Burn and Shock Trauma Institute
Burn Center
Loyola University Medical Center
Maywood, IL, USA

**Folke Sjöberg, M.D., Ph.D.**
Department of Hand and Plastic Surgery and
Intensive Care
Linköping University Hospital, and
Department of Clinical and Experimental Medicine
Linköping University
Linköping, Sweden

**Mark D. Talon, M.D.**
Shriners Hospital for Children
Department of Anesthesiology
UTMB
Galveston, TX, USA

**Jorge-Leon Villapalos, M.D., FRCS (Plast)**
Chelsea and Westminster Hospital Burns Service
London, UK

**Steven E. Wolf, M.D., FACS**
Professor and Vice Chairman for Research
Betty and Bob Kelso Distinguished Chair in Burn
and Trauma Surgery
University of Texas Health Science Center at San
Antonio
San Antonio, TX, USA

**Lee C. Woodson, M.D., PhD**
Shriners Hospital for Children
Department of Anesthesiology
UTMB
Galveston, TX, USA

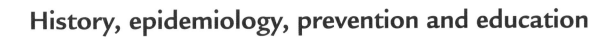

History, epidemiology, prevention and education

# A history of burn care

Leopoldo C. Cancio[1], Steven E. Wolf[2]

[1] MD, FACS, Colonel, Medical Corps, U. S. Army, Clinical Professor of Surgery, U. S. Army Institute of Surgical Research, Fort Sam Houston, TX, USA

[2] MD, FACS, Professor and Vice Chairman for Research, Betty and Bob Kelso Distinguished Chair in Burn and Trauma Surgery, University of Texas Health Science Center at San Antonio, San Antonio, TX, USA

*The opinions or assertions contained herein are the private views of the authors, and are not to be construed as official or as reflecting the views of the Department of the Army or the Department of Defense.*

## "Black sheep in surgical wards"

If one uses the incontrovertible index of postburn mortality, it is evident that our ability to care for burn patients has improved markedly since World War II. This can be quantified by the lethal area 50% (that burn size which is lethal for 50% of a population), which in the immediate postwar era was approximately 40% of the total body surface area (TBSA) for young adults in the U. S., whereas it increased to approximately 80% TBSA by the 1990s [1]. Furthermore, the mortality rate at the Galveston Shrine for children with 80% TBSA or greater (mean 70% full-thickness burn size) during 1982–96 was only 33% [2]. What has been responsible for these improved outcomes in burn care? What practices were essential to this growth, and what are the major problems that remain unsolved? In this chapter, we will take as our focal point the fire disaster at the Cocoanut Grove Night Club which took place in Boston in 1942, less than a year after Pearl Harbor. The response to that disaster, and the monograph written in its aftermath, serves as a useful benchmark for the burn care advances which followed. To fully appreciate those advances, however, we must go back in time to an earlier era.

A wide variety of therapies for burns have been described since ancient times [3], but the idea of collecting burn patients in a special place is relatively new, and emerged in Scotland during the 19th century. James Syme established the first burn unit in Edinburgh in 1843. He argued that mixing burn patients with postoperative patients would make him "chargeable with the highest degree of culpable recklessness." This logic motivated the Edinburgh Royal Infirmary leadership to set aside the former High School Janitor's House for burn patients. This experiment was relatively short-lived, however, since burn patients were transferred to one of the "Sheds" in 1848 to make way for an increased number of mechanical trauma casualties from railway accidents [4].

Another Scottish hospital, the Glasgow Royal Infirmary, had by 1933 accumulated 100 years of experience with over 10,000 burn patients, having established a separate burn ward midway through that period in 1883. In Dunbar's report on these patients, he commented:

> *Burn cases have until recently been looked upon as black sheep in surgical wards, and have been almost entirely treated by junior members of the staff, who have not had any great clinical experience from which to judge their results (…) In the pre-antiseptic era only the worst burns would come to the hospital. The state of the hospitals was well known to the public, who also knew that a burn of slight or moderate severity had a better chance of recovery at home.*

He documented the steady rise in the number of admissions to this hospital, a biphasic mortality pattern (with the highest number of deaths between postburn hours 12 and 24), the high incidence of streptococcal wound infection, the infrequency of skin grafting, and a frustratingly high mortality rate of 20–30% despite the introduction of antisepsis [5].

## Toxaemia, plasmarrhea, or infection?

Against this background, the founders of modern burn care must be credited with considerable clinical courage and intellectual foresight. Although the era of growth which they introduced is often dated to World War II, its roots were in earlier fire disasters and in World War I. This period featured a debate about the cause of postburn death and accordingly the appropriate treatment. A prevailing theory attributed death to the release of toxic substances from the burn wound: "The reaction of the body to a burn strongly resembles the clinical state described by the term 'toxaemia,' which implies the presence in the circulation of some toxic agent. The more serious cases usually present early in the course a clinical picture commonly described by such terms as shock or exhaustion." [6]. Treatments were widely employed to prevent this from happening. The most important such treatment was tannic acid, popularized by Davidson in 1925 [6]. Tanning of eschar, or of animal leather, involves collagen cross-linking and the formation of lipid-protein complexes in the remaining dermis. This generates a brown, supple, leather-like eschar [7]. Davidson asserted ambitiously that tannic acid not only lessens toxemia, but also provides analgesia, prevents loss of body fluid, limits infection, decreases scar formation, and generates a scaffold for healing [6].

By contrast, in 1930 Frank Underhill published seminal observations on the pathophysiology of burn shock based on experience gained following the Rialto Theater fire of 1921 in New Haven, CN. These included the concepts of "anhydremia" and "hemoconcentration". Here is his description:

*When loss of water from the blood becomes great, the circulatory deficiency becomes magnified. The thick, sticky blood . . . finds great difficulty in passing through the capillaries . . . the blood is quickly robbed of its oxygen by the tissues . . . the tissues in general suffer from inadequate oxygenation . . . the heart pumps only a portion of its normal volume at each stroke [8].*

Underhill then points out that his thinking on this process began during World War I, when he noted that inhalation of chemical warfare agents (chlorine, phosgene, and chlorpicrin) produced both massive pulmonary edema and hemoconcentration. Applying this concept to thermally injured skin led to our basic understanding of burn shock: "fluid rushes to the burned skin with great rapidity and is lost to the body . . . or the part affected becomes edematous with great celerity." The fluid lost is similar to plasma–implying increased capillary permeability–whereas in cholera it is a dilute salt solution. Measurement of the blood hemoglobin percentage is proposed as an index of resuscitation, and resuscitation aimed at preventing hemoconcentration is required for 24–36 hours postburn. Intravenous sodium chloride solutions should be used, supplemented by oral, rectal, and subdermal solutions [8].

In 1931, Alfred Blalock reported laboratory confirmation of Underhill's theory. Dogs underwent burns to one third of the body surface area, limited to one side of the body. After death, animals were sagittally bisected, and the difference in weight between the halves was estimated to be the amount of fluid lost into the tissues as a consequence of injury. This weight difference was on average 3.34% of the initial total body weight, indicating a loss of approximately one half of the circulating plasma volume. He also noted that the fluids collected in the subcutaneous tissues had a protein concentration similar to that of plasma, and that the blood hemoglobin content increased markedly [9].

But plasma loss was an incomplete description of the biphasic death pattern documented for burn patients. Shortly thereafter, Aldrich introduced the treatment of burn wounds with gentian violet, a coal-tar derivative which kills Gram-positive organisms. He argued against the toxemia theory, and attributed postburn toxic symptoms not to the eschar, but to streptococcal wound infection. Early use of gentian violet would prevent this, whereas tannic acid did not. He distinguished this delayed infectious process from "primary shock", downplaying the latter's importance: "it is sufficient to say that if it is combated early and adequately, with heat, rest, fluids, and stimulants, it can be overcome in the majority." [10].

## The Guinea Pig Club

The transformation of burn care required not only the above observations, but also an institutional commitment. In 1916, Sir Harold Gillies returned from service in France to lead the first plastic and oral-maxillofacial surgery service in the UK at Cambridge Military Hospital, Aldershot, later moving to Queen's Hospital in Sidcup, Kent. Gillies and team treated over 11,000 casualties with facial injuries by the end of the war, to include burns [11, 12]. The Spanish Civil War (1936–9) convinced the British leadership that the next war would involve air combat, and asked Gillies to establish plastic surgery units around London [12]. At that time, there were only 4 plastic surgeons in the country, including Gillies' cousin, Sir Archibald McIndoe, who had joined Gillies in 1930 after training at the Mayo Clinic [13]. During 1939, McIndoe established the burn unit for the Royal Air Force at East Grinstead, UK, which persists to this day. Beginning in summer 1940, approximately 400 RAF personnel (mainly fighter pilots) were seriously burned during the Battle of Britain, revealing both aircraft design limitations and the intensity of aerial combat. The focus of the new unit was on the reconstruction and rehabilitation of these patients. McIndoe assembled a team of nurses, anesthetists, microbiologists, orderlies, and others to undertake this journey into the unknown:

> *Historically there was little to guide one in this field apart from the general principles of repair perfected by British, Continental and American surgeons. There had until then been no substantial series of cases published and none in which a rational plan of repair had been proposed. At most, individual cases appeared . . . in which only too often the end result seemed to convert the pathetic into the ridiculous. [13]*

Soon, 4 more units were established in the UK, which together with East Grinstead served the hundreds of casualties who followed from operations such as Royal Air Force's strategic bombing campaign.

McIndoe's work underscores several important points about burn care. First, the impetus for a breakthrough in the organization and delivery of burn care was the catastrophic nature of modern warfare, the large number of casualties therefrom, and both a national and an individual commitment to care for these casualties. Second, the experimental nature of burn care was recognized, and a scientific approach based on clinical evidence was espoused. Among the East Grinstead unit's contributions were the condemnation of tannic acid as coagulation therapy for acute burn wounds; perfection and description of a methodology for burn wound reconstruction; and, in collaboration with Leonard Colebrook (see below), early experience with penicillin therapy for Gram-positive infections. Third, the East Grinstead unit became a hub for new UK burn units, as well as a training center for scores of surgeons and nurses in the principles of the emerging specialty. Fourth, the psychological and social needs of the patients were highlighted. At East Grinstead, this was embodied in the "Guinea Pig Club," a social network for burn survivors whose membership totaled 649 people. The longevity of both the needs of burn survivors, and the strength of this network, is exemplified that the last issue of *The Guinea Pig* magazine was published in 2003 [13]. Clearly, none of these steps–the scientific approach to improving burn care, the emphasis on clinical expertise on the part of all members of the multidisciplinary team, and the creation of a mechanism for effective psychosocial support–would have been possible without the concentration of patients at a center dedicated to overcoming a seemingly insurmountable problem.

The origin of infection control in burn patients, however, belongs not to McIndoe but to Leonard Colebrook, a physician, bacteriologist, and colleague of Alexander Fleming [14]. In an era dominated by multidrug-resistant gram-negative and methicillin-resistant *Staphylococcus aureus* infections, it is important to recall the major role played by *Streptococcus pyogenes* infections before the introduction of antibiotics. Colebrook confirmed Domagk's 1935 "startling success" on the efficacy of the sulfanilamide parent drug, Prontosil, using a murine model of streptococcal peritonitis, and reported lifesaving treatment of 38 patients with puerperal fever [15, 16]. Turning his attention to burns at the Glasgow Royal

Infirmary, he studied dressings impregnated with sulfanilamide and penicillin creams [14, 17] and the use of serum and plasma for burn shock resuscitation [18]. (The problem of Gram-negative burn wound infection remained to be recognized and solved at another time, since "coliform bacilli, *B. proteus* and *Ps. pyocyanea*, when present in the wounds, were apparently not affected" by these drugs.) [17]. He then established a new burn unit at the Birmingham Accident Hospital [19]. In contrast to the toxemia theory, Colebrook and others proposed that that burn wounds became infected with bacteria and that strict infection control practices could prevent infection by reducing transfer of these organisms; these concepts were incorporated into both the design and practices of the new burn unit [20, 21].

## Burns and sulfa drugs at Pearl Harbor

In the U. S., the attack on Pearl Harbor on 7 December 1941 served a function similar to that of the Battle of Britain by energizing burn care research. Fortuitously, the U. S., anticipating the likelihood of war, had already made two major national commitments to supporting medical research of military relevance. The first such effort was the creation by the National Research Council's (NRC) Division of Medical Sciences of Advisory Committees to the Surgeons General in April 1940 [22]. Critical among these for the burn care in the U. S. were the Committee on Chemotherapeutic and Other Agents, and the Committee on Surgery (which included, among others, Subcommittees on Surgical Infections and on Burns).

The second such effort was the creation by the federal government of the Committee on Medical Research (CMR) of the Office of Scientific Research and Development (OSRD) in June 1941 [23, 24]. The purpose of the CMR was to identify problems of military medical importance and to fund university research to solve these problems. These two activities (the NRC Advisory Committees and the CMR) were collocated at NRC headquarters, and the NRC advised the CMR on how best to expend federal funds [22]. In brief, by the time of Pearl Harbor the U. S. had the framework in place for academic, military, and federal collaboration in pursuit of solutions for combat casualty care.

For the NRC and the CMR, Pearl Harbor highlighted the importance of burns in modern warfare. About 60 percent of the over 500 casualties admitted to the Pearl Harbor Naval Hospital were thermally injured. Many of these wounds were contaminated by fuel oil or complicated by fragment injuries. Care was variable, and included some sort of topical tanning agent, delayed debridement, infusion of available intravenous fluids, and treatment of fractures [25]. "At the Naval Hospital, ordinary flit guns were used to spray tannic acid solution upon the burned surfaces," indicating the persistence of the toxemia theory in clinical care. On the other hand, both plasma and saline solution were used for fluid resuscitation, and sulfa drugs were given to patients with infected wounds–indicating a conglomeration of the competing theories of burn pathophysiology. In response to Pearl Harbor, the NRC rapidly dispatched Perrin Long, the chairman of the Committee on Chemotherapeutic and Other Agents, and surgeon I. S. Ravdin to Hawaii, in order to evaluate the use of sulfa drugs and other aspects of care. They submitted their report to the War Department on 18 January 1942, emphasizing the lifesaving characteristics of sulfa drug use and the value of plasma for resuscitation:

*We have been impressed again and again with the incalculable value of sulfonamide therapy in the care of many of the casualties . . . We believe that it is highly important that physicians–both civilian and military–become familiar with the general and specific considerations which govern the oral and local use of the sulfonamides in the treatment of wounds and burns . . . [25, 26].*

Despite this impression and the fact that the sulfa drugs were the only antibiotics available in significant quantities in 1941, their indications and limitations were unknown. Accordingly, the Subcommittee on Surgical Infections, chaired by Frank Meleney, defined this question as a major objective at its initial meeting in June 1940 [22]. Wound study units were set up at 8 U. S. hospitals and a multicenter trial was conducted of both local and systemic sulfa use. Meleney, in his report on this study, lamented that

*The original plan was altered to a considerable extent by the reports which came back from Pearl*

*Harbor. Observers who saw the casualties there were profoundly impressed by the low incidence of wound infection, which they believed to be due to the copious application of sulfanilamide to the wounds. Our original plan called for observation on control cases without drugs and other controls receiving treatment with local bacteriostatic agents other than the sulfonamides. But, said the Pearl Harbor observers: "You cannot withhold from these patients the benefit of the sulfonamide drugs." [27]*

By the end of 1942, 1,500 patients (with soft tissue injuries, fractures, and burns) had been enrolled. In his report on this study, Meleney concluded that neither local nor systemic sulfonamides were effective at controlling local wound infection, and that inadequate surgical treatment predisposed to infection. The antibiotics were effective at preventing systemic sepsis, but were not a panacea [27]. An awareness of these limitations, and emerging experience with *Staphylococcus* and *Clostridium* resistance to sulfa drugs [22], set the stage for research on penicillin.

## Penicillin and the burn projects

Although Alexander Fleming discovered penicillin in 1929, its clinical utility was not appreciated until 10 years later, when Howard W. Florey, Ernest Chain, and others (the "Oxford Team") performed murine and human experiments demonstrating the new drug's lifesaving potential against *Streptococcus*, *Staphylococcus*, and *Clostridium* infections [28, 29]. Since British pharmaceutical firms were overwhelmed with wartime production of other drugs, Florey went to the U.S. in summer 1941 to obtain support for large-scale manufacturing, ultimately meeting with and convincing the chairman of the CMR, Alfred N. Richards [24]. Once a method of mass-producing the drug had been developed, the CMR turned in January 1942 to the Committee on Chemotherapeutic and Other Agents, headed by Perrin Long, for help in organizing clinical trials [30]. Long appointed Champ Lyons at the Massachusetts General Hospital (MGH), Chester Keefer, and colleagues to accomplish this [30]. This was the origin of

one of the two burn-related research programs in place at the MGH at the time of the Cocoanut Grove fire in 1942 [31].

The second MGH research program dealt specifically with thermal injury [31]. On 7 January 1942, the NRC sponsored a pivotal conference on burns, chaired by I. S. Ravdin [32, 33]. The conference proceedings recommended plasma, topical tannic acid, and oral sulfadiazine. Henry Harkins presented the available formulas for resuscitation of burn patients. His own method (the "Method of Harkins") was based on hemoconcentration: give 100 cc of plasma for each point that the hematocrit exceeds 45. For wartime, when lab facilities are unavailable, he recommended the "First Aid Method": slowly give 500 cc of plasma for each 10 percent of the total body surface area (TBSA) burned [34, 35]. The latter is the first formula based on TBSA. The NRC report from the conference advocated 1000 cc of plasma for each 10 percent TBSA over the first 24 hours, in divided doses [32].

The Subcommittee on Burns was organized under Allen Whipple in July 1942 [22], and was charged with determining the best therapies for acute burns and whether tanning was appropriate. The wound study units of the Subcommittee on Surgical Infections were finding that tanned burns had a high wound infection rate, and the Subcommittee on Burns soon recommended against use or further procurement of tannic acid in October 1942–less than one year after it was liberally used at Pearl Harbor. Nevertheless, "it cannot be said that unanimous agreement was ever attained on the choice of the best local agent." [22]. Another early contribution by Whipple was stating for the first time the importance of well-organized 'burn teams':

*By burn team we mean a group made up of a general surgeon, interested in problems of infection and wound healing, a physician or technician, thoroughly trained in problems of fluid, protein and electrolyte imbalance, a general plastic surgeon... with experience in skin grafting large granulating areas, a group of trained nurses and orderlies, able and willing to stand the stress and strain of caring for severely burned patients [36].*

## The Cocoanut Grove fire of 1942, and beyond

The fire at the Cocoanut Grove (CG) nightclub in Boston, MA on 28 November 1942 was one of the worst civilian fire disasters in U. S. history, killing 492 of the estimated 1000 occupants [37]. Oliver Cope, editing the monograph published on the MGH's response, felt that they were well prepared in large part because of the war:

> Had such a catastrophe taken place before Pearl Harbor, the hospital would have been swamped. As it was, the injured found the staff prepared, for the war had made us catastrophe minded. (...) A plan of therapy for burns, suited to use in a catastrophe, was developed and decided upon. When the victims of the Cocoanut Grove fire arrived, the treatment was ready and it was applied to all. [31]

Specific preparations for war that were already in place at the time of this fire included organization of personnel, publication of a disaster manual, preparation of sterile supplies for 200 operations, acquisition of wooden i. v. poles and of saw horses to support stretchers, establishment of a blood bank, and training of Red Cross volunteers and of Harvard students as orderlies [38].

The CG monograph contains the first detailed description of a scientific approach to multidisciplinary burn care [37]. As such, it serves as an invaluable point of departure for understanding subsequent changes and current practice.

### Burn center concept

Although the MGH did not have a dedicated burn unit in 1942, the 39 CG patients were all hospitalized on a single ward. "In a disaster of this type, where the injuries were all of the same kind, the importance of concentration of casualties in one group in one ward or floor where they can be under concentrated medical treatment and where isolation procedures can be set up if needed, was clearly demonstrated." [39] The first permanent unit in the U. S. was established in Richmond, VA by Everett Evans, who had become chairman of the NRC Committee on Burns [40]. In

1947, the Army Wound Study Unit was moved from Halloran General Hospital to Fort Sam Houston, Texas by Edwin Pulaski–an Army surgeon who had trained under Meleney–and renamed the Surgical Research Unit (SRU) [41]. At that unit, patients with infected burns and other wounds were treated on a special ward at the U. S. Army's Brooke General Hospital. Two years later, growing concerns about the possibility of nuclear war with the Soviet Union, and recognition that such a war would generate thousands of burn survivors, refocused the SRU to the treatment of burns, and the second U. S. burn unit was formally established [40].

The U. S. Army Burn Center at the SRU (later renamed as the U. S. Army Institute of Surgical Research, USAISR) was at the forefront of many of the advances in burn care described below. Also critical for improving care in the U. S. was the unit's commitment to training surgeons, many of whom became directors of civilian burn centers [42–44]. Designation of the unit as the single destination for all U. S. military burn casualties, as well as for civilians in the region, provided the number of patients needed both to maintain clinical competence and to support the research mission during war and peace. Another major factor in the development of burn care in the U. S. was the decision in 1962 by the Shriners Hospitals for Crippled Children privately to fund the construction and operation of 3 pediatric burn units– in Cincinnati, Ohio; Boston, Massachusetts; and Galveston, Texas. These units opened during 1966–8, and like the U. S. Army Burn Center, became centers of excellence in care, teaching, and research [45, 46].

### Shock and resuscitation

The MGH used a version of the NRC First Aid Formula for resuscitation of the CG casualties. All but 10 patients were given plasma intravenously.

The initial dosage of plasma was determined on the basis of the surface area of the burns. For each 10 percent of the body surface involved, it was planned to give 500 cc in the first 24 hours. Because the plasma delivered by the Blood Bank during the first 36 hours was diluted with an equal volume of physiologic saline solution, the patient was to receive 1000 cc of fluid for each 10 percent burned. The plasma dosage was modified subsequently on the basis of repeated hematocrit and serum protein determinations [47].

Cope and Moore, in a follow-on paper in 1947, described a refinement of the NRC formula called the Surface Area Formula: 75 ml of plasma and 75 ml of isotonic crystalloid solution per TBSA, with one-half given over the first 8 hours, and one-half over the second 16 hours. The urine output was to be used as the primary index of resuscitation [33]. Subsequent revisions of this basic concept included the following formulas:

▶ **Evans Formula:** incorporation of body weight; colloid 1 ml/kg/TBSA and crystalloid 1 ml/kg/TBSA [48]
▶ **Brooke Formula:** decrease in colloid content to 0.5 ml/kg/TBSA, with crystalloid 1.5 ml/kg/TBSA; replacement of plasma with 5% albumin because of hepatitis risk [49]
▶ **Parkland Formula:** elimination of colloid; increase in crystalloid to 4 ml/kg/TBSA [50]
▶ **Modified Brooke Formula:** elimination of colloid during first 24 hours; crystalloid 2 ml/kg/TBSA [51]

Despite their differences, employment of these formulas reduced early deaths due to burn shock to about 13% of postburn deaths, and made acute renal failure due to burn shock distinctly unusual. Today, the hazards of "fluid creep" mandate a continued search for an approach to resuscitation that decreases the rate of edema formation [52, 53].

## Wound care and infection

By the time of the CG fire, tannic acid had fallen into disfavor: "A bland, protective ointment dressing is indicated in the treatment of skin burns since the chemical agents currently recommended are believed to be injurious to otherwise viable epithelium and delay wound healing." [54]. Attention turned to use of i. v. antibiotics for prevention of infection. Hemolytic streptococcal infection responded to sulfa drugs: "an effective blood level of sulfonamide offers the most certain control of systemic infection due to the hemolytic streptococcus." [55]. Meanwhile, Champ Lyons, the surgeon in charge of penicillin research at MGH, received enough of the experimental drug from Chester Keefer to treat 13 CG patients. The

doses given were too low and the experience was inconclusive, although he did not observe toxic side effects [55]. From there, Lyons undertook larger studies of penicillin at Bushnell General Hospital, Brigham City, Utah (April 1943) and at a new Wound Study Unit at Halloran General Hospital, Staten Island, New York (June 1943) [56, 57]; the latter was the forerunner of the U. S. Army SRU. These studies constituted the first large-scale studies of penicillin, documented efficacy against staphylococcal and streptococcal combat wound infections [57], and convinced the Army of the need for large-scale production of the drug [24]. Lyons next obtained a commission as an Army Major in August 1943, deploying to the North African theater to facilitate the introduction of penicillin into battlefield care under Edward Churchill [56].

Penicillin, however, was only a partial answer to the problem of late postburn death. In 1954, the SRU noted that effective fluid resuscitation now kept many patients with greater than 50% TBSA burns alive past the 2-day mark, only to succumb at a later date [58]. The conquest of hemolytic *Streptococcus* now revealed the role of Gram-negative organisms, and the presence of positive blood cultures, particularly in patients with large full-thickness burns, pointed at bacteremia of burn-wound origin [58]. The natural history of this "burn wound sepsis" was not clear, however, until a model of invasive *Pseudomonas* burn-wound infection in rats was conceived and characterized by Walker and Mason at the SRU [59–61]. At that time, however, no effective topic or intravenous therapy had been identified.

Pruitt et al. at the SRU achieved a dramatic improvement in postburn mortality in 1964, with the introduction into clinical care of a topical antimicrobial effective against Gram-negative burn wound infection, mafenide acetate (Sulfamylon) cream [62]. This drug had been first synthesized in the 1930s and evaluated by Domagk, but abandoned, interestingly, because of lack of efficacy against *Streptococcus* [63]. It was rediscovered by U. S. Army researchers at Edgewood Arsenal, who demonstrated efficacy in an otherwise lethal caprine model of *Clostridium perfringens* infection following extremity blast injury [64]. Because it penetrates deeply, it appeared particularly effective in wounds with devitalized tissue, a feature which also made it attractive for the treatment of full-thickness burns. Lindberg et al. at the SRU had similar success in the Walker-Mason *Pseudomonas* model [65]. In thermally injured patients, death from invasive burn wound infection declined from 59% (pre-mafenide) to 10% (post-mafenide) [62]. Meanwhile, Moyer and Monafo confirmed the effectiveness of 0.5% silver nitrate soaks in preventing burn-wound infection [66]. Charles Fox subsequently developed silver sulfadiazine to combine the advantages of a sulfonamide with the silver ion [67]. Silver sulfadiazine, the recently developed silver-impregnated fabrics [68], and mafenide acetate are the commonly employed antimicrobials used in burn care today.

*Burn surgery*

Surgeons accustomed to early excision of the burn wound should bear in mind that at the time of the CG fire, burn surgery was performed after the separation of eschar: "The first graft was applied on the twenty-third day... and the last at four months to several small areas" [69]. Originally, the surgical treatment of burn wounds, if performed, was limited to contracture release and reconstruction after the wound had healed by scar formation. In patients with larger wounds or burns of functional areas, this was wholly unsatisfactory. The creation of burn units committed to care for these patients led to the development of more effective techniques for wound closure. Artz noted that one should "wait until natural sequestration has occurred and a good granulating barrier has formed beneath the eschar... After removing the eschar... skin grafting should be performed as soon as the granulating surface is properly prepared [70]. Debridement to the point of bleeding or pain during daily immersion hydrotherapy (Hubbard tanks) was used to facilitate separation of the eschar [71]. Then, cadaver cutaneous allografts (homografts) were often used to prepare the granulating wound bed for autografting [72].

In patients with larger (>50% TBSA) burns and in the absence of topical antimicrobials, this cautious approach did not prevent death from invasive burn wound infection, leading some to propose a more radical solution: that of primary excision of the burn wound. Surgeons at the SRU suggested that a "heroic" practice of early excision, starting postburn

day 4, should be considered for patients with large burns. This would reduce the "large pabulum" of dead tissue available for microbial proliferation; immediate coverage with a combination of autograft and cadaver allograft would further protect the wound [61]. Several authors during the 1950s and 1960s demonstrated the feasibility of this approach, but not an improvement in mortality [73].

In 1968, Janzekovic described the technique of tangential primary excision of the burn wound with immediate grafting; operating in post-war Yugoslavia, she recalled that "a barber's razor sharpened on a strap was the pearl among our instruments." [74, 75] In a retrospective study, Tompkins et al. reported an improvement in mortality over the course of 1974–84 which they attributed to excision [76]. William F. McManus and colleagues at the Army Burn Center compared patients who underwent excision with those who did not during 1983–5, noting that an improvement in mortality could not be attributed to excision because preexisting organ failure precluded surgery in many unexcised patients. However, only 6 of the 93 patients (6.5%) who died in this study had invasive bacterial burn wound infection, whereas 54 of the 93 (58%) had pneumonia–indicating a shift from wound to non-wound infections [77].

In McManus' study, excision was performed a mean of 13 days postburn. By contrast, David Herndon et al. at Galveston implemented a method of excision within 48–72 hours of admission, which relied on widely meshed (4:1) autograft covered by allograft. In a small study of children during 1977–81, these authors noted a decrease in length of stay but not in mortality with this technique [78]. During 1982–5, adults were randomized to undergo early excision, vs. excision after eschar separation 3 weeks later. Young adults without inhalation injury and with burns >30% TBSA showed an improvement in mortality [79]. A recent metaanalysis found a decrease in mortality but an increase in blood use in early excision patients without inhalation injury [80].

Despite the limitations of the early studies, early excision is today performed in most U. S. burn centers – controversy remains about the definition of "early" and the feasibility of performing radical, total excision at one operation, especially in adults. We now understand excision and definitive closure of the burn wound as fundamental for patients with massive injuries; the "race" to achieve this before sepsis and other causes of organ failure supervene is the main effort; patients whose grafts fail repeatedly ("wound failure") will not, in the authors' experience, survive. To facilitate massive excision for patients with the largest wounds and limited donor sites, new methods of temporary and permanent closure have been sought. Burke and Yannas developed the first successful dermal regeneration template (Integra®), composed of a dermal analog (collagen and chondroitin-6-sulfate) and a temporary epidermal analog (Silastic) [81]. Cultured epidermal autografts provide material for wound closure for patients with the most extensive burns, although the cost is high and final take rates are variable [82–84]. The ultimate goal of an off-the-shelf bilaminar product for permanent wound closure, with a take rate similar to that of cutaneous autografts, has not yet been achieved.

### Inhalation injury and pulmonary care

Pulmonary problems were a significant cause of mortality after the CG fire, and options for diagnosis and treatment were limited. 114 patients were brought to the MGH, some alive, some dead; it is clear that many of these casualties died of carbon monoxide poisoning or early airway obstruction. Of the 39 patients who survived long enough to be admitted, 7 died, all of whom had evidence of inhalation injury. The authors noted: "Although intubation and tracheotomy were not highly successful in our cases, we believe that they fulfill a definite function in relieving labored breathing and in facilitating the delivery of oxygen, and should be resorted to in patients with acute cyanosis and in those with severe upper respiratory lesions." On the other hand, "the resuscitation of patients in acute attacks of edema was difficult and unsatisfactory" and "the pulmonary complications were bizarre and characterized by extreme variability, with areas of lung collapse and emphysema..." [85].

Subsequent improvements in inhalation injury required the development of positive-pressure mechanical ventilators. Forrest Bird, V. R. Bennett, and J. Emerson built mechanical positive-pressure venti-

lators towards the end of WWII, all inspired by technology developed during the war to deliver oxygen to pilots flying at high altitudes [86]. The availability of these and similar machines, and the Scandinavian polio epidemic of 1952, spurred the creation of separate intensive care units (ICUs) within hospitals [87]. Today, in one model of burn care, burn units are separate from ICUs, and the two types of units are run by different personnel. At the U. S. Army Burn Center and several other centers, by contrast, ICU beds have been located within the burn unit and have been directed by surgeon-intensivists–ensuring continuity of multidisciplinary care and of clinical research.

Once accurate diagnosis of inhalation injury by bronchoscopy and xenon-133 lung scanning became available, it was apparent that smoke-injured patients had greatly increased risk of pneumonia and death [88]. Large animal models were developed and the pathophysiology of the injury was defined [89, 90]. Unlike ARDS due to mechanical trauma or alveolar injury due to inhalation of chemical warfare agents, smoke inhalation injury was found to damage the small airways, with resultant ventilation-perfusion mismatch, bronchiolar obstruction, and pneumonia [91]. This process featured activation of the inflammatory cascade, which in animal models was amenable to modulation by various anti-inflammatory agents [92]. Practically, however, the most effective interventions to date have been those directly aimed at maintaining small airway patency and at avoiding injurious forms of mechanical ventilation. These include high-frequency percussive ventilation with the Volumetric Diffusive Respiration ventilator developed by Bird [93], and delivery of heparin by nebulization [94].

### Nutrition and the "Universal Trauma Model"

Bradford Cannon described the nutritional management of the survivors of the Cocoanut Grove fire: "All patients were given a high protein and high vitamin diet... it was necessary to feed [one patient] by stomach tube with supplemental daily intravenous amogen, glucose, and vitamins." [69] But it soon became apparent that survivors of major thermal injury evidenced a hypermetabolic, hypercatabolic state which lasted at least until the wounds were closed, and often resulted in severe loss of lean body mass.

Burns thus epitomize what David Cuthbertson, summarizing work done with orthopedic injuries, identified as the biphasic response to injury: an initial "ebb" period (shock) was followed by a longer "flow" period (inflammation) [95]. Thus, burns constitute "the universal trauma model," as described by Dr. Pruitt in the 1984 Scudder Oration on Trauma:

*The burn patient in whom a local injury (the severity of which can be readily and reproducibly quantified) evokes a global systemic response (the magnitude and duration of which are proportional to the extent of injury) meets the criteria for a useful clinical model (…) Among all trauma patients, the burn patient should perhaps be regarded as a metabolic caricature, since the metabolic rate in patients with burns of more than 50 percent of the body surface exceeds that encountered in any other group of patients.*

Cope et al. reported measurements of metabolic rate of up to 180% of normal in the early postburn period, ruled out thyrotoxicosis as an etiology, and recognized a relationship between wound size and metabolic rate [96]. Wilmore et al. identified the role of catecholamines as mediators of the postburn hypermetabolic state [97]. Wilmore et al. also demonstrated the feasibility of providing massive amounts of calories by a combination of intravenous and enteral alimentation [98]. Curreri published the first burn-specific formula for estimating caloric requirements: calories/day = 25(wt in kg) + 40(TBSA) [99]. Provision of adequate calories and nitrogen failed to arrest hypermetabolism and reduced, but did not eliminate, erosion of lean body mass in these patients. Three approaches have recently been taken to address this problem with modest success: use of anabolic steroids such as oxandrolone [100]; blockade of catecholamines with propranolol [101]; and insulin [102], insulin-like growth factor [103, 104], or human growth hormone [105, 106].

## Rehabilitation

As postburn mortality decreased, the problems of burn survivors, particularly those with deep and extensive injuries, became paramount [107–109]. The scientific study of rehabilitation of the thermally in-

jured patient is a relatively young field. The CG monograph briefly states:

*Six patients who received severe burns to the dorsum of the hands and wrists were referred to the Physical Therapy Department either while in the hospital or at the time of discharge to be treated as out-patients… In all cases surface healing was complete before beginning treatment… The first patient… was referred to this department 51 days after the fire… [110]*

This method, which conceives of rehabilitation as a "phase" which begins after resuscitation and reconstructive surgery phases, may be acceptable in patients with minor injuries. But it soon became apparent that wound healing is so prolonged in patients with major thermal injuries that these 3 phases must be conducted concurrently rather than sequentially, to avoid the catastrophic effects of chronic bed rest, extremity immobilization, and contracture formation [108]. In the 1950s, Moncrief began rehabilitation soon after admission, and resumed it 8–10 days after skin grafting [111, 112]. The advent of heat-malleable plastic (thermoplastic) material made it possible to fabricate increasingly complex and effective positioning devices [113]. This was followed by the introduction of pressure to treat hypertrophic scars, and the development of customized pressure garments [114]. Others reduced or eliminated the delay between skin grafting and ambulation, without deleterious effects on graft take [115, 116]. New frontiers for physical, occupational, and neuropsychiatric rehabilitation of burn patients include the following:

- ▶ Optimizing pain control; use of novel techniques such as virtual reality [117]
- ▶ Documentation of long-term outcomes [118, 119]
- ▶ Definition of barriers of return to work and community [120, 121]
- ▶ Diagnosis and treatment of posttraumatic stress disorder [122]
- ▶ Management of scar formation [123]

## Conclusions

This review indicates that the advances in burn care achieved since WWII were not accidental, but depended on integrated laboratory and clinical research; generous national funding; centers of excellence focused on comprehensive burn care; highly skilled multidisciplinary clinical teams; and committed leadership. Reflecting on recent progress in the 1976 American Burn Association presidential address, Colonel Basil Pruitt noted the importance of a tight working relationship between clinicians and basic scientists, working together to solve problems of clinical significance [124]. This paradigm should be strengthened and expanded, since we have entered an era in which the number of large burns has declined nationwide [125]. As a result, we are challenged with the need for multicenter trials if we are to continue to make progress. Fortunately, the creation of the American Burn Association (ABA) Multicenter Trials Group, and federal funding of several proposals under ABA leadership, has created the framework and the opportunity for such collaboration. In a manner reminiscent of events in the UK and US during WWII, the recent conflicts in Iraq and Afghanistan [126] and the attacks of 11 September 2001 [127] have highlighted the importance of thermal injury as a national problem. As a result, the following multicenter trials are currently being initiated:

▶ Outcomes after burn injury, using the National Burn Repository database
▶ Transfusion triggers
▶ Impact of occupational and physical therapy on outcomes
▶ High-volume hemofiltration in burn patients with septic shock and renal failure
▶ Rapid polymerase chain reaction (PCR) test for *Staphylococcus aureus* infection
▶ Community-based exercise
▶ Enteral glutamine effect on infections
▶ Inhalation injury scoring

The spirit of collaboration and inquiry embodied by these projects is the surest guarantee that they will bear fruit in the years to come.

## References

[1] Pruitt BA, Goodwin CW, Mason AD Jr (2002) Epidemiological, demographic, and outcome characteristics of burn injury. In: Herndon DN (ed) Total burn care. W. B. Saunders, London, pp 16–30

[2] Wolf SE, Rose JK, Desai MH et al (1997) Mortality determinants in massive pediatric burns. An analysis of 103 children with > or = 80% TBSA burns (> or = 70% full-thickness). Ann Surg 225(5): 554–565; discussion 565–569

[3] Artz CP (1970) Historical aspects of burn management. Surg Clin N A 50(6): 1193–1200

[4] Wallace AF (1987) Recent advances in the treatment of burns–1843–1858. Br J Plast Surg 40(2): 193–200

[5] Dunbar J (1934) Burn cases treated in Glasgow Royal Infirmary. Glasgow Medical Journal 122: 239–255

[6] Davidson EC (1925) Tannic acid in the treatment of burns. Surg Gynecol Obstet 41: 202–221

[7] Hupkens P, Boxma H, Dokter J (1995) Tannic acid as a topical agent in burns: historical considerations and implications for new developments. Burns 21(1): 57–61

[8] Underhill FP (1930) The significance of anhydremia in extensive superficial burns. JAMA 95: 852–857

[9] Blalock A (1931) Experimental shock. VII () The importance of the local loss of fluid in the production of the low blood pressure after burns. Arch Surg 22: 610–616

[10] Aldrich RH (1933) The role of infection in burns: the theory and treatment with special reference to gentian violet. N Engl J Med 208–309: 299

[11] Battle R (1978) Plastic surgery in the two world wars and in the years between. J Roy Soc Med 71(11): 844–848

[12] Mills SMH (2005) Burns down under: lessons lost, lessons learned. J Burn Care Rehab 26(1): 42–52

[13] Mayhew ER (2004) The Reconstruction of Warriors: Archibald McIndoe, the Royal Air Force and the Guinea Pig Club. Greenhill Books, London

[14] Jackson D (1978) Thirty years of burn treatment in Britain–where now? Injury 10(1): 40–45

[15] Colebrook L (1936) Treatment of human puerperal infections, and of experimental infections in mice, with prontosil. Lancet i:1279–1286

[16] Lerner BH (1991) Scientific evidence versus therapeutic demand: the introduction of the sulfonamides revisited. Ann Intern Med 115(4): 315–320

[17] Clark AM, Gibson T, Colebrook L et al () Penicillin and propamide in burns: elimination of haemolytic streptococci and staphylococci. Lancet 1943: 605–609

[18] Colebrook L, Gibson T, Todd JP et al (1944) Studies of burns and scalds. (Reports of the burns unit, Royal Infirmary, Glasgow, 1942–43). Medical Research Council Special Report Series No. 249. London: His Majesty's Stationery Office

[19] Lawrence JC (1995) Some aspects of burns and burns research at Birmingham Accident Hospital 1944–93: A.B. Wallace Memorial Lecture, 1994. Burns 21: 403–413

[20] Colebrook L (1945) A burns unit at the Birmingham Accident Hospital and Rehabilitation Centre. Nursing Times 6: 4–6

[21] Turk JL (1994) Leonard Colebrook: the chemotherapy and control of streptococcal infections. J Roy Soc Med 87(12): 727–728

[22] Lockwood JS (1946) War-time activities of the National Research Council and the Committee on Medical Research; with particular reference to team-work on studies of wounds and burns. Ann Surg 124: 314–327

[23] Stewart IP (1948) Organizing Scientific Research for War: The Administrative History of the Office of Scientific Research and Development. Little, Brown and Company, Boston

[24] Neushul P (1993) Science, government, and the mass production of penicillin. J Hist Med Allied Sci 48(4): 371–395

[25] Administrative History Section A, Bureau of Medicine and Surgery (1946) Pearl Harbor Navy Medical Activities (The United States Navy Medical Department at War, 1941–1945, vol. 1, parts 1–2. United States Naval Administrative History of World War II #68-A). Bureau of Medicine and Surgery, Washington, D. C.

[26] Lesch JE (2007) The First Miracle Drugs: How the Sulfa Drugs Transformed Medicine. Oxford University Press, Oxford

[27] Meleney FL (1943) The study of the prevention of infection in contaminated accidental wounds, compound fractures and burns. Ann Surg 118: 171–183

[28] Chain E, Florey HW, Gardner AD et al (1940) Penicillin as a chemotherapeutic agent. Lancet ii:226–228

[29] Ligon BL (2004) Penicillin: its discovery and early development. Semin Pediatr Infect Dis 15(1): 52–57

[30] Richards AN (1964) Production of penicillin in the United States (1941–46). Nature 4918: 441–445

[31] Cope O (1943) Forward. In: Aub JC, Beecher HK, Cannon B et al (eds) Management of the Cocoanut Grove Burns at the Massachusetts General Hospital. J .B. Lippincott Company, Philadelphia, pp 1–2

[32] National Research Council Division of Medical Sciences (1942). Treatment of burns. War Medicine 2: 334–339

[33] Cope O, Moore FD (1947) The redistribution of body water and the fluid therapy of the burned patient. Ann Surg 126: 1010–1045

[34] Harkins HN (1942) The treatment of burns in wartime. JAMA 119: 385–390

[35] Harkins HN (1942) The Treatment of Burns. Baillere, Tindall and Cox, London

[36] Whipple AO (1943) Basic principles in the treatment of thermal burns. Ann Surg: 187–191

[37] Saffle JR (1993) The 1942 fire at Boston's Cocoanut Grove nightclub. Am J Surg 166(6): 581–591

[38] Follett GP (1943) The Boston fire: a challenge to our disaster service. Ann J Nurs 43: 4–8

[39] Faxson NW (1943) The problems of the hospital administration. In: Aub JC, Beecher HK, Cannon B et al (eds) Management of the Cocoanut Grove Burns at the Massachusetts General Hospital. J.B. Lippincott Company, Philadelphia, pp 3–8

[40] Artz CP (1969) Burns in my lifetime. J Trauma 9(10): 827–833

[41] Pruitt BA Jr (1984) Forces and factors influencing trauma care: 1983 A.A.S.T. (American Association for the Surgery of Trauma) Presidential address. J Trauma 24(6): 463–470

[42] Heimbach DM (1988) American Burn Association 1988 presidential address "we can see so far because . . .". J Burn Care Rehab 9(4): 340–346

[43] Pruitt BA Jr (1995) The integration of clinical care and laboratory research. A model for medical progress. Arch Surg 130(5): 461–471

[44] Pruitt BA Jr (2000) Centennial changes in surgical care and research. Ann Surg 232(3): 287–301

[45] Artz CP (1979) History of burns. In: Artz CP, Moncrief JA, Pruitt BA Jr (eds) Burns: A Team Approach Philadelphia: W.B. Saunders 1979. pp 3–16

[46] Dimick AR, Brigham PA, Sheehy EM (1993) The development of burn centers in North America. Journal of Burn Care & Rehabilitation 14(2 Pt 2): 284–299

[47] Cope O, Rhinelander FW (1943) The problem of burn shock complicated by pulmonary damage. In: Aub JC, Beecher HK, Cannon B et al (eds) Management of the Cocoanut Grove Burns at the Massachusetts General Hospital. J. B. Lippincott, Philadelphia, PA, pp 115–128

[48] Evans IE, Purnell OJ, Robinett PW et al (1952) Fluid and electrolyte requirements in severe burns. Ann Surg 135: 804–817

[49] Reiss E, Stirman JA, Artz CP et al (1953) Fluid and electrolyte balance in burns. JAMA 152: 1309–1313

[50] Baxter CR, Shires T (1968) Physiological response to crystalloid resuscitation of severe burns. Ann N Y Acad Sci 150(3): 874–894

[51] Pruitt BA Jr, Mason AD Jr, Moncrief JA (1971) Hemodynamic changes in the early postburn patient: the influence of fluid administration and of a vasodilator (hydralazine). J Trauma 11(1): 36–46

[52] Saffle JR (2007) The phenomenon of "fluid creep" in acute burn resuscitation. J Burn Care Res 28: 382–395

[53] Pruitt BA, Jr (2000) Protection from excessive resuscitation: "pushing the pendulum back". J Trauma 49(3): 567–568

[54] Cope O (1943) The treatment of the surface burns. In: Aub JC, Beecher HK, Cannon B et al (eds) Management of the Cocoanut Grove Burns at the Massachusetts General Hospital. J.B. Lippincott Company, Philadelphia, pp 85–93

[55] Lyons C (1943) Problems of infection and chemotherapy. In: Aub JC, Beecher HK, Cannon B et al (eds) Management of the Cocoanut Grove Burns at the Massachusetts General Hospital. J. B. Lippincott Company, Philadelphia, pp 94–102

[56] Dalton ML (2003) Champ Lyons: an incomplete life. Ann Surg 237(5): 694–703

[57] Lyons C (1943) Penicillin therapy of surgical infections in the U.S. Army: a report. JAMA 123: 1007–1018

[58] Liedberg NC, Reiss E, Artz CP (1954) Infection in burns. III. Septicemia, a common cause of death. Surg Gynecol Obstetr 99: 151–158

[59] Teplitz C, Davis D, Mason AD, Jr., Moncrief JA (1964) Pseudomonas burn wound sepsis. I () Pathogenesis of experimental pseudomonas burn wound sepsis. J Surg Res 4: 200–216

[60] Teplitz C, Davis D, Walker HL et al (1964) Pseudomonas burn wound sepsis: II Hematogenous infection at the junction of the burn wound and the unburned hypodermis. J Surg Res 4: 217–222

[61] Walker HL, Mason AD, Jr, Raulston GL (1964) Surface infection with Pseudomonas Aeruginosa. Ann Surg 160: 297–305

[62] Pruitt BA, Jr., O'Neill JA, Jr, Moncrief JA, Lindberg RB (1968) Successful control of burn-wound sepsis. Jama 203(12): 1054–1056

[63] Jelenko Cd, Jelenko JM, Mendelson JA, Buxton RW (1966) The marfanil mystery. Surg Gynecol Obstetr 122(1): 121–127

[64] Mendelson JA, Lindsey D (1962) Sulfamylon (mafenide) and penicillin as expedient treatment of experimental massive open wounds with C () perfringens infection. J Trauma 2: 239–261

[65] Lindberg RB, Moncrief JA, Mason AD Jr (1968) Control of experimental and clinical burn wound sepsis by topical application of sulfamylon compounds. Ann N Y Acad Sci 150(3): 950–960

[66] Moyer CA, Brentano L, Gravens DL et al (1965) Treatment of large burns with 0.5% silver nitrate solution. Arch Surg 90: 812–867

[67] Fox CL Jr (1968) Silver sulfadiazine–a new topical therapy for Pseudomonas in burns. Therapy of Pseudomonas infection in burns. Arch Surg 96(2): 184–188

[68] Tredget EE, Shankowsky HA, Groeneveld A, Burrell R (1998) A matched-pair, randomized study evaluating the efficacy and safety of Acticoat silver-coated dressing for the treatment of burn wounds. J Burn Care Rehabil 19(6): 531–537

[69] Cannon B (1943) Procedures in rehabilitation of the severely burned. In: Aub JC, Beecher HK, Cannon B et al (eds) Management of the Cocoanut Grove Burns at the Massachusetts General Hospital. J. B. Lippincott Company, Philadelphia, 1943, pp 103–110

[70] Artz CP, Soroff HS (1955) Modern concepts in the treatment of burns. JAMA 159: 411–417

[71] Dobbs ER (1999) Burn therapy of years ago. J Burn Care Rehabil 20(1 Pt 1): 62–66; discussion 61

[72] Jackson D (1954) A clinical study of the use of skin homografts for burns. Br J Plast Surg 7: 26–43

[73] Jackson D, Topley E, Cason JS, Lowbury EJL (1960) Primary excision and grafting of large burns. Ann Surg 152: 167–189

[74] Janzekovic Z (2008) Once upon a time ... how West discovered East. J Plast Reconstr Aesthet Surg 61: 240–244

[75] Janzekovic Z (1972) Early surgical treatment of the burned surface. Panminerva Medica 14(7–8): 228–232

[76] Tompkins RG, Burke JF, Schoenfeld DA et al (1986) Prompt eschar excision: a treatment system contributing to reduced burn mortality. A statistical evaluation of burn care at the Massachusetts General Hospital (1974-1984). Ann Surg 204(3): 272–281

[77] McManus WF, Mason AD Jr, Pruitt BA Jr (1989) Excision of the burn wound in patients with large burns. Arch Surg 124(6): 718–720

[78] Herndon DN, Parks DH (1986) Comparison of serial debridement and autografting and early massive excision with cadaver skin overlay in the treatment of large burns in children. J Trauma 26(2): 149–152

[79] Herndon DN, Barrow RE, Rutan RL et al (1989) A comparison of conservative versus early excision. Therapies in severely burned patients. Ann Surg 209(5): 547–552; discussion 552–553

[80] Ong YS, Samuel M, Song C (2006) Meta-analysis of early excision of burns. Burns 32(2): 145–150

[81] Burke JF, Yannas IV, Quinby WC Jr et al (1981) Successful use of a physiologically acceptable artificial skin in the treatment of extensive burn injury. Ann Surg 194(4): 413–428

[82] Gallico GG 3rd, O'Connor NE, Compton CC et al (1984) Permanent coverage of large burn wounds with autologous cultured human epithelium. N Engl J Med 311(7): 448–451

[83] Rue LW, III, Cioffi WG, McManus WF, Pruitt BA Jr (1993) Wound closure and outcome in extensively burned patients treated with cultured autologous keratinocytes. J Trauma 34(5): 662–667

[84] Barret JP, Wolf SE, Desai MH, Herndon DN (2000) Cost-efficacy of cultured epidermal autografts in massive pediatric burns. Ann Surg 231(6): 869–876

[85] Aub JC, Pittman H, Brues AM (1943) The pulmonary complications: a clinical description. In: Aub JC, Beecher HK, Cannon B et al (eds) Management of the Cocoanut Grove Burns at the Massachusetts General Hospital. J.B. Lippincott Company, Philadelphia, pp 34–40

[86] Morris MJ (2006) Acute respiratory distress syndrome in combat casualties: military medicine and advances in mechanical ventilation. Mil Med 171: 1039–1044

[87] Rosengart MR (2006) Critical care medicine: landmarks and legends. Surg Clin North Am 86: 1305–1321

[88] Shirani KZ, Pruitt BA Jr, Mason AD Jr (1987) The influence of inhalation injury and pneumonia on burn mortality. Ann Surg 205(1): 82–87

[89] Shimazu T, Yukioka T, Hubbard GB et al (1987) A dose-responsive model of smoke inhalation injury. Severity-related alteration in cardiopulmonary function. Ann Surg 206(1): 89–98

[90] Herndon DN, Traber DL, Niehaus GD et al (1984) The pathophysiology of smoke inhalation injury in a sheep

model. Journal of Trauma-Injury Infection & Critical Care 24(12): 1044–1051

[91]  Shimazu T, Yukioka T, Ikeuchi H et al (1996) Ventilation-perfusion alterations after smoke inhalation injury in an ovine model. J Appl Physiol 81(5): 2250–2259

[92]  Traber DL, Hawkins HK, Enkhbaatar P et al (2007) The role of the bronchial circulation in the acute lung injury resulting from burn and smoke inhalation. Pulmonary Pharmacology & Therapeutics 20(2): 163–166

[93]  Cioffi WG, Jr., Rue LW, 3d, Graves TA et al (1991) Prophylactic use of high-frequency percussive ventilation in patients with inhalation injury. Ann Surg 213(6): 575–582

[94]  Enkhbaatar P, Herndon DN, Traber DL (2009) Use of nebulized heparin in the treatment of smoke inhalation injury. J Burn Care Res 30(1): 159–162

[95]  Cuthbertson DP (1942) Post-shock metabolic response. Lancet i:433–437

[96]  Cope O, Nardi GL, Quijano M et al (1953) Metabolic rate and thyroid function following acute thermal trauma in man. Ann Surg 137: 165–174

[97]  Wilmore DW, Long JM, Mason AD Jr et al (1974) Catecholamines: mediator of the hypermetabolic response to thermal injury. Ann Surg 180(4): 653–669

[98]  Wilmore DW, Curreri PW, Spitzer KW et al (1971) Supranormal dietary intake in thermally injured hypermetabolic patients. Surg Gynecol Obstet 132(5): 881–886

[99]  Curreri PW, Richmond D, Marvin J, Baxter CR (1974) Dietary requirements of patients with major burns. Journal of the American Dietetic Association 65(4): 415–417

[100]  Wolf SE, Edelman LS, Kemalyan N et al (2006) Effects of oxandrolone on outcome measures in the severely burned: a multicenter prospective randomized double-blind trial. J Burn Care Res 27(2): 131–139; discussion 140–141

[101]  Herndon DN, Hart DW, Wolf SE et al (2001) Reversal of catabolism by beta-blockade after severe burns. N Engl J Med 345(17): 1223–1229

[102]  Sakurai Y, Aarsland A, Herndon DN et al (1995) Stimulation of muscle protein synthesis by long-term insulin infusion in severely burned patients. Ann Surg 222(3): 283–294; 294–297

[103]  Cioffi WG, Gore DC, Rue LW 3rd et al (1994) Insulin-like growth factor-1 lowers protein oxidation in patients with thermal injury. Ann Surg 220(3): 310–319

[104]  Spies M, Wolf SE, Barrow RE et al (2002) Modulation of types I and II acute phase reactants with insulin-like growth factor-1/binding protein-3 complex in severely burned children. Crit Care Med 30(1): 83–88

[105]  Wilmore DW, Moylan JA Jr, Bristow BF et al (1974) Anabolic effects of human growth hormone and high caloric feedings following thermal injury. Surg Gynecol Obstet 138(6): 875–884

[106]  Hart DW, Wolf SE, Chinkes DL et al (2002) Beta-blockade and growth hormone after burn. Ann Surg 236(4): 450–6; discussion 456–457

[107]  Pereira C, Murphy K, Herndon D (2004) Outcome measures in burn care. Is mortality dead? Burns 30: 761–771

[108]  Richard RL, Hedman TL, Quick CD et al (2008) A clarion to recommit and reaffirm burn rehabilitation. J Burn Care Res 29(3): 425–432

[109]  Esselman PC, Thombs BD, Magyar-Russell G, Fauerbach JA (2006) Burn rehabilitation: state of the science. Am J Phys Med Rehabil 85(4): 383–413

[110]  Watkins AL (1943) A note on physical therapy. In: Aub JC, Beecher HK, Cannon B et al (eds) Management of the Cocoanut Grove Burns at the Massachusetts General Hospital. J. B. Lippincott Company, Philadelphia, pp 111–114

[111]  Moncrief JA (1958) Complications of burns. Ann Surg 147: 443–475

[112]  Moncrief JA (1958) Third degree burns of the dorsum of the hand. Am J Surg 96: 535–544

[113]  Willis B (1969) The use of orthoplast isoprene splints in the treatment of the acutely burned child: preliminary report. American Journal of Occupational Therapy 23(1): 57–61

[114]  Larson DL, Abston S, Evans EB et al (1971) Techniques for decreasing scar formation and contractures in the burned patient. J Trauma 11(10): 807–823

[115]  Schmitt MA, French L, Kalil ET (1991) How soon is safe? Ambulation of the patient with burns after lower-extremity skin grafting. J Burn Care Rehabil 12(1): 33–37

[116]  Burnsworth B, Krob MJ, Langer-Schnepp M (1992) Immediate ambulation of patients with lower-extremity grafts. Journal of Burn Care & Rehabilitation 13(1): 89–92

[117]  Carrougher GJ, Hoffman HG, Nakamura D et al (2009) The effect of virtual reality on pain and range of motion in adults with burn injuries. J Burn Care Res 30(5): 785–791

[118]  Yoder LH, Nayback AM, Gaylord K (2010) The evolution and utility of the burn specific health scale: a systematic review. Burns 36: 1143–1156

[119]  Klein MB, Lezotte DL, Fauerbach JA et al (2007) The National Institute on Disability and Rehabilitation Research burn model system database: a tool for the multicenter study of the outcome of burn injury. J Burn Care Res 28(1): 84–96

[120]  Esselman PC, Askay SW, Carrougher GJ et al (2007) Barriers to return to work after burn injuries. Archives of Physical Medicine & Rehabilitation 88(12 Suppl 2): 50–56

[121]  Esselman PC, Ptacek JT, Kowalske K et al (2001) Community integration after burn injuries. J Burn Care Rehabil 22(3): 221–227

[122]  Gaylord KM, Holcomb JB, Zolezzi ME (2009) A comparison of posttraumatic stress disorder between combat casualties and civilians treated at a military burn center. Journal of Trauma-Injury Infection & Critical Care 66(4 Suppl): 191–195

[123]  Kwan P, Hori K, Ding J, Tredget EE (2009) Scar and contracture: biological principles. Hand Clinics 25(4): 511–528

[124] Pruitt BA Jr (1977) Multidisciplinary care and research for burn injury: 1976 presidential address, American Burn Association meeting. J Trauma 17(4): 263–269

[125] Latenser BA, Miller SF, Bessey PQ et al (2007) National Burn Repository 2006: a ten-year review. J Burn Care Res 28(5): 635–658

[126] Kauvar DS, Cancio LC, Wolf SE et al (2006) Comparison of combat and non-combat burns from on-going U.S. military operations. J Surg Res 132(2): 195–200

[127] Anonymous (2002) Rapid assessment of injuries among survivors of the terrorist attack on the World Trade Center–New York City, September 2001. MMWR – Morbidity & Mortality Weekly Report 51(1):1–5

Correspondence: Dr. L. Cancio, USAISR, Ft. Sam Houston, TX 78234-6315, USA, E-mail: Lee.cancio@us.army.mil

# Epidemiology and prevention of burns throughout the world

Michael D. Peck

Director of International Outreach Programs, Arizona Burn Center, Phoenix AZ, USA; Clinical Professor of Surgery, University of Arizona College of Medicine-Phoenix, USA; Adjunct Professor, Division of Community, Environment and Policy, Mel and Enid Zuckerman College of Public Health, University of Arizona Health Sciences Center, Tucson AZ, USA

## Introduction

Injury is the physical damage that results when a human body is suddenly subjected to energy in amounts that exceed the threshold of physiological tolerance [23]. Injury is public health problem – out of every ten deaths in the world, one is due to injury [232]. Injuries are the fourth leading cause of death in men throughout the world (nearly 12 % of total deaths) after cardiovascular, infectious and neoplastic diseases. For example, injuries are the leading cause of death in men aged 15 – 59 in Latin America and the Caribbean [232]. Although progress is being made against many illnesses, the incidence of injuries is decreasing at rate slower than the reduction in illness in high-income countries (HIC). In low- and middle-income countries (LMIC), both death and disability from injuries is increasing very rapidly. In LMIC of Americas, Europe and Eastern Mediterranean Regions, more than 30 % of DALYs among men aged 15 – 44 years was from injury.[1] [232]

Injury is a burden on the young, taking more productive life-years than cancer or heart disease. Fire-related burns are among the leading causes of DALYs lost in LMIC [232]. For example, burns under 20 %

are approximately 6 % of all unintentional injuries in children under 15 years of age [232]. Injuries are also the most common cause of DALYs (Disability-Adjusted Life Year – the loss due either to death or disability of the equivalent of one year of good health) lost worldwide: injuries accounted for 17 % of disability-adjusted life years (DALY's) lost in adults aged 15 – 59 in 2004 [232].

Burns fall within this spectrum of mechanism of injury. Unintentional injuries include not only burns but traffic incidents, drowning, poisonings, and falls. Intentional injuries result from homicide, suicide, legal interventions, and conflicts; burns and fires are occasionally the mechanism for assault or self-harm. Without question, burns cause a significant proportion of the morbidity and mortality attributed to injuries throughout the world.

A burn is an injury to the skin or other organic tissue primarily caused by thermal or other acute trauma, according to the International Society of Burn Injuries. It occurs when some or all of the cells in the skin or other tissues are destroyed by hot liquids (scalds), hot solids (contact burns), or flames (flame burns). Injuries to the skin or other organic tissues due to radiation, radioactivity, electricity, friction or contact with chemicals are also identified as burns.

In 2004, incidence of burns severe enough to require medical attention was nearly 11 million people [232], fourth in all injuries behind road traffic acci-

---

1 Income categories for 2004 as defined by the World Bank by 2004 gross national income per capita. Low US$285 or less; lower middle US$285-3255; upper middle US$3256-10,065; high US$10,066 or more.

dents, falls, and interpersonal violence – this is higher than the combined incidence of tuberculosis and HIV infections, and just slightly less than the incidence of all malignant neoplasms. Burns under 20 % of the body surface area occur to 153 per 100,000 population of children aged 0–15 years, making them the fifth most common cause of non-fatal childhood injuries after intracranial injury, open wounds, poisoning, and forearm fractures [232]. Five percent of disabilities at all ages in Nepal are due to burns and scalds [213].

When confronted with the story of a burn survivor, the first picture that comes to mind is that of the agonizing open wounds, followed by resolution into undeniably obvious burn scars. But the thickened, non-compliant skin tells only part of the story. Much of the impact of burns is emotional, psychological and spiritual. Studies of recovery from burn injury in the US show clearly that the ability to adjust following injury is less dependent on the physical characteristics of the burn (such as burn size, burn depth or location), and more on pre-injury adjustment. Coping skills, family and community support, and general psychological health have more impact on recovery from burns than the burn itself [39].

In HIC, this means that burn survivors from struggling family backgrounds are likely to have problems reassimilating into school and community. In LMIC, the consequences are direr, with isolation from or even abandonment by the family, social segregation, unemployment and extreme poverty. Although burn victims from affluent families in LIC have a chance of recuperation, the vast majority of burn survivors will start from living situations that deny them the opportunity to recover from even a small burn.

Additionally, the sequelae of non-fatal burn injuries are often severe enough to cause permanent disability. In the Global Childhood Unintentional Injury Surveillance pilot study done among children (0–12 years of age) in Bangladesh, Colombia, Egypt and Pakistan, 17 % of survivors had long term (greater than six weeks) temporary disability, and 8 % had permanent disability [167]. The incidence of long-term temporary disability was highest in children surviving burns and traffic injuries. Only near-drowning victims had a higher rate of permanent disability. Permanent disability was eight times more common in burn survivors than in those children recovering from falls.

Thus comes the wisdom of one of the founding fathers of burn care in India, Dr. M. H. Keswani: "The challenge of burns lies not in the successful treatment of a 100 % burn, but in the 100 % prevention of all burn injuries." [112]

## Epidemiology

Although burns and fires account for over 300,000 deaths each year throughout the world, the vast majority of burn injuries are fortunately not fatal [232]. In 2008 there were 410,149 non-fatal burn injuries in the US, giving an age-adjusted rate of 136 per 100,000 each year [47]. A higher estimate comes from data collected from the National Hospital Ambulatory Medical Care Survey during the period of 1993 to 2004 in the US, in which the average annual emergency department visit rate for treatment of burns was 220 per 100,000 population [73]. The vast majority of these burns were treated and released from the emergency department; only 5 % were hospitalized or transferred. In comparison, only 45 % of non-fatal firearm injuries and near-drowning were treated and released, suggesting that the severity of most burns requiring medical treatment is low compared to other types of injury [47].

Epidemiological studies from LIC lend insight into the true impact burns have in communities. A cross sectional survey of nearly 1400 households in Tigray, Ethiopia, showed that 1.2 % of the population is burned each year. Over 80 % of these burns occurred at home, and 90 % healed without any complications. Only 1 % of the burn victims died [148]. A population-based survey of over 170,000 households representing nearly 350,000 children and 470,000 adults during 2003 in Bangladesh showed that the overall incidence of non-fatal burn injuries was 166 per 100,000, and that about 173,000 Bangladeshi children suffer moderate to severe burns each year, which is an annual rate of 288 burns per 100,000 children. Similar to the study in Ethiopia, 90 % of the burns occurred at home. The rate of permanent disability due to burns in childhood was 5.7 per 100,000, and the mortality rate was 0.6 per 100,000 [126, 127, 129].

Other studies confirm the relative infrequency with which burn patients require hospitalization. In a recent study of patients treated for burns at emergency departments in North Carolina in a recent study, 4 % were admitted and only 4 % were transferred to burn centers [57]. Based on the incidence of burns treated at emergency departments and the proportion of those patients requiring admission, it appears that anywhere from 5 to 16 burn patients per 100,000 population require admission for treatment of their injuries. In Pennsylvania in 1994, the rate of hospitalizations for treatment of burn injuries was 26.3 per 100,000, based on hospital discharge records [78].

Global data are even more elusive, but an estimate of the frequency with which children are hospitalized throughout the world for treatment of burns is a rate of 8 per 100,000 [44]. In a rural community survey in Ethiopia, burns were the second most common injury to children under 15 years of age. The annual incidence of burns severe enough to restrict activity for one or more days was 80 per 1000 children [58]. Burns were therefore the leading cause of admission for injury to pediatric hospitals in Ethiopia, and ranked third as a source of outpatient visits [210, 212].

There has been a decrease in emergency department visits for burn injury in the US from 1993 to 2004 [47]. The absolute number of burn injuries in the US may be declining, or the severity of those injuries decreasing, or both [43]. Fortunately a similar trend is being observed overseas. For example, the number of burn patients admitted annually to the Burn Unit of Lok Nayak Hospital and Maulana Azad Medical College, New Delhi, India, from 1993 to 2007 has declined from 1276 to 724 patients [7].

In parallel with the decline in emergency department visits and hospitalizations for burns, there has been a decline in mortality due to fire and flames across the world. The two decades from 1982 to 2002 have witnessed a decrease in fire and burn mortality in many countries. During this period of time, for instance, fire and burn mortality in Australian men declined from 1.5 to 0.7 per 100,000. Similarly the fire death rate in Brazilian women went from 1.1 to 0.5 per 100,000. Other countries observing reduction in fire and burn mortality from 1982 to 2002 include

Canada, France, Mexico, Panama, Thailand, the United Kingdom, and Venezuela [233]. In the US, the age-adjusted death rate from fire and burns has dropped from 2.99 per 100,000 in 1981 to 1.2 per 100,000 in 2006 [47]. Even in just the brief period of time between 2000 and 2004, the Global Burden of Disease Project noted a 6 % decline worldwide in fire and burn deaths from 5.1 to 4.8 per 100,000 (GBD 2008).

Yet not all countries have experienced a simple linear decline in the incidence of burn deaths during the last three decades. Significant political and economic upheaval in the nations which used to belong to the Union of Soviet Socialist Republics (USSR) has left its mark on trends in fire and burn deaths. Following a gentle decline through the early 1980's, fire and burn deaths began to rise before and just after the dissolution of the USSR in 1991. By the late 1990's, as capitalism and democracy began to replace communism, deaths rates again began to decline [164]. National variations in injury-related mortality may be related to individual factors, such as alcohol consumption and risk-taking behavior, as well as alterations in social, political and environmental factors [154].

## The inequitable distribution of burns

As noted by Mock and associates in a recent editorial in the *Bulletin of the World Health Organization*, injuries and violence cause disability and death to tens of millions of people across the globe each year, and this burden is unfairly borne primarily by those in LMIC where prevention programs are uncommon and the quality of acute care is inconsistent [142]. Burn injuries are dramatic examples of the inequity of injury.

The majority of burn deaths (90 %) occur in lower middle or low income countries. Slightly more than 7 % occur in high middle-income countries. Only 3 % of burn deaths across the world occur in HIC (Fig. 1; [232]). The rate of child injury death from fire and flames is nearly 11 times higher in LIC than in HIC (Table 1; [232]). Although in HIC the death rate in children from fire and flames is only 3 % of the overall rate of death from unintentional injuries of all kinds, it is over 10 % the death rate of all unintentional injuries in LIC [232]. In ab-

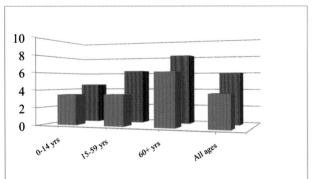

**Mortality Rates from Fire: World Total**
Deaths/100,000 population

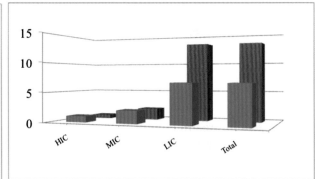

**Mortality Rates from Fire: Income Category**
Deaths/100,000 population

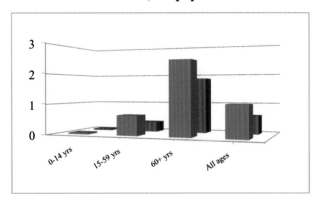

**Mortality Rates from Fire: HIC**
Deaths/100,000 population

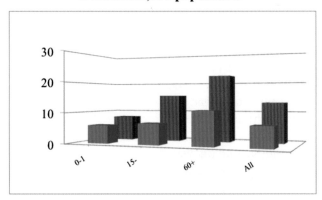

**Mortality Rates from Fire: LIC**
Deaths/100,000 population

**Fig. 1.** Low-income countries (LIC) disproportionately suffer the impact of fire deaths and burn injuries throughout the world, according to statistics from the Global Burden of Disease project [232]. In this figure, blue represents males and red represents females

solute numbers, the proportion of childhood deaths due to fire and flames in LIC is twice that in HIC (Table 2).

Even in HIC's, burn injuries disproportionately occur to racial and ethnic minorities in which socioeconomic status – more than cultural or educational factors – account for most of the increased susceptibility to burns. In the Republic of Korea (South Korea), for instance, the severity of burn injury is highest in the lowest socioeconomic groups [161]. For another example, the proportion of African-American infants requiring hospitalization at US

**Table 1.** Unintentional injury death rates per 100,000 children (0–20 years of age) by cause and country income level [232]

|  | Road traffic | Drowning | Fire & Burns | Falls | Poisoning | Other | Total |
|---|---|---|---|---|---|---|---|
| HIC | 7.0 | 1.2 | 0.4 | 0.4 | 0.5 | 2.6 | 12.2 |
| LMIC | 11.1 | 7.8 | 4.3 | 2.1 | 2.0 | 14.4 | 41.7 |
| World | 10.7 | 7.2 | 3.9 | 1.9 | 1.8 | 13.3 | 38.8 |

**Table 2.** Unintentional injury deaths (in millions) in children (0–14 years of age) by cause and country income level [232]

|  | Road traffic | Drowning | Fire & Burns | Falls | Poisoning | Other | Total |
|---|---|---|---|---|---|---|---|
| HIC | 6 | 2 | 1 | 1 | 0 | 5 | 14 |
| MIC | 53 | 71 | 10 | 11 | 9 | 137 | 292 |
| LIC | 108 | 62 | 62 | 23 | 23 | 120 | 399 |

burn centers for treatment is double the proportion of African-Americans in the general population [16]. Similarly, the standardized mortality ratio for fire deaths in 1981–1982 among aboriginals in Manitoba was 4.3 times that of the population of the entire province [79]. Indeed, in many aboriginal communities in North America and Greenland, the third most common cause of unintentional fatal injury is house fires [38, 145].

At the time of burn injury, all patients – young and old – experience shock, horror, pain and anxiety. The events that follow the injury may confuse the victims, and lead them to believe (sometimes correctly) that their death is imminent. Because few burn victims in LMIC receive appropriate first aid or immediate acute care, the medical mismanagement of the burn is likely to lead the survivor to the hopeless conclusion that little or nothing can be done to sooth the pain and relieve suffering. As a result, burn survivors become emotionally overwhelmed and typically withdraw. They lose interest in food and activity, and retreat to dark corners where they may lay motionless for hours. Unfortunately, this lack of activity compounds the speed with which the healing burn wound causes wound contractures to occur, and heightens the survivor's disability. For these reasons, the distribution of burn morbidity is also imbalanced. The prevalence of moderate and severe disability due to unintentional injuries in people under 60 years of age is 35.4 million in LMIC, 12.5 times higher than in HIC [232].

## Cost of fires and burns

A variety of features characteristic to burns lead to prolonged and expensive hospital stays. In addition to pain management and wound care, burn patients require attention to nutritional deficiencies, to the consequences of suppression of the immune system, and to rehabilitation therapy. In the US, the average hospital charge for care of a child (age 5–16 yrs) with extensive third degree burns requiring skin grafting is over US$140,000 [16]. In one state alone in 1994, hospital charges for treatment of burn injuries were over $93 million [78]. Yet in spite of this lavish medical care, many burned children leave hospitals in the US with permanent physical and psychological scars.

During the decade from 1999–2008, patients at burn centers in the US stayed a mean of 10 days in the hospital. The dominant predictors of hospital stay in burn patients are burn size and burn depth [162, 201]. Patients in US burn centers from 1999–2008 accumulated an average hospital charge of just over $58,000 per patient-stay. However, the charges for patients who died were nearly three times that for survivors. Hospital charges per day were over $4000 for survivors and nearly $12,000 for fatal cases.

Loss from burns and fires includes not only health care expenditures and property damage, but destruction of human resources as well. In 2006 there were nearly 70,000 years of potential life lost in the US because of burn fatalities [47]. The indirect costs of such loss of productive years of life arise from absence of useful employees from the workplace and lack of wage earners in families.

### Cost by age

When charges are viewed as a surrogate for intensity of care, certain trends are apparent. The presence of comorbid medical conditions typical in the elderly increases the need for more complex services and longer hospitalizations. Thus whereas the mean hospital charge per day for survivors was only $2900 for children aged one to five years, it was $4700 for elderly adults 60 years of age or older. Elderly patients admitted to a New York City burn center from 2000–2004 for treatment of scald burns had mean hospital charges of $113,000 per patient, even though the burns were relatively small (mean 7 % TBSA) [10]. On the other hand, mean hospital charges per day for fatal cases in US burn centers from 1999–2008 was $8850 for children one to five, compared to only $9400 for elderly adults, suggesting more intense utilization of resources used in attempts to salvage dying children [16].

As the proportion of the US population above 60 years of age grows, there will be shifts in expenditures for burn care. From 1999 to 2008 in the US, the percentage of patients admitted to burn centers who used Medicaid for health insurance stayed the same at nearly 13 % of all patients. However, with the aging of the population the percentage of Medicare-insured patients rose in the same time period from 9 % to 12 %. During that time period the proportion of Workers Compensation patients sank from 13 % to 8 %, reflecting the departure of working adults into retirement [16].

Children are also particularly impacted by thermal injuries and smoke inhalation. Fire and burn injuries resulted in the deaths of 1461 children in the US in 1985. There were 440,000 children treated for burns, of which nearly 24,000 were hospitalized. The society losses from these childhood burn injuries and deaths were estimated at approximately $3.5 billion [135].

Fortunately, the majority of young children have small burns requiring short hospitalizations. Seventy-five percent of children between the ages of one and five years in the US from 1999–2008 were burned over less than 10 % of their body surface area. These young children with small burns spent an average of only 3.6 days in the hospital [16]. Aside from the fact that prior to injury, children are healthier than their older counterparts, children are also more likely to be injured by hot liquids than by flames, and there are significant cost differences between the two mechanisms.

Using the Healthcare Cost and Utilization Project Kids' Inpatient Database for 2000 in the US, retrospective data analysis of pediatric burn-associated hospitalizations was done.[2] This analysis permitted an estimate that 10,000 children younger than 18 years were hospitalized for burn injuries during that year, and that the total charges for these hospitalizations were over $211 million. The mean length of stay was 6.6 days, and only 10 % of admissions lasted longer than 14 days. Because the predominance of short lengths of stay, mean charges were only $21,840 per patient, and only 10 % of patients accumulated charges in excess of $47,000. More than half of admissions were children younger than two years, and males outnumbered females at all ages. Children under two were more likely to suffer from scald burns, whereas older children were more likely burned by fire or flame [201].

## Cost by mechanism

Fire and flames are responsible for the bulk of the cost of burns. In 2008 fire departments in the US responded to nearly 1.5 million fires. There were 16,705 fire injuries, 3,320 fire deaths, and nearly $15.5 billion direct property losses. There was a fire death every 158 minutes in the US in 2008 [109]. The majority of the lost years of life are due to fire and flames (66,272), with only 1218 years of life lost due to scalds or contact burns [47].

The hospital charges per day in Pennsylvania in 1994 for treatment of flame burns from conflagrations were $4102, compared to $2187 for scald burns. This difference reflects the difference in depth of burn (flame burns are more likely to be third degree in depth than scald burns) and the subsequent additional intensity of resources needed to treat third degree flame burns and smoke inhalation injury, including intensive care, surgery, blood transfusions and antibiotics [78].

---

2   The Healthcare Cost and Utilization Project (HCUP) is a family of healthcare databases and related tools for research and decision making sponsored by the Agency for Healthcare Research and Quality. The four Shriners hospitals for burned children do not generally contribute data to their respective states' HCUP databases, and thus approximately 10% of the estimated 10,000 children admitted for burn care in the US each year were not included in this study. Therefore the collective incidence and related charges of pediatric burn admissions may be underestimated by approximately 10% in this study [201].

Data from LMIC regarding cost of burn treatment are scarce, but there are studies that corroborate the US experience that flame burns are expensive. For example, the cost of care for patients injured by kerosene stoves is high in LMIC. In 2003 in Cape Town, South Africa, the mean total cost per patient was US$6410. Extrapolating these costs to South Africa nationwide gives an estimated annual expense of US$26,250,000, which is more than 50 times the amount expended annually for kerosene in South Africa [216].

Nonetheless, because of the frequency with which scald burns occur, the cost of care for scalds is significant. Annual charges for treatment of scald burns in US children under 14 years is approximately $2.1 billion. Sixty percent of these charges are for children under the age of five years [149]. Again, indirect costs are difficult to quantify, but are no doubt significant because each day a child is hospitalized or home ill with burn injuries, that is a day that one of the parents or caregivers has to miss work. In addition, the cost of burn wound dressings is frequently not covered by most insurance policies, leaving the parents responsible for purchasing supplies out-of-pocket.

## Limitations of data

The majority of uncertainty in estimates of death in the Global Burden of Disease reports is associated with the assessment of systematic errors in primary data. That is, information about prevalence, incidence and mortality from injuries is generally fragmented, partial, incomparable and diagnostically uncertain [131]. To estimate uncertainly for regional mortality, a simulation approach was used to create uncertainty ranges that take into account uncertainty in the expected number of total deaths, uncertainty in the diagnosis of underlying cause of injury, and uncertainty arising from miscoding of cause, among others. Based on these estimates of uncertainty, the range of uncertainty for fire deaths is 3,000 to 5,000 deaths lower or higher than the estimates for fire deaths in East Asia, the Pacific, Europe and Central Asia. Even more uncertain are the estimates in South Asia and Sub-Saharan Africa, where the range of uncertainty surrounding the stated estimates is 10,000 to 14,000 deaths lower or higher. Thus the real number of fire deaths each year may be almost 30,000 higher than the estimate of 310,000. Sources of uncertainty for estimating burden of injury in the Global Burden of Disease reports include [131],

▶ Incomplete information
▶ Biases in information
▶ Disagreement among heterogeneous information sources
▶ Model uncertainty
▶ The data generation process itself.

The foundation for assigning disability weights to specific sequelae rests on an agreed definition and on an accepted method for measuring disability. First, there needs to be delineation of the health states among those living with the particular sequelae (such as burn scars), where a health state is defined by the levels on the various dimensions that constitute health. Second, there needs to be a valuation function that provides a systematic way to aggregate across multiple dimensions of health in order to arrive at a single index value that captures the overall level of health associated with a given health state [198]. Clearly the challenge is to find universal definitions for disability and tools for disability assessment. Accordingly, as many as half a million more DALYs may be lost each year to fires [131].

Routine reporting of fatal burns may be poor in LMIC. Special surveys or demographic surveillance by verbal autopsy and lay reporting may be needed to obtain trustworthy information. Community surveys, such as performed by Mashreky and associates (2008) in Bangladesh, will determine the incidence, circumstances, agent and mechanism, severity and consequences of burns, both fatal and non-fatal. The prevalence of disability and disfigurement, as well as the economic impact on the household, probably cannot be obtained except from comprehensive and thorough community surveys [34].

Much of the published literature on burn epidemiology characterizing etiology, severity and outcomes arises from studies of populations of patients treated at burn centers. Because of their design, these studies cannot enumerate the incidence and prevalence of important factors and variables that typify the burns that are commonly treated either at home or in primary care settings. Community surveys and examination of data from emergency rooms or clinics are preferable methods for establishing the magnitude of the burden of burn injuries throughout a district or region.

Other limitations arise in the interpretation of data from the US. Although the variable race is often studied, the limitations of racial and ethnic designations commonly used are subject to misinterpretation [163]. There are also pitfalls associated with use of length-of-stay as an outcome variable [169]. In one retrospective study of length of stay in burn patients, the variance unexplained by the studied variables was very high, with a coefficient of variance of nearly 100 % [162]. Patients admitted on Fridays may have longer lengths of stay for the same severity of injury as those admitted early in the week because of limited resources for discharge planning over the weekend. Excision and grafting of even small burns will lead to longer length of stay for pain control, immobilization, rehabilitation therapy, and assistance with activities of daily living than treatment of burns with topical antimicrobials only. Administration of intravenous medications, especially antibiotics and narcotics, will increase length of stay. Smoke inhalation injury and high-voltage electrical injury will also increase length of stay beyond the range noted for any given burn size. Lack of social support systems lead to longer hospital stays in the absence of medical factors necessitating continued in-patient care.

## Risk factors

### Socioeconomic factors

Household income and home value are correlated with fire deaths and burn injuries. In metropolitan Oklahoma City in 1987–90 the fire-related hospitalization and death rate was 3.6/100,000 [29]. However, when the examination of data from Oklahoma City was focused on an area characterized by lower median household income, lower property values, and poorer quality of housing, the fire injury rate was much higher, 15.3/100,000 [122]. Additionally, census tracts with low median incomes in Dallas had the highest rates of injury related to house fires, over 8 times that in tracts with high incomes [104]. Although there are a multitude of risk behaviors in low-income neighborhoods, such as alcohol and drug abuse that put those communities at risk for residential fires, clearly one important factor is the frequent absence of functioning smoke detectors. From 1991 through 1997 in Dallas, TX, the prevalence of operational smoke detectors was lowest in houses in the census tracts with the lowest median incomes [104].

Fire injuries also show the steepest social class gradient among all childhood injuries in England and Wales, with a 16-fold increase in death from fire and flames in the lowest socioeconomic class compared to the highest [181]. Non-fatal smoke inhalation injuries in an impoverished, multiethnic area of inner-city London in 1996–97 occurred at an incidence of 25/100,000 persons per year, over 30 times higher than the mortality from smoke inhalation in this series [60]. In this same quarter of London, the hospitalization rate for unintentional fire and flame injuries (8.2 per 100,000) was 1.75 times that in the southeastern United Kingdom, which includes urban, suburban and rural neighborhoods (DiGiuseppi 2000a).

Longitudinal observations of patients admitted to a single burn center in New Delhi suggest that overall socioeconomic improvements lead to a reduction in the frequency of injuries severe enough to require admission to a burn center. In 1993, the per-capita income in Delhi was US$450/year and 1276 patients were admitted that year; by 2005 the per-capita income in Delhi had risen to US$1542 and the number of admissions declined to 695 [7]. Although unproven, compelling is the hypothesis that the gradual decline in fire and burn deaths across the world is following improvements in living conditions and income.

### Race and ethnicity

In the US there are striking differences in susceptibility to burn injury by race. From 1991 through 1997, African-Americans in Dallas were 2.8 times more likely to be injured in house fires than whites [104]. In 2008 in the US the rate of non-fatal burns was 161 per 100,000 African-Americans, much higher than the observed rate of 109 per 100,000 in white non-Hispanics. In fact, in black Americans aged 35 to 39 years, the rate was 221 per 100,000 blacks, remarkably higher than the rate in whites in the same age group, which was 135 per 100,000 whites [47]. The emergency department visit rate for burn injuries from 1993 to 2004 in the US was 62 % greater among black than white subjects (340 vs. 210 per 100,000, respectively) [73].

The age-adjusted death rate from burns of all causes in the US in 2006 was highest in blacks (2.43 per 100,000) and lowest in Asians (0.44 per 100,000). Intermediate rates were noted among Native Americans (1.45), white non-Hispanics (1.11), and Hispanics (0.77 per 100,000). [47] Amongst children, there is a striking disparity in fire death rates between black and white children under the age of 15 years, with African-American children dying in residential fires at a rate nearly three times that of white children. However, by the teenage years of 15–19 years, this difference between the races is no longer present [47]. However, older African-Americans had 4.6 times the death rates of white seniors [87]. In Alabama from 1992 to 1997 the fire fatality rate was highest among older African-Americans [133]. Intriguingly, as household income increases, differences in fire death rates between blacks and whites diminish[137].

Racial differences in burn admissions occur by age group in data collected by the American Burn Association for the National Burn Registry.[3] Whereas for children under five years of age, 22 % of admissions to burn centers were black children and 44 % were white children, only 15 % of seniors aged 60 years or older were black and nearly 75 % were white (Table 3). In parallel with the decline of prevalence of blacks in the hospitalized burn population as age increases, Hispanic representation at burn centers was only 4 % of the elderly, compared to nearly 20 % of children under five

(Table 3). Hospital discharge rates for treatment of burns in Pennsylvania in 1994 showed that blacks were hospitalized for burns more than twice as frequently as whites (46.6 vs. 20.6 per 100,000, respectively) [78].

## Age-related factors: children

Despite their remarkable resilience, children across the world are commonly seriously injured, with pain and suffering, disability and occasionally death as the outcome. The highest fire-related death rates in children across the world occur in infants and children under four years of age. After age 15, death rates begin to climb again, presumably because of greater exposure to hazards, experimentation and risk-taking, as well as employment [232]. In the US, fires and burns were the third leading cause of unintentional injury death in the US in 2006 for children one to nine years of age [47].

Non-fatal burns in children are extremely common as well. In 2008 in the US, the crude rate of non-fatal burns was 156 per 100,000 in children under the age of 18 [47]. Strikingly, the rate for children up to three years of age was a staggering 358 per 100,000, and the fifth leading cause of unintentional non-fatal injury in US infants is burns [47]. The fact that 93 % of these young children were treated and released from emergency rooms suggests that the burns were probably minor scald and contact burns. In fact in the US, 67 % of the children hospitalized for burn injuries sustained burns of less than 10 % TBSA [201].

Compared to HIC, children under five years of age in LMIC have a disproportionately higher rate of burns [170]. For example, in Brazil, Côte d'Ivoire and India, nearly half of all childhood burns occur in infants [89, 189, 225]. Even in HIC, children who live in poor districts are at high risk of residential fire related injuries [105].

Various issues impact the likelihood that a child will be burned. These include literacy among mothers, knowledge of the risk of burns and of the means to secure health care, ownership of the house, kitchens separated from other living areas, use of fire-retardant chemicals in fabrics and upholstery, installation of smoke alarms and residential water sprinklers, appropriate first-aid and emergency response systems, and the existence of good quality health care services

---

3 The 2009 report of the National Burn Repository reviews the combined data set of acute burn admissions for the period 1999 – 2008. Seventy-nine hospitals (including 51 verified by the ABA as centers of excellence) from 33 states plus the District of Columbia contributed to this report, totaling 127,016 records. Sixty-two hospitals contributed more than 500 cases. Data were not dominated by any single center and appeared to represent a reasonable cross section of US hospitals.

**Table 3.** Summary of data from the National Burn Repository of the American Burn Association 1999–2008

| Age in years | White | Hispanic | Black | Scald | Flame | Contact | Electrical | Chemical | Burns >10% TBSA | Mortality |
|---|---|---|---|---|---|---|---|---|---|---|
| 0–0.9 N=3675 | 42% | 17% | 24% | 55% | 6% | 22% | >1% | >1% | 67% | >1% |
| 1–1.9 N=9387 | 42% | 21% | 22% | 57% | 4% | 20% | >1% | >1% | 67% | >1% |
| 2–4.9 N=7987 | 47% | 20% | 20% | 46% | 16% | 13% | 2% | >1% | 60% | 1% |
| 5–15.9 N=13,457 | 57% | 14% | 18% | 23% | 38% | 6% | 2% | >1% | 54% | >1% |
| 16–19.9 N=7230 | 66% | 12% | 13% | 17% | 40% | 4% | 2% | 2% | 50% | 2% |
| 20–29.9 N=19,033 | 60% | 13% | 16% | 18% | 35% | 4% | 4% | 3% | 47% | 2% |
| 30–39.9 N=17,657 | 61% | 13% | 15% | 18% | 36% | 4% | 5% | 4% | 45% | 3% |
| 40–49.9 N=18,421 | 64% | 9% | 17% | 17% | 38% | 4% | 5% | 4% | 46% | 4% |
| 50–59.9 N=12,523 | 66% | 8% | 17% | 16% | 39% | 5% | 4% | 3% | 44% | 6% |
| 60–69.9 N=6987 | 69% | 6% | 16% | 16% | 40% | 4% | 2% | 2% | 43% | 9% |
| 70–79.9 N=4825 | 72% | 4% | 14% | 15% | 42% | 4% | >1% | >1% | 40% | 16% |
| 80+ N=3594 | 77% | 3% | 13% | 16% | 38% | 6% | >1% | >1% | 36% | 25% |
| (Census 2000) | (70%) | (6%) | (12%) | | | | | | | |

[170]. Compared with children in the state of Tennessee (1980–1995) whose mothers had a college education, children whose mothers had less than a high school education had nearly 20 times greater risk of dying in a fire. Similarly, children whose mothers had three or more other children had over six times greater risk of dying in a fire when matched with children whose mothers had no other children. Likewise, when contrasted with children whose mothers were 30 years or older, children whose mothers were younger than 20 years of age had almost four times increased risk of dying in a fire. Fortunately, children characterized thusly comprise only 1.5% of the population. Nonetheless, the fatal fire rate for this high-risk group was 28.6 per 100,000, far exceeding the national norms for fire fatalities [197].

Children are more susceptible to burns than adults. The curiosity and desire to experiment of children is matched neither by their capacity to understand the potential of danger nor by their ability to respond to it [180]. Beginning at six months of age, children start reaching for objects and crawling, and are fully mobile by 18 months. This escalation in motor skills and activity increases the chance that children will encounter hot liquids and solids, electrical cords, candles, fireplaces, microwaves, treadmills, hair curlers and curling irons, ovens and stoves, chemicals, and other harmful agents. For instance, the majority of scald burns in children between the ages of six and 36 months are from hot foods and liquids spilled in the kitchen or dining room [149].

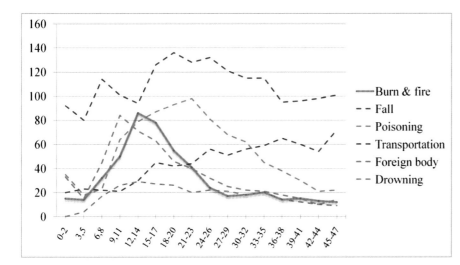

**Fig. 2.** Rates of injury hospitalization and death per 100,000 for children under four years of age in California 1996–1998 [5]. Rates are illustrated by three month intervals for the major categories of injury. The rate of burn and fire injuries peak between 12 and 18 months, similar to the pattern seen with foreign bodies in the airway and gastrointestinal tract. Rates of poisoning are begin to rise at the same period of childhood as burns, but do not decrease until after 27 months of age, nearly ¾ year later than the onset of the decrease in burns

Hot liquid and vapor injuries were the leading specific causes for children 12 to 17 months in a review of injuries in Californian children under the age of four years (Fig. 2). This age coincides with developmental achievements such as independent mobility, exploratory behavior, and hand-to-mouth activity. Although the child is able to gain access to hazards, he or she has not yet developed cognitive hazard awareness and avoidance skills [5]. Just as poisoning is linked to grasping and drinking behavior of children one to three years of age, scald burns are more common in children between one and five years of age than in any other age group [16].

Once risks are encountered, the child may lack the ability to escape danger. And because their cognitive development is not as advanced as motor development, they are not aware of the potentially damaging consequences of their behavior. For example, fires resulting from children's play are the leading cause of residential fire deaths in children under 10 years [149]. Therefore developmental stage becomes a risk factor for burn injuries [201].

Although the home is full of hazards, the young child views his or her dwelling as the centerpiece of their physical existence, in which they must eat, sleep, play, and resolve conflicts. Most home environments were not configured by architects to minimize the risk of injury to children. The space set aside for preparing and consuming food is such an example. Most women (mothers, grandmothers, aunts, nieces and older female children) find themselves involved in multiple tasks while preparing meals, including caring for the younger children. It is not surprising that low-income families are functioning in overcrowded conditions with only basic utilities and utensils, throughout which they are stressed by hunger, fatigue, frustration and fear. The prevention of scald or flame burns may be the last item on the agenda of the teenage sister charged with making dinner and caring for her younger siblings while her parents are away at work. In this regard, there is little difference between impoverished families in LMIC and HIC, thus explaining why scald burns in young children are universally common.

However, the presence of adults does not eliminate risk to children. In Greece the incidence of burns from contact with hot exhaust pipes while riding motorcycles 17 per 100,000 per year; many of these burns occur in children, who are passengers on the rear of the motorcycle. The responsibility of assuring safety to the child passenger rests with the motorcycle operator; the presence of contact burns from the exhaust pipe suggests negligence of this responsibility [130]. Similarly, review of childhood injuries treated at a large urban hospital in the US from 1972 through 1993 showed that adults were present 54 % of the time that children were injured by fireworks; for whatever reason, the presence of adults did not protect the children from harm [206]. Nonetheless, parents are aware of the importance of their responsibility of protecting children from the risk of burns, and consider lack of supervision around the home to be negligence, as noted in a survey of parents, students and teachers in rural Bangladesh [128].

## Age-related factors: the elderly

The elderly are at higher risk of injury than the younger age groups because they are more prone to injury due to deterioration of judgment and coordination as well as to the alterations in cognition and balance secondary to medications, and are more susceptible to the pathophysiological consequences of the physical insults of injury. Deaths from fires are the fourth leading cause of unintentional injury death (behind falls, motor vehicle incidents, and suffocation) among people aged 65 years or older in 2006 [47]. The elderly are at higher risk of dying in a residential fire than any other age group except for the very young [124]. Mortality data from 1984 collected by the National Center for Health Statistics showed that 29 % of the residential fire deaths were victims older than 65 years, although older people only represented 12 % of the US population at this time [87].

Even small, shallow burns are poorly tolerated by seniors. Elderly burn patients treated for scald burns had relatively small burns (mean 7 % TBSA) but high mortality (22 %). In addition, two-thirds who were living independently before the burn injury were forced into skilled nursing facilities after hospitalization for burn care [10].

Behavior patterns exacerbate the risk to the elderly. The elderly who smoke are more likely to die in residential fires than younger people who smoke [92]. Smoke detectors were absent in 75 % of the fatal fires involving the urban African-American elderly in Alabama from 1992 to 1997, and were completely absent in all of the fires leading to death of the rural African-American seniors. The cause of fire ignition was most often heating devices, which are used more commonly by the elderly and often with inadequate attention to the safe functioning of the device. Interestingly, alcohol was a factor in only 29 % of deaths of the elderly, compared with 74 % of the middle-aged [133].

Not only are the elderly more likely to die in residential fires, they are also more likely to succumb to complications following thermal injury. In US burn centers during the decade 1999–2008, in-hospital mortality was 9 % for the seventh decade of life, 16 % for the eighth, and 25 % for those over 80 years. These rates are even more striking when compared to the mortality rates for adults from 20 to 50 years (3 %) and especially to those for children under 16 years (less than 1 %) (Table 3).

In addition to their increased susceptibility to infectious and metabolic complications, the elderly are at higher risk for death after burns also because the burns for which they are admitted are larger in area. For example, although two-thirds of children under two years of age are hospitalized for treatment of burns less than 10 % of their body surface area, nearly 60 % of the elderly over 60 years of age are hospitalized for burns greater than 10 % BSA (Table 3). One study in Pennsylvania noted that patients 75 years and older had significantly more severe fire and burn injuries than younger patients (using the MedisGroups© morbidity score assigned during hospital stay) [78].

Indeed, age (along with burn size and presence of smoke inhalation injury) is one of the three most powerful predictors of outcome following thermal injury. Whereas the percentage of body surface area burned at which 50 % of cases will be fatal ($LA_{50}$) is over 90 % in children under two years of age, the $LA_{50}$ for elderly in the seventh decade of life is under 40 % TBSA, and is under only 20 % TBSA for those 80 years and older [16].

## Regional factors

The burden of burns is also unevenly distributed throughout regions of the world. For instance, the incidence of burn injuries severe enough to require medical care is nearly 20 times higher in the Western Pacific (including China) than in the Americas [232] (WHO regions of the world are graphically depicted in Fig. 3; specific lists of countries within each region can be found at http://www.who.int/about/regions/en/index.html.)

Burn fatalities are more like to occur in some regions of the world, even when gender and national income status are considered. Infants in Africa also have an incidence of fire-related burns which is three times the world average for this age group [103]. Specifically, the 2004 fire mortality rate in infant girls in Africa was 35 per 100,000, considerably higher than that in LMIC in Europe (3.5/100,000), the Americas (2.2/100,000), or the Western Pacific

**WHO Regions**

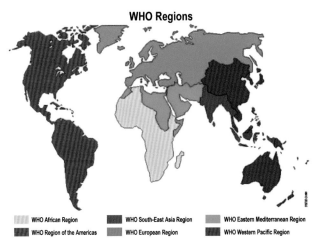

WHO African Region    WHO South-East Asia Region    WHO Eastern Mediterranean Region
WHO Region of the Americas    WHO European Region    WHO Western Pacific Region

**Fig. 3.** WHO Member States are grouped into six regions. Each region is further subdivided into low-income (LIC), middle-income (MIC), and high-income (HIC) countries. Both Africa and South-East Asia have no high-income countries. Listings of the countries in each region can be found at http://www.who.int/about/regions/en/index.html

(0.4/100,000) (Peden 2009). Similarly, fire death rates in boys 1–4 yrs in the Eastern Mediterranean LMIC were nearly twice that of those in boys 1–4 yrs in European LMIC. Moreover, fire mortality in South-East Asia was nearly six times that in the Western Pacific LMIC for boys under the age of four years.

Cold climates may be associated with a higher incidence of burn injury. Fatal residential fires in rural North Carolina that were not associated with smoking materials were caused primarily by heating appliances [186]. Lack of electricity mandates the use of hazardous flammable fuels, including open wood fires and kerosene heaters. Because children spend a great deal of time huddled together around open fires to keep warm, flame burns are common in Nepalese children (Thapa 1990). Older children are often responsible for lighting and tending fires, stoves and lamps, thus increasing their vulnerability to burns [114, 165].

On the other hand, the colder Northeastern region of the US had a lower fire and burn mortality rate in 2006 (0.97 per 100,000) than the more temperate South (1.49 per 100,000). In fact, the fire and burn mortality rate in some of the coldest states in the US were lower than the average national fire and burn mortality rate (1.23 per 100,000). For instance, the fire and burn mortality rate in New Hampshire and Ver-

mont was 0.5 per 100,000, and in Minnesota it was 0.7 per 100,000. Nonetheless, Alaska had the highest fire and burn mortality rate in the US, 2.72 per 100,000. Although temperate climates are not protective, warmer climates in the US seem to have lower fire and burn death rates, as noted in Arizona with 0.87 and Florida with 0.84 per 100,000 [47]. Even though it is tempting to associate fire and death mortality rates with alcohol use, data from the Substance Abuse and Mental Health Services Administration (SAMHSA) do not suggest any correlation between the two variables at a state level [102]. More discerning inspection of data from districts, cities and neighborhoods will be necessary to establish the association between burns and environmental or behavioral variables.

## Gender-related factors

Gender differences in injury rates begin to appear within the first year of life for many injuries. Sex differences in behavior appear about the same time as differences in injury rate and correlate with injury type. Boys are 70 per cent more likely to die by injury than girls in OECD[4] countries [222]. For children under 15 years of age, there are 24% more injury deaths among boys than among girls [232].

Burn death patterns follow a slightly different pattern. In the US in 2006 the mortality rates for burn deaths for children under 20 years of age was nearly identical (0.7 per 100,000 for boys and 0.65 per 100,000 for girls). However, in the youngest age group (infancy through four years) the fire death rate for boys was 1.24 that of girls [47].

There are several theories about why boys are more likely to be injured than are girls. Boys are socialized differently: parents are more likely to allow boys to roam further with fewer limits and to play

---

4   The Organisation for Economic Cooperation and Development (OECD) are 29 countries which produce two-thirds of the world's goods and services. The OECD member countries, as at December 2000, are: Australia, Austria, Belgium, Canada, the Czech Republic, Denmark, Finland, France, Germany, Greece, Hungary, Iceland, Ireland, Italy, Japan, the Republic of Korea, Luxembourg, Mexico, the Netherlands, New Zealand, Norway, Poland, Portugal, Spain, Sweden, Switzerland, Turkey, the United Kingdom of Great Britain and Northern Ireland, and the United States of America [222].

alone [40, 74, 189]. Boys are also engaged in more risk taking and higher activity levels and behave more impulsively than girls [67, 184]. However, in a study done in 1978 of injuries in children reported to the Consumer Product Safety Commission [179], the gender differences were not explained by exposure to risk.

The gender difference is observed in adults as well. The emergency department visit rate for burn injuries from 1993 to 2004 in the US was 50 % greater among men than women (270 vs. 180 per 100,000, respectively) [73]. In Pennsylvania in 1994, the overall hospital discharge rate for treatment of burns in men was over twice that in women (37 vs. 16.5 per 100,000, respectively) [78]. The age-adjusted rate of non-fatal burns in the US in 2008 was 143 per 100,000 in men, higher than the rate of 128 per 100,000 seen in women [47]. However, in the US from 2001 to 2006, non-fatal scald burns were more common among elderly women than elderly men (age 65 years or older) [48].

Nonetheless, elderly males have higher fire death rates in the US than elderly females [87]. However, the difference is most prominent in the 20 to 44 age group, in which the ratio of fire mortality in men is nearly twice that in women [47].

Additionally, males shoulder a higher proportion of the disability associated with injury. Men account for 78 % of the DALY's lost from injuries to adults 15–44 years of age in Australia [37].

Occupational activities put people at risk for work-related injuries. During the time period 1993 to 2004 in the US, 23 % of emergency department visits for burn injury were work-related [73]. From 1999 to 2008, 11 % of admissions to US burn centers were for occupational injuries [16]. US workers in the mining, transportation and public utilities industries had the highest rate of death from thermal injury in 1992 to 1999. Occupations with the highest risk of death by fire include truck drivers, firefighters, miners, airline pilots, and operators of ovens, furnaces and kilns [171]. Because the majority of these high-risk occupations are held by men, adult males will have higher rates of burn injuries in countries which offer them these roles. Men were seen nearly twice as often as women for work-related burns in US emergency departments 1993–2004 [73].

Gender differences in burn incidence may vary by age, region and national income category. For instance, in rural Ethiopia burns occur more often to boys than girls, but it is women who are more frequently burned than men [54].

Gender differences in HIC and LIC fire deaths are polar opposites. Rates of death by fire in HIC are twice as high in males as in females in the 15 to 59 year age group. However, in this same age group in LIC, female deaths from burns occur at a rate 2.3 times that in males. The discrepancy is greatest in WHO South-East Asia and Eastern Mediterranean Regions [232]. Nine percent of all deaths among Egyptian women of reproductive age were caused by burns [193].

However, the gender distribution of non-fatal burns differs between countries. Although some countries such as Egypt and India have a greater proportion of burns among girls, a higher number of cases in boys have been reported in Angola, Bangladesh, China, Côte d'Ivoire, Kenya and Nigeria [2, 35, 80, 82, 98, 126, 150, 225, 234].

The gender discrepancy in LMIC fire death rates is present but less pronounced in young children. However, between the ages of 15 and 19 women begin to suffer a disproportionate share of fire deaths. Women between the ages of 15 and 59 in LIC have an astonishingly high fire death rate of 15.6 per 100,000 [232]. In India, approximately 65 % of burn deaths occur to women, most often caused by kitchen accidents, self-immolation and domestic violence [195].

The increasing proportion of burns among girls as they enter adolescence can be explained in some cases by the changing activities as they approach the responsibilities of adulthood. In the Ardabil province of Iran in 2006, teenage girls were three times as likely to be burned in the kitchen as teenage boys. In Ardabil, 21 % to 37 % of children are involved in kitchen jobs such as lighting the oven, preparing tea and carrying hot food; the mean age for starting to help in the kitchen is approximately 8 years [18].

*Intent*

The vast majority of burn injuries in the world are unintentional. In US burn centers from 1999–2008, 2 % of admissions were for assault-by-burning (including child abuse), and less than 1 % for self-harm or attempted suicide [16]. Similarly, in 1994 in Pennsylvania, 2 % of burn admissions were for self-inflicted injuries, and another 2 % for assault-by-burning; 95 % were unintentional [78]. Only 2.4 % of admissions to burn centers in Taiwan, ROC, from 1997 to 2003 were for self-inflicted injuries [217].

India has the highest number of cases of intentional self-harm by burning in the world. The majority of victims are young women, as opposed to Europe, where they are more often men in their fourth or fifth decade of life [88, 116].

### Comorbidity

Because epilepsy is often untreated in LMIC, it is a frequent initiating factor in many severe burns [139]. During a seizure the epileptic may fall into an open fire or onto a stove. The severity of injury is sometimes and unfortunately exacerbated by traditional beliefs that epilepsy is contagious; victims in Ethiopia are often left to burn because of fear by potential rescuers of contacting the disease by touching the victim [211]. Burns precipitated by epileptic seizures occurred in 44 % of adult burn injuries in a community survey in rural Ethiopia, and 29 % of adult burns admitted to the hospital were precipitated by epileptic seizures [54]. Epilepsy was the most common personal risk factor, other than age, in remote subsistence village of the highlands of Papua New Guinea during 1971 to 1986, where the mortality rates from fire and flames were nearly 15 per 100,000, many times higher than reported rates from other countries [33]. In rural Bangladesh, 0.7 % of all deaths to women (15–44 years of age) were caused by falls into fires during seizure activity; this is an annual rate of approximately 2 per 100,000 [75].

Many Muslim epileptics insist on fasting during the holy month of Ramadan and hence miss their anti-epileptic medications. Therefore, burns in epileptics are commonly seen during Ramadan in Islamic populations. These burns are typically sustained during seizures while in the kitchen or falling on the hot ground (which can reach temperatures over 115 °F). In a prospective study of burns in epileptics in Saudi Arabia, 40 % of injured patients sustained the burn while fasting because they did not take their anti-epileptic medications [11, 12].

Peripheral neuropathy is a disorder commonly caused by leprosy and diabetes mellitus, and results in sensory loss of the extremities. People with sensory peripheral neuropathy are vulnerable to burn injuries, especially hot water scalds [110]. Handling hot cooking utensils or warming neuropathic feet too close to a fire can also cause deep burns.

One of the reasons that the elderly are at higher risk of sustaining injuries is because of coexisting medical conditions. Seventy-seven percent of burn center patients aged 59 years or older in a single-center study had one or more preexisting medical conditions at the time of injury, and in 57 % of patient's judgment, mobility or both were impaired [132]. In another study, 50 % of octogenarians admitted for burn treatment sustained injury because of a cerebrovascular accident [45]. Physical or cognitive disabilities are distinct risk factors for burns, especially for scald burns or for death from residential fires. Thirty-seven patients with disabilities were admitted to a burn center in Toronto between 1984 and 1992; the majority of them (84 %) were admitted for scald burns in the home. Although some were elderly as well (median age was 58 years), the extent of disability was significant in all cases, including spinal cord disorders or injuries, epilepsy or other neurological disorders. Given the relatively small size of burn (mean was 10 % TBSA), the mortality rate was 22 %, which is high compared to 4 % in the general burn population. The average length of stay for disabled burn patients was 2.8 days per percent body surface area burned, in comparison to the general population of burn patients in whom length of stay is approximately one day per percent burn [16, 22]. Although the relative risk of burns in the elderly with dementia has not yet been established, expert opinion among burn centers is that dementia is a significant risk factor for burns. Indeed, elderly patients with dementia tend to have poorer outcomes from burns injuries, and rehabilitation is very limited [9].

### Agents

Flame burns and scalds occur at approximately the same frequency in children under the age of 18 years in some LMIC, including China and Iran [117, 234]. In general, however, and particularly in younger children, scald burns are more common than flame burns in children. For example, three pediatric hospitals in Mexico noted that the majority of emergency room visits for burns in children under 10 years of age was because of exposure to boiling liquids, most commonly overly hot bath water [99]. Over 75 % of children under the age of 18 hospitalized for treatment of burns in Taiwan, Republic of China, were injured by scalding liquids [221]. In burn centers in the US, scald burns account for nearly half the admissions of children under five years of age. For very young children under two years, flame burns cause only 5 % of admissions; contact burns are more common in this age group, involving over 20 % of admissions (Table 3).

Even when older children up to the age of 18 years are included in analysis, scald burns still outnumber fire and flame injuries by a ratio of 1.6:1 in US burn centers and 5:1 in all US hospitals [201, 16]. Nonetheless, older children and young teenagers between five and 16 years of age experience fewer scald burns than their younger siblings: only 23 % of admissions are for scalds, compared to 38 % for flame burns (Table 3).

Scald burns are very common in adults as well. A study of discharges from all hospitals in Pennsylvania in 1994 (including hospitals without burn centers as well as the six hospitals with burn centers) showed that 56 % of admissions were for treatment of scald burns [78].

Nonetheless, flame burns overall cause more admissions to US burn centers than any other single cause of thermal injury. Through the adult decades, flame burns continue to be the cause for 35 % to 42 % of admissions, and scalds for 15 % to 18 % (Table 3).

Fortunately, the majority of burns of any etiology are small to moderate in size: 86 % of burns admitted to US burn centers 1999–2008 involved less than 20 % of the body surface area [16].

Clothing ignition is a common cause of severe flame burns. Although conflagrations caused 78 % of the deaths in the elderly in the US in 1984, 11 % of fatalities were from clothing ignitions [87]. Women of the Indian subcontinent wearing loose flammable saris (made of cotton or synthetic textiles) are vulnerable to fire deaths when their clothing is ignited while cooking near open flames, particularly if the cooking source is an open fire pit or a small kerosene stove on the ground [66]. Ninety-three percent of burn injuries in rural Ethiopia occurred inside the home where open fires were used in the common room and often ignite clothing [58]. Likewise, ignition of grass skirts in warm coastal areas of Papua New Guinea account for nearly half of hospitalizations for burns [32].

Flammable fuels are often the agents of fire acceleration or heat production in incidents that result in flame burns. The unsafe use of gasoline was implicated in 87 % of patients in whom the cause of the burn could be identified at single-site retrospective study of burns admitted from 1978 to 1996 in the US [28]. Liquefied petroleum gas (LPG) has replaced kerosene in many households in LMIC as per-capita income has risen and availability of smaller and more affordable LPG cylinders has improved. In Delhi, LPG-related burns were responsible for over 10 % of admissions from 2001 to 2007 [7].

Electrical and chemical burns are rarely reasons for admission in children, occurring less than 2 % of the time, but account for 4 % to 5 % of admissions of adults from 20 to 60 years of age (Table 3). The frequency of admissions for contact burns declines precipitously with age: although one-fifth of admissions of children under two years are for contact burns, only about 5 % of adult admissions are for contact burns (Table 3).

## Residential fires

The products of combustion consist of fire gases, heat, visible smoke, and toxicants. The hazards created by these products of combustion include effects of heat on the upper airway, toxicant damage to the sub-glottic respiratory system, impaired vision due to smoke density or eye irritation, and narcosis from inhalation of asphyxiants. These effects lead contribute to restricted vision, loss of motor coordination, impaired judgment, disorientation, physical incapacitation and panic. The resultant delay or prevention of escape from the burning structure leads to injury and death from inhalation of toxic gases and from thermal burns. Extricated survivors may go on to die later in the hospital from complications such as respiratory failure, septic shock, and multiple organ system failure, all of which are rooted in the initial exposure to products of combustion [94].

Smoke is defined as the airborne solid and liquid particulates and fire gases created during combustion and when materials undergo decomposition or transformation by heat [20]. Pyrolysis is the decomposition of a material from heat and does not require the normal atmospheric level of oxygen, leading to incomplete combustion. The toxicant gases produced in a fire can be categorized into separate classes: the asphyxiants which induce unconsciousness, and the irritants which inflame the eyes and respiratory tract. The major threat in most fire atmospheres is carbon monoxide, an asphyxiant produced by incomplete combustion.

The vast majority of deaths due to fires in the US each year occur because of exposure to products of combustion in structure conflagrations. From 1992 to 2001, two-thirds of fire deaths in the US occurred in residential fires [76]. (Although residential fires are the primary cause of fire mortalities, they account for only half of structure fire injuries and less than one-third of the dollar loss for fires.) Residential fires accounted for 76 % of the years of life lost in 2006 in the US due to flame burns [47].

Although most victims of fatal fires die from smoke inhalation, a few will die of thermal injury directly. Temperatures higher than 300 °F are reached within five to ten minutes in building fires, and in an aircraft cabin the temperatures near 500 °F in just five to six minutes [69, 98]. Flashover[5] can occur in less than 10 minutes in even a slowly progressing residential fire, at which time temperatures soar from 1100 °F to over 2000 °F in seconds, creating an environment in which survival is unprecedented. In the absence of inhalation of products of combustion and pyrolysis, death can be caused by heat-induced laryngospasm or by vagal-reflex mediated cardiac arrest [202].

Although a well-burning fire produces much more carbon dioxide than carbon monoxide (CO), materials in most structure fires smolder because of rapid depletion of oxygen in the interior of the building. Although the pathophysiology of CO poisoning is well-under-

stood, there remains no readily apparent explanation for the observation that the range of carboxyhemoglobin (COHb) tolerated is very wide. Although COHb saturation greater than 35 % can cause death in some people, others have survived COHb saturations as high as 64 % [94]. The average COHb level in fire fatalities is 60 %, with a range of 25 to 85 % [202]. About 10–15 % of CO binds to myoglobin and cytochrome A3, blocking production of ATP and causing muscular weakness, thus exacerbating the difficulties the victim encounters during escape maneuvers [229].

Unfortunately, COHb levels rise rapidly in house fires. When the CO level in inspired air reaches 5 %, COHb rises to 10 % in 10 seconds and to 40 % (a fatal level in some people) in only 30 seconds [209]. A study in East Denmark from 1982–1986 demonstrated that the blood alcohol concentration averaged about 190–200 mg/dl in fatalities from residential fires, and the mean COHb was about 60 % [214]. However, it is clear that some people with pre-existing functional impairments are at risk for increased CO toxicity at lower COHb levels, including children and the elderly, the physically disabled, and those impaired by alcohol, drug or medication intoxication [60, 104]. Largely for this reason, children under age five years and the elderly over 65 years account for 45 % of home fire deaths [108]. Patients with coronary artery disease cannot increase coronary blood flow when COHb rises above 10 % [25]. In addition to inhibiting cognitive responses, ethanol also potentiates the effects of CO such that lower levels of COHb are associated with fatality [46].

Although hydrogen cyanide (HCN), which is produced by the combustions of materials that contain nitrogen such as wool, silk, acrylonitrile polymers, nylons, and polyurethanes, is 20 times more toxic than CO, its role as a causative agent in human fire fatalities is less clear than that of CO. For example, in many fire deaths, COHb is in the toxic range, but cyanide levels are not toxic [119]. Nonetheless, low levels of COHb in other fire fatalities suggest that other toxic gases such as HCN may play a role in causing death [8].

Because oxygen is consumed during combustion, the oxygen level in the inspired air ($O_2$) can drop from 21 % to levels that affect coordination, mentation and consciousness. When $O_2$ drops to 17 %, coordination is impaired, when it drops to 14 %

---

5   Flashover is defined as a transitional phase in the development of a compartment fire in which surfaces exposed to thermal radiation reach ignition temperature more or less simultaneously and fire spreads rapidly throughout the space resulting in full room involvement or total involvement of the compartment or enclosed area. (NFPA 921 - 1992, Guide for Fire and Explosion Investigations, National Fire Protection Association, Quincy, MA, (1992).)

judgment becomes faulty, and below 6% unconsciousness occurs [94].

Acrolein is formed from the smoldering of all plant materials (including wood and the natural fibers used in decorations and furnishings), and is a potent sensory and pulmonary irritant. It is extremely irritating to the eyes at concentrations as low as a few parts per million [170].

Level of consciousness and thus ability to escape are affected by drugs and alcohol [8]. One-third to one-half of victims of fatal fires have ingested alcohol [81, 133, 207]. Ethanol intoxication significantly impairs the ability to escape from fire and smoke and is a contributory factor in smoke-related mortality. Whereas victims found near escape exits had blood alcohol levels (BALs) averaging 88 mg/dl, the mean BAL was 268 mg/dl in those found dead in bed, presumably having made no attempt to escape [27]. Moreover, if even one person in the house is impaired by alcohol or drug usage, others in the dwelling are at increased risk of death from fire as well [190].

Perhaps the most deadly combination leading to fatal fires is alcohol and cigarettes. Not only in higher socioeconomic neighborhoods is smoking in bed while inebriated one of the most common causes of death by fire, but also in indigenous communities in North America. Seventy-six percent and 90% of the adult victims of residential fires in Canadian Indians in Manitoba and Alberta, respectively, were under the influence of alcohol at the time of death [79, 106].

Risk factors for fatal and non-fatal house fire injuries include young or old age, male gender, non-white race, low income, disability, smoking and alcohol use [227]. Single, detached mobiles homes had the highest rate of fire deaths of all types of residences [227]. In rural areas, risk of death from a residential fire in a mobile (manufactured) home is 1.7 times the risk in a single- or multiple-family home [190]. In addition, the presence of an able-bodied adult who is not impaired by alcohol or drugs will significantly the odds of survival in a house fire [124]. Burn injuries and fire fatalities are more common in older homes and from fires started in the bedroom or living room from heating equipment, smoking or children playing with fire [104].

## Non-electric domestic appliances

In many households in LMIC, especially in rural areas lacking electrification, open flames are common, including floors of huts with open hearths which are used for cooking and warmth, candles, and small kerosene and naphtha stoves and lanterns. The fire risk from these sources are contributed by lack of enclosure for open fires, floor-level location of fires and stoves, instability of appliances, nearby storage of volatile and flammable fuels, flammable clothing and housing materials, and lack of exits [34].

A large number of burn injuries and fire deaths in LMIC are related to the nature of non-electric domestic appliances that are used for cooking, heating, lighting or all three. The incidence of injuries is largely associated with the use of stoves and lamps, and from kerosene (termed paraffin in some countries) and petroleum as well as butane, liquid petroleum gas and alcohol. Associated problems include appliance design and construction, fuel combustion and instability, and mechanical inefficiency. Ignorance of safe usage techniques is also contributory. Industry and government regulations and standards are either nonexistent or not adequately enforces [165].

Informal settlements in densely populated urban areas are often scenes for fires that lead to incalculable property damage and horrific loss of life. From 2002 to 2004, approximately 12% of households in South Africa were "shacks", living quarters assembled from highly combustible and toxic materials and usually assembled close to one another on uneven ground. Kerosene is used as fuel for small stoves; the more inexpensive the stove, the more likely it is to tip over or malfunction. During a simulated shack fire triggered by a kerosene stove that was knocked over while burning, the temperature in the shack reached an excess of 1670°F in less than four minutes [159]. Shack fire burns are the second most common reason for admission to burn centers in Cape Town, and the most common cause of shack fires in these cases is the use of kerosene stoves [83].

Serious injuries from kerosene stoves have been documented in Egypt, Ethiopia, India, Nigeria, Pakistan and other LMIC [6, 70, 85, 90, 120, 123, 148, 196]. The underlying problem of kerosene stove-related fires often lies with design issues. Poor design allows for fuel leakage, which is especially common when stove reservoirs are being filled. Kerosene can leak onto clothing, or if heat or flames are present nearby during fueling, vapors can ignite. Ignorance of safe techniques in using fuel and appliances will also lead to catastrophic explosions if gasoline contaminates or is substituted for kerosene. In addition, these small, portable stoves are often very unstable, easily tipping over while being moved or even when resting in place. On occasion, the small stove is used as a weapon, thrown by the assailant at the victim, igniting his or her clothing on fire [165].

The essential issue is that families at greatest risk because of poverty, ignorance, and overcrowding, lack the resources needed to purchase stoves of safe and dependable design. The most affordable stoves in South Africa are little over US$3 each, but these flame or wick stoves are notorious for rapidly fluctuating flame size, instability, and explosions. In addition, the impoverished housing conditions lead to poor air circulation, and incomplete combustion of kerosene in flame stoves produces significant levels of toxicants such as carbon monoxide. Even in dwellings supplied with electricity, low-income families will often choose to use kerosene stoves for cooking because of cost savings.

## War, mass casualties, and terrorism

Military personnel are at high risk for burn injury in wartime. In general, however, the distribution of burn size in combat is similar to that observed in the US community: 80 % of burns are less than 20 % TBSA in size [173]. Many burn casualties occur during combat at sea. In the Falkland Islands campaign (1982), for instance, 34 % of all British Navy casualties were burns [50]. Personnel in armored fighting vehicles are also at relatively high risk for burn injuries and fire deaths. For example, the proportion of burn casualties during the Yom Kippur War (1973) was nearly 11 %, higher than that of less than 5 % seen during the Israeli Six-Day War (1967) because there was greater saturation of the battlefield with tanks and anti-tank weaponry [156]. Subsequent to the Yom Kippur War, the Israeli army enforced use of flame retardant garments and installed automatic fire extinguishing systems within tanks. These changes led to a decrease in incidence to less than 9 % of military burn casualties

during the Lebanon War (1982). Those modifications have also been credited with reduction of burn size in those who were injured [71].

Fire, flames and explosions have caused mass burn casualties over the centuries. In 1190, a fire in Clifford's Tower, York, UK, took the lives of 150 Jews who had been besieged by an anti-Semitic mob [63]. A theater fire in Canton, China, claimed the lives of 1670 in 1845. In Santiago, Chile (1863), between 2000 and 3000 lives were lost when a gas lamp near the main altar ignited veils on the walls of *la Iglesia de la Compañía de Jesús* (the Church of the Company of Jesus) [151]. On April 27, 1865, *USS Sultana*, a steamboat returning Union prisoners-of-war to their homes in the North, caught fire when one of its boilers exploded on the Mississippi River near Memphis and sank, taking with her approximately 1800 casualties from burns and drowning [101].

Throughout the twentieth century in the US, there have been several fire or burn disasters in which more than 100 people were killed, including the Iroquois Theater fire in Chicago (1903) with 602 fatalities and 220–250 injuries, forest fires near Cloquet and Moose Lakes in Minnesota (1918) with 800 fatalities and 85 injuries, and the Cocoanut Grove Nightclub fire in Boston (1942) with 492 fatalities and 166 injuries [31]. More recent examples include fire disasters at the Beverly Hills Supper Club in Kentucky (1977) with 165 fatalities, the MGM Grand Hotel in Las Vegas (1980) with 84 fatalities, the Alfred P. Murrah building explosion in Oklahoma City (1995) with 168 fatalities, and the attacks on the Pentagon Building and the World Trade Center (2001) with 189 and 2750 deaths, respectively. The last three mass-casualty incidents were the result of terrorism, and casualties were caused not only by smoke inhalation and thermal injuries, but by blast, crush and fall injuries.

Indeed, most of the mass-casualty terrorist attacks in the US have employed conventional explosives or incendiary agents (such as jet fuel). A bomb placed under the staircase in the 16th Street Baptist Church in Birmingham, AL, in 1963 caused the death of four young girls; the motivation was anger over public integration of the races [203]. The first attack by foreign terrorists on American soil came in 1993 when a truck bomb with conventional explosives was detonated in the underground parking garage of the World Trade Center, taking the lives of six persons. The uses of ammonium nitrate and fuel oil in Oklahoma City, and of jet fuel delivered by commercial airliners at the Pentagon and World Trade Center have escalated the toll from such deadly terrorist attacks.

Terrorist attacks have dominated regions of religious, cultural and political conflict since the latter half of the twentieth century. Sectarian violence in Northern Ireland has resulted in nearly 3000 deaths since 1968, much of them from explosions. Progress in negotiations between Israelis and Palestinians has been hampered by the frequency of terrorist incidents; between 2000 and 2002, Israel sustained two bombings per month. Before they were neutralized in Sri Lanka in 2009, the Liberation Tigers of Tamil Eelam conducted approximately 200 suicide bombings since the late 1980's. The armed conflicts in Iraq, Afghanistan and Pakistan have all been marked by frequent suicide bombings. Clearly, preparation for any terrorist event in the future must take into account the inevitability of burn injuries as a result of explosive devices [55].

## Interventions

A priority in LMIC must be to improve the provision of health care for burns to all in the population so that inequity in acute treatment is eliminated. This includes the training of doctors and nurses in acute burn care management as well as those in the allied services (such as physiotherapists, nutritionists, occupational therapists, psychologists and social workers). However, the reality is that social, political and fiscal challenges make this goal many years distant in the future.

Thus the conclusion to be drawn is that prevention is the key to alleviation of suffering from burns. Truly the best way to treat a burn is to prevent it from happening in the first place. In reality, effective prevention programs will face similar barriers to implementation as those faced by efforts to improve acute care, but in many ways prevention is much more cost-effective, and will clearly reach vastly greater numbers of people. People of LMIC will be best protected from the horrors of burn injuries by expanding the global effort to eliminate burns.

Prevention works. The number of child deaths by injury in OECD nations fell by about 50 % between 1970 and 1995 [218]. According to research in Israel 1998–2000, injury prevention programs were effective in reducing burn-related hospitalizations among infants and toddlers, especially from more affluent communities [168]. In Harstad, Norway, in 1987, a comprehensive community-based injury prevention program characterized by strengthening of public participation and the enhancement of community empowerment achieved by recording and actively using the local burn injury data, resulted in a reduction in burn injuries in children [235].

Aside from the reduction in pain and suffering, prevention efforts are cost-effective as well. It has been estimated that for every dollar spent on smoke alarms, $69 in fire-related costs are saved [147].

The traditional approach to injury prevention involves the three E's: education, engineering and enforcement. However, although many resources are expended on community education, the beneficial effects are not clear. Two reviews have not identified evidence of beneficial effects from community, school, or clinic based fire safety education on fire injuries [61, 228]. Counseling and educational interventions had only a modest effect on the likelihood of owning a smoke alarm (odds ratio [OR] 1.3) or having a functional alarm (OR = 1.2), but these effects were enhanced in the setting of primary child health care surveillance (OR 1.9 and 1.7, respectively) [61, 62]. Similarly, review of the effectiveness of school education programs in reducing the incidence of burns in Israel noted a lack of efficacy [168].

Engineering (modification of agents or environment) and enforcement (creation and implementation of guidelines, codes and laws) require more resources, but are more effective. There are several examples of successful approaches to reduction of incidence or severity of burns [21].

### Smoke detectors

During combustion, the combined hazards of heat and smoke intensify over time to a point at which environmental conditions are incompatible with life. Between the time the fire is discovered and the critical time at which point escape is impossible, is a period during which actions can be taken to minimize or prevent injury. The role of early detection systems is to lengthen this interval. (In some cases, when victims

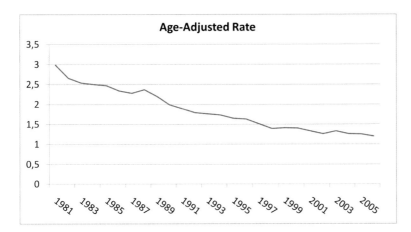

**Fig. 4.** Deaths from fire and burns in the US have declined from a rate of 2.99 per 100,000 in 1981 to 1.2 per 100,000 in 2006, according to the Web-based Injury Statistics Query and Reporting System of the Centers for Disease Control and Prevention (http://webappa.cdc.gov/sasweb/ncipc/mortrate.html). (CDC 2009) Residential fire deaths cause the majority of deaths due to fire and burns in the US, ranging from 70–80% each year from 1981 through 2006. Age-adjusted death rates from residential fires declined an average of 20% every five years from 1981 to 1991. The decrease in residential fire death rates recently has been less remarkable, with only a 10% decrease from 2001 to 2006

are overcome by hypoxia and CO poisoning while asleep or intoxicated, there is effectively no interval time period for action.) Data from the United Kingdom, which tracks the interval between the time of ignition and the time of discovery, confirm that smoke alarms result in quicker fire discovery. Sixty-three percent of the home fires in which the alarm was raised by the smoke alarm were discovered within five minutes of ignition, and the fire was confined to the item of origin in 62% of these incidents [59].

Early detection systems include different types of fire warning equipment such as sprinklers and devices that detect heat or smoke.[6] From 1977 to 1982 there was rapid increase in the number of homes protected by smoke alarms, followed by a slower but continual rise in installation through 1993. Although the prevalence of usage has leveled since then, 96% of homes surveyed by telephone reported having at least one working smoke alarm

[3, 223]. The death rate per 100 reported home structure fires from 2003 to 2006 in the US was twice as high when no working smoke alarm was present (that is, either no smoke alarm was present or an alarm was present but did not operate) compared to the rate with working smoke alarms (1.16 vs. 0.59). Having a working smoke alarm cuts the chances of dying in a residential fire in half [4].

Inversely correlating with the rise in usage of smoke detectors has been the decline in residential fire and flame deaths. The age-adjusted death rate in 1981 from residential fires was 2.28; by 1997 that rate was reduced by almost 50% (Fig. 4; CDC 2009). Although smoke alarms have contributed significantly to this reduction in mortality, other factors have been beneficial as well, including safer heating and cooking appliances, child resistant lighters, flame resistant mattresses, furniture, and clothing, and improvement in acute care of burn victims.

Many states and the District of Columbia have laws that require smoke alarms to be installed in both new and existing buildings. Other states have laws for specific conditions, such as new home construction, multi-family dwellings, or rental properties. As a result, burn injuries have decreased 26% and deaths decreased 31% [149].

These efforts to promote smoke detectors are best combined with accompanying educational efforts so that building occupants develop and rehearse escape plans in advance. Likewise, plans should be made as to whether ancillary devices, such as escape ladders might be necessary [13]. Installing, testing and maintaining smoke alarms are critical for protection from a residential fire, but

---

6   Photoelectric detectors pass a beam a light above a sensor. Under normal conditions, the light beam passes above the sensor with no deflection of light to the sensor, which is positioned at 90 degrees from the light beam. However, when smoke particles in the air cause some of the light to scatter, some of the light is dispersed to the sensor, which then triggers the alarm. Photoelectric alarms respond sooner to fires that begin with a long period of smoldering without flames. Ionizing detectors contain a small amount of Americium-241, which emits *alpha* particles. The Americium ionizes the oxygen and nitrogen in the air of the ionization chamber, causing a small current to flow between the two plates in the chamber. The presence of smoke in the chamber disrupts this current flow, which is then detected and triggers the alarm. Ionizing detectors respond quickly in flaming fires.

they are not enough. A smoke alarm merely sounds the warning, but it cannot by itself remove people from harm. Unfortunately, many households have not developed the escape plans that would allow them to use to best advantage the extra warning time smoke alarms provide. Escape plans will identify obstacles to secondary exits if the main door is blocked, establish a meeting place outside the home for household members to gather, and make provisions for disabled, young or old household members [4].

Almost two-thirds of home fire deaths resulted from fires in properties without sounding smoke alarms. In 2003–2006, smoke alarms were present in roughly two-thirds (69 %) of reported home fires and sounded in roughly half (47 %) of the home fires reported to U. S. fire departments. Forty percent of home fire deaths resulted from fires in which no smoke alarms were present at all. Twenty three percent of the deaths were caused by fires in properties in which smoke alarms were present and but failed to operate [4].

Despite the dissemination of smoke detectors into homes, 2704 people died in 2006 from residential fires [47]. Although the death rate in residential fires is doubled if smoke alarms are either not installed or not functional, the presence of functional alarms does not eliminate the risk of death. Functional smoke alarms were found in 34 % of residential fire deaths from 2000–2004, and the mortality rate in residences with functional smoke alarms was 0.55 per 100,000 [3]. The households with smoke alarms that don't work now outnumber the households with no alarms by a substantial margin [4]. Any program to ensure adequate protection must include smoke alarm maintenance. In one-fifth of all homes with smoke alarms, none were working [4].

In reality, people do not always evacuate when fire alarms sound. Fire alarms are intended to meet four objectives: 1) warning occupants, 2) stimulating them to respond immediately, 3) initiating the evacuation process, and thus 4) providing enough time to escape. In truth, however, rather than assuming that a fire is occurring, people who hear a fire alarm tend to seek the reason for the alarm, such as the smell of smoke. Once they do recognize a fire, instead of calling the fire department and evacuating, they may engage in other activities such as fighting the fire or collecting belongings. People often fail to respond for a variety of reasons: 1) sometimes the signal is not recognized as a fire alarm, being misinterpreted as a burglar, elevator, or security door alarm, 2) sometimes people do not know what they should do, particularly if they are outside the home environment such as in a commercial space, 3) because of nuisance alarms, people may not believe the smoke alarm signals a real danger, and 4) because of distance from the alarm, background noise, or individual characteristics, they may not hear the signal [172].

Studies of unwanted alarms have consistently shown that smoke alarms produce far more nuisance activations than real alarms. A study of Veterans Administration hospitals found one unwanted activation for every six devices per year and 15.8 unwanted activations for every real alarm [64]. The 2000 New Zealand smoke alarm installation follow-up study found that smoke alarms provided warnings of actual fires in 7 % of the households, but 38 % of the households reported problems with nuisance alarms [65].

Regrettably, the stress of nuisance alarms outweighs the benefit of smoke alarm protection to some people. A study in the UK during 1999–2002 conducted group and individual interviews with adults and children to explore perceptions of fire risk, the benefits and problems associated with smoke alarms, and whether they would recommend smoke alarms to others. Some adults described feeling very stressed by false alarms, and expressed resentment about the smoke alarm going off during what was perceived as normal cooking. The perception of some children was that smoke alarms activated any time someone was cooking. As a consequence, smoke alarm activations were not viewed as emergencies. The authors remarked, "In a population already managing a range of health risks, a public health intervention that makes mealtime more, rather than less, stressful, where noise can threaten leisure or relationships with fellow occupants, alarms could pose a threat to immediate wellbeing." [182]

A Cochrane review of interventions to promote residential smoke alarms and to assess their effect on the prevalence of owned and working smoke alarms and on the incidence of fires and burns was done of controlled (randomized or non-randomized) trials published between 1969 and 2007. Of 26 completed trials, 17 were randomized. Counseling and educational interventions, with or without allocation of free or discounted smoke alarms, only modestly increased the likelihood of owning an alarm (OR 1.36) and having an installed, functional alarm (OR 1.29). Only one randomized controlled trial reported injury outcomes, and no effect was found on injuries, hospitalizations or deaths from a smoke alarm donation program. Two trials showed that smoke alarm installation programs increase the likelihood of having a working smoke alarm, and one of these studies also noted a reduction in fire-related injuries. The conclusions of the reviewers were that (1) programs to promote smoke alarms have only a modest beneficial effect on ownership and function, (2) programs to promote smoke alarms have no demonstrated beneficial effects on fires or fire-related injuries, (3) community smoke alarm donation programs neither increase smoke alarm prevalence or reduce fires and injuries, and (4) community smoke alarm installation programs increase the prevalence of functional alarms and decrease injuries [62]. There is a paucity of the type of data needed by practitioners and policymakers who are seeking to implement smoke alarm promotion interventions [17].

In 2003–2006, smoke alarms were present but did not sound in 23% of the home fire deaths (Ahrens). When smoke alarms were not present on all floors of the residence, they sounded in only 4% of the fires and alerted occupants in only 2% of the fires (Ahrens). On the other hand, when interconnected smoke alarms are present on all floors, they sounded in half the fires and alerted occupants 26% of the time (Ahrens). Whereas hardwired alarms operated 91% of the time, battery-powered alarms sound in only 75% of fires (Ahrens). Of the alarms that failed to operate, 75% had missing, disconnected or dead batteries (Ahrens).

In a study in Dallas from 1991–1998, smoke alarms showed no protective efficacy in preventing burn injuries or fire deaths in fires started by arson or by children playing with matches or lighters, although they conferred protection against injuries and deaths from all other causes [105]. In rural North Carolina in 1988, the absence of a smoke alarm was relatively more lethal in the case of fires in which children were present, and when no one in the house was impaired by alcohol or drug use. Moreover, the presence or absence of a smoke alarm had no correlation with the risk of death when a person with either a cognitive impairment or physical disability was present [190].

In 1998 the Centers for Disease Control and Prevention (CDC), the US Fire Administration, the Consumer Product Safety Commission and several other national organizations combined efforts to develop the Smoke Alarm Installation and Fire Education (SAIFE) Program. The plan includes recruiting local communities and community partners, hiring a local coordinator, canvassing neighborhood homes, installing long-lasting lithium-powered smoke alarms, and providing general fire safety education and 6-month follow-up to determine alarm functionality. This program has demonstrated 90% functional alarms in follow-up surveys (of those the program installed), potentially saving 610 lives in the 16 states involved [24].

Unfortunately, there are scarce data from LMIC on utilization of smoke alarms. In Mexico, only 9% of homes in the upper socioeconomic stratum had smoke alarms, and none of the homes in the poorest stratum had alarms. An injury prevention educational campaign that included promotion of smoke alarm installation and use had no effect on the use of smoke alarms. However, this was not surprising, considering that smoke alarms could not be purchased in any of the nearby retail stores [140]. Clearly, more work is needed in LMIC, starting with an analysis of the impact of residential fires on injury and mortality.

An Alaskan study compared photoelectric and ionization smoke alarms in rural Eskimo Inupiat villages and ionization smoke alarms where home area averaged roughly 1,000 square feet or less. At the time of follow-up after installation, 81% of the ionization homes had working smoke alarms compared to 96% of the homes with photoelectric devices. Ninety-two percent of the ionization homes but only 11% of the photoelectric homes had experienced at least one false alarm. Ninety-three percent of the 69 ionization false alarms were due to cooking as were four of the six of the photoelectric false alarms. False alarms were more common in homes that were smaller, that used wood fuel for heat and in which the smoke alarms were located near the cooking areas. Thus photoelectric alarms may be the preferred choice for homes with limited living space, an observation that is relevant as smoke alarm installation programs are advanced in LMIC [215].

The following are recommendations for use of smoke alarms from the National Fire Protection Association (www.nfpa.org/smokealarms):

► Ensure that smoke alarms are working by testing monthly, replacing batteries at least yearly, and performing maintenance as instructed by the manufacturer. (Use of lithium batteries assures that the alarm will function for several years. All alarms should be replaced every eight to ten years, because of dust and moisture accumulation, clouding of the receptor and lens of photoelectric devices, and degradation of Americium-421 in ionization alarms.)
► Smoke alarms should be installed on every level of the home, outside each sleeping area, and inside each bedroom.
► Smoke alarms should be interconnected so that a fire detected by any of them will trigger the other alarms to sound.
► Develop an escape plan so that all occupants know what to do when a smoke alarm sounds.
► Use both ionization and photoelectric alarms because their effectiveness varies with how much flame is present in the fire.
► Install smoke alarms at a safe distance from nuisance sources, such as kitchen stoves, to minimize the number of nuisance alarms. Under no circumstances should an alarm be disabled because of repeated nuisance alarms – it should be replaced or repositioned.

## Residential sprinklers

Prevention of burn injuries and fire deaths, as well as amelioration of fire damages, is effectively and efficiently accomplished through the combined use of smoke detectors and sprinkler systems [53]. Smoke detectors are triggered in the initial moments of the fire event; sprinklers act throughout the event to minimize spread of the fire and in some cases extinguish it. The National Fire Protection Association estimates that the fire death rate in 2003–2006 was

80 % lower in structures protected by sprinklers. In homes with both smoke detectors and sprinklers, the chance of surviving a residential fire is nearly 97 % [93].

However, neither smoke detectors nor sprinklers nor a combination of the two will work effectively to protect certain individuals, such as,

► victims who act irrationally, who return to the fire after safely escaping, or who are unable to act to save themselves, such as people who are physically disabled, bedridden or under restraint;
► victims whose clothing is on fire and sustain fatal fire injuries from fires too small to activate smoke detectors or sprinklers; and
► victims who are unusually vulnerable to fire effects, such as older adults, and those impaired by alcohol or drugs.

Unfortunately, fewer than 2 % of US single-family dwellings are fitted with sprinkler systems [16]. San Clemente, California, was the first US jurisdiction to mandate installation of sprinklers in all new residential structures. The cost of installation of sprinkler systems in new houses is approximately $1 to $2 per square foot; retrofitting sprinklers in existing building is somewhat more expensive, but is comparable to the cost of purchasing and installing new carpeting.

## Hot water temperature regulation

Although scald burns are nearly as common as flame burns, particularly in children, across the globe in 2002 only 5.4 % of all burn deaths were attributed to scalds; 93 % of deaths were fire-related [170]. Hot tap water causes nearly one quarter of all pediatric scald burns, and most of these occur in the bathroom. The damage caused by hot tap water burns tends to be more severe than that by other types of scald burns [149]. Experiments on human subjects have shown that partial- or full-thickness burns occur only after six hours of exposure if water is 111 F (44 C). Yet if the temperature of the water is increased to 140°F (60 °C), burns occur within three seconds of exposure [144]. Because water at 120°F (49 °C) takes 10 minutes to cause significant thermal injury to the skin, hot water heaters are ideally set at this temperature to give people time to escape the damaging effects in time.

Children under the age of five years are at highest risk for hospitalization for burns in HIC among all childhood age groups, and nearly 75 % of these burns are from hot liquid, hot tap water or steam [170]. For instance, 100 % of children admitted from 1994 through 2004 to two burn centers in Finland were the result of hot water scalds [157]. A hospital-based survey in France during 1991–1992 noted that 17 % of childhood burn injuries were due to scalds [136]. However, a large proportion of scald burns in children are cared for in clinics and emergency rooms without need for hospitalization.

In 1977 in Washington state, 80 % of homes had tap water temperatures greater than 129 °F (54 °C). In 1983 a Washington State law was passed, requiring new water heaters to be preset at 120 °F (49 °C). Five years later, 77 % of homes (84 % of homes with postlaw and 70 % of homes with prelaw water heaters) had tap water temperatures of less than 129 °F (54 °C). Mean temperature in 1988 was 122 °F (50 °C) compared with 142 °F (61 °C) in 1977. Few people increased their heater temperature after installation. Compared with the 1970s, numbers of patients admitted for treatment of scald burns, as well as total body surface area burned, mortality, grafting, scarring, and length of hospital stay for scald burns were all reduced. The combination of education and legislation seems thus resulted in a reduction in frequency, morbidity, and mortality of tap water burn injuries in children [72].

In the mid-1980's in Wisconsin, an educational campaign, which included free thermometers mailed with utility bills, resulted in reduction in the temperature of an estimated 20,000 hot water heaters [111]. A similar study in Dunedin, New Zealand, of a national media campaign combined with educational interventions to households with young children noted a reduction of 50 % in the number of households with hot water heater temperatures over 158 °F (70 °C). However, the majority of households still had temperatures above 131 °F (55 °C) at the end of the intervention [226].

The first state legislation regulating water temperatures was a bill passed in Florida in May, 1980, which mandated preset water heater temperatures to no higher than 125 °F (52 °C). Legislation now exists within the administrative code concerning the regulation of tap water temperature for the District of Columbia and 47 states. In addition, hospitals and related healthcare facilities often have building codes that limit the temperature of hot water supplied to the patients. The majority of states have also adopted a model plumbing code developed by a standards organization, such as the International Code Council (ICC) or International Association of Plumbing and Mechanical Officials (IAPMO), and amend the code to fit their regional needs. These codes not only differ in their individual content, but by their differing editions as well. Different editions of each code can be adopted by different jurisdictions, making plumbing legislation even less uniform across the US. Besides having several different codes to choose from, the application of the code differs from state to state. Some states enforce a state-wide code, while others allow the code to be amended by individual counties. Moreover, different states may apply the code only toward certain buildings. Thus there is no uniform national standard for tap water temperature regulation. Instead, there is a system in the US of state and local jurisdictions adopting a variety of codes and applying them inconsistently across counties and cities. These codes and regulations attempt to reduce scald burns, but because of the lack of uniformity, tap water scalds still remain a serious issue [49].

Building services engineers are directed to store and operate hot water systems at a temperature of 140 °F (60 °C) to prevent outbreaks of Legionnaires' disease. To prevent scald burns from direct exposure to water at this temperature, mixing valves can be installed in the hot water supply pipe work to provide hot water at safe temperatures for bathing, showering and washing. Thermoscopic or thermostatic mixing valves were developed and first marketed in 1979. Following this, the UK Department of Health and Social Security issued a recommendation that the suitable reduction in water temperature from the heating source (recommended 60 °C) to the tap (recommended 52 °C) should be achieved by a "suitable mixing arrangement" [146]. Electricity Association Technology Ltd. (EATL) investigated the performance of automatic mixing valves in 1992 in the UK. EATL found that although the valves studied all performed equally well at mixing hot and cold water when the supply was constant, there was clear differ-

**Table 4.** Haddon Matrix applied to the problem of residential fires in LMIC due to non-electric domestic appliances [166]

| | Host/human factors | Object/substance | Physical environment | Sociocultural environment |
|---|---|---|---|---|
| Pre-event | • Wear tight clothing<br>• Keep water and dry sand at hand<br>• Teach consumers safe techniques for use | • Identify safer fuels<br>• Change appliance design<br>• Provide pictograms with operating instructions<br>• Safer containers for kerosene<br>• Teach safe fuel use techniques | • Store fuels in clearly marked, red containers<br>• Teach consumers how to assess kerosene for quality before purchase<br>• Place stoves on stable surfaces, away from flammable substances and out of reach of children | • Prevent kerosene contamination<br>• Create political or economic leverage for adoption of design improvement<br>• Legislate for design regulations and enforcement<br>• Use evidence-based research to support advocacy and programs<br>• Implement building codes<br>• Develop safety curricula in schools<br>• Train caregivers and health workers<br>• Train volunteers to observe risky behaviors and unsafe practices |
| Event | • "Stop, drop and roll" when clothing catch fire<br>• Use blankets to smother clothing flames<br>• Use water or sand to extinguish structure fires | • Turn off device if possible when fire starts | • Have emergency contact information nearby | • Prepare neighbors to intervene in putting out fires and assisting victims |
| Post-event | • Appropriate first aid<br>• Acute care for burns<br>• Rehabilitation for injuries | • Discard faulty equipment | • Clean and retrofit environment with regard to future prevention | • Educate community using event as an example |

ences in function amongst the valves when there was loss of cold water supply (as might occur in the household during bathing or showering when another water appliance, such as toilet or washing machine, is turned on) [208].

### Lamps and stoves

Although there is slow progress in providing electricity to residences, less than one-quarter of Africans had access to electricity in 2005 [231]. The global use of kerosene in lamps and stoves will no doubt continue for years to come. Unfortunately, many low-income families use makeshift lamps from wicks placed in discarded beverage or medicine bottles, and even from burnt-out light bulbs [170]. Burns caused by homemade bottle lamps or commercial wick lamps are common in LMIC [6, 115].

Prevention of lamp burns in LMIC includes three approaches. The first is educational campaigns that promulgate safe behavior with kerosene lamps, including avoiding replenishment of the fuel reservoir while the wick is lit and placing the lamps on stable surfaces. One study in low-income South African communities demonstrated limited but demonstrable success in educating those at highest risk [198]. Another is to use safer oil, such as vegetable oils (e. g. coconut and sesame oils). Unfortunately, these oils are too heavy to rise to the top of the wick, and do not perform well.

The third option is to provide impoverished families with an inexpensive lamp that is designed with safety in mind. Such a lamp is currently being produced and marketed in Sri Lanka. It is short and heavy, so that it does not easily tip over, and has two flat sides that prevent it from rolling if it does tip over. The screw-top lid averts fuel spillage, and the thick glass with which it is made avoids breakage if it falls. It is produced from recycled glass at the low cost of only US$ 0.35 each, and its production provides a boost to the local economy. Its use has been credited with a significant reduction in burn injuries and fires in Sri Lanka [190].

The use of kerosene stoves is even more widespread than homemade lamps, and the magnitude of injury, death and destruction that accompanies them places a tremendous burden on low-income communities. The conceptual framework for prevention of these injuries lends itself to the Haddon Matrix [187]. Table 4 is an inventory of options for interventions in all three time dimensions (pre-event, event, and post-event) including education programs, environmental modifications, and enforcement of existing or creation of new legislation.

Many options outlined in this table appear to be suitable for application in many LMIC. Clearly much could be accomplished by addressing issues of verification of fuel quality, safety of fuel storage and usage, and dispersion of appropriately designed appliances. Compulsory standards covering the performance, safety and homologation requirements for non-pressure paraffin fuelled cooking stoves and heaters intended primarily for domestic use were effected by the South African government on January 1, 2007 [84]. These standards were developed after evaluation of nine commonly used stove designs in 2003 showed that not one of the designs met the current national standards. Currently, the SANS 1906:2006 standard for non-pressure stoves and heaters is the only compulsory standard in place. Only one heater has a license to trade under this standard – the Goldair Heater model RD85A (Fig. 5). The new PANDA stove holds a temporary license under this standard. The standard for pressurized kerosene-fuelled appliances (SANS 1243:2007) is currently voluntary and none of the pressure appliances on the market have applied for approval from South Africa Bureau of Standards Commercial against this standard [160].

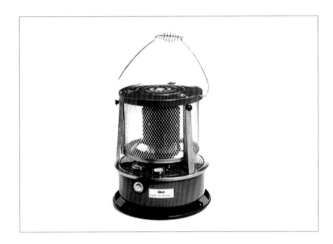

**Fig. 5.** The only heater that has a license to trade under the South African standard for non-pressure stoves and heaters is the Goldair Heater model RD85A. It has a three-liter fuel tank, giving it approximately 16 hours of operation. Currently it can be purchased for US $ 84, making it out of the reach of acquisition by most low-income families

Feasibility and cost of implementation of such regulations are often the final barrier to improvements in burn prevention. Enforcement of regulations and codes depends not only upon government commitment but also upon consumer investment in the plan. It is essential that consumers are informed and use their purchasing power to insist that manufacturers, distributors and suppliers of appliances adhere to existing safety standards. Local and regional government health departments should use their influence to support the standards and their enforcement. The public and government should insist on appropriate standards approval before purchasing appliances destined for domestic use regardless of whether the relevant applicable standard is voluntary or compulsory. Such an approach requires intensive educational campaigns both for the community and for relevant government agencies.

## Fireworks legislation

Nearly 10,000 people were treated in US emergency rooms in 2007 for fireworks-related injuries. Boys between the ages of five and 15 years have the highest injury rates. Nearly 4,200 children under the age of 15 years were admitted to emergency rooms in the US in 2002 for treatment of fireworks-related injuries [149, 230]. Similarly, the association between boys and fireworks injuries has been noted in other countries, such as Australia and Greece [1, 224]. Almost 33,000 fires were started by fireworks in 2006 in the US, resulting in six deaths, 70 injuries, and $ 34 million in property damages [92].

The injuries caused by fireworks can be very severe because of heat production (temperatures of ignited devices may exceed 1200 °F) and blast effect. Only approximately 50 % of treated fireworks injuries in the US are burns; approximately one-third are contusions or lacerations, and one-quarter affect the eyes [92, 206]. In Northern Ireland, over half of the patients present with blast injuries to the hand [77]. The use of illegal fireworks accounts for only 8 % of the injuries; most injuries in the US occur while using fireworks approved by Federal regulations. Sparklers and small firecrackers cause 40 % of fireworks injuries. The risk of fire death relative to exposure makes fireworks one of the riskiest consumer products available in the US [92].

Fireworks are associated with national and cultural celebrations throughout the world [12]. On Independence Day in the US each year, more fires are reported than on any other day of the year [92]. As a prelude to the arrival of spring, Persians since at least 1700 BCE have celebrated Chahārshanbe-Sūri on the last Wednesday night of each year. The festivities include participants jumping over bonfires in the streets and setting off fireworks, both hazardous activities. Despite the ubiquity of these practices in Persia and their persistence since ancient times, only 1 % of surveyed families acknowledged having any education on the safe use of fireworks in 2007 in Tehran, Iran; over 98 % of families were ignorant of fireworks safety standards [188].

Fireworks have been regulated in the United Kingdom since 1875, starting with laws covering the manufacture, storage, supply and behavior in the presence of gunpowder. In particular, the last decade has seen the passage of several pieces of fireworks legislation in the UK [68]. The US Consumer Product Safety Commission has regulated consumer fireworks safety since the 1970's. Current regulations prohibit the sale of the most dangerous types of fireworks, including large reloadable shells, "cherry bombs", aerial bombs, M-80's, "silver salutes", and aerial fireworks containing more than two grains (130 mg) of powder. Other firecrackers and ground devices are limited to only 50 mg of powder, which is the pyrotechnic composition designed to produce an audible effect ("bang"). Also regulated are the composition of the materials (hazardous materials such as arsenic and mercury are proscribed), the length of time fuses must burn (at least three but no more than nine seconds), and the stability of the bases [220].

Access to all fireworks is banned in the US states of Delaware, Massachusetts, New Jersey, New York and Rhode Island. Arizona allows the exclusive use of novelty fireworks, and only sparklers are permitted in Illinois, Iowa, Maine, Ohio, and Vermont [222]. The impact of legislation on the incidence of fireworks-related injuries is unclear. Presumably because of proliferation of fireworks legislation, the number of fireworks injuries in the UK dropped from 707 in 2001 to 494 in 2005 [68]. Another opportunity for studying the efficacy of fireworks legislation occurs when restrictions are neutralized. After repeal of a law banning private fireworks in Minnesota, there was an increase in the number of children suffering fireworks-related burns [183]. However, this was not observed after liberalization of fireworks laws in Northern Ireland [77].

Reduction in fireworks-related injuries has been observed elsewhere as a result of focused campaigns. In Denmark, where fireworks are commonly used at New Years' celebrations, prohibition of the sale of firecrackers coupled with school education programs led to a reduction in the number of children treated for fireworks injuries at two Danish burn centers from 17 in 1991–1992 to only three children in 1993–1994 [200].

Passage and enforcement of legislation in LMIC is often challenging, and education programs may currently be the only option for injury prevention in some cases. In India fireworks injury commonly occur during Diwali (Festival of Lights). The experience at one hospital in Mumbai from 1997 through 2006 was that the prevalence of fireworks injuries was decreasing, due to aggressive education campaigns by government and non-government organizations. Forty-one injuries were treated at the beginning of the study period; only three injuries were treated in 2006 [175].

## Fire-safe cigarettes

There were over 140,000 smoking-material (lighted tobacco products) fires in the US in 2006 which caused 780 deaths, 1600 injuries and $606 million in property damage. One-fourth of all structure fire deaths in the US involved smoking materials in 2006 [91]. Most fire deaths are associated with ignition of upholstered furniture, mattresses and bedding by dropped cigarettes. Sadly, one-quarter of fatalities from smoking-material fires were not the smokers whose cigarettes started the fires. There has been a reduction in smoking-material fires of 57% from 1980 to 2006. Both the decline in cigarette consumption as well as standards and regulations that have made mattresses and upholstered furniture more resistant to ignition have contributed to this trend [91].

Smoking-material fires result from the intersection of human behavior, a source of ignition, and a supply of fuel. Prevention of such fires requires modifications of one or more of these factors. Fortunately, cigarette consumption has decreased over 40% since 1980. Modification of smoking behavior includes emphasis on smoking out-of-doors, but efforts to modify smoking behavior are hampered by the relatively high prevalence of alcohol use among those at highest risk for death from residential fires. Newer furniture, mattresses and bedclothes are more fire resistant, but older models will be more prevalent in low-income housing where the risk of fire is greater. Because cigarettes are the most common source of ignition in fatal residential fires, US consumer safety movements since the 1970's have focused on legislating mandatory production of fire-safe cigarettes [30].

The first bill was introduced by Rep. Joseph Moakley (D-MA) in 1978, who continued his efforts in the US House of Representatives for another two decades. By the end of the 20th century, it was clear that passage of Federal laws was progressing too slowly, so the emphasis was redirected toward state laws. In 2003, the first state law requiring all cigarettes to be low-ignition was passed in the state of New York. By the end of 2010, all states had either passed or enacted fire-safe cigarette legislation [51].

A fire-safe cigarette has a reduced tendency to burn when left unattended. To achieve this, most manufacturers wrap cigarettes with two or three thin bands of less-porous paper. These bands act as "speed bumps" to slow down the rate at which the cigarette burns. If a fire-safe cigarette is left unattended, the burning tobacco will reach one of these speed bumps and extinguish itself. Fire-safe cigarettes meet an established cigarette fire safety performance standard (based on ASTM E2187, Standard Test Method for Measuring the Ignition Strength of Cigarettes) [91].

One year after the New York State law went into effect, researchers from the Harvard School of Public Health compared the physical properties of cigarettes sold in New York with cigarettes sold in Massachusetts and California. Although nearly 100% of cigarettes purchased in MA and CA burned to the end, only 10% of cigarettes in New York had a full burn. The quantity and quality of toxins present in cigarette smoke was not different amongst the products. Consumer acceptance was acceptable, as evidenced by the observation that tobacco tax income in New York State did not change after implementation of the law [52].

## Children's sleepwear

Regulation of the manufacture of children's sleepwear exemplify the power of coalitions – including health care experts, safety advocacy groups, technical experts, and government agencies – in responding to the needs of the public. An all-too common cause of severe burn injury in children in the 1960's was ignition of sleepwear[7] (most often by stoves and matches) [99], leaving the young survivors with the scars and complications of third degree burns. One study found that the average sleepwear fire caused burns over nearly one-third of the child's body surface, two-thirds of which was third degree in depth [134].

In 1971, the U.S. Secretary of Commerce delivered a flammability standard for children's sleep-

---

7    "Sleepwear" is defined as any article of clothing intended to be worn primarily for sleeping or activities related to sleeping. "Daywear" is defined as clothing designed to be worn during the day. However, it is now common to see daywear used at night in place of pajamas, nightgowns or other traditional night clothes.

wear in the Flammable Fabrics Act. In 1973 the responsibility for administration and enforcement of this act was passed to the U.S. Consumer Product Safety Commission (CPSC). The primary aim of the standard was to minimize the risk of ignition of children's sleepwear; the secondary aim was to diminish the extent of injury by reducing the speed at which fire would spread after ignition occurred. The mandatory resistance to flammability was applied to all children's sleepwear garments, sizes 0–6 × and 7–14. T meet the children's sleepwear standard, the dry garment had to char fewer than seven inches on its bottom edge after exposed to flame for three seconds [118].

By requiring that children's sleepwear be flame-resistant, these standards helped protect children from burns. A retrospective study of children admitted to the Shriners Burns Institute of Boston during the eight-year period 1969 through 1976 showed that the promulgation of flammability standards reduced the incidence of flame burns from the ignition of sleepwear (Fig. 6; [134]). The National Fire Protection Association (NFPA) estimated that the enactment of the flammability standards for sleepwear in 1971 resulted in a ten-fold decrease in childhood deaths caused by ignition of sleepwear [138].

However, in 1996 amendments to these standards allowed exemption of tight-fitting children's sleepwear and infant garments sized 9 months or smaller.[8] The rationale for relaxation of the standards was that there were decreased sales of sleepwear because daywear was being used for night clothes.[9] CPSC was subsequently challenged by an alliance of stakeholders (Safe Children's Sleepwear Coalition) with a mutual interest in the health and safety of children, including the NFPA's Center for High-Risk Outreach, the American Burn Association and the Shriners Hospitals for Children [56]. In response to this challenge, the CPSC resolved to collect data prospectively using a National Burn Center Reporting System (NBCRS) starting in 2003. The NBCRS was a

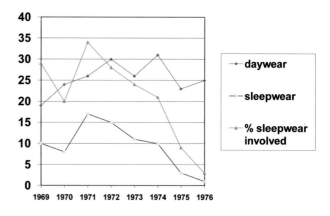

**Fig. 6.** Sleepwear involvement in flame burns at the Boston Shriners Burns Institute 1969–76 [134]

surveillance system focused on clothing-related burn injuries to children treated in the U. S. in which children were injured by the ignition, melting or smoldering of clothing. Ninety-two burn centers in the U. S. participated.

The first report was issued in September 2004 [19]. This analysis scrutinized the cases of 213 victims of 209 incidents, which were submitted by 44 burn centers. Of the 209 reported incidents, only 36 involved clothing worn for sleeping, most of which was daywear.[10] Of those incidents involving sleepwear, none involved tight-fitting sleepwear or infant garments sized 9 months or smaller.

Results from the second report were distributed in a memo dated January 12, 2007. These data were provided by 33 burns centers about 261 children injured in 253 incidents. In only 33 of these incidents were the children injured while wearing clothing that at some point was worn for sleeping. Nineteen of these 33 incidents involved daywear which was being worn for sleeping. Only 14 incidents involved sleepwear subject to the Standards for the Flammability of Children's Sleepwear. As in the first report, there were no incidents involving tight-fitting sleepwear or infant garments sized 9 months or smaller.

The conclusion reached by the author of this memo, Patricia K. Adair in the Directorate for Engin-

---

8   Current requirements are published in the Code of Federal Regulations, Title 16, Parts 1615 and 1616.

9   Although difficult to quantify, the clothing industry's perception of consumers was that sleepwear treated for reduction in flammability was less comfortable (and therefore less popular) than untreated cotton, such as that found in T-shirts.

---

10  Daywear is subject to the Standard for the Flammability of Clothing Textiles, but is not subject to the flame-resistant requirements of the Standards for the Flammability of Children's Sleepwear.

eering Sciences for CPSC, was that the analysis of data from March 2003 through December 2005 revealed no deaths or injuries attributable to the exempted infant size and tight-fitting sleepwear.

Thus the CPSC allowed remain the modifications to the standards. However, there are marketing responsibilities for retailers, distributors, and wholesalers who sell children's sleepwear [219].

(1) They should not advertise, promote, or sell as children's sleepwear, any garment which another party has indicated does not meet the requirements of the children's sleepwear flammability standards and/or are not intended or suitable for use as sleepwear.

(2) They should place or advertise fabrics and garments covered by the children's sleepwear standards in different parts of a department, store, catalog, or web site, from those in which fabrics and garments which may resemble but are not children's sleepwear are sold or marketed.

(3) They should use store display signs, and/or catalog or web site notations that point out the difference between different types of fabrics and garments, for example, by indicating which are sleepwear items and which are not.

(4) They should avoid advertising or promoting garments or fabrics that do not comply with the children's sleepwear standards in a manner that may cause consumers to view those items as children's sleepwear or as being suitable for making such sleepwear.

In a letter dated January 4, 2007, Dr. Russell Roegner, Associate Executive Director of Epidemiology at the U. S. Consumer Product Safety Commission, noted that the study on clothing-related burn injuries to children had ended. The result of data analysis led the CPSC staff to conclude that because more than half of children's clothing fires involved flammable liquids, they had initiated a new project on flammable liquids. To date, the results of the new project on flammable liquids have not been distributed, aside from the publication on Sept 20, 2008, of a public information safety alert on the dangers of flammable liquids [221].

In summary, the chronicle of Standards for the Flammability of Children's Sleepwear has ups and downs. Clearly, the institution of these standards back in the early 1970's led to a dramatic reduction in a devastating form of childhood injury. The relaxation of these standards twenty years later shows the effects of the erosion of consumer support as well as the power of industry pressure. The inability of the US burn care community to demonstrate convincingly that the relaxation of standards left no mark on the incidence of childhood burns was indeed an illustration of the need for comprehensive, accurate national databases.

*Acid assaults*

Although most burns are unintentional injuries, a small proportion occur because of assaults [86]. Chemical attacks have been reported in several countries, including Bangladesh, Cambodia, China, India, Jamaica, Nepal, Nigeria, Pakistan, Saudi Arabia, South Africa, Uganda, UK, and US. Across the world, male victims are more commonly reported; many of these are associated with robbery or violent crime. Alkali is the agent most commonly used in the US, but elsewhere the injuries sustained are due to acids [125].

The highest incidence of chemical burns in the world is in Bangladesh [26]. The perpetrators are often scorned suitors, but disagreements over property boundaries and animal ownership are also common instigations. Acids are favored over alkalis because they can be easily obtained from car batteries, jewelry workshops and leather tanneries [199]. The face and eyes are the usual target, with the intent being to disfigure or blind or both. Because of the scarcity of treatment options available to the victims, they often unfortunately suffer permanent mutilation, physical disability, psychological devastation, abandonment, and destitution. In the districts wherein such attacks occur, disempowerment of women and gender discrimination are common. Sadly, few perpetrators are punished for their crimes.

One shining light of an effective prevention program for these horrifying injuries is the Acid Survivors Foundation (ASF) of Bangladesh which has been working to reduce acid attacks on children and women since 1999. ASF has been raising public awareness, building institutional capacity and lobbying, working with other nongovernmental organizations, the media, celebrities and student groups to elevate community consciousness. It has also fos-

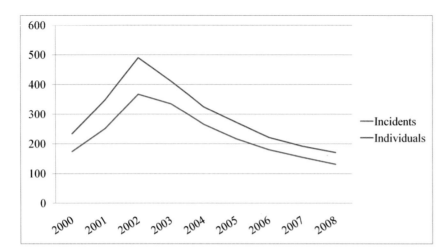

**Fig. 7.** The Acid Survivors Foundation (ASF) of Bangladesh has involved all sectors of society, including students, media, celebrity groups, and non-governmental organizations, to address the root cause of acid violence, which is gender discrimination and disempowerment of women. ASF and its partners have successfully worked to develop and enforce laws, policies and procedures for combating acid violence. As a result, Bangladesh has seen a decrease in the incidence of acid attacks. (http://www.acidsurvivors. org/index.html)

tered advocacy and lobbying efforts with the government to ensure the passage and enforcement of laws and to create systems to provide service to acid survivors. As a result, the number of victims has dropped from 490 in 2002 to 171 in 2008 (Fig. 7). Based on the success of ASF, similar organizations have been formed in Cambodia, India, Pakistan and Uganda.

### Burns first aid treatment

The goal of injury prevention is to reduce the burden of injuries upon a community. Primary prevention seeks to do this by preventing the injuries from occurring in the first place. However, even with the most effective primary prevention programs in place, burn injuries will continue to occur. Secondary prevention, therefore, is designed to minimize the damage done when a burn occurs.

Appropriate first aid treatment of burns plays a role in determining outcome by limiting tissue damage and therefore curtailing the depth of the burn. In some cases, particularly with scald burns, appropriate first aid may avert the need for surgical excision and grafting [152, 204]. Appropriate first aid treatment of burns is cool, running water within the temperature range of 50 °F to 60 °F as soon as possible after the injury has occurred. Colder water, particular in victims with larger body surface area burns, may induce hypothermia. Application of ice causes vasoconstriction of the dermal plexus and exacerbates the depth of thermal injury [41, 42, 100, 155, 176, 177].

However, the knowledge of appropriate first aid treatment of burns is widespread neither in the community nor among health care workers. Fewer than 40 % of admissions to a regional burn center in Western Australia were treated appropriately following the burn injuries. Twenty per cent used no first aid techniques, and the remainder applied substances such as honey and toothpaste [178]. Similar surveys in Hungary and Vietnam revealed that only approximately one-quarter of patients had received appropriate burns first aid [153, 158]. A survey of understanding of appropriate burns first aid treatment among health care workers showed even more disheartening results, with fewer than 20 % of those surveyed able to answer correctly all questions put to them about burns first aid [178].

Nonetheless, appropriate burn first aid can be successfully taught. Public information campaigns in Vorarlberg, Austria, and Jamshedpur, India, have led to an improved understanding of appropriate burns first aid in the community [36, 82]. A multimedia educational campaign about burns first aid in Auckland, New Zealand, resulted in a reduction of in-patient admissions and surgical procedures [205]. Although such public education campaigns are at least temporarily effective, their long-term results are not yet known.

### Burn care systems

Systems for care of injuries within communities is yet another component of secondary prevention. For example, establishment of trauma care systems in the US has successfully reduced mortality from blunt and penetrating injuries [121]. Although burn centers have been functioning for nearly six decades, there is unfortunately a dearth of evidence that supports their effectiveness at reducing morbidity and mortality. Nonetheless, the bulk of expert opinion defends the need to establish within each region a tertiary care center that can provide acute and rehabilitative care for burn victims, as well as interaction with community and pre-hospital primary care systems that are responsible for prevention and first aid [191].

Nearly half a million burns are treated by licensed health care providers each year in the US [14]. There are approximately 4000 deaths a year in the US from residential fires (3500) and due to other causes (500 from motor vehicle and aircraft crashes, scalds, chemical and electrical injuries). The majority of deaths (75 %) occur at the scene, typically from smoke inhalation; however, 40,000 burn patients are admitted to hospitals in the US each year. These injured patients live within a population of over 300 million people scattered over more than 3.5 million square miles. There has to be a system in place to provide regional care for burn injuries throughout the US, whether that be with numerous small burn units that are geographically close to the patients they serve, or with large regional centers that function efficiently and effectively because of economy of scale [95].

Although emergency care for serious burns is available to most residents of the US, the care of minor burns is often provided at primary care facilities. In North Carolina in a recent study, 92 % of burn injuries were treated by Emergency Physicians; 4 % were admitted and only 4 % were transferred to burn centers [57]. Alternatively, specialty hospitals that lack burn centers may provide care to burn patients in consultation with the nearest burn center [192].

In 2008, there were 128 burn centers in the United States including 51 centers verified by the American Burn Association. Over 45 % of the US population lives within two hours by ground transport of a verified burn center. Nearly 80 % of the population lives within two hours of a verified center. Regional variation in access to verified burn centers by both ground and rotary air transport was significant. The greatest proportion of the population with

access was lowest in the southern United States and highest in the northeast region [113].

Fortunately, even at US burn centers the proportion of patients with life-threatening burns is relatively low. The average mortality rate throughout the 62 US burn centers contributing to the ABA NBR was only 4 % during the decade 1999–2008 [16]. Seventy-seven percent of patients at burn centers were hospitalized for care of burns less than 10 % of their body surface area; the mortality in this subset of patients was only 0.6 % [16]. This is true in other HIC, such as Taiwan, ROC, where the overall mortality rate among hospitalized burn patients from 1997 to 2003 was only 3 % and the $LA_{50}$ was 80 % TBSA [221].

However, the profile of injury severity and mortality is distinctly different in LMIC. For instance, during the years 1992 to 2000, the mean burn size of over 11,000 patients admitted to a single burn center in Delhi was 50 % TBSA, much greater than the 12 % TBSA mean burn size of patients whose records were recorded in the ABA NBR during a similar period. Additionally, mortality was also 50 % during this period of time in Delhi, compared to only 5 % at US burn centers [7, 13]. Such contrasts reflect more on the socioeconomic differences between LMIC and HIC, as well as on the limitation of resources available to burn centers in developing countries. Nonetheless, it is notable that this same burn center in Delhi has reduced the mortality rate from 50 % down to 40 % during the subsequent time period 2001 to 2007 [7]. Although the improvement in survival may be related to the rising economic status of India, it is also a tribute to the devotion and dedication of doctors and nurses at resource-restricted burn centers.

The ability of health care systems to provide burn care to a region depends on the availability of human resources (staff and training) and physical resources (infrastructure, supplies and equipment). Resources essential for burn services at all facilities (including out-patient clinics and care provided by non-medical providers) consist of training necessary to assess burn wound depth and capability (training and supplies) to apply clean or sterile dressings. Other resources are essential for higher levels of facilities (such as specialist or tertiary care centers), involving the capacity for debridement and skin grafting (Table 5; [141]).

## Role of the World Health Organization

A Consultation Meeting on the Prevention and Care of Burns was held at WHO Headquarters in Geneva, CH, on April 3–4, 2007. The goal was to promote the development of the spectrum of burn control measures, to include improvements in burn prevention and strengthened burn care, as well as better information and surveillance systems, and more investment in research and training. A broad-based strategic plan was created and published in a document that describes what is seen as the important steps towards the global goal of decreasing the rates of burn injuries and death, as well as the minimizing the sequelae of burns, such as disfigurement and disability [143]. This Burn Plan is organized into seven main components which correspond to the challenges in burn prevention and care:

For each component, there are full descriptions of areas of work needing to be done, expected products and output, and timeline. The full document can be accessed on-line at http://whqlibdoc.who. int/publications/2008/9789241596299_eng.pdf.

For example, the goal for the Policy Component is to increase the enactment and implementation of effective, sustainable burn prevention and care policies worldwide, including action plans, legislation, regulations and enforcement. The first area of work includes incorporating burn prevention and care into national and local health plans and injury control plans, as well as supporting the development of appropriate policy and legislation for burn prevention and care by countries. The expected products and outputs for these areas of work are policy statements and guidelines on burn prevention legislation, regulations, and enforcement, and appropriate information to support policy recommendations, such as estimates of cost-effectiveness of burn prevention and treatment strategies.

The next area of work for the Policy Component is to increase the number of countries that have and are implementing legislation and policies on burn prevention. To this end, the expected products and outputs are increased number of countries with national health insurance plans that include burn prevention and care and that receive and utilize guidance from WHO on policies, strategies and regulations on burn prevention and care.

To further these goals, the International Society of Burn Injuries is currently advocating for a resolution on the Prevention of Burn Injuries and Fire Deaths to the World Health Assembly, whose passage would ensure that burn prevention would be given priority among other health concerns at the WHO. In addition, the Department of Violence and Injury Prevention and Disability is currently creating a Best Practices manual demonstrating the most effective burn prevention programs known throughout the world.

## Conclusions and recommendations

### Surveillance

The approach to injury prevention includes four stages: surveillance, analysis, intervention and evaluation. Precise description of the problem(s) is the basis to planning effective interventions, yet in many LMIC, data on burns are scarce, inaccurate, or both. In some countries, a lack of reliable data on risk factors further hampers the development and enactment of effective burn prevention strategies, while in others, incomplete description of burn incidents leads to underassessment of the magnitude of the public health problem. There is a need for better surveillance with formal epidemiologic studies, which will more accurately assess the true incidence in vulnerable populations. A model for such a system can be found in Taiwan, ROC, where the support of the Childhood Burn Foundation provides resources to all 43 hospitals in the country to collect data on hospitalized burn patients. This comprehensive database, which utilizes the Internet for data entry, captured information on over 12,000 patients from 1997 to 2003 [221].

### Smoke alarms

The effectiveness and reliability of smoke alarms can be improved through improvements in technology, including 1) greater waking effectiveness for certain populations, 2) quicker, more certain responses to the range of fire types coupled with reduced nuisance alarms, 3) more cost-effective ways to interconnect alarms in existing homes. In addition, continued research is needed to improve measurement and performance of smoke alarms. Improvements must be made in educational approaches that change behavior in regards to home escape planning, inspection and maintenance of smoke alarms, and developing safe options for dealing with nuisance alarms. Human behavior in residential fires requires more research to determine effective cues, increase in the perception of the value of immediate escape, development of exit skills under stress, and strategies to reduce the learned irrelevance of alarms [174].

## Transition away from open fires and kerosene appliances

There is an assumption held by some that the inevitable transition from open fires and kerosene appliances toward more sophisticated devices for cooking, heating and lighting will result in a diminution of burn injuries in LMIC. However , the current experience suggests that this transition period is not without hazard. In Delhi, for example, LPG-related burns accounted for less than 1 % of admissions to a single burn center from 1993 to 2000, but from 2001 to 2007 were responsible for over 10 % of admissions [7]. Electrification can certainly reduce the risk of disasters caused by malfunctioning kerosene stoves, but can also lead to a whole new set of haz-

ards from electrical injury because of substandard wiring techniques, unsafe practices, illegal poaching of power and scavenging copper from overhead lines, and inadequate barriers around high-voltage poles and towers. Thus as developing communities convert to more common use of LPG and electricity, steps must be taken to ensure the safety of the residents.

## Gender inequality

In LIC the burden of burns falls mostly on women and female children, who are at risk of "occupational" injuries while they tend fires and prepare food. Sadly, they are also selected as victims of horrific assaults, such as acid throwing or "bride burning" [86]. The latter is a phenomenon related often to the dissatisfaction of the husband with the wife's dowry, and may occur either as self-immolation or as assault by the husband's family [107]. Clearly these particularly tragic events deserve focus above and beyond usual burn prevention efforts. Elimination of acid attacks and bride burning require a multitude of coordinated actions involving passage and enforcement of protective legislation, education of men and boys about appropriate behavior toward women, and resources for women in need of shelter or care.

**Table 5.** Burns and wounds [141]

| Resources | Basic | GP | Specialist | Tertiary |
|---|---|---|---|---|
| Burn depth assessment | E | E | E | E |
| Sterile dressings | D | E | E | E |
| Topical antimicrobials | D | E | E | E |
| Physiotherapy | I | E | E | E |
| Debridement | I | PR | E | E |
| Escharotomy | I | PR | E | E |
| Skin graft | I | PR | E | E |
| Reconstructive surgery | I | I | D | E |
| Early excision & grafting | I | I | D | D |

Designation of priorities: "E"–essential; "D"–desirable; "PR"–possibly required; "I"–irrelevant.
Range of health facilities: "Basic"–outpatient clinics and non-medical providers; "GP"–district hospitals and primary health centers without specialty care; "Specialist"–hospitals with operating rooms and limited surgical personnel; "Tertiary"–hospitals with broad range of subspecialists.

| A WHO Plan for Burn Prevention and Care |
| --- |
| **1. Advocacy** |

- Raising awareness
- Promoting and supporting action
- International, multisectoral cooperation

| **2. Policy** |
| --- |

- Effective and sustainable burn prevention and care policies
- Action plans, legislation, regulations, enforcement

| **3. Data and measurement** |
| --- |

- Magnitude and burden
- Risk factors

| **4. Research** |
| --- |

- Set agenda of priorities
- Promote and foster trials of promising interventions

| **5. Prevention** |
| --- |

- Stronger, more effective burn prevention programs
- More countries with national burn strategies

| **6. Services** |
| --- |

- Strengthen treatment services available
- Acute care
- Rehabilitation
- Recovery

| **7. Capacity building** |
| --- |

- Sufficient knowledge and skill to effectively carry out all of the above components of the Burn Plan

## Community surveys

Community surveys are needed in the US to establish the degree to which Hispanics utilize the health care system for treatment of burns. The very low incidence of non-fatal burns in Hispanics treated at US hospital emergency departments suggests that many burns are being treated by families with home remedies. The few population-based surveys that have been done in Bangladesh have demonstrated the tremendous utility of this approach, outlining clearly not only the true incidence of burns within the community, but also the extent of disability and death that accompany burns [126–129]. Only with an accurate appreciation of the burden of burn injuries within a region can effective lobbying efforts move forward in funding agencies and government health departments.

## Acknowledgements

The author wishes to express his gratitude to the following for their help in preparing this chapter: Amy Acton, David Barillo, Peter Brigham, Ernest Grant, Carol Runyan, and Fiona Wood.

## References

[1] Abdulwadud O, Ozanne-Smith J (1998) Injuries associated with fireworks in Victoria: an epidemiological review. Inj Prev 4: 272–275

[2] Adamo C et al (1995) Epidemiological data on burn injuries in Angola: a retrospective study of 7230 patients. Burns 21: 536–538

[3] Ahrens M (2008) Home smoke alarms: the data as context for decision. Fire Technology 44: 313–327

[4] Ahrens M (2009) Smoke alarms in US home fires. National Fire Protection Association, Fire Analysis and Research Division, September 2009. http://www.nfpa.org/assets/files//PDF/OS.SmokeAlarms.pdf

[5] Agran PF et al (2003) Rates of pediatric injury by 3-month intervals for children 0 to 3 years of age. Pediatrics 111;e683-e692. http://www.pediatrics.org/cgi/content/full/111/6/e683

[6] Ahuja RB, Bhattacharya S (2002) An analysis of 11,196 burn admissions and evaluation of conservative management techniques. Burns 28: 555–561

[7] Ahuja RB et al (2009) Changing trends of an endemic trauma. Burns 35: 650–656

[8] Alarie Y (2002) Toxicity of fire smoke. Crit Rev Toxicol 32: 259–289

[9] Alden NE et al (2005) Burn injury in patients with dementia: an impetus for prevention. J Burn Care Rehabil 26: 267–271

[10] Alden NE et al (2007) Tap water scalds among seniors and the elderly: socio-economics and implications for prevention. Burns 33: 666–669

[11] Al-Qattan MM (2000) Burns in epileptics in Saudi Arabia. Burns 26: 561–563

[12] Al-Qattan MM, Al-Zahrani K (2009) A review of burns related to traditions, social habits, religious activities, festivals and traditional medical practices. Burns 35: 476–481

[13] American Burn Association (2006) National Burn Repository, 2006, v. 2.0. http://www.ameriburn.org/NBR2005.pdf

[14] American Burn Association (2007) Burn incidence and treatment in the US: 2007 fact sheet. http://www.ameriburn.org/resources_factsheet.php

[15] American Burn Association (2009) National Burn Repository, 2009, v.5.0. http://www.ameriburn.org/2009NBRAnnualReport.pdf

[16] American Housing Survey 2007 (2008) U. S. Department of Commerce and U. S. Department of Housing and Urban Development, Table 1C-4, 2–4, and 2–25.

[17] Arai L et al (2005) It might work in Oklahoma but will it work in Oakhampton? Context and implementation in the effectiveness literature on domestic smoke detectors. Inj Prev 11: 148–151

[18] Arshi S et al (2006) Prevention oriented epidemiologic study of accidental burns in rural areas of Ardabil, Iran. Burns 32: 366–371

[19] Ascone DS (2004) U. S. Consumer Product Safety Commission National Burn Center Reporting System. CPSC Division of Hazard Analysis. http://www.cpsc.gov/CPSCPUB/PREREL/prhtml05/05 028.pdf

[20] ASTM (1982) Standard terminology relating to fire standards. American Society for Testing and Materials, Philadelphia, E176–182

[21] Atiyeh BS et al (2009) Burn prevention mechanisms and outcomes: pitfalls, failures and successes. Burns 35: 181–193

[22] Backstein R et al (1993) Burns in the disabled. Burns 19: 192–197

[23] Baker S et al (1992) The injury fact book, 2nd edn. Lexington Books, Lexington, MA

[24] Ballesteros M et al (2005) Working toward the elimination of residential fire deaths: the Centers for Disease Control and Prevention's Smoke Alarm Installation and Fire Safety Education (SAIFE) Program. J Burn Care Res 26: 434–9

[25] Balraj EK (1984) Atherosclerotic coronary artery disease and "low" levels of carboxyhemoglobin: report of fatalities and discussion of pathophysiologic mechanisms of death. J Forensic Sci 29: 1150–1159

[26] Bari SM et al (2002) Acid burns in Bangladesh. Ann Burns Fire Disasters 14: 115–118

[27] Barillo DJ et al (1986) Is ethanol the unknown toxin in smoke inhalation injury? Am Surg 52: 641–645

[28] Barillo DJ et al (1998) Preventable burns associated with a misuse of gasoline. Burns 24: 439–443

[29] Barillo DJ et al (1996) Fire fatality study: demographics of fire victims. Burns 22: 85–88

[30] Barillo DJ et al (2000) The fire-safe cigarette: a burn prevention tool. J Burn Care Rehabil 21: 164–170

[31] Barillo DJ, Wolf S (2006) Planning for burn disasters: lessons learned from one hundred years of history. J Burn Care Res 27: 622–634

[32] Barss P, Wallace K (1983) Grass skirt burns in Papua New Guinea. Lancet 1 (8327): 733–734

[33] Barss P (1991) Health impact of injuries in the highlands of Papua New Guinea: a verbal autopsy study (dissertation). Johns Hopkins School of Hygiene and Public Health, Baltimore, MD

[34] Barss P et al (1998) Injury prevention: an international perspective. Oxford University Press, New York

[35] Bawa Bhalla S et al (2000) Burn properties of fabrics and garments worn in India. Accident Analysis and Prevention 32: 407–420

[36] Beer GM, Kompatscher P (1996) Standardization of the first aid treatment of burn injuries in Vorarlberg, Austria. Burns 22: 130–134

[37] Begg S et al (2007) The burden of disease and injury in Australia 2003. PHE 82. Australian Institute of Health and Welfare, Canberra

[38] Bjerregaard P (1992) Fatal non-intentional injuries in Greenland. Art Med Res 51[Suppl 7]: 22–26

[39] Blakeney P et al (1993) Social competence and behavioral problems of pediatric survivors of burns. J Burn Care Rehabil 14: 65–72

[40] Block J (1983) Differential premises arising from differential socialization of the sexes: some conjectures. Child Development 54: 1335–1354

[41] Blomgren I et al (1982) Effect of cold water immersion on oedema formation in the scalded mouse ear. Burns 9: 17–20

[42] Boykin JV et al (1980) Histamine-mediated delayed permeability response after scald burn inhibited by cimetidine or cold-water treatment. Science 209: 815–817

[43] Brigham PA, McLoughlin E (1996) Burn incidence and medical care use in the United States: estimates, trends, and data sources. J Burn Care Rehab 17: 95–107

[44] Burd A, Yuen C (2005) A global study of hospitalized pediatric burn patients. Burns 31: 432–438

[45] Cadier MA, Shakespeare PG (1995) Burns in octogenarians. Burns 21: 200–204

[46] Caplan YH et al (1986) Accidental poisonings involving carbon monoxide, heating systems, and confined spaces. J Forensic Sci 31:117–121

[47] Centers for Disease Control (2009) Web-based injury and statistics query and reporting system (WISQARS©) http://webappa.cdc.gov/sasweb/ncipc/mortrate9.html

[48] Centers for Disease Control (2009a) Nonfatal scald-related burns among adults aged ≥ 65 years – United States, 2001–2006. MMWR 58: 993–996

[49] Peck M et al (2010) Hot tap water legislation in the United States. J Burn Care Res 31: 918–925

[50] Chapman CW (1983) Burns and plastic surgery in the South Atlantic campaign 1982. J Royal Navy Med Serv 69: 71–79

[51] Coalition for Fire-Safe Cigarettes™ (2009) State-by-state efforts. National Fire Protection Association. http://www.firesafecigarettes.org/itemDetail.asp?categoryID=93&itemID=1295&URL=Legislative%20updates/State-by-state%20efforts#oregon

[52] Connolly GN et al (2005) Effect of the New York State cigarette fire safety standard on ignition propensity, smoke constituents, and the consumer market. Tob Control 14: 321–327

[53] Council on Scientific Affairs (1987) Preventing death and injury from fires with automatic sprinklers and smoke detectors. JAMA 257: 1618–1620

[54] Courtright P et al (1993) The epidemiology of burns in rural Ethiopia. J Epidemiol Community Health 47: 19–22

[55] Crabtree J (2006) Terrorist homicide bombings: a primer for preparation. J Burn Care Res 27: 576–588

[56] Cusick JM et al (1997) Children's sleepwear: relaxation of the Consumer Product Safety Commission's flammability standards. J Burn Care Res 18: 469–476

[57] DeKoning EP et al (2009) Epidemiology of burn injuries presenting to North Carolina emergency departments in 2006–2007. Burns 35: 776–782

[58] Demamu S (1991) Community-based study of childhood injuries in Adamitulu District, Ethiopia (thesis). Addis Ababa University, Department of Community Health

[59] Department for Communities and Local Government (2008) Fire Statistics, United Kingdom, 2006, London, U. K., pp 35–42. http://www.communities.gov.uk/documents/fire/pdf/firestats2006.pdf

[60] DiGuiseppi C et al (2000) Urban residential fire and flame injuries: a population based study. Inj Prev 6: 250–254

[61] DiGuiseppi C et al (2000a) Systematic review of controlled interventions to promote smoke alarms. Arch Dis Child 82: 341–348

[62] DiGuiseppi C et al (2001) Interventions for promoting smoke alarm ownership and function. Cochrane Database of Systematic Reviews, Issue 2. Art. No.: CD002 246

[63] Dobson RB (1995) Clifford's tower and the jews of Medieval York. English Heritage, London

[64] Dubivsky PM, Bukowski RW (1989) False Alarm Study of Smoke Detectors in Department of Veterans Affairs Medical Centers (VAMCS), NISTIR 89–4077, Gaithersburg, MD: National Institute of Standards and Technology, p 45

[65] Duncanson M et al (2000) Follow-up Survey of Auahi Whakatupato Smoke Alarm Installation Project in the Eastern Bay of Plenty, New Zealand Fire Service Commission Research Report Number Seven, University of Otago. http://www3.fire.org.nz/CMS_media/pdf/98ae995639dd13b93f3af49e08d73bac.pdf

[66] Durrani KM, Raza SK (1975) Studies on flammability of clothing of burn victims, changes therein, and their wearability after a borax rinse. J Pakistan Med Assoc 25: 99–102

[67] Eaton W (1989) Are sex differences in child motor activity level a function of sex differences in maturational status? Child Development 60: 1005–1011

[68] Edwin AFL et al (2008) The impact of recent legislation on paediatric fireworks injuries in the Newcastle upon Tyne region. Burns 34: 953–964

[69] Einhorn IN (1975) Physiological and toxicological aspects of smoke produced during the combustion of polymeric materials. Environ Health Perspect 11:163–189

[70] El-badawy A, Mabrouk AR (1998) Epidemiology of childhood burns in the burn unit of Ain Shams University in Cairo. Egypt Burns 24:728–732

[71] Eldad A, Torem M (1990) Burns in the Lebanon War 1982: "the Blow and the Cure." Military Medicine 155: 130–132

[72] Erdmann TC et al (1991) Tap water burn prevention: the effect of legislation. Pediatrics 88: 572–577

[73] Fagenholz PJ et al (2007) National study of emergency department visits for burn injuries, 1993 to 2004. J Burn Care Res 28: 691–690

[74] Fagot B (1978) The influence of sex of child on parental reactions to toddler children. Child Development 49: 459–465

[75] Fauveau U, Blanchet T (1989) Deaths from injuries and induced abortion among rural Bangladeshi women. Soc Sci Med 29: 1121–1127

[76] Federal Emergency Management Agency (2004) Fire in the United States 1992–2001, 13 th edition. National Fire Data Center, Emmitsburg, MD

[77] Fogarty BJ, Gordon DJ (1999) Firework related injury and legislation: the epidemiology of firework injuries and the effect of legislation in Northern Ireland. Burns 25: 53–56

[78] Forjuoh SN (1998) The mechanisms, intensity of treatment, and outcomes of hospitalized burns: issues for prevention. J Burn Care Rehabil 19: 456–460

[79] Friesen B (1985) Haddon's strategy for prevention: application to Native house fires. Circumpolar Health. University of Washington Press, Seattle 84: 105–109

[80] Gali BM et al (2004) Epidemiology of childhood burns in Maiduguri, north-eastern Nigeria. Nigerian j Med 13: 144–147

[81] Gerson L, Wingard D (1979) Fire deaths and drinking: data from the Ontario fire reporting system. Am J Drug Alcohol Abuse 6: 125–133

[82] Ghosh A, Bharat R (2000) Domestic burns prevention and first aid awareness in and around Jamshedpur, India: strategies and impact. Burns 26: 605–608

[83] Godwin Y et al (1996) Shack fires: a consequence of urban migration. Burns 23: 151–153

[84] Government Gazette (2006) Compulsory specification for non-pressurized paraffin stoves and heaters. Government Notice No. R 1091. https://www.sabs.co.za/content/uploads/files/VC9089.pdf

[85] Grange AO et al (1988) Flame burns disasters from kerosene appliance explosions in Lagos, Nigeria. Burns 14: 147–150

[86] Greenbaum AR et al (2004) Intentional burn injury: an evidence-based, clinical and forensic review. Burns 30: 628–642

[87] Gulaid JA et al (1989) Deaths from residential fires among older people, United States, 1984. J Am Geriatr Soc 37: 331–334

[88] Gupta RK et al (1988) Study of fatal burn cases in Kanpur (India). Forensic Sci Int 37: 81–89

[89] Gupta M et al (1992) Paediatric burns in Jaipur, India: an epidemiological study. Burns 18: 63–67

[90] Gupta M et al (1996) The kerosene tragedy of 1994, an unusual epidemic of burns: epidemiological aspects and management of patients. Burns 22: 3–9

[91] Hall JR (2008) U. S. smoking-material fire problems. National Fire Protection Association Fire Analysis and Research Division. National Fire Protection Association, Quincy, MA. http://www.nfpa.org/assets/files//PDF/OS. Smoking.pdf

[92] Hall JR (2009) Fireworks. National Fire Protection Association Fire Analysis and Research Division. National Fire Protection Association, Quincy, MA. http://www.nfpa.org/assets/files/pdf/os.fireworks.pdf

[93] Hall JR (2009a) U. S. experience with sprinklers and other fire extinguishing equipment. National Fire Protection Association Fire Analysis and Research Division. National Fire Protection Association, Quincy, MA. http://www.nfpa.org/assets/files//PDF/OSsprinklers.pdf

[94] Hartzell GE (1991) Combustion products and their effects o life safety. In: Cote AE (ed) Fire protection handbook. National Fire Protection Association, Quincy, pp 3–3 to 3–14

[95] Heimbach DM (2003) Regionalization of burn care – a concept whose time has come. J Burn Care Rehabil 24: 173–174

[96] Hemeda M et al (2003) Epidemiology of burns admitted to Ain Shams University Burns Unit, Cairo, Egypt. Burns 29: 353–358

[97] Híjar-Medina MC et al (1992) Accidents in the home in children less than 10 years of age. Causes and consequences. Salud Pública de México 34: 615–625

[98] Hill IR (1990) An analysis of factors impeding passenger escape from aircraft fires. Aviat Space Environ Med 61: 261–265

[99] Horrocks AR et al (2004) The particular flammability hazards of nightwear. Fire Safety J 39: 259–276

[100] Hudspith J et al (2004) First aid and treatment of minor burns. Br Med J 328: 1487–1489

[101] Huffman A (2009) Sultana: the worst maritime disaster in American history. Harper Collins

[102] Hughes A et al (2008) State Estimates of Substance Use from the 2005–2006 National Surveys on Drug Use and Health. Substance Abuse and Mental Health Services Administration, Office of Applied Studies, Rockville, MD. http://oas.samhsa.gov/2k6state/2k6State.pdf

[103] Hyder AA et al (2004) Review on childhood burn injuries in Sub Saharan Africa: a forgotten public health challenge. African Safety Promotion: A Journal of Injury and violence Prevention 2: 43–49

[104] Istre GR et al (2001) Deaths and injuries from house fires. NEJM 344: 1911–1916

[105] Istre GR et al (2002) Residential fire related deaths and injuries among children: fireplay, smoke alarms, and prevention. Inj Prev 8: 128–132

[106] Jarvis GK, Boldt M (1982) Death styles among Canada's Indians. Soc Sci Med 16: 1345–1352

[107] Jutla RK, Heimbach D (2004) Love burns: an essay about bride burning in India. J Burn Care Rehabil 25: 165–170

[108] Karter MJ, Miller AL (1990) Patterns of fire casualties in home fires by age and sex, 1983–1987. NFPA Fire Analysis and Research Division, Quincy, MA

[109] Karter MJ (2009) Fire loss in the United States 2008. FPA Fire Analysis and Research Division, Quincy, MA

[110] Katcher ML, Shapiro MM (1987) Lower extremity burns related to sensory loss in diabetes mellitus. J Fam Pract 24: 149–151

[111] Katcher ML (1987a) Prevention of tap water scald burns: evaluation of a multi-media injury control program. Am J Public Health 77: 1195–1197

[112] Keswani MH (1986) The prevention of burning injury. Burns 12: 533–539

[113] Klein M et al (2009) Geographic access to burn center hospitals. JAMA 302: 1774–1781. http://jama.ama-assn.org/cgi/reprint/302/16/1774

[114] Laditan AAO (1987) Accidental scalds and burns in infancy and childhood. J Trop Pediatr 33: 199–202

[115] Laloë V (2002) Epidemiology and mortality of burns in a general hospital of Eastern Sri Lanka. Burns 28: 778–781

[116] Laloë V (2004) patterns of deliberate self-burning in various parts of the world. Burns 30: 207–215

[117] Lari AR et al (2002) Epidemiology of childhood burns in Fars province, Iran. J Burn Care Res 23: 39–45

[118] Liao CC, Rossignol AM (2000) Landmarks in burn prevention. Burns 26: 422–434

[119] Lundquist P et al (1989) The role of hydrogen cyanide and carbon monoxide in fire casualties: a prospective study. Forensic Sci Int 43: 9–14

[120] Mabrouk A et al (2000) Kerosene stove as a cause of burns admitted to the Ain Shams burn unit. Burns 26: 474–477

[121] MacKenzie EJ et al (2006) A national evaluation of the effect of trauma-center care on mortality. NEJM 354: 366–378

[122] Mallonee S et al (1996) Surveillance and prevention of residential-fire injuries. NEJM 335: 27–31

[123] Marsh D et al (1996) Epidemiology of adults hospitalized with burns in Karachi, Pakistan. Burns 22: 225–229

[124] Marshall SW et al (1998) Fatal residential fires: who dies and who survives? JAMA 279: 1633–1637

[125] Mannan A et al (2007) Cases of chemical assault worldwide: a literature review. Burns 33: 149–154

[126] Mashreky SR et al (2008) Epidemiology of childhood burn: yield of largest community based injury survey in Bangladesh. Burns 34: 856–862

[127] Mashreky SR et al (2008a) Consequences of childhood burn: findings from the largest community-based injury survey in Bangladesh. Burns 34: 912–918

[128] Mashreky SR et al (2009) Perceptions of rural people about childhood burns and their prevention: a basis for developing a childhood burn prevention programme in Bangladesh. Public Health 123: 568–572

[129] Mashreky SR et al (2009a) Non-fatal burn is a major cause of illness: findings from the largest community-based national survey in Bangladesh. Inj Prev 15: 397–402

[130] Matzavakis I et al (2005) Burn injuries related to motor-cycle exhaust pipes: a study in Greece. Burns 31: 372–374

[131] Mathers CD et al (2006) Sensitivity and uncertainly analyses for burden of disease and risk factor estimates. In: Lopez AD et al (eds) Global burden of disease and risk factors. Oxford University Press and the World Bank, New York, pp 399–426

[132] McGill V et al (2000) Outcome for older burn patients. Arch Surg 135: 320–325

[133] McGwin G et al (2000) The epidemiology of fire-related deaths in Alabama, 1992–1997. J Burn Care Rehabil 21: 75–83

[134] McLoughlin E et al (1977) One pediatric burn unit's experience with sleepwear-related injuries. Pediatrics 60: 405–409

[135] McLoughlin E, McGuire A (1990) The causes, cost, and prevention of childhood burn injuries. Am J Dis Child 144: 677–683

[136] Mercier C, Blond MH (1996) Epidemiological survey of childhood burn injuries in France. Burns 22: 29–34

[137] Mierley MC, Baker SP (1983) Fatal house fires in an urban population. JAMA 249: 1466–1468

[138] Miller GD (1995) Falling through the safety net. National Fire Protection Association Journal 6:xi-xv

[139] Minn YK (2007) Who burned and how to prevent? Identification of risk for and prevention of burns among epileptic patients. Burns 33: 127–128

[140] Mock C et al (2003) Injury prevention counseling to improve safety practices by parents in Mexico. Bull WHO. 81: 591–8

[141] Mock C et al (2004) Guidelines for essential trauma care. World Health Organization, Geneva, 2004. http://whqlibdoc.who. int/publications/2004/9241546409.pdf

[142] Mock C et al (2008) Child injuries and violence: the new challenge for child health. Bull World Health Organ 86: 420

[143] Mock C et al (2008a) A WHO plan for burn prevention and care. World Health Organization, Geneva, CH. http://www.who.int/violence_injury_prevention/media/news/13_03_2008/en/index.html

[144] Moritz AR, Henriques FC (1947) Studies of thermal injury: the relative importance of time and surface temperature in the causation of cutaneous burns. Am J Pathol 23: 695–720

[145] Muir BL (1991) Health status of Canadian Indians and Inuit-1990. Ottawa, Canada: Indian and Northern Health Services, Medical Services Branch, Health and Welfare Canada, pp 1–58

[146] Murray JP (1988) A study of the prevention of hot tap-water burns. Burns 14: 185–193

[147] National Center for Injury Prevention and Control (2001) Injury fact book 2001–2002. Centers for Disease Control and Prevention, Atlanta, GA

[148] Nega KE et al (2002) Epidemiology of burn injuries in Mekele Town, Northern Ethiopia: a community based study. Ethiop J Health Dev 16: 1–7

[149] NSKC (National SAFE KIDS Campaign) (2004) Burn Injury Fact Sheet. Washington (DC): NSKC. http://www.preventinjury.org/PDFs/BURN_INJURY.pdf

[150] Ndiritu S et al (2006) Burns: the epidemiological pattern, risk and safety awareness at Kenyatta National Hospital, Nairobi. East African Medical Journal 83: 455–460

[151] New York Times (1863) Terrific tragedy in Chili: two thousand five hundred persons roasted to death in a church. Dec 14, 1863

[152] Nguyen NL et al (2002) The importance of immediate cooling – a case series of childhood burns in Vietnam. Burns 28: 173–176

[153] Nguyen NL et al (2008) First aid and initial management for childhood burns in Vietnam – an appeal for public and continuing medical education. Burns 34: 67–70

[154] Notzon FC et al (1998) Causes of declining life expectancy in Russia. JAMA 279: 793–800

[155] Ofeigsson OJ et al (1972) Observations on the cold water treatment of cutaneous burns. J Pathol 108: 145–150

[156] Owen-Smith MS (1977) Armoured fighting vehicle casualties. J Royal Army Med Corps 123: 65–76

[157] Papp A et al (2008) Paediatric ICU burns in Finland 1994–2004. Burns 34: 339–344

[158] Papp T et al (1978) The health education of inpatients on the prevention and first aid of burns. Burns 1: 92–93

[159] Paraffin Safety Association of Southern Africa (2003) 2003 SABS stove test report. www.psasa.org

[160] Paraffin Safety Association of Southern Africa (2008) The status of paraffin appliances in South Africa – October, 2008. Paraffin Safety Association of Southern Africa, Cape Town, SA. http://www.pasasa.org/files/documents/programmes/safer-systems/20081112-The_status_of_paraffin_appliances_in_South_Africa.pdf

[161] Park JO et al (2009) Association between socioeconomic status and burn injury severity. Burns 35: 482–490

[162] Peck MD et al (1996) Comparison of length of hospital stay with mortality rate in a regional burn center. J Burn Care Rehabil 17: 39–44

[163] Peck MD et al (2007) Invited critique: National study of emergency department visits for burn injuries, 1993–2004. J Burn Care Res 28: 691–693

[164] Peck MD et al (2007a) Trends in injury-related deaths before and after dissolution of the Union of Soviet Socialist Republics. International J of Injury Control and Safety Promotion 14: 139–151

[165] Peck MD et al (2008) Burns and fires from non-electric domestic appliances in low and middle income countries. Part I: the scope of the problem. Burns 34: 303–311

[166] Peck MD et al (2008a) Burns and fires from non-electric domestic appliances in low and middle income countries. Part II: a strategy for intervention using the Haddon matrix. Burns 34: 312–319

[167] Peden M et al (2008) World Report on Child Injury Prevention. World Health Organization, Geneva, pp 78–98. http://whqlibdoc.who.int/publications/2008/9789241563574_eng.pdf

[168] Peleg K et al (2005) Burn prevention programs for children: do they reduce burn-related hospitalizations? Burns 31: 347–350

[169] Pereira C et al (2004) Outcome measures in burn care: is mortality dead? Burns 30: 761–771

[170] Potts JW et al (1978) A study of the inhalation toxicity of smoke produced upon pyrolysis and combustion of polyethylene foams. J Combustion Toxicology 5: 408–433

[171] Quinney B et al (2002) Thermal burn fatalities in the workplace, United States, 1992 to 1999. J Burn Care Rehabil 23: 305–310

[172] Proulx G (2007) Response to Fire Alarms. Fire Protection Engineering, Winter pp 8–11

[173] Pruitt BA et al (2007) Epidemiological, demographic, and outcome characteristics of burn injury. In: Herndon DN(ed) Total Burn Care, third edition. Saunders Elsevier, Philadelphia, PA, pp 14–32

[174] Public/Private Safety Council (2006) White Paper: home smoke alarms and other fire detection and alarm equipment. http://www.nfpa.org/assets/files//PDF/Research/SmokeAlarmsWhitePaper0406.pdf

[175] Puri V et al (2009) Fireworks injuries: a ten-year study. J Plast Reconstruc Aesthet Surg 62: 1103–1111

[176] Raghupati N (1968) First-aid treatment of burns: efficacy of water cooling. Br J Plast Surg 21: 68–72

[177] Raine TJ et al (1981) Cooling the burn wound to maintain microcirculation. J Trauma 21: 394–397

[178] Rea S et al (2005) Burn first aid in Western Australia – do healthcare workers have the knowledge? Burns 8: 1029–1034

[179] Rivara F et al (1982) Epidemiology of childhood injuries: II. Sex difference in injury rates. Am J Dis Child 136: 502–506

[180] Rivara F (1995) Developmental and behavioral issues in childhood injury prevention. J Developmental Behavior Pediatrics 16: 362–370

[181] Roberts I. (1997) Cause specific social class mortality differentials for child injury and poisoning in England and Wales. J Epidemiol Common Health 51: 334–5.

[182] Roberts H et al (2004) Putting public health evidence into practice: increasing the prevalence of working smoke alarms in disadvantaged inner city housing, J Epidemiol Community Health 48: 280–285. http://jech.bmj.com/cgi/reprint/58/4/280

[183] Roesler JS, Day H (2007) Sparklers, smoke bombs, and snakes, oh my! Effect of legislation on fireworks-related injuries in Minnesota, 1999–2005. Minnesota Med J 90: 46–47

[184] Rosen BN, Peterson L (1990) Gender differences in children's outdoor play injuries: a review and integration. Clin Psychol Rev 10: 187–205

[185] Rossi LA et al (1998) Childhood burn injuries: circumstances of occurrences and their prevention in Ribeirão Preto, Brazil. Burns 24: 416–419

[186] Runyan CW et al (1992) Risk factors for fatal residential fires. NEJM 327: 859–863

[187] Runyan CW (2003) Introduction: back to the future-revisiting Haddon's conceptualization of injury epidemiology and prevention. Epidemiol Rev 25: 60–64

[188] Saadat S et al (2009) Safety preparedness of urban community for New Year fireworks in Tehran. Burns 35:719–722

[189] Saegert S, Hart R (1990) The development of sex differences in the environmental confidence of children. In: Burnett P (ed) Women in society. Maaroufa Press, Chicago, pp 157–175

[190] Safe Bottle Lamp Foundation (2009) http://www.safebottlelamp.org/

[191] Saffle JA (2001) Organization and delivery of burn care. In: Practice guidelines for burn care. American Burn Association, Chicago: pp 18–57. http://www.ameriburn.org/PracticeGuidelines2001.pdf

[192] Sagraves SG (2007) A collaborative systems approach to rural burn care. J Burn Care Res 28: 111–114

[193] Saleh S et al (1986) Accidental burn deaths to Egyptian women of reproductive age. Burns 12: 241–245

[194] Salomon JA et al (2003) Health State Valuations in Summary Measures of Population Health. In: Murray JL, Evans D (eds) Health Systems Performance Assessment: Debate, Methods, and Empiricism, World Health Organization, Geneva, pp 409–36

[195] Sanghavi P et al (2009) Fire-related deaths in India in 2001: a retrospective analysis of data. Lancet 373: 1282–1288

[196] Sawhney CP (1989) Flame burns involving kerosene pressure stoves in India. Burns 15: 362–364

[197] Scholer SJ et al (1998) Predictors of mortality from fires in young children. Pediatrics 101:E12–16

[198] Schwebel DC et al (2009) An intervention to reduce kerosene-related burns and poisonings in low-income South African communities. Health Psychology 28: 493–500

[199] Shahidul B, Choudhury I (2001) Acid burns in Bangladesh. Ann Burns Fire Disasters 14: 1–9

[200] Sheller JP et al (1995) Burn injuries caused by fireworks: effect of prophylaxis. Burns 21: 50–53

[201] Shields BJ et al (2007) Healthcare resource utilization and epidemiology of pediatric burn-associated hospitalizations, United States, 2000. J Burn Care Res 28: 811–826

[202] Shkrum MJ, Ramsay DA (2007) Forensic pathology of trauma. Humana Press, Totowa, NJ

[203] Sikora F (1991) Until justice rolls down: the Birmingham Church bombing case. University of Alabama Press, Tuscaloosa, AL

[204] Skinner A, Peat B (2002) Burns treatment for children and adults: a study of initial burns first aid and hospital care. NZ Med J 115:U199

[205] Skinner A et al (2005) Reduced hospitalization of burns patients following a multi-media campaign that increased adequacy of first aid treatment. Burns 30: 82–85

[206] Smith GA et al (1996) The rockets' red glare, the bombs bursting in air: fireworks-related injuries to children. Pediatrics 98: 1–9

[207] Squires T, Busuttil A (1997) Alcohol and house fire fatalities in Scotland, 1980–1990. Med Sci Law 37: 321–325

[208] Stephen FR, Murray JP (1993) Prevention of hot tap water burns – a comparative study of three types of automatic mixing valves. Burns 19: 56–62

[209] Stewart RD et al (1976) Rapid estimation of carboxy-hemoglobin level in fire fighters. JAMA 235: 390–392

[210] Tamrat A (1981) Accidents and poisoning in children. Ethiop Med J 24: 39–40

[211] Tekle-Haimanot R (1993) Neurological disorders. In: Kloos H et al (eds) The ecology of health and disease in Ethiopia. Westview Press, Boulder, CO, pp 483–491

[212] Tekle Wold F (1973) Accidents in childhood. Ethiop Med J 11: 41–46

[213] Thapa NB (1989) Report of injury survey in Bhumisthan Village Panchayat Dhadhing and in Bir Hospital Kathmandu. National Programmes on Accident and Injury Prevention. National Board of Health and Welfare, Stockholm

[214] Theilade P (1990) Carbon monoxide poisoning. Five years' experience in a defined population. Am J Forensic Med Pathol 11: 219–225

[215] Thomas M (2000) Ionization and photoelectric smoke alarms in rural Alaskan homes. West J Med 173: 89–92. http://www.pubmedcentral.nih.gov/picrender.fcgi?artid=1071008&blobtype=pdf

[216] Thorpe T (2004) Critical cost based analysis of inclusive expense to the South African Government of patients with burn injuries sustained from non-pressurised paraffin stoves. Fincore Financial, South Africa

[217] Tung KY et al (2005) A seven-year epidemiology study of 12,381 admitted burn patients in Taiwan – using the Internet registration system of the Childhood Burn Foundation. Burns 31S: S12–S17

[218] UNICEF (2001) A league table of child deaths by injury in rich nations. Innocenti Report Care No. 2, UNICEF Innocenti Research Centre, Florence. http://www.unicef-irc.org/publications/pdf/repcard2e.pdf

[219] US Consumer Product Safety Commission Office of Compliance (2001) Summary of Children's Sleepwear Regulations, 16 C. F. R. Parts 1615 & 1616. http://www.cpsc.gov/businfo/regsumsleepwear.pdf

[220] US Consumer Product Safety Commission Office of Compliance (2001a) Summary of Fireworks Regulations, 16 C. F. R. Parts 1500 & 1507. http://www.cpsc.gov/BUSINFO/regsumfirework.pdf

[221] US Consumer Product Safety Commission (2008) Flammable Liquids Safety Alert, CPSC Publication 5140. http://www.cpsc.gov/CPSCPUB/PUBS/5140.pdf.

[222] US Consumer Product Safety Commission (2009) Fireworks. Publication #12. http://www.cpsc.gov/cpscpub/pubs/012.pdf

[223] US Fire Administration (1983) Residential Smoke and Fire Detector Coverage in the United States: Findings from a 1982 Survey. Washington, DC: Federal Emergency Management Agency

[224] Vassilia K et al (2004) Firework-related childhood injuries in Greece: a national problem. Burns 30: 151–153

[225] Vilasco B et al (1995) Burns in Adidjan, Côte d'Ivoire. Burns 21: 291–296

[226] Waller AE et al (1993) An evaluation of a program to reduce home hot tap water temperatures. Australian J Public Health 17:116–123

[227] Warda L et al (1999) House fire injury prevention update. Part I. A review of risk factors for fatal and non-fatal house fire injury. Inj Prevention 5: 145–150

[228] Warda L et al (1999a) House fire injury prevention update. Part II. A review of the effectiveness of preventive interventions. Inj Prev 5: 217–225

[229] Weaver LK (1999) Carbon monoxide poisoning. Crit Care Clin 15: 297–317

[230] Witsaman RJ et al (2006) Pediatric fireworks-related injuries in the United States: 1990–2003. Pediatrics 118: 296–303

[231] World Bank (2009) Africa results and monitoring system: improve access to and the reliability of clean energy. http://web.worldbank.org/WBSITE/EXTERNAL/COUNTRIES/AFRICAEXT/EXTAFRRES/0,,menuPK:3506948~pagePK:64168427~piPK:64168435~theSitePK:3506896,00.html.

[232] World Health Organization (2008) The Global Burden of Disease: 2004 Update. World Health Organization, Geneva. http://www.who.int/healthinfo/global_burden_disease/GBD_report_2004update_full.pdf.

[233] World Health Organization (2009) WHO mortality database. http://www.who.int/healthinfo/morttables/en/index.html. Accessed December 22, 2009.

[234] Yongqiang F et al (2007) Epidemiology of hospitalized burn patients in Shandong Province, 2001–2005. J Burn Care Res 28: 468–473

[235] Ytterstad B, Sogaard AJ (1995) The Harstad injury prevention study: prevention of burns in small children by a community-based intervention. Burns 21: 259–266

Correspondence: Michael D. Peck, M.D., Sc.D., FACS, Arizona Burn Center, Maricopa Medical Center, 2601 East Roosevelt Street, Phoenix, AZ 85008, USA, Tel: +1 602 344 5624, Fax: +1 602 344 5705, E-mail: michael_peck@medprodoctors.com

# Prevention of burn injuries

Anna Arno[1,2], Judy Knighton[1]

[1] Ross Tilley Burn Centre, Sunnybrook Health Sciences Centre, Department of Surgery, Division of Plastic Surgery, University of Toronto, Toronto, Canada
[2] Burn unit and Plastic Surgery Department, Vall d'Hebron University Hospital, Autonomous University of Barcelona, Barcelona, Spain

## Introduction

Prevention means anticipation. In modern medicine, prevention has become the goal of all healing strategies. It has been shown that prevention is key for maintaining health and having the highest quality of life, despite increasing age. Furthermore, prevention is the more efficient way to treat an illness, since it reduces, not only hospital stay, but also drug use and cost of complications. However, prevention can also be expensive and it has until recently been considered a luxury and sometimes impractical, especially in the developing world.

Like other injury mechanisms, the prevention of burns requires epidemiology and risk factors studies. In fact, the complete care of any illness or injury implies epidemiology (measurement of risk factors, frequency and distribution of the injury), prevention, injury biomechanics (physical and functional responses of the victim to the energy), treatment and rehabilitation.

Although burns represent a small number of all traumatic injuries, they are responsible for significant morbidity and mortality worldwide, leading to chronic devastating sequelae, not only physical, but also psychological and social. As a result, burn prevention is particularly important and should be a major focus of attention.

## Burns prevalence and relevance

To measure the frequency and risk of a disease, epidemiologists, health care providers, government agencies and insurers calculate the prevalence and incidence of a disease, respectively. Whereas the prevalence is the total number of cases of a disease in a population at a given time, the incidence is the number of new cases in that population in a given time period.

A burn injury represents one of the most severe forms of trauma, and occurs in more than two to three million people in North America each year. In the United States, an estimated 500,000 people seek medical attention for burn injury per year, but burns incidence and severity is decreasing recently. However, the exact incidence of burns differs between countries; the reported is 31.2 per 100,000 persons/year referred to a specialized unit for definitive treatment. According to the World Health Organization (WHO), an estimated 330,000 deaths per year worldwide are related to thermal injury, and most of them are due to fire-related burns. More than 90% of these fatal, fire-related burns occur in the developing world, in particular South-East Asia (Table 1). On average in the United States in 2003, a fire death occurred about every 2 hours and someone was injured every 29 minutes. At present, burns are the fourth leading cause of death from unintentional injury. A severe burn represents a devastating injury,

**Table 1.** Estimated number of deaths and mortality rates due to fire-related burn by WHO region and Income group, 2002

| REGION | Africa | America | | South-East Asia | Europe | | Eastern Mediterranean | | Western Pacific | | World |
|---|---|---|---|---|---|---|---|---|---|---|---|
| Income group | L/M | H | L/M | L/M | H | L/M | H | L/M | H | L/M | |
| Number of burn deaths (thousands) | 4.3 | 4 | 4 | 184 | 3 | 21 | 0,1 | 32 | 2 | 18 | 312 |
| Death rate (per 100 000 population) | 6.2 | 1.2 | 0.8 | 11.6 | 0.7 | 4.5 | 0.9 | 6.4 | 1.2 | 1.2 | 5 |
| Proportion global mortality due to fires (%) | 13.8 | 1.3 | 1.3 | 59 | 1 | 6.7 | 0.02 | 10.3 | 0.6 | 5.8 | 100 |

L = Low, M = Middle, H = High.
From: WHO Global Burden of Disease Database, 2002 (Version 5)

affecting nearly every organ system and leading to significant morbidity and mortality. In order to maintain a morbidity and mortality statistics database for burns, the ABA/TRACS (Trauma Registry of the American College of Surgeons) Burn Patient Registry was created in the US in the 1990s. However, there is still a strong need for homogeneous national and international burn registration systems.

Although mortality has declined over the past few years due to improved medical care and promotion of burn prevention, management of major burns still remains a challenge, even in modern, developed countries. The increasing number of burn survivors are at risk for developing long-term psychological and physical sequelae, with potentially devastating consequences to them, their families and society in general. Furthermore, burns have important human and material costs. Providing adequate hospital care to a burn patient costs approximately US$ 1000 per day and major burns usually require admission to intensive care units, which are very resource-intensive expensive.

In most developing countries, the same standard of care is not possible due to limited resources and inaccessibility to sophisticated skills and technologies, leading to a higher morbidity and mortality. Although these countries are in special need of burn prevention, the reality is often the opposite, where there is a lack of government-funded burn prevention programmes. In these countries, some health authorities consider injury prevention to have a much lower priority than disease prevention. Despite mounting evidence that injury is largely preventable, burn prevention has been forgotten in the past by public health authorities as these injuries are believed to be random accidents. While natural disasters are unavoidable, accidents can be prevented and represent a public health problem that requires government and community involvement. A key to keep in mind is that the best care for burns is prevention, which takes time, energy and money. Eventually, it is likely the most effective solution to the world's burn problem.

## Burn injury risk factors

Burn risk is linked with poverty, lack of running water, crowding, illiteracy, unemployment, lapses in child supervision – mostly in large and single-parent families, recent pregnancies or mothers' being away from home, prior history of a sibling being burned-, presence of pre-existing physical/emotional challenges in a child and lack of education (although in some societies, higher education of individuals is associated with increased risk of immolation rituals involving burns, for example).

With these risk factors in mind, one can ascertain why burns are more common in the developing world and how low socioeconomic status has been linked to increased risk of unintentional injury and mortality.

Another important risk factor for burns is drug use. Medications, such as sleeping pills, narcotics, synthetic stimulant drugs, such as methamphetamines, alcohol and/or smoking are usually the prodrome of flame burns in many teenagers and adults. For instance, in South Korea it is not unusual to see groups of teenagers in a room engaging in butane gas abuse, which causes euphoria and hallucinations. Facial burns result from sniffing the flammable gas, in addition to potentially severe systemic effects, such as pulmonary oedema, gastritis and cardiac dysrhythmias. Sniffing nitrous oxide also causes confusion; in this case, the cold gas results in frostbite to the cheek.

In a large European review, risk factors for death from a burn were found to be older age, higher total body surface area burned and previous comorbidity in the form of chronic diseases. Multiorgan failure and sepsis were the most frequent leading causes of death. Burn shock and inhalation injury were responsible for most of the early deaths (<48h). Half of the burns were suffered by children <16 years old and 60% occurred in men (but in elderly people, women were more frequently burned).

When dealing with burn risk factors, it is important to analyze the who, how and where factors in order to design an effective prevention plan.

## WHO?

Regarding the age of the individual, children under 5 years of age comprise the highest risk group for burn injuries. Causative factors in all incidents involving babies are a mixture of imprudence, impulsiveness, curiosity, lack of experience and a desire to imitate adults. Furthermore, this age group lacks a sense of danger and awareness and they hardly understand cause-and-effect relationships.

At the other end of the age continuum, elderly people over 64 years are also a high risk population. Their risk of dying in a fire is 2.5 times greater than the general population. The main causes of burn injuries in the elderly are flame burns due to smoking and cooking (Table 2). Additional risk factors include medical conditions associated with physical or mental impairment: stroke, poor eyesight, decreased hearing and mobility, diabetes (peripheral neuropathy with decreased or no lower extremity pain perception), dementia (such as Alzheimer's, with confusion and forgetfulness), depression and suicide.

**Table 2.** Elderly burn prevention tips

| FLAME burns | 1. Ask a relative or neighbour to routinely check for gas leak odor.<br>2. Use large ashtrays. Smoke only while upright. Never smoke in bed or when drowsy.<br>3. Never use flammable liquids to start a fire or prime a carburetor or as a cleaning solvent.<br>4. Never store flammable liquids near a pilot light or other heat source.<br>5 Check the smoke detector battery once a month. Use a broom handle to perform the check or ask a friend to do so.<br>6 Have a flashlight, keys, eyeglasses and whistle at the bedside to summon help if needed.<br>7. Wear close-fitting clothes while cooking or near any potentially dangerous heat source (fireplace, campfire, wood-burning stove). Garments that are flame resistant are recommended.<br>8. Use the back burners of the stove and turn handles inward.<br>9. Avoid throw rugs in the kitchen area and keep the floor clean to avoid falls.<br>10. Use a cooking timer with an audible alarm.<br>11. If using a speace heater, ensure that the automatic shut off is in working order should the heater accidentally tip over.<br>12. Never lay anything on or near a heating device (e.g., space heater, wood-burning stove, kitchen stove, baseboard heater). |
|---|---|
| CONTACT burns | 1. Use all heating devices that are placed on or near the skin with caution (e.g., heating pad, hot water bottles, space heaters). |
| SCALD burns | 1. Place a nonskid mat and handrails in the bathtub or shower to prevent accidental falls and to allow easy access in and out of the area.<br>2. Check the temperature on the hot water heater; the recommended setting is 120°F (48.8°C). Install antiscald devices in bathroom plumbing. |

Adapted from: Thompson RM, Carrougher GJ (1998) Burn prevention. In: Carrougher GJ (ed) Burn care and therapy. Mosby, St. Louis, pp 497–524 [18]

**Table 3.** Burn prevention tips at home: in the kitchen, living room and bathroom

| KITCHEN | 1. Keep hot items in the centre of the table and away from children. |
|---|---|
| | 2. Keep food away from the stove, so no one will be tempted to reach across hot stove elements. |
| | 3. Keep young children away from the cooking area. |
| | 4. Use place mats instead of tablecloths (young children use tablecloths to pull themselves up) |
| | 5. Roll up electrical cords and unplug appliances when not in use. |
| | 6. Use pot holders, not towels. |
| | 7. Turn pot handles, inward, toward the back of the stove; use back elements of stove for cooking. |
| | 8. Store pot holders, paper towels and seasonings, candy or toys away from the stove top. |
| | 9. Avoid full or puffy sleeves while cooking. |
| | 10. Use a large lid or baking soda to put out small grease fires in pans. |
| LIVING-ROOM | 1. Do not use extension cords in place of permanent wires. |
| | 2. Cover unused electrical outlets with safety plugs. |
| | 3. Use fireplace matches to light a fireplace. |
| | 4. Keep matches and lighters away from children. |
| | 5. Soak cigarettes in water before placing in garbage to ensure they are fully extinguished. |
| BATHROOM | 1. Run hot and cold water together. |
| | 2. Set the hot water heater thermostat to low 50°C. |
| | 3. Never leave children alone in the bathroom. |
| | 4. Use a "no slip" plastic mat in the bathtub to prevent falls. |

In India, young women (16–35 years old) are the most prone to suffer burns at home, due to the tradition of cooking at floor level or over an open fire, compounded by the wearing of loose fitting clothing made from non-flame retardant fabric. In the least developed European countries, there is also female burn predominance and a higher proportion of electrical burn injuries comparing with western Europe, with a male predominance.

## WHERE?

Most childhood burns occur in the home, in developed as well as in developing countries. The modern home can contain a number of harmful substances and pieces of equipment, such as electricity, gas and chemicals (Table 3). Lapses in child supervision, such as forgetting to turn off the oven or stove element at bath time lead to a higher risk of unintentional burn injuries.

Adult burns are reported to have a more variable location, with almost equal frequencies in the home, outdoors and in the workplace. For all age groups, the kitchen is the most common scene of burns, followed by the bathroom and the outdoors (i. e. backyard, garage).

## HOW?

Burns in children are caused usually by scald, flame and contact burns, in order of most to least frequency (although in some countries, such as Australia, contact burns are the second cause after scalds, and, in the developing world, flame burns are the most common). It has been shown that when the child becomes older, flame injury predominates, becoming the most common cause of burns in children aged 6–17 years old.

Not only are young children more prone to suffer contact burns, but also the elderly, the physically impaired people, patients with diabetes, all of whom may have some inability to withdraw from heated objects or who have limited sensation to their extremities (Table 10).

In the developing world, the commonest cause of injury is a flame burn. Most such accidents are related to malfunctioning kerosene pressure stoves and homemade kerosene lamps used for lighting, or from domestic appliances using flammable fuel. On the other hand, many households are made of highly combustible and toxic materials, such as wood and plastics, which burn easily, leading to high mortality rates due to severe smoke inhalation injury.

In the developed world, fire is sometimes related, not only to accidental burns, but also to homi-

**Table 4.** Vectors leading to burns related to cultural and social traditions or festivities

1. Tanning
2. Aesthetic skin branding
3. Steel chopsticks use (Korea)
4. Barbecues, flambé food, fondues
5. Primus stoves
6. Kerosene oil for lighting
7. Sandal burns (heating device)
8. Ember or "brasas" (Mediterranean countries)
9. "Kangari" burns
10. "Dowry" and "sati" burns (India)
11. Drug abuse or use
12. The "street soccer" game.
13. "Shabbes" burns (Jewish orthodox children)
14. "Friday" mass and pilgrimage to Mecca and extremely hot temperatures and barefeet
15. "Camphor" burns of the plam (India)
16. Garlic burns (traditional medicine practice)
17. Self-mutilation by burning (Buddhist community)
18. Fireworks
19. Halloweeen "Egyptian mummy" burn (United Kingdom).
20. Chinese mid-autumn festival burns
21. Cupping (Middle East)
22. The Turkish "flying toy balloon" burn
23. Coining (Vietnam)

Adapted from: Al-Quattan MM, Al-Zahrani K (2009) A review of burns related to traditions, social habits, religious activities, festivals and traditional medical practices. Burns 35: 476–481 [2]

cide or suicide attempts. Self-inflicted burns tend to be more extensive and have 14 times higher mortality than accidental burns due to the use of accelerants. In the developing world, some flame-related burns are the result of social traditions and religious rituals (Table 4).

## Burn prevention types

We can classify burn prevention in two ways:

### A) Primary, secondary and tertiary prevention

Focusing on the time elapsed since injury; this classification is similar to the one published by Haddon in 1968, with the phases pre-event (primary prevention), actual event (secondary prevention) and post-event (tertiary prevention) and the nine-cells matrix combination (Table 5).

**A1) Primary burn prevention** aims to avoid the injury from occurring at all. Primary burn prevention strategies include automatic protection, legislation/regulation and education.

**A1. 1) Automatic protection** represents the most effective primary preventive strategy. It involves elimination of environmental hazards or more accurate product design.

**A2. 2) Legislation/regulation:** Community, state, national or international governmental regulations and laws are in place to reduce injury. For instance, local ordinances that require apartment buildings to have working smoke detectors or installation of antiscald devices; regulation of exits and fire escapes from buildings where people work or congregate, as well as laws, not only for the installation but more importantly for the maintenance of equipment for fire control; regulations of fire drills in educational institutions; regulations of handling and disposition of any kind of flammable materials, etc.

**A2. 3) Education:** Educational programs focus on providing information about an identified area of concern and seek to make the public aware of the

**Table 5.** The Haddon matrix for burn control

| | Agent or vector | Host | Environment | |
| | | | Physical | Social |
|---|---|---|---|---|
| PRE-event | Fire-safe cigarette | Control seizure | Non-slip tub surface | Legislation: factory preset water heater thermostats |
| EVENT | Sprinklers, smoke detectors | Flame-retardant clothes | Fire escapes | Fire drill education |
| POST-event | Water | First aid antibiotics | Emergency Medical Services | Emergency and rehabilitation services |

From: Hunt JL, Arnoldo BD, Purdue GF (2007) Prevention of burn injuries. In: Herndon DN (ed) Total burn care. Saunders Elsevier, Galveston, pp 33–39

dangers and to teach appropriate preventive strategies. They also inform people about the medical and social consequences of burn injuries; i. e. parents are taught to insert plastic plugs to cover the electrical outlets to prevent electrical burns in small children.

While burn prevention educational campaigns have reduced the incidence of burn injuries, they have not eliminated the injuries entirely. Education may increase knowledge, but does not always lead to behavioural and/or lifestyle change needed to diminish or eliminate incidence or severity of burn injuries.

Probable causes of failure of burn education primary prevention programmes may be the brevity of the campaign, multiplicity of messages and separation of the interventions. It has been postulated that the prevention program needs to be repeated several times to be effective. In some US states, burns education in public schools is mandated by law. In fact, school children constitute the largest high-risk group to suffer burn injuries. Although similar prevention methods may be used to reach both children and adults, it has been shown that the amount of time required to adequately convey a burn injury prevention curriculum is age-dependent, and that extracurricular school activities are very important. For children 6–12 years of age, games would be an effective educational prevention tool. Family education is also crucial. Posters, mass media and multimedia strategies are effective means of disseminating the burn prevention message in general.

**A2) Secondary burn prevention** seeks to minimize the already-produced injury and consists of teaching early injury detection and treatment. For example, an individual whose shirt catches fire is taught to STOP, DROP to the ground and ROLL to extinguish the flames; other examples include "apply cool water to a burn" or "crawl under smoke" (see Table 6).

**A3) Tertiary burn prevention** involves avoiding impairment and maximizing functionality during the phase of rehabilitation after a burn. Indeed, not only secondary, but also tertiary burn prevention strategies aim at limiting the already- produced damage.

**Table 6.** First aid counselling after a burn (secondary prevention)

If your clothing catches fire:
 - STOP (don't run!)
 - DROP to the ground
 - ROLL to put the fire out

If a burn occur: COOL
 - Immediately pour cool water – not ice – on the burn
 - Cover burn with a clean sheet and seek medical attention

## B) Active versus passive prevention

Focusing on the three aspects of injury prevention: agent, environment and host.

**B1) Active burn prevention**: Active prevention requires individual effort. Education is the only active primary burn prevention strategy. For instance, teaching people to lower their tap water temperature through educational campaigns. Active prevention is the least effective and most difficult strategy to maintain, especially over a long period of time.

**B2) Passive burn prevention** includes legislation/regulation and product design/environmental change. Passive prevention strategies don't require "correct behaviour" by the individual and appear to be more successful than active prevention strategies. However, many of the more effective burn prevention programs contain both active and passive measures. Among the passive prevention methods, legislation appears to play a major role.

To sum up (Table 7), burn prevention involves not only physicians, nurses and other health care-providers but also engineers, legislators and inspectors.

**Table 7.** Strategies to reduce severity injury and parameters of injury occurrence

ACTIVE (Education)
 - Agent + Host + Environment

PASSIVE
 - Product engineering + Environmental change + Legislation
 - Agent + Environment

# Burn prevention: The basics to design a plan

Any injury prevention campaign should consider the following ABCDE steps:

A = Analyze the data.
B = Build a coalition.
C = Communicate the problem.
D = Develop the interventions.
E = Evaluate the program.

Efforts at burn prevention should target the population groups most at risk and should aim at minimizing the effects of specific risk factors and harmful actions. To achieve success, it is necessary for a leader, who has strong knowledge about the epidemiology, care and recovery of burn patients to guide colleagues, who are also well-informed and culturally sensitive to the specific population where the prevention is going to be conducted.

That is to say, that every burn prevention programme has to be population-specific and differ, depending on the country/ individual characteristics (education, socioeconomic status, geography, traditions, cultural or religious beliefs and social habits . . .); in other words, the who, where, when and how burns happen must be taken into consideration. For instance, in India, the task of educating students appears to be more worthy because they are more receptive and spread easily the educational messages to their parents and friends.

In conclusion, knowing the general risk factors –the vector or energy source, the host or victim and the environment- is essential for preventing and controlling any injury.

Any injury prevention plan is not valid until the results of its application are evaluated (Table 8). If a prevention plan fails to have success, possible solutions may be to:

a) change the technique to measure the burn incidence reduction. Mortality and, more importantly, morbidity data must be used for outcome measures.

b) modify the prevention program design to a more appropriate one.

Regarding this problem, however, some researchers found that patients who sustain burn injury use burn prevention strategies at similar rates, when compared with those who do not. They defend that those individuals with lower education and in-

**Table 8.** Autosurvey to evaluate oneself's burn prevention tools

- Do you put handles stick out from the stove?
- Do you leave children alone in the kitchen while food is cooking?
- Do your children play in the kitchen while you are cooking?
- Are appliance cords hang down from counters or tables?
- Do you rush to fix breakfast or dinner?
- Do you check for children before carrying hot liquid?
- Is hot coffee or tea left on the table when no adult is there?
- Are children alone in the bathroom when the tub is being filled?
- Do you forget to test the temperature of your child's bath water?
- Do you have long hair and wear it loose while cooking?
- Are matches and cigarette lighters lying around where children can find them?
- Are flammable liquids stored on a high, cool shelf, away from open flame in tightly sealed containers?
- Do you store children's snacks over the stove?
- Do you pour charcoal lighter fluid on coals after they have started burning?
- Do you smoke near gasoline?
- Do you wear a bathrobe while cooking?
- Do you spill lighter fluid on your clothes?
- Do you usually fall asleep while smoking?

come, remain more susceptible to burn injury, independently of the prevention strategy used.

## Target-specific burn prevention strategies

### Flame burns

Prevention of burns from residential fires

The use of smoke alarms has had the greatest impact in decreasing fire deaths in the US, but they have to be maintained –not only installed- to be really effective.

On the other hand, fire sprinklers complement smoke detectors and are the most effective tool to prevent the spread of fires in their early stages. In 1993, the National Fire Protection Association (NFPA) estimated smoke alarms alone could reduce fire deaths by 52%; sprinklers alone could decrease fire deaths by 69% and the combined use of them by 82%.

House fires account for most of the major burn injuries. Causes of injuries and burn prevention tips include:

*a) Careless cigarette smoking:* Canada was the first country to pass fire-safe cigarette legislation in 2004. People must be aware of practising safe behaviour while using any flammable materials. It is also recommended that one practice EDITH (Exit Drills in the Home), so that everyone will know the meeting place and how to escape in case of a fire.

A cigarette left unattended can burn for as long as 30 minutes. In 1993, 40% of residential fire deaths were caused by the careless use of cigarettes. Most smoking fires started in the bedroom or living room. Some severe COPD (Chronic Obstructive Pulmonary Disease) patients use home oxygen and then, at the same time, they go to light a cigarette, leading to facial burns. Furthermore, alcohol is often combined with cigarette smoking or other substance abuse, with the victim falling asleep. In fact, statistics have shown that it is quite common for burn patients to have higher blood alcohol levels.

*b) Heating equipment:* Never leave small children unattended next to a heat source. Also don't leave candles unattended.

In middle Asia, the "sandal" is an ancient heating device responsible for a high number of third degree foot burns in small children in Uzbekistan. The "sandal" is a table, around which people sit which has a hole in the floor underneath, where lit coals are placed. Unsupervised toddlers crawl and fall into the coals leading to severe burns.

During winters in Kashmir, people charcoal braziers, known as "kangari", between their legs to keep warm. Repeated exposure results in erythema to the inner thighs and lower abdomen and may also promote skin cancer.

*c) Electrical equipment malfunction:* You should install not only smoke, but also CO (carbon monoxide) detectors.

Whereas smoke alarms are now present in almost 100% of homes, CO detectors are largely absent, but they should also be present. CO inhalation is the main cause of fatal poisoning in the industrialized world and CO intoxication is present in flame injuries, especially those sustained indoors. CO is produced by open flames, whenever a carbon-based fuel, gas, oil, wood or charcoal is burned. Products

**Table 9.** Prevention tips for home burns in developing countries

1. Cooking should be done only on a platform, not on the floor.
2. Don't use a pressure stove.
3. Do not pour kerosene into a burning stove or lamp.
4. Do not adjust a rack for storing materials just above the cooking range.
5. Do not allow younger children to play with matchsticks, candles and electric switches.

include charcoal grills, gas water heaters, stoves and lanterns. Carbon monoxide-generating appliances, such as stoves, are often used during power outages or for financial reasons in low-income households. If the heating source is either used improperly or ventilation is inadequate, CO levels can become toxic and have fatal consequences.

*d) Cooking:* You should be very careful when cooking, avoid wearing loose clothing that could catch on fire, avoiding cooking when naked (especially in the summer and hot weather countries) and install smoke detectors and automatic sprinklers in the home and restaurants.

In many developing countries, cooking is still done using primus stoves, which are an important cause of burns, due to the presence of kerosene. Apart from the kitchen, Kerosene is also used as a nightly light source and contained in home-made chimneys, located in the living rooms or bedrooms in houses in the developing world (Table 9).

*e) Children playing with matches and lighters:* Matches and lighters must be kept out of the reach of children. Children should be taught, at an early age, that matches and lighters are tools and not toys.

## Prevention of outdoors flame-burns

In many dry and warm-climate countries, especially during the summer, forest fires caused by unattended fallen cigarettes or intentionally by individuals with psychiatric disorders who enjoy provoking fires. In some rural areas of Spain, farmers burn olive trees or timber to produce embers or "brasas", which leave incandescent residue. These residues remain alight and undergo slow combustion and, hence, are used for heating, but they may also produce flame burns.

Outdoor barbeques are commonly held in many countries during summer months. Instead of using an authorized carbon source of heat, some people use gasoline or alcohol to make the flames grow, causing flame burns. Other cooking-related burns involve the making of fondues flambéed food.

Outdoor, recreational fires are also a normal practice during the warmer months of the year and may cause severe burns. They involve mostly the hands, with a mean TBSA (Total Body Surface Area) of 3.5%, and the main mechanism is falling into the fire. Parents can play an important role in educating their children about campfire safety and the hazards of both active and extinguished fires.

In India, marital traditions are associated with "dowry" and "sati" burns, which both have high mortality rates. After marriage, if the gifts (known as "dowry") are not considered enough, the wife is put on fire (usually after pouring kerosene on her body) and this is known as "dowry burns". In "sati burns", the wife throws herself on the burning body of the deceased husband. Although the government has made efforts to prevent these burns by writing legislation and including it under the Penal Code, these type of injuries still occur and some families lie and report "dowry burns" as kitchen accidents.

In a similar manner, in the developing world, some religious activities involve self-inflicted ritual burns (especially in the Buddhist community) or promote unintentional burning (e. g. foot burns in Muslims who leave mosques barefoot where temperatures exceed 50 °C).

Also in India, a special type of fire-related burn (jaggery) causes severe and deadly pediatric burns. Jaggery is the non-industrial refinement of sugar cane into a sugar product and represents an important source of income and significant role in cooking and cultural rituals in rural India. Legislation aimed at improving dangerous work environments, establishing minimum age requirements and maximum hours of work, as well as with engineering or product design safety improvements, would be effective in reducing these types of injuries.

Fireworks are an important cause of burns in many countries around the world, due to its use during national holidays, traditional festivals or special events, such as New Year's Eve or other celebrations, such as the Olympic games, Independence day (US), Guy Fawkes Night (Commonwealth), Fallas (Valencia, Spain), Hari raya (Malaysia), Mawlid and Eid al-Adha (Muslim countries), Charshanbe-Soori (Iran) or Purim (jewish festivity). Contact hand burns from holding the fireworks, are most frequently seen accounted for largely by boys 10–14 years of age. However, in approximately 50% of the cases bystanders are injured. Eyes are affected in 18% of cases. Flame burns may also occur when the clothes catch fire. Complete firework bans are found in Hungary, Ireland, Australia and the northeast USA, at the present time.

A specific type of outdoor burn is seen during war. Combat-related thermal injuries generally affect the hands and head, mainly through improvised explosive devices, causing blast injuries and polytrauma. They generally involve less than 20% TBSA and have relatively low mortality rates (4% of all war deaths and 5–20% of all war-injuries). Preventive measures against war-related burn injuries include improvement in predeployment education to reduce noncombat injuries, flame retardant military clothing and decreased combat episodes.

## Prevention of clothing-ignition burns

Clothing burns result from a combination of 3 factors: flammability, the behaviour of the wearer and the heat source. In the 1940s, many children in the US suffered leg burns as a result of the ignition of a particular cowboy suit or chaps, made of highly flammable brushed rayon. This initiated research interest in clothing flammability, leading to the following findings:

a) Wool: Burns very slowly and does not ignite. It melts with a red glow and finally extinguishes itself.
b) Cotton: Burns like a torch and is completely destroyed in a matter of seconds. Cotton combined with wool burns less than either by itself.
c) Rayon: Ignates easily, but not as intensely as cotton.
d) Raised cut materials: Are very flammable.
e) Silk: Produces a red glow but usually extinguishes quickly.
f) Nylon: Melts but clings to the underlying surface.

Apart from the materials, what has been shown to be very important in terms of preventing clothing-ignition burns, is the fit of the clothes themselves. Closer-fitting outfits decrease the incidence and mortality of clothing-related burns. Loose-fitting clothing, particularly if the person is in an upright position, allows for greater airspace between the fabric and skin, allowing to oxygen promote the flame, thereby worsening the burn. These facts explain why the safest sleepwear for children is considered to be a snug-fitting cotton, flame-resistant garment. By definition, flame-resistant garments don't ignite easily and must self-extinguish quickly.

**Table 10.** Burn prevention tips for impaired people

| | |
|---|---|
| FLAME burns | 1. Use extreme caution when cooking. Wear close-fitting and flame-resistant clothes while cooking or near any heat source.<br>2. Avoid throw rugs in the kitchen area and keep the floor clean to avoid falls.<br>3. Use larger astrays. Smoke only while upright. Never smoke in bed or when drowsy.<br>4. Maintain smoke detectors, alarms and prinkler systems in good working order. Check the smoke detector battery once a month.<br>5. Determine emergency exit plans. Practice them routinely with household members. Keep all exit routes clear.<br>6. Have a flashlight, keys, eyeglasses and whistle at the bedside to summon help if needed.<br>7. Ensure that the local fire department is aware of any household members with special needs. |
| CONTACT burns | 1. With individuals with decreased sensation, use all heating devices that are placed on or near the skin with caution (e.g., heating pad, hot water bottles, space heaters). |
| SCALD burns | 1. For people cooking from a wheelchair, a mirror positioned over the stovetop allows one to see the contents of a pot during cooking. Avoid using heavy, large pans that may be awkward to use especially when filled with hot food.<br>2. Check the temperature on the hot water heater; the recommended setting is 120 °F (48.8 °C).<br>3. Install antiscald devices in bathroom plumbing. |

Adapted and modified from: Thompson RM, Carrougher GJ (1998) Burn prevention. In: Carrougher GJ (ed) Burn care and therapy. Mosby, St. Louis, pp 497–524 [18]

## Prevention of scald burns

Scald burns are responsible for the majority of non-fatal burn injuries in the world. Furthermore, scald burns are the main cause of burn injury in toddlers, involving mostly splash burns from spilled liquids. These injuries are difficult to prevent, and the exact incidence is unknown. These burns are not usually fatal, but unintentional injuries are the leading cause of deaths in children. Other populations at high risk for scald burns, while bathing, are the elderly and people with epilepsy, where there is a heightened risk of seizures and falls and, in the elderly, thinner skin.

Preventive strategies include reducing temperature of hot water heaters to a maximum of 49–54ºC (Table 11), installing anti-scald devices to shower heads and faucets or inserting shut-off valves in the water circuit to detect temperatures over a certain level, using large round handles or push-and-turn type handles to prevent young children from turning on the hot water or using liquid-crystal thermometers in bathtubs to alert the caregiver to the water temperature. In some US states, it is imperative, by law, to install appropriate tempering valves in all new domestic dwellings, and water from shower heads and bathtub inlets cannot exceed 46 °C. Small children and disabled people should be constantly supervised when close to hot water. Special caution should also be paid when removing warmed foods – especially liquids – from the microwave oven to avoid steam and scald burns.

**Table 11.** Time/Temperature relationships in scalds

| TEMPERATURE | TIME TO PRODUCE FULL-THICKNESS BURN |
|---|---|
| 48.8 °C = 120 °F | 5 minutes |
| 51.6 °C = 125 °F | 1.5–2 minutes |
| 54.4 °C = 130 °F | 30 seconds |
| 57.2 °C = 135 °F | 10 seconds |
| 60 °C = 140 °F | 5 seconds |
| 62.9 °C = 145 °F | 3 seconds |
| 65.5 °C = 150 °F | 1.5 seconds |
| 68.3 °C = 155 °F | 1 second |

**Table 12.** Pediatric burn prevention tips

| | |
|---|---|
| FLAME burn | 1. Store all matches and lighters securely so they are inaccessible to children.<br>2. Use only child-resistant lighters.<br>3. Never leave children unattended near a heat source.<br>4. Infants should wear flame-resistant sleepwear and costumes.<br>5. Teach children to STOP, DROP and ROLL on the ground if their clothing were to catch fire and to place cool water on a burn.<br>6. Install smoke detectors on each level of the house and outside all sleeping areas. (Be sure to read the manufacturer's instructions). Test the batteries once a month, and allow children to hear the alarm so that they will recognize the sound.<br>7. Practice EDITH (Exit Drills In The Home).<br>8. Install a fire escape ladder in all bedrooms above the first floor.<br>9. Review the home fire exit plan with all home childcare providers.<br>10. If a child engages in fire play or fire-setting behaviour, contact the local fire department or burn center for educaton and counselling recommendations. |
| CONTACT burns | 1. Use curling irons, irons and glue guns with caution when small children are present.<br>2. If the outside temperature is high, use caution when placing children in car seats or using metal buckles. They should be examined by an adult before use by a child.<br>3. Caution children about touching heated radiators, space heaters and floor furnace grates.<br>4. Never leave a child unattended near a campfire. Make sure the child wears shoes to prevent injury from contact with hot coals. |
| SCALD burns | 1. Check the temperature on the hot water heater; the recommended setting is 120 °F (48.8 °C).<br>2. Install antiscald devices in bathroom plumbing.<br>3. Never leave young childen unattended in the bathtub or in the kitchen while cooking; restrict a child's access to the kitchen when cooking.<br>4. Face children away from the bathtub faucet to reduce the likelihood of the child turning on the hot water.<br>5. Double-check the temperature of the bath water before placing a child in the tub (recommended temperature is 36.1–37.8 °C or 97–100 °F)<br>6. Review bathtub safety tips with all home childcare providers.<br>7. When carrying or holding children, be sure to keep hot beverages away from the child.<br>8. When cooking, use the back burners and always turn the pot handles inward.<br>9. Keep appliances toward the back of the countertop. Wind cords up and out of reach.<br>10. Avoid using tablecloths with young children present; they can pull them off easily.<br>11. Supervise children closely when hot foods are being served and carried.<br>12. Never microwave a child's bottle or allow young children to remove items from the microwave.<br>13. Take extra precautions when removing heated foods from the microwave oven when children are around.<br>14. Use cool mist (not steam) vaporizers. |
| CHEMICAL burns | 1. Keep all chemicals inaccessible to children and in their original container.<br>2. When finished with a chemical, recap and discard the container appropriately. |
| ELECTRICAL burns | 1. Make sure all electrical outlets are inaccesible to young children. Block outlets with heavy furniture and use outlet covers to prevent a child from attempting to insert things into them.<br>2. Never place an electrical appliance near a water source (e.g., bathtub, sink).<br>3. Use electrical extension cords with caution. Mouth burns have been associated with extension cords.<br>4. Teach children never to extend objects near high-power lines. |
| RADIATION burns | 1. Apply sunscreen to all exposed skin before sun exposure, reapply it as recommended and wear protective clothing. |

From: Thompson RM, Carrougher GJ (1998) Burn prevention. In: Carrougher GJ (ed) Burn care and therapy. Mosby, St. Louis, pp 497–524 [18]

## Prevention of contact burns

Contact burns, as well as chemical burns, can be avoided by adopting appropriate preventive measures. In developed countries, contact burns from the use of gas-fire places, domestic central heating radiators, irons and ovens have been identified. The surface temperature of the glass front on gas fireplace units can reach 200 °C, on average 6.5 minutes after ignition. A full-thickness burn may occur in less than 1 second with this temperature, and these contact burns can occur in both adults and children (Table 12). In toddlers and preschool children, domestic heating devices located too close to their beds have been found to be responsible for many hand contact burns.

## Prevention of chemical burns

Chemicals, used in the home, should be locked away and rendered inaccessible to children. All chemicals should be stored in their original containers. The Occupational Safety and Health Administration (OSHA) regulations require eyewash stations and showers in all facilities that use potentially injurious chemical products to allow for instant and copious irrigation following exposure.

## Prevention of electrical burns

Electrical injuries can be prevented by strict adherence to safety rules regarding household wiring, electrical outlets and appliance cords. The majority of high-voltage electrical injuries occur at work and may be fatal or lead to devastating sequelae such as amputations. In addition, bystanders are at risk for injury and should never touch someone, who is in direct contact with electricity until the current has been shut off. In the case of children, when the regional resistance (wet mouth) is low and the peripheral resistance is high (e. g. an ungrounded foot), then an oral burn results, but if this latter is also low (e. g. a grounded foot or hand), then electrocution results. Prevention must be directed to the female end of the extension cord. In 1976, the "Crikelair protective cuff" was described in the scientific literature; it consists of a plastic, transparent and non-conductive cuff which attacks

to the female end of the extension cord to prevent injuries.

In some developing and western-world countries, thieves can also suffer electrical burns during their attempts to steal the cupper wire.

In Korea, people eat using steel – not plastic or wood – chopsticks; children may insert the steel chopsticks into the wall socket, producing severe pediatric electrical burns. To prevent such injuries, they could be encouraged to use wooden chopsticks.

Lightning is a form of direct electrical current that kills approximately one hundred people each year in the US. Lightning injuries can be avoided by leaving the area or seeking shelter when a storm approaches.

## Conclusions

Although burns constitute a small number of casualties, they consume a disproportionate amount of resources and require specialized care. More importantly, burns are traumatic injuries with potentially chronic and devastating physical, mental and social sequelae, which occur in individuals who are less able to protect and care for themselves, such as children, the elderly or people under the effect of drugs or who have mental health concerns.

The vast majority of burns occur in the developing world, who do not have the same resources to care for these burn patients. Further, the victims in those countries are often amongst the poorest and most vulnerable. Most of the advances in burn prevention, care and recovery have been incompletely applied to the developing world. In order to ameliorate that, international support – such as that developed by the WHO (World Health Organization) and ISBI (International Society of Burn Injuries) – is strongly needed.

Burns are preventable and prevention should continue to be as important as proper treatment. Burn prevention campaigns should include active, as well as, passive tools, including education (with a focus on behavioural changes to be truly effective), product safety improvements and legislation. Prevention programmes should be population-specific and address the different risk factors, including age, gender, geography, comorbidities, culture and traditions. More accurate worldwide epidemiologic registries would be helpful in tracking the efficacy of programmes, with a goal of reducing burn injuries to lower levels than exist at currently.

## References

[1] Atiyeh BS, Costagliola M, Hayek SN (2009) Burn prevention mechanisms and outcomes: Pitfalls, failures and successes. Burns 35: 181–193

[2] Al-Quattan MM, Al-Zahrani K (2009) A review of burns related to traditions, social habits, religious activities, festivals and traditioal medicinal practices. Burns 35: 476–481

[3] Prasad Sarma B (2011) Prevention of burns: 13 years' experience in Northeastern India. Burns 37: 257–264

[4] Patil SB, Anil Kahre N, Jaiswal S et al (2010) Changing patterns in electrical burn injuries in a developing country: Should prevention programs focus on the rural population? J Burn Care Res 31: 931–934

[5] Taira BR, Cassara G PA, Meng H et al (2011) Predictors of sustaining burn injury: Does the use of common prevention strategies matter? J Burn Care Res 32: 20–25

[6] Crickelair GF, Dhaliwal AS (1976) The cause and prevention of electrical burns of the mouth in children: A protective cuff. PRS 58(2): 206–209

[7] Rimmer RB, Weigand S, Foster KN et al (2008) Scald burns in young children: A review of Arizona burn center pediatric patients and a proposal for prevention in the Hispanic community. J Burn Care Res 29: 595–605

[8] Kendrick D, Smith S, Sutton AG et al (2009) The effect of education and home safety equipment on childhood thermal injury prevention: meta-analysis and meta-regression. Inj Prev 15: 197–204

[9] Abeyasundara SL, Rajan V, Lam L et al (2011) The changing pattern of pediatric burns. J Burn Care Res 32: 178–184

[10] Parbhoo A, Louw QA, Grimmer-Somers K (2010) Burn prevention programs for children in developing countries require urgent attention: A targeted literature review. Burns 36: 164–175

[11] ABA (2011) Fire and Burn prevention news. March; 6(1): 1–5

[12] Hunt JL, Arnoldo BD, Purdue GF (2007) Prevention of burn injuries. In: Herndon DN (ed) Total burn care. Saunders Elsevier, Galveston, pp 33–39

[13] Light TD, Latenser BA, Heinle JA et al (2009) Jaggery: An avoidable cause of severe, deadly pediatric burns. Burns 35: 430–432

[14] WHO (2008) A WHO plan for burn prevention and care. WHO, Geneva

[15] Roeder RA, Schulman CI (2010) An overview of war-related thermal injuries. J Craniofac Surg 21(4): 971–75

[16] Brusselaers N, Monstrey S, Vogelaers D et al (2010) Severe burn injury in Europe: A systematic review of the incidence, etiology, morbidity and mortality. Crit Care 14: R188

[17] Wisee RPL, Bijlsma WE, Stilma JS (2010) Ocular firework trauma: A systematic review on incidence, severity, outcome and prevention. Br J Ophthalmol 94: 1586–91

[18] Thompson RM, Carrougher GJ (1998) Burn prevention. In: Carrougher GJ (ed) Burn care and therapy. Mosby, St. Louis, pp 497–524

[19] Neaman KC, DO VH, Olenzek EK et al (2010) Outdoor recreational fires: A review of 329 adult and pediatric patients. J Burn Care Res 31: 926–930

Correspondence: A. Arno, M.D., Burn Unit and Plastic Surgery Department, Vall d'Hebron University Hospital, Autonomous University of Barcelona, Passeig de la Vall d'Hebron 119–129, 08035, Barcelona, Spain, E-mail: aiarno@vhebron.net

# Burns associated with wars and disasters

Jonathan B. Lundy, Leopoldo C. Cancio

US Army Institute of Surgical Research, Fort Sam Houston, TX, USA

*Note: The opinions or assertions contained herein are the private views of the authors, and are not to be construed as official or as reflecting the views of the Department of the Army or the Department of Defense.*

## Introduction

Military operations and civilian mass casualty disasters provide among the most difficult scenarios in burn-patient management. At the same time, they historically have also led to changes in care. The purpose of this chapter is to review experience with burn care during current combat operations in Iraq and Afghanistan, and to highlight the lessons learned from a century of major peacetime fire disasters.

## Wartime burns

The historical incidence of thermal injury during conventional (non-nuclear) warfare ranges from 5 to 20 % [1, 2]. As with casualties from fire disasters, approximately 20 % of thermally injured combat casualties have burns of 20 % of the total body surface area (TBSA) or greater [3]. Burns have been responsible for 4 % of overall combat mortality since World War II [4]. During current operations, common causes of thermal injury in military personnel include incendiary devices, improvised explosive devices, or ignition of combustible material in armored personnel carriers or aboard ship [5]. Military personnel are also at risk of non-combat-related burns due to mishandling of munitions or carelessness during burning of waste material [6].

Unlike civilian care, military burn care uniquely requires transport of patients along multiple medical treatment facilities termed "echelons" or "roles"; the capabilities of these facilities increase as the casualty moves further from the battlefield (Table 1). During current operations, U. S. military casualties receive rapid initial care at the point of injury from non-medical personnel who receive additional first-aid training (Combat Lifesavers) and/or from combat medics (U. S. Army Healthcare Specialists, U. S Navy Hospital Corpsmen). These interventions include movement away from the source of thermal/chemical injury, intravenous (IV) or intraosseous line placement, initiation of fluid infusion, and pain management [7, 8]. This emergency, prehospital echelon is referred to as Role I care.

The American Burn Association (ABA) and the American College of Surgeons Committee on Trauma have established criteria for referral of burn patients to a burn center. In general, these criteria should be applied to combat casualties as well, but on the battlefield this may not be immediately possible. Thus, initial burn care to include fluid resuscitation, emergency procedures, and surgical management of concomitant traumatic injuries is currently performed in the Combat Zone by small, austere, highly mobile teams termed Role II-b facilities (U. S. Army Forward Surgical Team, U. S. Navy Forward Resuscitative Surgical System). From there, casualties go to Role III facilities (U. S. Army Combat

**Table 1.** USTRANSCOM guidelines for burn flight team transport of patients during conflict in Iraq and Afghanistan

| |
|---|
| Burns involving 20% or more of the total body surface area |
| Inhalation injury requiring intubation |
| Burn and/or inhalation injury with $PaO_2$-to-$FiO_2$ ratio less than 200 |
| High voltage electrical injury |
| Burns with concomitant traumatic injuries |
| Burn patients with injury/illness severity warranting Burn Flight Team assistance as determined by the attending, validating, or receiving surgeon |

Support Hospital, U. S. Air Force Theater Hospital, U. S. Navy Fleet Hospital or Hospital Ship). This is the first echelon at which definitive surgical care, to include some surgical specialties, is available. Alternatively, many will bypass Role II-b, going directly to Role III facilities. Long-term management of thermally-injured U. S.combat casualties requires evacuation, via a Role IV hospital in Germany, to the continental United States (CONUS). There, most thermally injured casualties are cared for at the U. S. Army Burn Center (U. S. Army Institute of Surgical Research, USAISR), Fort Sam Houston, TX. This Role V center, established in 1949, is the only burn center serving the U. S. Department of Defense [9].

The purpose of this section is to review recent US military experience with care of thermally injured combat casualties, from point of injury to definitive care at the USAISR. Topics pertinent to combat burn care include epidemiology, fluid resuscitation, evacuation, lessons learned from the current major theaters of combat operations (Iraq and Afghanistan), definitive care at the USAISR, and the care of host-nation burn patients.

## Epidemiology of burns sustained during combat operations

Between 2001 and 2008, during Operations Iraqi and Enduring Freedom, a total of 9.3% of all casualties sustained thermal injury, alone or in combination with other injuries of varying severity (Ms. Susan West, Joint Theater Trauma Registry, personal communication, 27 August 2010). A distinguishing feature of these conflicts has been the large number of injuries suffered as a result of improvised explosive devices (IEDs) [6]. These devices can be constructed from almost any material that can house an explosive charge. Kauvar et al. found that of 273 thermally injured U. S. military personnel injured in Iraq and Afghanistan and admitted to the U. S. Army Burn Center between March 2003 and May 2005, 62% were wounded as a direct result of hostile activity [5]. Of these, 52% sustained thermal injury as a result of the ignition of an explosive device. Over 70% of these explosive devices were IEDs or vehicle-borne IEDs. The remaining explosion-related burns were the result of landmines, mortars, or rocket-propelled grenades.

Explosions may cause thermal injury by one of two mechanisms: as a result of contact with the heat generated by the explosion itself (also known as "quaternary blast injury"), or as a result of the ignition of fuel or other combustible materials in close proximity to the explosion. The larger body surface area burns typically include burns to the lower extremities and trunk, and are seen more commonly in casualties confined to a burning vehicle [5, 10]. The smaller burns localized to the face and hands are seen more commonly in casualties injured by the explosion itself [5].

Burns to the hands and face comprise a significant portion of burned casualties. In Kauvar's study, the hands were burned in 80% of patients; the head (predominantly the face) was burned in 77%. Only 15% of casualties had burns isolated to the hands and head; 6% to the hands only. Burns to the hands and face require extensive treatment typically out of proportion to the TBSA burned, which impacts the return to duty rate [5].

Noncombat burns are also common during military operations, accounting for over half of the burns seen during the Vietnam War [10]. Of 102 noncombat burns sustained in the current theaters of operations by May 2005, burning waste (24.5%), ammunition and gunpowder mishaps (20.2%), mishandling of gasoline (17.3%), electrical injuries (8.2%), and scald burns (6.4%) were the leading causes [6]. As demonstrated by Kauvar, combat burns have significantly higher injury severity scores, a higher incidence of other injuries, and a higher incidence of inhalation injury [6]. Despite lower severity, noncombat burns still lead to evacuation of personnel from the theater of operations and a reduction in military readiness. Kauvar noted over 30% of noncombat burned patients and over 40% of combat burned patients were unable to return to full military duty.

Preventive measures may be effective on the battlefield. For example, the use of fire-retardant gloves by tank crew members during the 1982 Israeli war in Lebanon decreased the incidence of hand burns from 75 to 7% in the personnel who sustained burns [11]. Fire-retardant flight suits have been reported to decrease both the incidence and severity of thermal injury suffered after military helicopter accidents [12].

## Fluid resuscitation and initial burn care in theater

Thermal injury results in fluid shifts from the intravascular space into the interstitium in both burned and (in larger burns) unburned tissue. The goal of burn resuscitation is to replace these intravascular volume losses and to prevent end-organ hypoperfusion and damage, at the lowest possible physiologic cost. Fluid resuscitation of burned soldiers may be complicated by problems which are less frequently present in the civilian setting. Inhalation injury increases fluid resuscitation requirements and is present more frequently in combat casualties (up to 15%) [3]. In addition, the burned combat casualty may have multiple traumatic injuries in addition to burns, increasing the volume and complexity of fluid resuscitation. Meanwhile, lack of burn-specific experience on the part of many deployed providers; relatively austere field hospitals; and the diminution in care which necessarily occurs when casualties are placed aboard evacuation aircraft all compound the difficulty of initial resuscitation [3].

Early experience during current combat operations revealed a trend towards over-resuscitation of thermally injured casualties [3, 13]. Over-resuscitation may cause abdominal compartment syndrome, extremity compartment syndrome, pulmonary edema, airway obstruction, and/or progression of wound depth [3, 13, 14]. Together, these complications have been termed "resuscitation morbidity" [15]. As a result, a burn resuscitation guideline was developed and disseminated to all U. S. medical treatment facilities in theater [13]. The guidelines included a 24-hour burn resuscitation flow sheet (Fig. 1), as well as recommendations for the man-

agement of casualties with difficult burn resuscitations. After the implementation of the guideline, US casualties experienced a significant decrease in the combined endpoint of abdominal compartment syndrome and mortality [13].

Other steps taken by the USAISR to improve care of the burned casualty on the battlefield include predeployment training of providers in wartime burn care, the deployment of a burn surgeon to augment the busiest Combat Support Hospital in theater, and a weekly theater-wide video teleconference to communicate patient outcomes and provide feedback [3, 16]. A burn Clinical Practice Guideline was published on the Internet and includes instructions on the management of the difficult resuscitation, indications for and technique of escharotomy, initial wound care, and USAISR contact information.

The USAISR pioneered the modified Brooke formula for fluid resuscitation, which predicts the fluid requirements for the first 24 hours postburn as lactated Ringer's solution, 2 ml/kg/percent TBSA burned, with half of this volume programmed for delivery over the first 8 hours and half over the following 16 hours. Chung et al., in an attempt to simplify fluid resuscitation rate calculations for adults, developed the ISR Rule of 10s [17]. This rule initiates fluid resuscitation at a rate in ml/hr equal to TBSA X 10 for patients weighing 40 to 80 kg. For every 10 kg above 80, the intial fluid rate is increased by 100 ml/hr. Regardless of how the initial fluid infusion rate is determined, it must be adjusted during the first 48 hours postburn based on the patient's physiologic response. The primary index of the adequacy of fluid resuscitation is a target urine output of 30–50 ml/hr in adults. The lactated Ringer's rate is adjusted up or down by roughly 25% increments every hour or two to achieve this target.

Children weighing less than 40 kg cannot be resuscitated using the Rule of Tens. Rather, a weight-based formula such as the modified Brooke formula must be used. The target urine output for children is approximately 1–2 ml/kg/hr, and the lactated Ringer's infusion rate is adjusted up or down in order to achieve this target. To prevent hypoglycemia, *additional* glucose-containing fluids (such as D5W in ½ normal saline) must be given to children at a constant, maintenance rate which is not adjusted.

**JTTS Burn Resuscitation Flow Sheet**  Page 1

Date:

Initial Treatment Facility:

| Name | SSN | Pre-burn Est. Wt (kg) | %TBSA | Estimated fluid vol. pat. should receive | | |
|------|-----|------------------------|-------|-------------|-------------|----------------|
| | | | | 1st 8 hrs | 2nd 16th hrs | Est. Total 24 hrs |

Date & Time of Inury

BAMC/ISR Burn Team DSN 312-429-2876

| Tx Site/ Team | HR from burn | Local Time | Crystalloid (ml) Colloid | TOTAL | UOP | Base Deficit | BP | MAP (>55)/ CVP | Pressors (Vasopressin) 0.04 u/min) |
|---|---|---|---|---|---|---|---|---|---|
| 1st | | | | | | | | | |
| 2nd | | | | | | | | | |
| 3rd | | | | | | | | | |
| 4th | | | | | | | | | |
| 5th | | | | | | | | | |
| 6th | | | | | | | | | |
| 7th | | | | | | | | | |
| 8th | | | | | | | | | |
| Total Fluids 1st 8 hrs: | | | | | | | | | |
| 9th | | | | | | | | | |
| 10th | | | | | | | | | |
| 11th | | | | | | | | | |
| 12th | | | | | | | | | |
| 13th | | | | | | | | | |
| 14th | | | | | | | | | |
| 15th | | | | | | | | | |
| 16th | | | | | | | | | |
| 17th | | | | | | | | | |
| 18th | | | | | | | | | |
| 19th | | | | | | | | | |
| 20th | | | | | | | | | |
| 21st | | | | | | | | | |
| 22nd | | | | | | | | | |
| 23rd | | | | | | | | | |
| 24th | | | | | | | | | |
| 24 hr Total Fluids: | | | | | | | | | |

**Fig. 1.** Flow sheet used in theater for documentation of burn resuscitation

Initial burn wound care in the combat zone includes debridement and dressing of burn wounds in the operating room under sterile conditions. This is typically carried out at a level III facility. US military level II and III facilities have wound-care materials to include mafenide acetate, silver sulfadiazine, and silver-impregnated dressings [18]. Classically, burn wounds are treated at the USAISR by alternating mafenide acetate cream in the morning, with silver sulfadiazine cream in the evening. During transport, silver-impregnated dressings offer the advantage of less frequent wound care, but this supposes that the wounds are clean and that burned extremities are well perfused, thus decreasing the need for frequent dressing changes and wound inspection.

Escharotomies are performed during initial wound debridement, or later during resuscitation when indicated. The usual indication for escharoto-my of an extremity is the loss or progressive diminution of arterial pulsatile flow as determined by Doppler flowmetry. In the deployed setting, it may be prudent to perform escharotomies in patients with large burn size and circumferential (or nearly so) full-thickness burns of an extremity, since monitoring in flight is nearly impossible. This concern should be balanced by the need to obtain good hemostasis before flight, and the potential for escharotomy sites to bleed in flight.

### Evacuation of thermally-injured combat casualties

During the Vietnam war, thermally injured military personnel were evacuated to Camp Zama, Japan and remained at that facility for variable amounts of time (up to several weeks) before evacuation to the U. S. [19–22]. Injuries sustained during current operations have been evacuated more rapidly. Due to the urban environment in Iraq, evacuation times to a Role III Combat Support Hospital are typically less than 60 minutes. In Afghanistan, due to rural operations and difficult terrain, casualties may not arrive at a Combat Support Hospital for up to 4 hours after injury. Evacuation out of the theater of operations to a Role IV hospital takes about 8 hours, and is carried out by a US Air Force Air Evacuation (AE) crew for stable patients, or by an AE crew augmented by a US Air Force Critical Care Air Transport Team (CCATT) for critically ill patients. Landstuhl Regional Medical Center (LRMC) is the Role IV hospital in Germany which supports casualties arriving from both Iraq and Afghanistan. The flight from LRMC to CONUS requires an AE crew, often augmented by a CCATT or by the USAISR Burn Flight Team. The flight from LRMC to the USAISR is over 5,300 miles (8,600 km) and takes approximately 12 to 13 hours [23]. In sum, it is now feasible for a severely burned casualty to arrive at the Army Burn Center within 3–4 days of injury on the battlefield.

The USAISR Burn Flight Team pioneered the air evacuation/transportation of critically ill burn patients in 1951 [21, 22]. The guidelines for Burn Flight Team utilization are listed in Table 1 [23]. The highly specialized BFT crews are equipped and experienced in the management of severely burned, critically-ill casualties and are ideally suited to evacuate multiple casualties during a single mission (Fig. 2). Flights staffed by Burn Flight Teams have carried as many as 13 burned casualties on a single mission during the current conflicts [23]. Burn Flight Teams bring specialized equipment to perform emergency procedures en route such as fiberoptic bronchoscopy, escharotomy, fasciotomy, resuscitation, management of septic shock, decompressive laparotomy, emergency airway procedures, and tube thoracostomy.

Renz et al. conducted a retrospective analysis of the evacuation of war-related burn casualties that were treated at the USAISR [23]. The study encompassed a four-year period from March 2003 to February 2007 and included 540 burned US military casualties. The mean TBSA involved was 16.7% (range 0.1 to 95%) and 342 (63.3%) of casualties were burned as a result of an explosion. During the flight from LRMC to the USAISR, 160 (29.6%) burned casualties required only AE crews; CCATT augmented AE crews

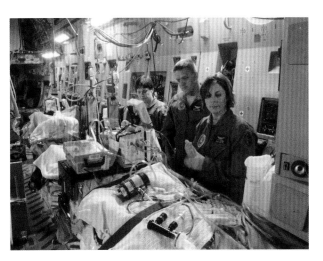

**Fig. 2.** U.S. Army Burn Flight Team members providing en route critical care to multiple thermally injured casualties

in the care of 174 (32.2%); and the Burn Flight Team cared for 206 (38.1%). Mean transit time for stable patients evacuated by AE crews was 7 days, and transit time for casualties evacuated by CCATT and Burn Flight Teams was less than 4 days [23].

Such rapid evacuation of patients with severe thermal injury carries both risks and benefits. The most notable risk is the inevitable degradation in care that occurs aboard the aircraft, despite the presence of CCATT or Burn Flight Teams. This is particularly important during the first 24 hours postburn, during which rapidly evolving burn shock may make fluid resuscitation difficult even in a U. S. burn center. The most notable benefits are the ability to complete excision and grafting of the burn wound within days of injury, and to place the patient in the burn center before complications such as pneumonia make transport more hazardous. Consideration of these risks and benefits argues in favor of a rather small "window" between hours 24 and 48, during which burn patient evacuation off the battlefield is ideally accomplished.

### Definitive management of burned casualties at USAISR

The management of thermally injured combat casualties follows standard principles of burn care. When possible, early burn wound excision (within the first 5–7 days of injury) with application of autograft is performed to close wounds. Cadaver allograft is used for temporary closure of excised burn wounds when adequate autograft is not available. In Chapman's review of long-term outcomes after combat-related burns, out of 285 combat-related burn patients, 35 % had an associated traumatic injury [24]. Fractures, large soft tissue defects, and traumatic amputations are some of the more common injuries. These associated injuries make definitive wound closure challenging, increase the open surface area at risk for infection, and complicate long-term rehabilitation.

Military burn casualties remain inpatients at the USAISR Burn Center until all wounds are closed, inpatient rehabilitation needs are met, and nonmedical attendants (typically family members) have been educated in wound care and activities of daily living. Military personnel are then assigned to the Fort Sam Houston Warrior Transition Unit and discharged to local housing. Many blast-injured casualties suffer traumatic amputations and require fitting and rehabilitation with extremity prostheses. The newly constructed Center for the Intrepid provides a state-of-the-art amputee rehabilitation center for these personnel.

Wolf et al. reviewed the outcomes of burned combatants and civilians treated at the USAISR between April 2003 and May 2005 [15]. The authors hypothesized that due to the delays in evacuation and associated traumatic injuries, outcomes would be worse for the military burned casualties. Of 751 total patients cared for at the USAISR during the period studied, 273 were military personnel. Overall, the mortality of the US military personnel sustaining burns in the combat theaters was no different from locally evacuated civilians. Of the 285 patients in Chapman's return to duty study mentioned above, 190 patients were categorized as having returned to duty [24]. A total of 95 burned military casualties were medically discharged. Patients who were medically discharged had larger TBSA and full thickness burn size, more frequently suffered inhalation injury and associated traumatic injuries, and had a higher injury severity score [24]. An earlier study by Kauvar et al. noted that 10 % (n=13) of military burn casualties that were able to return to duty required limitations due to their injuries [5].

## Care of host-nation burn patients

One challenging aspect of military medical care in the deployed setting is the care of host-nation casualties. Host-nation civilians and military personnel during wartime are frequently evacuated to US military medical treatment facilities on the battlefield. The impetus for caring for these patients at US facilities stems from several sources. Article 56 of the 4th Geneva Convention of 1949 states that "the Occupying Power has the duty of ensuring and maintaining, with the cooperation of national and local authorities, the medical and hospital establishments and services, public health and hygiene in the occupied territory." Similarly, U. S. Army FM 8–10–14, *Employment of the Combat Support Hospital,* states that "Only urgent medical reasons will determine priority in the order of treatment to be administered. This means that wounded enemy soldiers may be treated before wounded Americans or allies (…) Civilians who are wounded or become sick as a result of military operations will be collected and provided initial medical treatment in accordance with theater policies and transferred to appropriate civilian authorities as soon as possible." In practice, this means that host-nation patients presenting to U. S. forces with life-, limb-, or eyesight-threatening injuries have received initial care at U. S. medical treatment facilities.

Whereas resuscitation and lifesaving surgery might conceivably be completed within roughly two days of injury for patients with non-thermal injuries, in the case of burn patients the threat to life continues until the wounds are fully closed. Evacuation out of the combat zone (i. e., evacuation to echelons higher than Role III hospitals) has not been available to host-nation patients. Furthermore, host-nation facilities on the current battlefield, whether in Iraq or in Afghanistan, have not been equipped to provide burn care comparable to that available in U. S. Role III hospitals. This constellation of factors–the Geneva Convention moral imperative, the duration of the threat to life caused by thermal injury, and the discrepancy between U. S. and local capabilities–has made the disposition of host-nation burn patients problematic, and motivated U. S. Role III hospitals to provide definitive care. It would be incorrect to conclude that Role III hospitals were capable of providing the same level of care as a burn center in the U. S., however. Lack of experience on the part of many providers, absence of multidisciplinary burn team members, limitations with respect to supplies, equipment, and physical plant, and patient-related factors such as delays in presentation heightened the challenge.

Because burn patient care is very costly with respect to supplies, manpower, and length of stay, and because bed space is limited at Role III facilities, it was necessary to expedite such treatment. Several techniques evolved over time to accomplish this. Patients with burns of up to 50–60 % TBSA received definitive care at Role III hospitals. It became apparent that surgical care of patients with larger burns was futile; these patients were therefore triaged to comfort care. Excision and grafting of burns was performed at Role III hospitals within a day or two of admission (Fig. 3). Negative-pressure wound therapy (Vacuum-Assisted Closure) was frequently used to speed up engraftment or to help prepare wound beds for grafting. Topical wound therapies, such as artificial skin (Biobrane), silver-impregnated dressings (Silverlon; others), and gamma-irradiated homograft (Gammagraft) were used as appropriate. A small number of burned children were flown out of theater on commercial airlines by civilian charities for care at Shriners Institutes for Burned Children in the U. S. (Fig. 4) [25]. From these events, we can conclude that burn care, to include *definitive care of civilians of all ages* with major thermal injuries, is part of the usual workload of Role III hospitals on the modern battlefield; that these hospitals should have the supplies and equipment needed to provide definitive care to these patients; and that personnel should obtain experience with definitive burn care before deploying.

## Disaster-related burns

Mass casualties as a result of fire have occurred with some regularity in the US since the country was founded. The first large-scale fire occurred at Jamestown, Virginia in May 1607, decimating the colony [26, 27]. Worldwide, catastrophic fires have punctuated history due to their social and political implications. A recent development in the latter half of the twentieth century and specifically in the last two

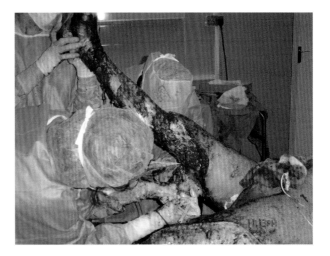

**Fig. 3.** Excision to fascia of infected lower extremity burns in an Iraqi male at the Combat Support Hospital (CSH) in Baghdad. Patient was transferred from a local facility 10 days after injury by an improvised explosive device (IED), and was successfully excised and grafted on day of admission to CSH

decades is the emergence of terrorism as a cause of mass casualty burns. Burn disasters are challenging because (1) burn victims are extremely resource- and time-intensive in their care needs and (2) burn expertise is normally concentrated in specialized centers, but local hospitals with no experience in the care of burns may be required to provide care of casualties for hours or days following a disaster.

Burn mass casualty incidents have provided unique opportunities for health care providers to

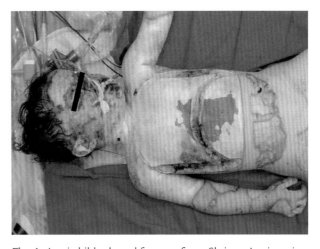

**Fig. 4.** Iraqi child selected for transfer to Shriners Institute in Boston, MA. Despite extensive full-thickness burns, patient was extubated and transitioned to oral medications before commercial flight

review the treatment of these patients and to develop improvements in care. An excellent example of this is the Cocoanut Grove nightclub fire that occurred in Boston, MA in 1942. As a result of the attack on Pearl Harbor in 1941 (where half of the casualties were burned), the Massachusetts General Hospital and Boston City Hospital were conducting research in burn care and had already developed guidelines for disaster preparedness which included the development of a blood bank, publication of a disaster manual, and accumulation of sterile supplies for multiple simultaneous operations [28]. The physicians that cared for victims of the Cocoanut Grove fire paved the way for the future management of burn victims [28]. More recently, since the terrorist attacks on the World Trade Center on 11 September 2001 in New York City and the bombing in Bali on 12 October 2002, awareness has increased regarding the importance of disaster preparedness. The purpose of this section is to outline the epidemiology of burns suffered by victims of mass casualty events, review techniques for triage, prehospital care, acute management and resuscitation, and other principles of care of multiple burn victims by burn centers.

## Epidemiology

Barillo performed a thorough review of historic US fire catastrophes during the twentieth century [9]. The largest number of significant fires were classified as "residential" and included fires in hotels, nursing homes, jails, and hospitals [9]. Fatally injured casualties from burn disasters typically die at the scene, during transport to a local hospital, or shortly after arrival to the hospital [30–39]. For example, the Iroquois Theater fire of 1903 in Chicago resulted in 602 deaths with a list of 571 fatalities published in the Chicago Tribune by the morning after the fire [30]. The Cocoanut Grove fire death toll was 492. Three hours after the fire occurred, the city mortuary had accounted for over 400 bodies in morgues around the city [31]. More recently, the 1990 Happy Land Social Club fire in Bronx, New York resulted in 87 deaths all identified at the scene, and the 1991 Imperial Foods plant disaster in Hamlet, North Carolina resulted in 25 deaths with 24 pronounced at the scene [32, 33]. The Station Nightclub fire in Warwick, Rhode

Island in 2003 occurred in a 1950s-era building that was not equipped with sprinklers when it ignited as a result of pyrotechnics during a concert [38]. Of the 439 people inside at the time of the fire, 96 people died at the scene and only an additional 4 died in surrounding area hospitals in the weeks following the incident. The Rhode Island hospital evaluated a total of 64 patients in their emergency department, admitting 47 to a converted trauma ward. A total of 28 of the 47 admitted had inhalation injury. 33 had less than 20% TBSA burns, 12 patients had burns of between 21 and 40%, and two had burns of 40% TBSA. The predominance of early deaths in indoor fire disasters points to the importance of asphyxia (hypoxia and inhalation of toxic gases) and upper airway injury.

By contrast, the Ringling Brothers Circus in 1944 at Hartford, Connecticut led to a predominance of fatalities due to severe burns from the heavy canvas that was engulfed by flames and fell onto the crowd [36]. The canvas had been coated with paraffin dissolved in gasoline to make it waterproof. The open air tent resulted in only a few patients suffering inhalation injury [37]. In Arturson's review, fires due to indoor disasters tend to cause smaller TBSA burns in survivors than casualties burned in outdoor catastrophic fires [40]. Experts suggest that in disaster-related fires, 80% of survivors will sustain burns of 20% or less of the TBSA [41].

Medical response at the scene of the attack on the World Trade Center towers on 11 September 2001 was complicated by the fact that both towers collapsed, making evacuation and survival the primary mission of first responders [43–45]. Had the towers not collapsed, many more thermally injured casualties may have survived and needed treatment at burn centers [46–48]. A total of 39 casualties sustained burns that required treatment. The New York-Presbyterian Weill Cornell Center, with a total burn bed capacity of 40, received 18 patients by the 27th hour after the disaster [48]. Nine were transferred directly from the scene and an additional nine were transferred from surrounding hospitals. The mean TBSA burned at that burn center was 52 +/– 7% (range 14 to 100%). Eight of the patients sustained burns involving more than 60% of the TBSA. Inhalation injury complicated the injuries of 14 patients admitted to the burn center.

The terrorist attack on a nightclub in Bali, Indonesia on 12 October 2002 resulted in the single largest loss of civilian life in Australia's history [49]. The disaster caused more than 200 fatalities at the scene. The burn center at the Repatriation General Hospital in Concord, Sydney received a total of 12 burn victims, 11 of them evacuated within 54 to 69 hours of the incident. The TBSA involvement ranged between 15 and 85%, mostly full thickness in depth.

## Treatment of disaster-related burns

### Prehospital

The scene of a burn catastrophe is best described as chaotic in the moments after the incident. In Arturson's review of the San Juanico, Mexico liquid petroleum gas explosion in 1984, the author notes that no evacuation plan was in place to remove casualties from the scene [50]. Poor evacuation management affects outcomes, evidenced by the analysis of the petroleum gas tanker truck explosion in Los Alfaques, Spain in 1978 [51]. The incident caused a highway blockage, presenting two evacuation routes for patients needing further care. The group of 82 patients that was transported south had no en route medical care, traveled 150 km, and had a survival rate of 43%. The 58 patients taken via the north evacuation route were provided care en route and experienced a 93% survival rate. A lack of field triage after the 1970 Osaka, Japan gas line explosion resulted in misutilization of hospital-based physicians [52]. Central to most recent US burn disasters has been the establishment of an onsite triage center. This is accomplished by both insightful on-scene responders as well as local emergency medical responders. After the MGM Grand Hotel fire in Las Vegas, Nevada in 1980, over 3000 patients were triaged on the scene, allowing for evacuation of only 726 patients to hospitals and movement of 1700 minimally injured casualties to an off-site treatment center [52]. In order to prevent overwhelming of the regional burn center that will provide care for victims of a burn catastrophe, care should be provided on or close to the scene to both minimally injured victims as well as casualties suffering non-survivable injuries [54]. Some have suggested that on site presence of a burn surgeon may facilitate triage of victims so that resources are optimized at receiving hospitals [39].

Guidance for initial triage of burned victims is different during a mass casualty situation. The lethality of a burn differs based on age and TBSA involved. The lethal area fifty percent ($L_A50$) for a young adult is 80% [29]. This means that of young adults suffering 80% TBSA burns, half of the patients receiving care at a US burn center can be expected to survive. During a burn disaster, providers performing triage may be required to triage patients in this age group with burns over 80% TBSA into the expectant category. The presence of inhalation injury, concomitant traumatic injuries, and advanced age decrease the $L_A50$. The ABA has published an age/TBSA survival grid that can be used to guide on-scene providers triaging burn victims (Fig. 5) [42]. This grid should only be used in the setting of a burn catastrophe, however. Ultimately, the burn center's outpatient clinic will be responsible for the long-term wound care and rehabilitative needs of minimally burned victims not needing inpatient treatment.

A three-level method can be used for on-scene triage in catastrophic fires [29]. Level 1 includes sorting patients as acute or non-acute. Level 2 triage categorizes patients into immediate, delayed, minimal, and expectant. Level 3 triage sorts based on priority of evacuation. If a burn provider is not available on the scene of a fire, burn triage should occur before casualties enter the emergency department as to not overwhelm the facility with patients, most of whom will need outpatient care. Following catastrophic fires, "secondary triage" may be necessary in hospital to select patients for transfer to hospitals distant from the admitting burn facility [55].

International support is another way to enhance a region's ability to care for mass casualty survivors. After the café fire in Volendam, Netherlands in 2001, 182 burn victims required hospital admission [58]. Due to the overwhelming number of acutely ill burn victims, some patients were transferred to burn centers in Belgium and Germany. The USAISR Burn Flight Team has assisted in several international burn disasters since its inception in 1951 [16]. Days after the Bashkirian gas pipeline explosion in 1989, 17 personnel from the USAISR arrived in Ufa, Russia and assisted with excision and autografting of burn wounds and rehabilitation [57].

# Appendix

## Age/TBSA Survival Grid

Provided by Jeffrey R. Saffle, MD
Director, Intermountain Burn Center
Salt Lake City, UT

CAVEAT: This grid is intended only for mass burn casualty disasters where responders are overwhelmed and transfer possibilities are insufficient to meet needs.

**This table is based on national data on survival and length of stay.**

Triage Decision Table of Benefit-to-Resource Ratio based on Patient Age and Total Burn Size

Burn Size (%TBSA)

| Age/ years | 0 – 10% | 11-20% | 21-30% | 31-40% | 41-50% | 51-60% | 61-70% | 71-80% | 81-90% | 91+% |
|---|---|---|---|---|---|---|---|---|---|---|
| 0-1.99 | High | High | Medium | Medium | Medium | Medium | Low | Low | Low | Expectant |
| 2-4.99 | Outpatient | High | High | Medium | Medium | Medium | Medium | Low | Low | Low |
| 5-19.9 | Outpatient | High | High | High | Medium | Medium | Medium | Medium | Medium | Low |
| 20-29.9 | Outpatient | High | High | High | Medium | Medium | Medium | Medium | Low | Low |
| 30-39.9 | Outpatient | High | High | Medium | Medium | Medium | Medium | Medium | Low | Low |
| 40-49.9 | Outpatient | High | High | Medium | Medium | Medium | Medium | Low | Low | Low |
| 50-59.9 | Outpatient | High | High | Medium | Medium | Medium | Low | Low | Expectant | Expectant |
| 60-69.9 | High | High | Medium | Medium | Medium | Low | Low | Low | Expectant | Expectant |
| 70+ | High | Medium | Medium | Low | Low | Expectant | Expectant | Expectant | Expectant | Expectant |

**Fig. 5.** American Burn Association age/survival grid for triage during burn disasters resulting in multiple casualtiest

Expansion of both hospital personnel and bed space is necessary. After the Station nightclub fire, physicians from the Rhode Island Hospital fortunately began receiving casualties during a shift change when two sets of staff were in house and available [38]. The trauma ward was cleared of inpatients, and burn bed capacity was increased by utilizing extra suction and oxygen mounts already present in the trauma ward rooms. This allowed rapid expansion and enabled admission of a large number of burn casualties. Bedside paper charting may be more efficient than complex computer-based charting, especially if outside providers are brought in to assist [22]. Delegation of care can be performed, such that a burn surgeon and senior burn nurse provide oversight and managerial support and non-burn providers carry out daily care to include wound care, pain management, resuscitation, and rehabilitation [29]. The stress on the hospital staff must be alleviated by implementation of a rotation schedule, a meal service, and a counseling program [59]. Supply and equipment lists should be generated including standard and portable mechanical ventilators, monitoring devices, resuscitative equipment, surgical supplies, wound-care items, and rehabilitation equipment [29]. Harrington et al. reported that established protocols for burn care (e. g. resuscitation, wound care, ventilator management, donor site care, rehabilitation) streamlined the management of multiple burn patients and allowed for inexperienced providers to manage casualties effectively [38]. Yurt et al. noted that surgical management of multiple burn victims requires early and frequent coordination to maintain a smooth flow of patients into and out of the operating room [46].

## Command and control, communication

The city, region, state, and nation should have established plans for disaster management. These plans should be enacted early after a catastrophe and should dictate a means and location for triage, a command center, evacuation plans for casualties, the roles of hospitals in the area, and means of communication. Redundant methods of communication should link all of the above sites [29]. Communication should be maintained between the local burn center and neighboring and national burn centers to coordinate for evacuation and discuss bed availability. Current methods of communication that may be helpful include satellite telephones, international cellular phone, and Internet access. In any given disaster, some of these resources may not be functional.

## The American Burn Association (ABA) disaster management plan

Burn care delivered by a burn center remains the optimal treatment plan for any burn victim including victims injured in a mass casualty incident. Currently, the US has 123 burn centers, 56 of which are ABA verified, and approximately 1793 burn beds nationwide [60]. Burn centers are recognized by the US Department of Health and Human Services in legislation outlining the federal response to terrorist acts [42]. Any event that results in more burned victims than the local burn center is organized to manage is defined as a mass casualty burn disaster. Triage from the scene should result in arrival of burn victims from a burn catastrophe within 24 hours of the incident. Under the ABA disaster management plan, each burn center has a defined "surge capacity", defined as the ability to handle up to 50 % more patients than the maximum number normally listed as capacity. Once surge capacity is reached, individual burn directors should begin triage of burn victims to burn centers with available beds, ideally centers that are ABA verified. This should occur within the first 48 hours after the disaster.

The US disaster response system is tiered so that limits are placed on federal involvement in local affairs during and after a disaster. The levels of response include a local and state response, followed by a civilian Federal response, and finally Military Support to Civil Authorities. The National Disaster Medical System (NDMS), now part of the Department of Health and Human Services (DHHS), is charged with coordinating medical care during Federal disaster response. NDMS functions include medical response to the site, movement of victims from the site to unaffected areas, and assistance with definitive medical care in unaffected areas. An essential component of NDMS's medical response to the disaster site is Disaster Medical Assistance Teams (DMATs). DMATs are sponsored by a local major medical center, are comprised of 35 personnel each to include physicians, nurses, and administrative staff, and are tasked with providing care during a disaster. In addition, there are 4 Burn Specialty Teams (BSTs) whose role is to augment local capabilities in burn care in the event of a disaster [42]. BSTs provide assistance with acute management to include resuscitation as well as directing triage and transfer of burn victims [42]. The final tier in the national disaster plan incorporates the use of Military Support for Civil Authorities.

## Summary

Military operations and civilian mass casualty disasters confront providers with both tragedy and with the potential for strengthening the scientific and organizational foundation of burn care. Table 2 provides a list of advances that occurred following some of the major wars and fire disasters of the last 100 years. These advances were possible not only because of the galvanizing effect of the events, but also because committed multidisciplinary team members worked together to care for patients, to learn from their experiences, and to document those experiences in a disciplined fashion.

**Table 2.** Relationship between wars or disasters and advances in burn care

| Event | Date | Examples of Advances Made | References |
|---|---|---|---|
| Rialto Theater Fire | 1921 | Concept of burn shock as plasma loss | Underhill [61] |
| Battle of Britain | 1940 | Burn reconstruction techniques | Mayhew [62] |
| Pearl Harbor | 1941 | U. S. government burn research program | Lockwood [63] |
| Cocoanut Grove Nightclub fire | 1942 | Fluid resuscitation formulas; comprehensive description of care; fire code changes | Cope and Moore [64] Saffle [65] |
| Cold War | 1949 | U. S. Army Burn Center | Artz [66] |
| Vietnam War | 1966 –72 | Topical antimicrobial therapies; metabolic support | Moreau et al. [67] Pruitt et al. [68] Wilmore et al. [69] |
| Gulf War | 1990 –91 | National collaboration for burn bed reporting in U. S. | Shirani et al. [70] |
| World Trade Center and Pentagon attacks | 2001 | Improved regional disaster response plans | Yurt et al. [46] |
| Iraq and Afghanistan Wars | 2001 – present | Rapid aeromedical evacuation; ABA-DOD multicenter research collaboration | Renz [23] |

ABA, American Burn Association; DOD, Department of Defense.

## References

[1] Cancio LC, Horvath EE, Barillo DJ et al (2005) Burn support for Operation Iraqi Freedom and related operations, 2003–2004. J Burn Care Rehabil 26: 151–161

[2] Champion HR, Bellamy RF, Roberts CP, Leppaniemi A (2003) A profile of combat injury. J Trauma 54[Suppl]: S13–19

[3] Chung KK, Blackbourne LH, Wolf SE et al (2006) Evolution of burn resuscitation in Operation Iraqi Freedom. J Burn Care Res 27: 606–611

[4] Thomas SJ, Kramer GC, Herndon DN (2003) Burns: military options and tactical solutions. J Trauma 54[Suppl]: S207–218

[5] Kauvar DS, Wolf SE, Wade CE et al (2006) Burns sustained in combat explosions in Operations Iraqi and Enduring Freedom (OIF/OEF explosion burns). Burns 32: 853–857

[6] Kauvar DS, Cancio LC, Wolf SE et al (2006) Comparison of combat and non-combat burns from ongoing US military operations. J Surg Res 132: 195–200

[7] Black IH, McManus J (2009) Pain management in current combat operations. Prehosp Emerg Care 13: 223–227

[8] Tactical Combat Casualty Care Guidelines, November2009, accessed from Military Health Systems website, http://www.health. mil/Education_And_Training/ TCCC. aspx, 26 August 2010

[9] Barillo DJ, Wolf SE (2006) Planning for burn disasters: lessons learned from one hundred years of history. J Burn Care Res 27: 622–634

[10] Allen BD, Whitson TC, Henjyoji EY (1970) Treatment of 1963 burned patients at 106th general hospital, Yokohama, Japan. J Trauma 10: 386–392

[11] Eldad A, Torem M (1990) Burns in the Lebanon War 1982: "the blow and the cure". Mil Med 155: 130–132

[12] Voisine JJ, Albano JP (1996) Reduction and mitigation of thermal injuries: what can be done? Mil Med 161: 54–57

[13] Ennis JL, Chung KK, Renz EM et al (2008) Joint theater trauma system implementation of burn resuscitation guidelines improves outcomes in severely burned military casualties. J Trauma 64[Suppl]: S146-152

[14] Markell KW, Renz EM, White CE et al (2009) Abdominal complications after severe burns. J Am Coll Surg 208: 940–947

[15] Wolf SE, Kauvar DS, Wade CE et al (2006) Comparison between civilian burns and combat burns from Operation Iraqi Freedom and Operation Enduring Freedom. Ann Surg 243: 786–795

[16] Barillo DJ, Cancio LC, Hutton BG et al (2005) Combat burn life support: a military burn-education program. J Burn Care Rehabil 26: 162–165

[17] Chung KK, Salinas J, Renz EM et al (2010) Simple derivation of the initial fluid rate for the resuscitation of severely burned adult combat casualties: in silico validation of the rule of 10. J Trauma 69[Suppl]: S49-54

[18] D'Avignon LC, Saffle JR, Chung KK, Cancio LC (2008) Prevention and management of infections associated

with burns in combat casualty. J Trauma 64[Suppl]: S277–286

[19] Anonymous (1967-1972) Annual Research Progress Reports. Fort Sam Houston, TX: US Army Institute of Surgical Research

[20] Grissom TE, Farmer JC (2005) The provision of sophisticated critical care beyond the hospital. Crit Care Med 33[Suppl]: S13–21

[21] Kirksey TD, Dowling JA, Pruitt BA Jr et al (1968) Safe expeditious transport of the seriously burned patient. Arch Surg 96: 790–794

[22] Treat RC, Sirinek KR, Levine BA et al (1980) Air evacuation of thermally injured patients: principles of treatment and results. J Trauma 20: 275–279

[23] Renz EM, Cancio LC, Barillo BJ et al (2008) Long range transport of war-related burn casualties. J Trauma 64[Suppl]: S136–145

[24] Chapman TT, Richard RL, Hedman TL et al (2008) Military return to duty and civilian return to work factors following burns with focus on the hand and literature review. J Burn Care Res 29: 756–762

[25] Lundy JB, Swift CB, McFarland CC et al (2010) A descriptive analysis of patients admitted to the intensive care unit of the 10th combat support hospital deployed in Ibn Sina, Iraq from October 19, 2005 to October 19, 2006. J Intensive Care Med 25: 156–162

[26] Smith D (1978) History of firefighting in America. Dial Press, New York

[27] Goodman EC (2001) Fire! The 100 most devastating fires and the heroes who fought them. Black Dog and Leventhal Publishers, New York

[28] Follett GP (1943) The Boston fire: a challenge to our disaster service. Am J Nurs 43: 4–8

[29] Cancio LC, Pruitt BA (2005) Management of mass casualty burn disasters. Int J Disaster Medicine 2005;1–16

[30] Cowan D (2001) Great Chicago fires: historic blazes that shaped a city. Lake Claremont Press, Chicago

[31] Moulton RS (1962) The Cocoanut Grove fire. National Fire Protection Association, Boston

[32] National Fire Protection Association (1990) Fire investigations: nursing home fire, Norfolk, VA, October 5, 1989. National Fire Protection Association, Quincy, MA

[33] Klem TJ (1992) 25 die in food plant fire. NFPA J 86: 29–35

[34] Finland M, Davidson CS, Levenson SM (1946) Clinical and therapeutic aspects of the conflagration injuries in the respiratory tract sustained by victims of the Cocoanut Grove disaster. Medicine 25: 215–283

[35] Schorow S (2005) The Cocoanut Grove fire. Commonwealth Editions, Beverly, MA

[36] Kimball WY (1944) Hartford city holocaust. NFPA Q 1944;9–21

[37] O'nan S (2000) The circus fire. Anchor Books, New York

[38] Harrington DT, Biffl WL, Cioffi WG (2005) The Station nightclub fire. J Burn Care Rehabil 26: 141–143

[39] Mackie DP, Koning HM (1990) Fate of mass burn casualties: implications for disaster planning. Burns 16: 203–206

[40] Arturson G (1992) Analysis of severe fire disasters. In: Masselis M, Gunn SWA (eds) The management of mass burn casualties and fire disasters: Proceedings of the First International Conference on Burns and Fire Disasters. Kluwer Academic, Dordrecht, The Netherlands, pp 24–33

[41] Pruitt BA Jr (2001) Aeromedical transport and field care of burn patients in disaster situations. In: Haberal MA, Bilgin N (eds) Burn and fire disaster in the Middle East. Haberal Education and Research Foundation, Ankara, Turkey, pp 229–243

[42] ABA Board of Trustees (2005) Committee on Organization and Delivery of Burn Care. Disaster management and the ABA plan. J Burn Care Rehabil 26: 102–106

[43] Simon R, Teperman S (2001) The World Trade Center attack: lessons for disaster management. Crit Care 5: 318–320

[44] Asaeda F (2002) The day that the START triage system came to a stop: observations from the World Trade Center disaster. Acad Emerg Med 255–256

[45] Bradt DA (2003) Site management of health issues in the 2001 World Trade Center disaster. Acad Emerg Med 10: 650–660

[46] Yurt RW, Bessey PQ, Bauer GJ et al (2005) A regional burn center's response to a disaster: September 11, 2001, and the days beyond. J Burn Care Rehabil 26: 117–124

[47] Centers for Disease Control and Prevention (2002) Rapid assessment of injuries among survivors of the terrorist attack on the World Trade Center-New York City, September 2001. Morbid Mortal Wkly Rep 51: 1–5

[48] Centers for Disease Control and Prevention (2002) Deaths in World Trade Center terrorist attacks-New York City, 2001. Morbid Mortal Wkly Rep 51: 16–18

[49] Kennedy PJ, Haertsch PA, Maitz PK (2005) The Bali burn disaster: implications and lessons learned. J Burn Care Rehabil 26: 125–131

[50] Arturson G (1987) The tragedy of San Juanico-the most severe LPG disaster in history. Burns 13: 87–102

[51] Arturson G (1981) The Los Alfaques disaster: a boiling liquid, expanding-vapour explosion. Burns 7: 233–251

[52] Ishida T, Ohta M, Sugimoto T (1985) The breakdown of an emergency system following a gas explosion in Osaka and the subsequent resolution of problems. J Emerg Med 2: 183–189

[53] Buerk CA, Batdorf JW, Cammack KV, Ravenholt O (1982) The MGM Grand Hotel fire: lessons learned from a major disaster. Arch Surg 117: 641–644

[54] Sharpe DT, Foo IT (1990) Management of burns in major disasters. Injury 21: 41–44

[55] Wachtel TL, Dimick AR. Burn disaster management. In: Herndon DN (ed) Total burn care. WB Saunders, London, pp 19–31

[56] Shirani KZ, Pruitt BA Jr, Mason AD Jr (1987) The influence of inhalation injury and pneumonia on burn mortatlity. Ann Surg 205: 82–87

[57] Becker WK, Waymack JP, McManus AT et al (1990) Bashkirian train-gas pipeline disaster: the American military response. Burns 16: 325–328

[58] Kuijper EC (2004) The 2003 Everett Idris Evans memorial lecture: every cloud has a silver lining. J Burn Care Rehabil 24: 45–53

[59] Cushman JG, Pachter HL, Beaton HL (2003) Two New York City hospitals' surgical response to the September 11, 2001, terrorist attack in New York City. J Trauma 54: 147–154

[60] American Burn Association website, http://www.ameriburn.org/, accessed 26 August 2010

[61] Underhill FP (1930) The significance of anhydremia in extensive superficial burns. JAMA 95: 852–857

[62] Mayhew ER (2004) The reconstruction of warriors: Archibald McIndoe, the Royal Air Force and the Guinea Pig Club. Greenhill Books, London

[63] Lockwood JS (1946) War-time activities of the National Research Council and the Committee on Medical Research; with particular reference to team-work on studies of wounds and burns. Ann Surg 124: 314–327

[64] Cope O, Moore FD (1947) The redistribution of body water and the fluid therapy of the burned patient. Ann Surg 126: 1010–1045

[65] Saffle JR (1993) The 1942 fire at Boston's Cocoanut Grove nightclub. Am J Surg 166: 581–591

[66] Artz CP (1969) Burns in my lifetime. J Trauma 9: 827–833

[67] Moreau AR, Westfall PH, Cancio LC, Mason AD Jr (2005) Development and validation of an age-risk score for mortality prediction after thermal injury. J Trauma 58: 967–972

[68] Pruitt BA Jr, O'Neill JA Jr, Moncrief JA, Lindberg RB (1968) Successful control of burn-wound sepsis. JAMA 203: 1054–1056

[69] Wilmore DW, Curreri PW, Spitzer KW et al (1971) Supranormal dietary intake in thermally injured hypermetabolic patients. Surg Gynecol Obstet 132: 881–886

[70] Shirani KZ, Becker WK, Rue LW et al (1992) Burn care during Operation Desert Storm. J UW Army Medical Dept PB 8–92–1/2: 37–39

Correspondence: Jonathan B. Lundy, M.D., US Army Institute of Surgical Research, Fort Sam Houston, 78234 Texas, USA, E-mail: Jonathan.lundy1@amedd.army.mil

# Education in burns

Kunaal Jindal, Shahriar Shahrokhi

Ross Tilley Burn Center, Sunnybrook Health Sciences Centre, Department of Surgery, Division of Plastic Surgery, University of Toronto, Toronto, ON, Canada

## Introduction

Education and team building in burn care can be broken down into three main components: surgical education, mentorship, and interprofessional education. This brief chapter will highlight these in order to provide a framework for current trends and the future of education in this field. These ideas are not novel and they have been successfully implemented in other fields. Our goal is to harness this knowledge for implementation in burn care, thus not only improving education, but also enabling recruitment and retention of health care providers in this field.

## Surgical education

### Background

Historically, the traditional method of educating a resident in the practice of surgery has been centered on the hospital-based, apprenticeship model, initially described by William Halsted over 100 years ago [22]. Skill acquisition has been reliant on observation, assisting and subsequently performing the task [6]. This is what many residents have come to understand as the classic "see one, do one, teach one" mentality. Within this template, residents learn principles and gain experience while caring for real patients, and are given increasing amounts of responsibility to prepare them to practice independently. The skills and knowledge acquired during their training is contingent on exposure to the disease conditions and procedures encountered by their faculty, rather than curricular needs [47]. Given the varied patient population and practice patterns of each program, experience based training in surgery does not ensure standardization of skills [56].

Scrutiny of the conventional framework has caused a significant "paradigm shift" towards a more objective standardized approach to education. With the progression of technology in surgery, patient safety and medical error have created a demand for innovation in surgical education [58]. Attendance by way of case logs insufficiently comments on surgical competence [38]. The institution of work hour restrictions has reduced operative experience and thus, surgical skill procurement. Over the past decade, efforts to address these issues have been successful in augmenting Halsted's original ideals. The shifting dynamics of surgical education is both challenging and exciting for residents and educators alike, as it provides the foundation to alter the future of this craft.

### Simulation

The learning curve associated with new procedures carries inherent patient morbidity, as they require a level of technical skill and confidence normally gained through practice [62]. For example, the donor site morbidity of an improperly harvested split thickness skin graft is significant, especially if a second site is eventually required. Simulators are an objective and reproducible medium that can allow technology to ease the transition from beginner to expert, while standardizing education, decreasing costs, reducing patient risk and improving outcomes [56]. The efficacy of simulators has been reported in the literature [10], and their widespread application is seen in General Surgery [32], Urology [24], Gynecology [13] and endoscopy [51]. Increasing prevalence of simulation in medical training has prompted the Accreditation Council for Graduate Medical Education (ACGME) and the American College of Surgeons (ACS), to implement a phased approach to formally require their use in surgical education.

The advent of simulators has forged a new era of excellence in surgery. The low-stress environment alleviates the anxiety of the operating room and enhances resident learning, while allowing for mistakes and improvement without compromising patient care [6]. The skills gained in this practical learning atmosphere have been proven to enrich performance in live operative models and therefore, can be transferable to the operating room [53]. The concept that "physical and mental skills are learned through a long process of persistent and dedicated efforts with repetition to reinforce the activity" [6], is fundamental to the development of a successful surgeon. Fitts and Posner described the 3 stages of skill acquisition in 1967. The student must first intellectualize the process, second develop the proper motor behavior, and third subsequent repetition gradually results in smooth performance through muscle memory [17]. The notion of 'practice before the game' holds true for musicians and athletes, and similarly, simulation has been shown to be effective in surgical motor skill acquisition [5].

Time is the key challenge faced by most programs establishing a skills lab. Resident workload and responsibility is demanding and often prohibits dedication to practice. Similarly, the commitments of academic faculty, limits their time to supervise and provide necessary feedback. In order for a skills curriculum to achieve optimal results, sufficient time allocation is imperative. Simulation training is a pivotal tool in surgical education, which should be adopted into the armamentarium of any residency program.

Although the use of simulation in burn training is limited (STSG models), there is great educational potential for its utilization.

## Education in the internet era

The evolution of the World Wide Web has become one of the most important accomplishments in history. It has revolutionized the dissemination of information and the propagation of knowledge. Over 220 million people (73%) in the United States use the Internet [58] for the purposes of education, research, business, news and entertainment. The Internet possesses an incredible opportunity for the growth of surgical education, and to overcome several of its current challenges. The widespread availability of online materials has permitted the shift of education away from the operating room. The issues of time constraints, patient safety and geographical limitations have been greatly attenuated with the initiation of web-based learning. The Internet has also facilitated the development of global collaboration of medical education [58].

Currently, e-learning has been successfully integrated into surgical programs for instruction in areas including anatomy [11], course curriculum [29], procedural skills [12] and problem-based learning [15]. There are endless implementation strategies to supplement training. Individual programs can dictate the published content they wish to provide, ranging from links to journal articles and seminars, to modules and videos [58]. Online simulators are also becoming ubiquitous, creating a reusable, accurate and self-directed model for the accession of knowledge and skills.

## Rotations as courses

In Halsted's model of surgical education, each rotation served as the primary route by which residents built their knowledge base. At the conclusion of a given rotation an attending staff awards a pass, which inadequately examines the resident's mastery of clinical and intellectual content, and their ability to function autonomously [34]. The current teaching system must place greater accountability on the resident by formally assessing their attainment of objectives throughout residency. This approach will increase resident motivation in developing superior study habits while keeping abreast of pertinent topics. Qualifying and certification exam results have been shown to improve with weekly assigned readings and exams [16]. A study by Maddaus [34], in which rotations were restructured as courses with learning objectives, pre-tests, post-tests and oral exams, has revealed favorable preliminary results. Reorganizing burn rotations into discrete courses would be advantageous and beneficial by putting greater responsibility and liability on the resident.

Web-based learning is a promising resource with growing potential that must be considered in the development of any curricular program. It is however, important to view it as an augment to an educational program, unable to replace formalized teaching [58].

# Mentorship

Mentoring relationships have been well established as an essential element for achieving growth and success in business, politics and academia [46]. Within the healthcare system, although mentorship has clearly had a positive impact in nursing [52, 55], the literature in surgical training is limited. It is designed to provide support, encouragement and professional vision [21], and has been described as crucial in surgical training [18] and influential in career path selection [35]. Faculty members who were mentored have more confidence, more productive research endeavors and greater career satisfaction [31, 42, 57], while a lack of mentoring is considered an important factor hindering career progress in academic medicine [28].

## Peer mentorship

Peer mentoring is defined as a relationship in which mentors and mentees are similar in professional status and they help each other and themselves through teaching and collaborative learning [59]. This model provides support in a non-evaluative environment [26], while promoting collegiality and a nurturing climate for personal and vocational growth [55]. It has been successfully applied in nursing, resulting in a less stressful and more comfortable environment [3, 36]. Students report increased self-confidence

and social integration, mitigating much of the initial anxiety associated with a new rotation [55]. Mentors enjoy the satisfaction of service while honing their interpersonal and communication skills [37].

## Hierarchical mentorship

The classical model of mentorship involves a pupil learning skills and knowledge from a preceptor or established expert in the field. This allows for the transference of experience from one generation to the next. In addition to the obvious advantages to the resident, hierarchical mentoring encompasses many benefits for the staff. Mentors develop a sense of pride and privilege in fulfilling their role of shaping the successors of their field. Medicine is the pursuit of lifelong learning, and mentorship programs give the 'lions' a chance to learn from the 'cubs' in an effort to retool themselves in this progressively changing environment. This mutually beneficial relationship has also been shown to increase faculty retention [4].

## What is a mentor

A mentor is a trusted educator whose role extends far beyond the teaching of technical skills and clinical judgment in the clinics, operating room and on the wards. They are role models who provide direction and instill values, while demonstrating effective communication, time management and successful prioritization of multiple personal and professional commitments [39]. The relationship is dynamic and adapts over time to meet the needs of the mentee [63]. Although support is the primary principle, mentees need to be challenged and given both positive and negative feedback to enable professional development [43]. Successful execution of this role requires many important qualities that a mentor must possess. Competence, confidence and commitment are 3 essential attributes vital to knowledgeable mentors who are respected in their field [41].

The ingredients that produce an outstanding mentor are rarely innate. "Mentorship has been a casually acquired trait with varying levels of success, but it is clear that the face of medicine and surgical training in the 21st century requires deliberate cultivation of mentors" [39]. It would be beneficial to implement staff development programs, highlighting effective mentoring skills and mentor responsibilities [4].

## Implementation

Although informal mentoring occurs in the daily interactions with more senior surgeons, formal mentorship programs increase satisfaction and efficacy [18]. The success of the mentor relationship is significantly higher when mentees select their own mentors [18, 19]. Role preparation of both sides ensures a smooth introduction, as mentors need training, and mentees need objectives and reasonable expectations [52]. As with any new relationship, adequate meeting time is compulsory for the development of a trusting and fruitful alliance.

Mentorship primarily occurs because mentors consider it a rewarding feature of their profession. Increasing demands on faculty time and the current criteria for academic advancement have seriously threatened the future of mentorship. Scholarship over citizenship is currently the gauge for promotion in surgery; thus, mentoring descends to a lower priority being largely uncompensated and undervalued [31]. There is a need for novel ideas to enhance faculty participation in this cornerstone of surgical training. Institutional recognition and appreciation of mentors and publicly rewarding mentorship excellence will increase the prestige of the activity and faculty enrollment. Mentorship can also be adapted into the faculty evaluation process for promotion [31].

"Mentoring is a vital cog in the machinery of medical education" [43] and should be strongly considered in burn unit curricula.

## Interprofessional education

In medicine, physicians are largely educated in isolation of other health professionals, resulting in limited collaboration, communication and coordination of care [48]. Many surgeons have been educated in a culture that places value on individual accomplishments; however, the importance of teamwork in medicine is becoming increasingly evident in the delivery of quality care and reduction

of medical errors [7, 40, 44, 45, 54, 60]. In complex care settings like burn units, a single health care professional is not equipped to handle the diversity of their patients' needs. A strong, coherent team approach in a burn unit reduces mortality, shortens length of stay and improves rehabilitation [20]. The relationship with other health care professionals has become an emphasis of modern surgical professionalism [30].

### What is interprofessional education

Health Canada defines interprofessional education (IPE) as "socializing health care providers in working together, in shared problem solving and decision making, towards enhancing the benefits for patients; developing mutual understanding of, and respect for, the contributions of various disciplines; and instilling the requisite competencies for collaborative practice." The Centre for the Advancement of Interprofessional Education (CAIPE) similarly refers to IPE as instances when "two or more professions learn from and about each other to improve collaboration and the quality of care" [8]. IPE is a unique approach to learning, where knowledge is attained through social collaboration with other professions, and the learning process is equally as important as the content itself [48]. It improves the understanding of team member complementary skills and increases mutual accountability. The contact between professions is insufficient to build the communication, respect and trust necessary for effective team performance [49]. Learning 'as' a team, rather than simply 'in' a team, enhances the collective capability [2].

### Approaches to interprofessional education

There are numerous models to engage the members of the burn unit in interactive learning. These health professionals include students, residents, occupational therapists, physiotherapists, social workers, nurses, respiratory therapists, dieticians, intensivists, surgeons and any other specialists that are involved in the complex care of these patients. Exchange based learning can be achieved through seminars, workshop discussions and case study sessions, where members of the team can explore the realms of each other's roles in the setting of collaborative care [23]. Problem based learning is an effective example of the action based educational approach, as the team is actively involved in working together to determine the most suitable course of action. Simulation not only has educational merit in technical skill acquisition, it is also useful in the teaching of IPE when feedback is given in small instructor led groups simulating a real situation [27]. The growth of online resources has allowed asynchronous communication to overcome collaborative time scheduling and geographic constrainsts, while permitting practicing health care workers to learn together [1, 9, 25, 50]. This model has been shown to be effective in teaching IPE [33].

Student feedback reveals that interprofessional education, through learning outside one's disciplinary boundaries, forges mutual respect [14, 64]. Interprofessional education provides the tools necessary to reduce the gaps in current practices by forming a profound comprehension of the patient care team.

# References

[1]    Arias AA, Bellman B (1995) Networked collaborative research and teaching. In: Boschmann E (ed) The electronic classroom: a handbook for education in the electronic environment. Learned Information, Medford, pp 180–185

[2]    Barr H (2009) An anatomy of continuing interprofessional education. J Contin Educ Health Prof 29: 147–150

[3]    Becker MK, Neuwirth JM (2002) Teaching strategy to maximize clinical experience with beginning nursing students. J Nurs Educ 41: 89–91

[4]    Benson CA, Morahan PS, Sachdeva AK, Richman RC (2002) Effective faculty preceptoring and mentoring during reorganization of an academic medical center. Med Teach 24: 550–557

[5]    Boehler ML, Schwind CJ, Rogers DA, Ketchum J, O'Sullivan E, Mayforth R, Quin J, Wohltman C, Johnson C, Williams RG, Dunnington G (2007) A theory-based curriculum for enhancing surgical skillfulness. J Am Coll Surg 205: 492–497

[6]    Buscarini M, Stein JP (2009) Training the urologic oncologist of the future: where are the challenges? Urol Oncol 27: 193–198

[7]    Campbell SM, Hann M, Hacker J, Burns C, Oliver D, Thapar A, Mead N, Safran DG, Roland MO (2001) Identifying predictors of high quality care in English general practice: observational study. BMJ 2 001 323: 784–789

[8]    Centre for the Advancement of Interprofessional Education (CAIPE) (1997) Interprofessional education: a definition. CAIPE, London, Bulletin No. 13

[9]    Chen LLJ, Gaines B (1998) Modelling and supporting virtual cooperative interaction through the World Wide Web. In: Sudweeks F, McLaughlin M, Rafaeli S (eds) Network and netplay: Virtual groups on the Internet. AAAI Press/MIT Press, Menlo Park, pp 221–242

[10]    Chipman JG, Schmitz CC (2009) Using objective structured assessment of technical skills to evaluate a basic skills simulation curriculum for first-year surgical residents. J Am Coll Surg 209: 364–370

[11]    Choi AR, Tamblyn R, Stringer MD (2008) Electronic resources for surgical anatomy. ANZ J Surg 78: 1082–1091

[12]    Chenkin J, Lee S, Huynh T, Bandiera G (2008) Procedures can be learned on the Web: a randomized study of ultrasound-guided vascular access training. Acad Emerg Med 15: 949–954

[13]    Clevin L, Grantcharov TP (2008) Does box model training improve surgical dexterity and economy of movement during virtual reality laparoscopy? a randomised trial. Acta Obstet Gynecol Scand 87: 99–103

[14]    Cooper H, Spencer-Dawe E, McLean E (2005) Beginning the process of teamwork: design, implementation and evaluation of an inter-professional education intervention for first year undergraduate students. J Interprof Care 19: 492–508

[15]    Corrigan M, Reardon M, Shields C, Redmond H (2008) "SURGENT" – student e-learning for reality: the application of interactive visual images to problem-based learning in undergraduate surgery. J Surg Educ 65: 120–125

[16]    de Virgilio C, Chan T, Kaji A, Miller K (2008) Weekly assigned reading and examinations during residency, ABSITE performance, and improved pass rates on the American Board of Surgery examinations. J Surg Educ 65: 499–503

[17]    Fitts PM, Posner, MI (1967) Human performance. Brooks/Col, Belmont

[18]    Flint JH, Jahangir AA, Browner BD, Mehta S (2009) The value of mentorship in orthopaedic surgery resident education: the residents' perspective. J Bone Joint Surg Am 91: 1017–1022

[19]    Ford HR (2004) Mentoring, diversity, and academic surgery. J Surg Res 118: 1–8

[20]    Gibran NS, Klein MB, Engrav LH, Heimbach DM (2005) UW burn center. A model for regional delivery of burn care. Burns 31: S36–39

[21]    Gilmour JA, Kopeikin A, Douche J (2007) Student nurses as peer-mentors: collegiality in practice. Nurse Educ Pract 7: 36–43

[22]    Halstead WS (1904) The training of the surgeon. Johns Hopkins Hosp Bull 15: 267–275

[23]    Hammick M, Olckers L, Campion-Smith C (2009) Learning in interprofessional teams: AMEE guide no 38. Med Teach 31: 1–12

[24] Hammond L, Ketchum J, Schwartz BF (2005) Accreditation council on graduate medical education technical skills competency compliance: urologica surgical skills. J Am Coll Surg 201: 454–457

[25] Harasim L, Hiltz SR, Teles L, Turoff M (1995) Learning networks: a field guide to teaching and learning online. MIT Press, Cambridge

[26] Heinrich K, Scherr M (1994) Peer mentoring for reflective teaching. Nurse Educ 19: 36–41

[27] Issenberg SB, Mcgaghie WC, Petrusa ER, Gordon DL, Scalese RJ (2005) Features and uses of high-fidelity medical simulations that lead to effective learning: A BEME systematic review. Med Teac 27: 10–28

[28] Jackson VA, Palepu A, Szalacha L, Caswell C, Carr PL, Inui T (2008) "Having the right chemistry": a qualitative study of mentoring in academic medicine. Bull Am Coll Surg 93: 19–25

[29] Kalet AL, Coady SH, Hopkins MA, Riles TS (2007) Preliminary evaluation of the Web Initiative for Surgical Education (WISE-MD). Am J Surg 194: 89–93

[30] Kitto, SC, Gruen RL, Smith JA (2009) Imagining a continuing interprofessional education program (CIPE) within surgical training. J Contin Educ Health Prof 29: 185–189

[31] Levy BD, Katz JT, Wolf MA, Sillman JS, Handin RI, Dzau VJ (2004) An initiative in mentoring to promote residents' and faculty members' careers. Acad Med 79: 845–850

[32] Lin E, Szomstein S, Addasi T, Galati-Burke L, Turner JW, Tiszenkel HI (2003) Model for teaching laparoscopic colectomy to surgical residents. Am J Surg 186: 45–48

[33] Luke R, Solomon P, Baptiste S, Hall P, Orchard C, Rukholm E, Carter L (2009) Online interprofessional health sciences education: from theory to practice. J Contin Educ Health Prof 29: 161–167

[34] Maddaus MA, Chipman JG, Whitson BA, Groth SS, Schmitz CC (2008) Rotation as a course: lessons learned from developing a hybrid online/on-ground approach to general surgical resident education. J Surg Educ 65: 112–116

[35] McCord JH, McDonald R, Leverson G, Mahvi DM, Rikkers LF, Chen HC, Weber SM (2007) Motivation to pursue surgical subspecialty training: is there a gender difference? J Am Coll Surg 205: 698–703

[36] McKeachie W, Svinicki M (2006) Active learning: cooperative, collaborative and peer learning. In: Sommer S (ed) Teaching tips: strategies, research, and theory for college and university teachers. Houghton Mifflin Co, New York, pp 213–220

[37] Miller A (2002) Mentoring students and young people. Kogan Page Ltd, London

[38] Miller DC, Montie JE, Faerber GJ (2003) Evaluating the Accreditation Council on Graduate Medical Education core clinical competencies: techniques and feasibility in a urology training program. J Urol 170: 1312–1317

[39] Möller MG, Karamichalis J, Chokshi N, Kaafarani H, Santry HP (2008) Mentoring the surgeon. Bull Am Coll Surg 93: 19–25

[40] Morey JC, Simon R, Jay GD, Wears RL, Salisbury M, Dukes KA, Berns SD (2002) Error reduction and performance improvement in the emergency department through formal teamwork training: evaluation results of the MedTeams project. Health Serv Res 37: 1553–1581

[41] Morton-Cooper A, Palmer A (2000) Mentoring in practice. In: Morton-Cooper A, Palmer A (eds) Mentoring, preceptorship and clinical supervision. Blackwell Science, Oxford, pp 59–62

[42] Ramanan RA, Phillips RS, Davis RB, Silen W, Reede JY (2000) Mentoring in medicine: keys to satisfaction. Am J Med 112: 336–341

[43] Ramani S, Gruppen L, Kachur EK (2006) Twelve tips for developing effective mentors. Med Teach 28: 404–408

[44] Reeves S, Zwarenstein M, Goldman J, Barr H, Freeth D, Koppel I, Hammick M (2008) Interprofessional education: effects on professional practice and health care outcomes. In: Cochrane Review Cochrane Library Issue 1. Wiley, London

[45] Risser DT, Rice MM, Salisbury ML, Simon R, Jay GD, Berns SD (1999) The potential for improved teamwork to reduce medical errors in the emergency department. The MedTeams Research Consortium. Ann Emerg Med 34: 373–383

[46] Roche GR (1979) Much ado about mentors. Harv Bus Rev 1: 14–31

[47] Sachdeva AK, Bell RH Jr, Britt LD, Tarpley JL, Blair PG, Tarpley MJ (2007) National efforts to reform residency education in surgery. Acad Med 82: 1200–1210

[48] Sargeant J (2009) Theories to aid understanding and implementation of interprofessional education. J Contin Educ Health Prof 29: 178–184

[49] Sargeant J, Loney E, Murphy G (2008) Effective interprofessional teams: "Contact is not enough" to build a team. J Contin Educ Health Prof 28: 228–234

[50] Scardamalia M, Bereiter C (1996) Computer support for knowledge-building communities. In: Koschmann T (ed) CSCL: theory and practice of an emerging paradigm. Erlbaum, Mahwah

[51] Shirai Y, Yoshida T, Shiraishi R, Okamoto T, Nakamura H, Harada T, Nishikawa J, Sakaida I (2008) Prospective randomized study on the use of a computer-based endoscopic simulator for training in esophagogastroduodenoscopy. J Gastroenterol Hepatol 23: 1046–1050

[52] Sprengel AD, Job L (2004) Reducing student anxiety by using clinical peer mentoring with beginning nursing students. Nurse Educ 29: 246–250

[53] Stelzer MK, Abdel MP, Sloan MP, Gould JC (2009) Dry lab practice leads to improved laparoscopic performance in the operating room. J Surg Res 154: 163–166

[54] Stevenson K, Baker R, Farooqi A, Sorrie R, Khunti K (2001) Features of primary health care teams associ-

ated with successful quality improvement of diabetes care: a qualitative study. Fam Pract 18: 21–26

[55] Sweet S, Fusner S (2008) Social integration of the advanced placement LPN: a peer mentoring program. Nurse Educ 33: 202–205

[56] Rosen JM, Long SA, McGrath DM, Greer SE (2009) Simulation in plastic surgery training and education: the path forward. Plast Reconstr Surg 123: 729–738

[57] Palepu A, Friedman RH, Barnett RC, Carr PL, Ash AS, Szalacha L, Moscowitz MA (1998) Junior faculty members' mentoring relationships and their professional development in US medical schools. Acad Med 73: 318–323

[58] Pugh CM, Watson A, Bell RH Jr, Brasel KJ, Jackson GP, Weber SM, Kao LS (2009) Surgical education in the internet era. J Surg Res 156: 177–182

[59] Topping KJ (1996) The effectiveness of peer tutoring in further and higher education: a typology and review of the literature. Higher Ed 32: 321–345

[60] Unützer J, Katon W, Callahan CM, Williams JW Jr, Hunkeler E, Harpole L, Hoffing M, Della Penna RD, Noël PH, Lin EH, Areán PA, Hegel MT, Tang L, Belin TR, Oishi S, Langston C; IMPACT Investigators. Improving Mood-Promoting Access to Collaborative Treatment (2002) Collaborative care management of late-life depression in the primary care setting: a randomized controlled trial. JAMA 288: 2836–2845

[61] Walsh K (2007) Interprofessional education online: the BMJ learning experience. J Interprof Care 21: 691–693

[62] Watt DA, Majumder S, Southern SJ (1999) Simulating split-skin graft harvest. Br J Plast Surg 52: 329

[63] Wensel TM (2006) Mentor or preceptor: what is the difference? Am J Health Syst Pharm 63: 1597

[64] Wilcock PM, Janes G, Chambers A (2009) Health care improvement and continuing interprofessional education: continuing interprofessional development to improve patient outcomes. J Contin Educ Health Prof 29: 84–90

Correspondence: Dr. Shahriar Shahrokhi, Sunnybrook Health Sciences Centre, Sunnybrook Research Institute, Rm D704, 2075 Bayview Ave. Toronto, ON M4N 3M5, Canada, E-mail: Shar. Shahrokhi@sunnybrook. ca

# European practice guidelines for burn care: Minimum level of burn care provision in Europe

Pavel Brychta

Department of Burns and Reconstructive Surgery, University Hospital Brno, Czech Republic; European Burns Association (EBA), President

## Foreword

Clinical practice guidelines (CPG´s) are currently a regular part of a clinician's armamentarium in virtually all branches of medicine. These guidelines are constantly upgraded and expanded through the work of physicians around the world. GPG's in burn medicine also play an important role in successful burn treatment. European Burns Association (EBA) and namely its Executive Committee recognize the value of GPG's, but have identified duplicity and varying levels of quality in the different national and other *Practical Guidelines for Burn Care* [1–18].

Europe is a continent moving towards the unification of virtually all aspects of life, including medicine and burn care. Open borders allow European citizens to move freely between countries. In the same respect, health care personnel are seeking employment in counties other than where they have received their training. This brings into question the quality of education received in the home country in relation to the established level in a different land. In the case of injury or illness in a foreign country, European citizens may find themselves in a medical facility which does not meet the standards of their home country. This is a pressing issue among patients, insurance companies and national health care authorities.

This is the driving force behind the development of *European Guidelines for Burn Care Provision* which will recommend, among other things the *Minimum European Level of Burn Care Provision*.

*Guidelines for Minimum European Level of Burn Care Provision* could become an important tool in improving burn care in Europe.

## Background

### Introduction

Clinical Practice Guidelines (CPG's) for various medical fields first appeared in publications in the early 1990's. CPG's offer structured and highly qualified reviews of relevant literature, giving physicians the best available information gained from concrete clinical studies to improve treatment (evidence based medicine – EBM).

This concept has proven to be very useful and currently thousands of CPG's exist for a wide range of medical branches. CPG's have contributed significantly to the upgrading of many medical strategies and work is being done to further improve these guidelines.

At present "Guidelines or Recommendations" work with 3 categories of evidence and suggestions:
1. Standards
2. Guidelines
3. Options

## Standards

are generally accepted principles of treatment based on a very high degree of clinical certainty supported by Class I evidence (based on prospective, randomised controlled clinical studies)

Standards are rigorously applied rules. Some European countries have their own approved standards for some steps in clinical burn treatment.

## Guidelines

are strategies of treatment based on moderate clinical certainty supported by Class II evidence (retrospective studies with relatively clear results).

Guidelines should be followed and only broken if medically justified.

This level of clinical certainty (Class II evidence) is much more frequent and accessible.

*(Unfortunately, the word Guidelines is used in a more global sense for all 3 kinds of recommendations and also in a more specific sense for this middle category. This is unfortunately misleading, but routinely used.)*

## Options

are possible ways of treatment based on personal clinical observation and/or Class III evidence (clinical series, case reports, expert opinions, etc.)

Options should be put through future clinical studies.

## General outlining of the European Practice Guidelines for Provisional Burn Care

When speaking about the Practice Guidelines for Provisional Burn Care, the following questions should be answered:
1. What is burn injury and burn care in general?
2. Where should burn care be provided?
3. Who should be the subject providing burn care?
4. Who should be the object of burn care?
5. How should burn care be provided?
6. Which European countries are involved?

These questions will be discussed in the following chapters. There is more interest in the category *Organization of Burn Care delivery (where it is done, who is the object and who is the subject of the burn care)* than the others. Therefore, Definition of a Burn Centre and the Transferral Criteria to the Burn Centre are explained in detail.

There is an explanation for this fact. Whereas evidence based basal steps in burn treatment are the same in all over the world, the organisation of delivery differs regionally.

Consequently, EBA EC Committee will propose its own recommendations.

They should be used as guidelines for classification of medical facility as a burn centre, thus fulfilling the recommendations of the European Burn Association.

## Burn injury and burn care in general

A *Burn* is a complex trauma needing multifaceted and continuous therapy.

Burns occurs through intensive heat contact to the body which destroys and/or damages human skin (thermal burns).

In addition to thermal burns, there are electric, chemical, radiation and inhalation burns. Frostbite also comes under this category.

*Burn Care* is the complex and continuous care for burn patients.

▶ The main goal of this care is to ensure optimum resuscitation in the emergency period and then to reach re-epithelialization of injured or destroyed skin either by support of spontaneous healing or by surgical necrectomy and grafting with STSAG. Subsequent treatment is to ensure the optimum postburn quality of life.

▶ Burn care includes thermal as well as electric and chemical burns. Inhalation and radiation injury and frostbite also comes under this category.

▶ Developments over the last several decades have clearly shown that burn care treatment offered in specialised burn centres brings better results than in non-specialized centres.

▶ Through the gathering of experience and critical evaluation of relevant literature, recommendations have been made to facilitate the optimum delivery of burn care including specific diagnostic and therapeutic procedures.

Burn treatment as part of burn care aims to provide:
1. first aid
2. pre-hospital care

3. transportation to an appropriate medical facility
4. management of the emergency period (resuscitation)
5. renewal of damaged and destroyed skin in acute periods
6. prevention and treatment of all complications
7. main surgical reconstruction
8. somatic and psychosocial rehabilitation

## Burn care provision

(Recommendations for European minimum level of Provisional Burn Care)

The most important aspects of Burn Care Provision can be concentrated into two definitions:
1. The burn centre
2. Transfer criteria to the burn centre
These two topics are elaborated in detail.

## The burn centre

The Burn Centre is an organized medical system for the total (complex and continuous) care of the burn patient. It is the highest organized unit among the Burn Care facilities.

*The Burn Centre:*
1. Has appropriate spaces and spatial arrangement
2. Is situated inside a hospital
3. Is properly equipped for all aspects of the treatment of burn patients.
4. Treats adults and/or children with all kinds and extents of burns.
5. Includes a medical staff and an administrative staff dedicated to the care of the burn patient.
6. The Burn Centre is the highest form of Burn Care Facility
7. Sustains a very high level of expertise in the treatment of the burn patient.
8. Conducts a certain minimal number of acute procedures and consequent reconstructive surgical procedures per year.

### Burn Centre space and spatial arrangement
► Should have access to an operating room with at least 42 m², air conditioning, preferably laminar air flow and wide range temperature settings for acute surgical burn treatment.
► This operating room is equipped with all the needs for burn surgery and a respiratory assistance service on a 24-hour basis.
► A second theatre should be devoted to secondary burn reconstruction.
► Should have at least 5 acute beds specially equipped and designed for the care of a major burn patient, i. e. high room temperature, climate control, total isolation facilities, adequate patient surveillance, intensive care monitoring facilities, etc.
► Have an established current germ surveillance program.
► Include enough regular beds in the adult and/or children´s wards to meet current needs.
► Have enough specialised and equipped spaces for rehabilitation and occupational therapy.

### Burn Centre situated inside a hospital
► Should maintain or at least have access to a skin bank.
► Must have easy access and cooperate with other departments, especially with Radiology, Microbiology, Clinical Biochemisty, Clinical Haemathology, Immunology, Surgery, Neurosurgery, Internal Medicine, Neurology, ENT, Ophthalmology, Gynaecology, Urology, Psychiatry etc.
For these reasons, a Burn Centre should be situated inside the largest hospitals in each country.

### Is properly equipped for all aspects of the treatment of burn patients
The Burn Centre has equipment of sufficient quality and quantity for specialized burn care. This includes instruments currently found in surgical operating theatres, Intensive Care Units and Standard Care Wards in addition to specialised knives (Humby, Watson . . .) and dermatomes (either electric or air driven) mesh and or Meek dermatomes, etc.

### The Burn Centre includes a medical staff and an administrative staff dedicated to the care of the burn patient
The main features of the Burn Centre Personnel (Staff) are as follows:

*The burn centre director (chief of staff, leading burn specialist)*

▶ A medical specialist dedicated to and experienced in burn treatment, familiar with all aspects of complex and continuous burn care (with at least 10 years of clinical practice), taking responsibility for all activities at the Burn Centre.

▶ Formal education typically is: plastic surgeon, general surgeon, anaesthetist or intensivist. Surgical background is preferred, as the causal treatment of severe burns is done with surgery, but an intensivist with some surgical training and education is also acceptable.

*The burn centre director (chief of staff, leading burn specialist)*

▶ Typically, a post-graduate education lasting a minimum of 5 years.

▶ 2 years basal education in surgery (22 months in a surgical department, 2 months in an internal department.

▶ 3 subsequent years in a burn centre (including 1 year in a department of plastic surgery, 2 months in a department of anaesthesiology and intensive care for children/adults.

▶ After certification, another 5 years working in a burn centre is recommended.

*Staff physicians*

▶ Staff physicians must have a high level of expertise in burn treatment. This can be attained through two years of instruction in a burn centre which follows basic practices in surgical and internal skills. In centres treating children, paediatricians (incl. paediatric surgeon) must also be present.

▶ A burn centre must have at least one full time burn care surgeon (specialist) and one anaesthetist available in the centre on a 24-hour basis.

▶ The minimal number of staff physicians is one per 2 intensive beds.

▶ Acute surgical burn wound treatment is provided by the team recruited from the burn centre staff. This team must always consist of a burn surgeon plus 2 to 3 paramedics and an anaesthetist with his/her nurse.

▶ During surgery, at least one fully accredited burn specialist must be present in ICU.

*Staff nurses*

▶ led by a registered nurse with years of experience in burn care in a burn centre, also possessing managerial expertise.

▶ Patients should have 24 hour access to a registered, highly skilled nurse experienced in the care of burn patients.

▶ The centre should be equipped with a sufficient amount of nurses to meet modern standards of care of burn patients. At least one nurse per patient on a BICU bed.

▶ Nurses should be able to handle all types and degrees of severity in burn and critically ill patient cases, different types of cutaneous wounds and ulcers and all aspects of primary rehabilitation.

*Rehabilitation personnel*

▶ Burn centres should have permanently assigned physical and occupational therapists in the burn team.

▶ Rehabilitation personnel should have at least one year of experience in a burn centre.

▶ Rehabilitation personnel should deal with both in and out patients.

*Psychosocial work*

▶ Burn centres should have a psychologist and a social worker available on a daily basis.

*Nutritional services*

▶ A burn centre should have dietician service available for consultation on a daily basis.

*Other staff members*

▶ Specialists cooperating closely with the burn team but not necessarily being on staff: general, orthopaedic and cardiothoracic surgeons, neurosurgeons and neurologists, internists, ENT specialists, ophthalmologists, urologists, gynaecologists, psychiatrists, radiologists, biochemists, haematologists, microbiologists, immunologists and epidemiologists.

Having a well-educated and trained burn centre staff, along with appropriate space arrangement and medical equipment, is the key factor in improving burn care and its outcome.

## The Burn Centre is the highest form of Burn care facility

Lower organisation units other than a Burn Centre are:
1. Burn Unit
2. Burn Facility

These facilities provide only some aspects of Burn Care and are present in virtually all European countries. They are typically affiliated to surgical or paediatric departments and a unified European definition is currently not possible. Severe burn patients, as defined in the next chapter, should not be referred to Burns Units and/or Burns Facilities for definitive treatment.

## The Burn Centre sustains a very high level of expertise in the treatment of burn patients

To ensure the current high level of training and expertise in the treatment of all aspects of burns, the following items should be adhered to by a burn centre:
1. Provide complex and continuous burn care.
2. Be involved in teaching and research activities in addition to diagnostic and therapeutic activities.

## Conducts a certain minimal number of acute procedures and follow up reconstructive surgical procedures per year

- A burn centre should admit at least 75 acute burn patients annually, averaged over a three-year period.
- A burn centre should always have at least 3 acute patients admitted in the centre, averaged over a three-year period.
- A burn centre must have in place its own system of quality control.
- A burn centre should perform at least 50 follow-up reconstructive surgical procedures annually.
- In Europe, one burn centre is advisable for every 3–10 million inhabitants.
- Burn Centre treats adults and/or children with all kinds and extents of burns.

## Transferral criteria to a burn centre

It is very important to identify the patients who should be referred to a burn centre.

Patients with superficial dermal burns on more than:
- 5% of TBSA in children under 2 years of age
- 10% of TBSA in children 3–10 years of age
- 15% of TBSA in children 10–15 years of age
- 20% of TBSA in adults of age
- 10% of TBSA in seniors over 65 years of age

In addition:
- Patients requiring burn shock resuscitation.
- Patients with burns on the face, hands, genitalia or major joints.
- Deep partial thickness burns and full thickness burns in any age group and any extent.
- Circumferential burns in any age group.
- Burns of any size with concomitant trauma or diseases which might complicate treatment, prolong recovery or affect mortality.
- Burns with a suspicion of inhalation injury.
- Any type of burns if there is doubt about the treatment.
- Burn patients who require special social, emotional or long-term rehabilitation support.
- Major electrical burns
- Major chemical burns
- Diseases associated to burns such as toxic epidermal necrolysis, necrotising fasciitis, staphylococcal scalded child syndrome etc., if the involved skin area is 10% for children and elderly and 15% for adults or if there is any doubt about the treatment.

## Countries currently considering participation in the clarification of European Guidelines for Burn Care

The following European Countries and their population of over 500 million inhabitants are considering involvement into the clarification of European Guidelines for Burn Care:

| | | |
|---|---|---|
| Portugal | The Netherlands | Czech Republic |
| Spain | Luxemburg | Slovakia |
| France | Germany | Hungary |
| Ireland | Switzerland | Slovenia |
| UK | Austria | Serbia |
| Iceland | Italy | Croatia |
| Norway | Estonia | Bosnia and Herzegovina |
| Sweden | Latvia | Greece |
| Finland | Lithuania | Romania |
| Belgium | Poland | Bulgaria |

These countries, with the exception of Switzerland, are either members of EU or EEA (EFTA), or will

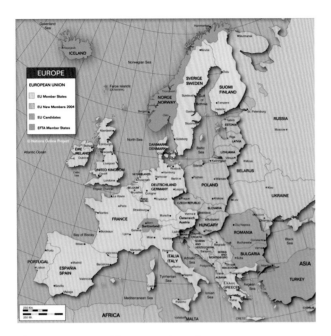

**Fig. 1.** Structure of European Countries

soon be joining one of these groups. In any case, these countries are already cooperating in the exchange of burn information.

The situation at present is unclear in several countries, which geographically are situated in Europe, but their level of cooperation, data exchange and/or other factors do not allow their involvement in the System of European Guidelines for Burn Care. These countries are Belarus, Ukraine, Moldova and Albania.

## Conclusion

This present theses does not, of course, have the form of standards and/or guidelines as mentioned at the beginning of this article. They must go through the process of "translation" or "conversion" to become standards and/or guidelines.

Because this process is quite sophisticated, expensive and time consuming, perhaps this article could be interesting for those involved in burn care in Europe.

## References

[1] American Burn Association & American College of Surgeons (1995) Guidelines for the operation of Burn Centres. Bull Am Coll Surg 80: 10, 34–41

[2] Childs C (1998) Is there evidence-based practice for burns. Burns 24: 29–33

[3] NSW Health Department (1996) Management guidelines for people with burn injury.

[4] Practice Guidelines for Burn Care (2001) American Burn Association. J Burn Care Rehabil

[5] NSW Health Department (2003) Selected speciality and statewide service plans. Numer 4 Severe Burn Service

[6] National Burn Care Review Committee Report (Ken Dun): Standards and Strategy for Burn Care (year not announced – 2002 or 2003)

[7] Allison K, Porter K (2004) Consensus on the pre-hospital approach to burns patient management. Injury 35(8): 734–738

[8] Disaster management and the ABA Plan (2005) ABA Board of Trustees; Committee on Organization and Delivery of Burn Care. J Burn Care Rehabil 26(2):102–106

[9] Küntscher MV, Hartmann B (2006) [Current treatment strategies for paediatric burns]. Handchir Mikrochir Plast Chir 38(3): 156–163. Review. German

[10] Haik J, Ashkenazy O, Sinai S, Tessone A, Barda Y, Winkler E, Orenstein A, Mendes D (2005) Practice Guidelines for burn care, 2006. Burn care standards in Israel: lack of consensus. Burns 31(7): 845–849

[11] Gibran NS (2006) Committee on Organization and Delivery of Burn Care, American Burn Association. J Burn Care Res 27(4): 437–438

[12] American Burn Association and Americal College of Surgeons Committee of Trauma (2007) Guidelines for the Operation of Burn Centers. J Burn Care Res 28(1)

[13] Alsbjörn B, Gilbert P, Hartmann B, Kazmierski M, Monstrey S, Palao R, Roberto MA, Van Trier A, Voinchet V (2007) Guidelines for the management of partial-thickness burns in a general hospital or community setting-recommendations of a European working party. Burns 33(2): 155–160

[14] New Zealand Guidelines Group. Management of Burns and Scalds in Primary Care June 2007

[15] Ennis JL, Chung KK, Renz EM, Barillo DJ, Albrecht MC, Jones JA, Blackbourne LH, Cancio LC, Eastridge BJ, Flaherty SF, Dorlac WC, Kelleher KS, Wade CE, Wolf SE, Jenkins DH, Holcomb JB (2008) Joint Theater Trauma System implementation of burn resuscitation guidelines improves outcomes in severely burned military casualties. J Trauma 64[2 Suppl]: S146–51; discussion S151–152

[16] Kamolz LP, Kitzinger HB, Karle B, Frey M (2009) The treatment of hand burns. Burns 35(3): 327–337

[17] Vogt PM, Krettek C (2009) [Standards of medical care for burn injuries]. Unfallchirurg 112(5): 461

[18] Carter JE, Neff LP, Holmes JH 4th (2010) Adherence to burn center referral criteria: are patients appropriately being referred? J Burn Care Res 31(1): 0 26–30

Correspondence: Pavel Brychta, Department of Burns and Reconstructive Surgery, University Hospital Brno, Jihlaská 20, CZ-62500 Brno, Czech Republic, E-mail: dr.brychta@seznam.cz

# Pre-hospital and initial management of burns

# Pre-hospital, fluid and early management, burn wound evaluation

Folke Sjöberg

Department of Hand and Plastic Surgery and Intensive Care, Linköping University Hospital, and Department of Clinical and Experimental Medicine, Linköping University, Linköping, Sweden

## Introduction

### Modern care

In the last 20 years large changes in burn care and in the background and logistics around the care for the burn injured has occurred which has implications for how burn care now should be administered and practically performed. Firstly the incidence of burn injuries has decreased in the Western world and a decrease of about 30 % is evident from e. g., since the eighties [1–2]. In parallel, length of stay in the burn care facilities for the injured has been reduced to about 40 % of what it was at that time [3–4]. Thirdly, the outcome of burns has been significantly improved over the same time period. This may be exemplified by the 50 % survival chance that was present for a 45 % total burn surface area burn (TBSA %) in a 21 year old in the late 70-ties, which is to be compared to the corresponding 50 % survival chance for 80–90 % TBSA % burn in the same age patient today [5-6]. Fourth, patients, with smaller burns, today are to a significant extent treated as outpatients and smaller injuries may have their surgery done as outpatients as well [7–9]. At the same time an increasing proportion of the patients are in the elderly age groups where the injury poses a larger treat as compared to in younger patients [10–11]. In this age group care is to a large extent influenced by co-morbidities [12].

Based on these changes the approach to burn care has been to centralize this type of care to larger burn units and centers. A process, that is ongoing in most countries, however with a variable intensity. The multidisciplinary approach to the care and the need to keep the care process unified for this patient group has lead to that the centralization process has been pursued and is most often successful. The latter exemplified by lower mortality rates and shorter lengths of stay [6, 13–14]. At the same time such organizational changes bring about important care implications for the general medical practitioners and medical organizations [13–14]. The decreased incidence and the centralized care reduce the magnitude of medical staff that have experience of these cases and that treats them on a regular basis. This then calls for good teaching programs and a good organized care. Especially the early management and stabilization of the patients needs to be well functioning at any level of care as this care is often provided at a non-burn center by personal with limited experience of burns. Importantly, as the outcome has been improved significantly in later times, the care to be provided needs to be optimized and the tolerance for any less successful results is low. It is relevant to note that there is an inherent risk in "over"- centralizing care even of small injuries that should be cared for at the local hospital [15]. Therefore continuous teaching programs are important. This early part of the treatment has therefore been the target of specially organized teaching programs initially started through the Advance trauma life support (ATLS) concept [16–17] followed by more specifically burn oriented programs such as: the American "Advanced Burn Care Life Support Course (ABLS; www.Ameriburn.org)" provided by the American Burn Association and which is also taught outside the US as e. g., in Japan [18] or Sweden. This course is also available on line on the web [19]; or the Australian and New Zeeland "Emergency Management of Severe Burns (EMSB; www.anzba.org. au)" course which also is provided in other countries such as Britain and South Africa [20–21]. The present chapter will therefore rely strongly on these principles as the strategies for the initial care is presented. These are important as they have implications for the success of the whole treatment process and the final outcome. As pointed out the final care of the burn patients is in cases of significant burns undertaken at burn centers and the improved early stabilization and transport care that today can be offered is one of the reasons why modern burn care provides successful results and increased survival. From a teaching perspective modern burn care in western countries may thus be described as most often provided at three locations, firstly, at the scene of the accident or very close by; secondly at a local hospital where also initial stabilization and the start of fluid therapy usually is undertaken and finally the transport to the final care level, a tertiary referral burn unit or center. In densely populated areas direct transport to the burn center is also an often employed alternative. Transport times are then usually in the range of less than 1 hour. The present chapter will review current principles for the care at these first two locations.

## Early management

### At the accident

The early and immediate care provided to a burn patient may vary depending on many factors most of all related to: the type of injury (thermal, chemical or electric); where the accident has occurred and its relation to different care levels and the available resources. The latter case, being relevant in situations with large number of injuries, such as in disaster settings or similar circumstances and where other approaches and strategies also will come into play to ascertain good outcome [22]. In far, distant places the care may be started and undertaken by a companion or a bystander, which may also be the case in other settings immediately after the injury. The more organized assessment and care in the very early stage is otherwise most often done, in the western world, by paramedics from an ambulance rescue team or at times from rescue squads comprising personal with higher medical education such as nurses and/or doctors or personal from a rescue groups arriving by e. g., helicopter. At all levels, a similar approach is undertaken based on early trauma rescue principles (ATLS/ABLS). This evaluation/care may mainly be divided into:

▶ primary assessment,
▶ secondary assessment

which is followed by transportation to the next level of care.

The knowledge gained and the treatments undertaken under way needs to be adequately registered and communicated properly to the next level, so that any important findings and interventions made, are properly extended further down in the treatment process.

Most urgently at the site of the fire or accident is to stop the fire process, electricity or chemical exposure and move the patient into a safe area. This may include getting the person out from a trapped situation in e. g., a vehicle. Stopping the fire in e. g., in clothing's is best done by suffocation of the fire (rolling and adding garments on the burning clothing's), if not water or other type of fire extinguishers are within reach. Flushing with properly tempered fluid is very good as it not only extinguishes the fire but also cools the wound and thereby reduces the convection of heat and it reduces pain. Be aware of the risk for hypothermia. At this point clothing, jewelry should be removed as they retain heat and may affect blood flow, as the extremities swell (e. g. jewelry/fingers). Early management also includes, if the exposure is based on chemicals, flushing with significant amounts of water and being aware of the contamination risk for others such as the rescue team, which shall take adequate precautions using gloves and gowns. If the eyes are involved flushing becomes even more important prior to having the eyes examined by an ophthalmologist. It is also important to stress that neutralizing agents are contraindicated as they induce heat. In cases of accidents involving electricity, there is also a need to stop the current/voltage or using an insulator prior to getting into contact with the patient.

At the site of the accident, in the immediate period after the injury, the patient is cared for by regular ATLS/ABLS/EMSB or other well organized trauma algorithms (ABC) and in their relevant order, i. e., A. Airway, B. Breathing, C. Circulation, D. Disability, E. Exposure – each specified in more detail below under primary/secondary assessment. Very important at this site is also to confirm or exclude other injuries that may be more important than the burn itself (see below the details for this under secondary survey). Pain treatment may be important in this setting especially if there is a somewhat longer initial transport. Pain relief is accomplished preferably by i. v., morphine in incremental doses in the larger burns if drugs are at this point available. It is also important to stress that there is an over representation of abuse, psychiatric disorders and criminality among burn injured patients. This may in certain circumstances have implications for the further care procedures. Most importantly at the site of the accident is to be aware of the risk of being infected/contaminated by Hepatitis B and C or HIV, which makes it important for the rescue personal to take appropriate precautions (glasses/glows/gowns).

Wound care at the site of the accident is rather uncomplicated. Burnt textiles may be removed and the patient covered by clean sheets, to reduce the risk of contamination of the wound and also to maintain body temperature. There is no need for ointments or other local treatments at this stage. At times commercially available burn wound coverings may be presented at the site of injury but the potential positive effects of these are yet undocumented why clean sheets may always be preferred.

In the case of isolated burn injuries there is little need to force an uncontrolled early transport unless there is other life threatening illnesses present. It has been suggested in guidelines of the ABA that if transport times are less than an hour – start of fluid treatment is not mandatory. Transport principles for the burn injured to the local hospital vary according to the local geographic situations, but often airborne transport (helicopter or fixed wing) in Europe is recommended when the transport time exceeds 2 hours or is more than 100 km.

## At a local hospital – stabilization prior to transport to the Burn Center

### Primary assessment

The primary assessment scheme follows a strict order scheduled according to how urgent the intervention is. It should be done as early as possible and repeatedly controlled during the care of the patient. Some parts may be performed less thorough at e. g., the site of the accident as more is gained by rapid transport to the next care level or there is a risk of hypothermia, e. g. a detailed burn extent determination outside in the cold.

### Airway

The airway is immediately assessed, evaluated and dealt with. A compromised airway may be cared for by small means such as bending the neck backwards or pulling the yaw forward. Facial burns or upper airway edema may compromise the airway as time passes from the time of the accident – making intubation necessary. Unconsciousness, very uncommon in the uncomplicated burn setting unless there is a significant carbon monoxide or cyanide exposure, or another injury, may be a reason for a compromised airway and will call for an early intubation. Provide, if possible oxygen at 100% by a non-rebreathing mask to optimize oxygenation and treat possible carbon monoxide/cyanide effects. At this point also evaluate the spine for any concomitant injuries and the need for fixation – not to cause spinal cord injuries.

### Breathing

In conjunction to the evaluation of the upper airway the breathing pattern should be assessed and the lungs examined for proper function and especially in the case of circular thoracic burns, as these may compromise breathing mechanics as edema develops in the thoracic wall, which calls for escharotomies (Fig. 1). This may be particularly important in small children as they rely more on auxiliary breathing muscles in their breathing.

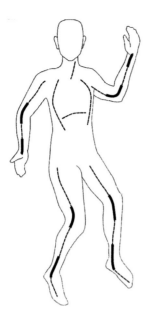

**Fig. 1.** Escharotomies. The lines indicate the location for escharotomies. Note that it is important that the cut is deep enough to accomplish a tissue release. This needs to be specifically addressed at the areas marked, as it is more difficult to assess the right tissue depth at these locations, i. e., close to the major joints

## Circulation

The circulatory status of the patient should be examined. It includes assessing the skin color, sensitivity, peripheral pulses and capillary refill. Heart rate and blood pressure should also be included to confirm adequate organ perfusion. Be aware that heart rate effects needs to be judged cautiously as it may also be affected by other reasons than hypovolemia, such as pain. Blood pressure monitoring when done may be difficult, be aware of the risk for faulty or compromised measurements by e. g., deep circumferential burns. In cases the peripheral circulation in the extremities is compromised consider early escharotomies (Fig. 1).

## Disability

The burn injured patient during "normal" conditions in the acute phase should not have an altered level of consciousness (LOC) even in cases of very severe burns. The LOC should be assessed, e. g., by the Glascow Coma Scale (GCS). If the Level of consciousness (LOC) is altered, suspect other underlying processes such as other trauma, carbon monoxide and/or cyan-

ide intoxication, hypoxia, or other medical conditions such as e. g., stroke or diabetes.

## Expose and examine

The patient should be thoroughly examined and in order to do this removal of the clothing is necessary. Be aware of the risk for hypothermia. Jewelry, especially such as rings etc. should be removed due to the risk of compromising extremity (finger) blood flow as tissue edema develops. At this occasion the important assessment of the burn injuries may be performed and evaluated. Important for the outcome is to initiate the fluid therapy, which may also be done at this point and when the extent of the burn injury becomes evident.

## Secondary assessment

The complementary second assessment is undertaken rapidly after the first assessment and it is aimed at examining the patient thoroughly from head to toe, mainly in order to rule out other more important injuries that may pose a danger to the patient. One important point is that this examination needs to be undertaken in detail as the burn injury often is the most prominent injury and it may lead to that other injuries may be overlooked.

Other issues to address, at this point is to get a good medical history. This is important from mainly two aspects, firstly, the circumstances around the burn injury as it may help in the determining the prognosis and may indicate the future burn treatment needs. Secondly, to assess the patients present co-morbidities and ongoing medical treatments.

1. *Circumstances of the burn.* Where and when did it happen – what were the injury mechanisms (scald, flame, chemical or electrical)? Especially the factors, heat level (degrees) and exposure time (seconds) may signal the risk for deep injuries. Indoor accident and risk for inhalation injuries. Are other injury mechanisms present and relevant?

2. *Medical history.* Previous or associated illnesses (diabetes, hypertension, other heart, lung or kidney disease) – Ongoing medical treatment, alcohol use or other (abuse), allergies. Time for last oral fluid or food intake. The tetanus immunization status, – need for complementary injections?

## Fluid treatment

A corner stone in the treatment of the burn injury is the fluid treatment. Usually i. v., fluid is provided to injuries larger than 15% total burn surface area % (TBSA %) [23–24]. In order to provide fluid treatment intravenously, i. v. lines are needed. These are most commonly applied in the extremities in non-injured tissue, but in cases of massive burns also burned areas may be used. In larger burns getting vascular access may prove difficult and central i. v. lines may be mandatory as may intraosseous, or cutdown strategies in children. The fluid treatment may be initiated early at the scene of the accident, but should not significantly delay transportation. If transport is planned for more than 1 hour starting the i. v. fluid is most often recommended. The background for the fluid needs for the burn patients is the rapid fluid loss to the injured tissue that is caused by the negative imbibition pressure, developing in the injured tissues secondary to the thermal injury and that "pulls" the fluid from the vascular space into the surrounding tissues. This effect is at its maximum after approximately two hours. Also a generalized permeability increase in the vascular tree is developing in parallel and that is due to the generalized inflammatory reaction that develops in the body after the burn injury. This effect is added to the effect by the imbibition pressure and they constitute the reason for the fluid needs of the burn injured [25]. The permeability change is claimed to subside at 24 hours and it is therefore most often recommended that the fluid provided are based on crystalloids until this time point [26–28]. In the US fluids are based on lactated Ringer solutions whereas many countries else were do use acetated Ringer. In cases of refractory situations despite extensive fluid volume provided, the addition of colloids and/or vasoactive drugs may be relevant and needed [29–30]. For most injuries this is however uncommon. There are several fluid protocols in use world wide today (Table 1) and the most commonly used is the one first presented by Dr. Baxter in the 60-ties, called the Parkland formula as it was used initially at the Parkland Memorial Hospital in Dallas (Table 2) [31]. This scheme recommends in adults 2–4 ml/kg/TBSA% of crystalloids (ringers solution (lactate/acetate) for the first 24 hours, 50% provided during the first 8 hours and 50% during the

**Table 1.** Alternative fluid protocols (Modified from Warden GD [32])

| Crystalloid based protocols | |
| --- | --- |
| Parkland | Ringerlactate/acetate 2–4 ml/kg/TBSA%; half of the fluid during first 8 h |
| | Children: Ringer lactate/acetate 3–4 ml/kg/TBSA% + the regular 24h maintenance fluid needs |
| Modified Brooke | Ringerlactate/acetate 2 ml/kg/TBSA% |
| **Colloid based protocols** | |
| Evans | NACl 1 ml/kg/TBSA% +colloid 1 ml/kg/TBSA%+ 2 000 ml glucose solution (5%) |
| Brooke | Ringerlactate/acetate 1.5 ml/kg/TBSA% +Colloid 0,5 ml/kg %+ 2 000 ml glucose solution (5%). |
| Slater | Ringerlactate/acetate 2 000 ml/24 + fresh frozen plasma 75 ml/kg/24h |
| **Dextran based protocols** | |
| Demling | Dextran 40 in NaCl (2 ml/kg/h in 8h) + Ringerlactate/acetate in sufficient amounts to induce a urine volume of 30 ml/h + fresh frozen plasma (0,5 ml/kg/h from 8–26h post burn) |
| **Hypertonic protocols** | |
| Monafo | 250 mEq Na/l. Amounts provided to induce a urine output of 30 ml/h |
| Warden | Ringerlactate + 50 mEq Sodium bicarbonate (total 180 mEq) during the first 8h to induce a urine output of 30–50 ml/h. Thereafter Ringerlactate with the same urinary output goal |

following 16 hours. In children the corresponding fluid volume need is larger, that is 3–4 ml/kg/TBSA% and to this the normal 24 hour fluid needs are added (Table 2). It is important to stress that the fluid volume suggested is to be closely adjusted according to endpoints, – that is mainly urine output. In order to maintain perfusion of internal organs the endpoint and goal is for a urine output of 30 ml/h (or 0.5 ml/kg/h) in adults and 1 ml/kg/h in children. If insufficient urine output, a 30% increase in the fluid volume per hour provided is recommended. Alternatively, if urine output is too large a corresponding decrease is suggested.

**Table 2.** The Parkland protocol

| Adults |
| --- |
| Ringerlactate/acetate 2–4 ml/kg/TBSA%. 50% provided during the first 8 h. the remaining fluid during the following 16 h. |

| Children |
| --- |
| Ringerlactate/acetate 3–4 ml/kg/TBSA%. 50% provided during the first 8 h. the remaining fluid during the following 16 h. Normal 24 h fluid needs are added to this as glucose solution. |

It is important to stress that neither too little fluid nor to large fluid volumes in relation to the needs should be provided as it will lead to less successful results [33]. The needs vary largely between injuries and patients underlining the need for close surveillance and follow up. In general and presently, in cases of less successful fluid resuscitations most often too large fluid volumes have been provided [30]. Too large fluid volumes will lead to deepening of the burn wound and secondary complications from other body compartments such as generalized large edema including cerebral, pulmonary edema and compartment situations, most importantly abdominal compartment syndrome [33]. Especially if using central circulatory endpoints rather than urine output during the first 12–18 hours such risk is higher [34]. Using the parkland formula the patients appear "hypovolemic" as examined by central circulation techniques. e. g., echocardiography in the very early part of the resuscitation period [35–36].

There are situations where larger fluid needs may be present. In general it has been claimed especially for inhalation or electrical injuries and in cases of a delayed start of fluid treatment. In the case of inhalation injuries the data supporting larger fluid needs are older and in newer investigations smaller effects of inhalation injury on the fluid needs have been seen [30]. In electrical injuries the total tissue damage may be larger despite that the skin burn is less extensive. Other instances where larger fluid volumes are called for are in cases of high voltage electrical injuries or crush injures or when myo- och hemoglobinemia is present. Under these circumstances an increased diuresis and alkalinisation of the urine is recommended. The diuresis should reach 1–2 ml/kg/h

(adults) and the pH of the urine should be kept alkaline preferably around or above 7. This is accomplished by adding sodium bicarbonate solution to the resuscitation fluids. This strategy should be continued as long as the pigments are present in the urine.

## Burn wound evaluation

Most often the first burn wound evaluation is made under the heading "exposure" in the primary survey, at e. g. the accident. A more thorough examination is then made during the second survey. In evaluating the wound it is important to have it adequately exposed and cleaned from debris and blisters, the latter situation calls for good analgesia or is done during general anesthesia. The risk of hypothermia should always be addressed. The wound evaluation is done mainly in two aspects, to determine, the depth and total percent surface area injured (TBSA %). The depth is mainly important as it affects the treatment (surgical excision or not) and the TBSA % is important for the prognosis. TBSA% (including depth) is together with the age of the patient and the prevalence of inhalation injury the most important prognostic factors for the injury. This will govern prognosis and also the fluid treatment.

### Burn wound depth

How deep into the skin the injury progresses is dependent on several factors. Firstly, it depends on the thermal energy transferred to the tissue. This depends on the temperature and the exposure time, high temperature and longer exposure times increases the risk for significant injuries. The energy transfer process is further affected by the type of transfer, e. g., convection transfers more energy, and this is counteracted by the ability of the tissue to withstand the temperature (thicker skin – better resistance) or dissipate the heat (higher blood flow reduces the injury). In practice this is exemplified by the lover risk for injuries on the back, in palms and soles with their thicker nature and the higher risk in elderly and children with their generally thinner skin.

Burn wound depth (Fig. 2) has traditionally been divided into three levels according to anatomy, first degree – epidermal injury, second degree – dermal and third degree sub dermal burns. Today a two level

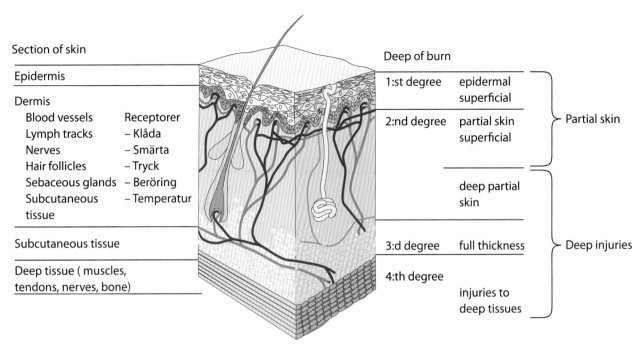

**Fig. 2.** Burn wound. Skin anatomy in relation to burn wound depth terminology

nomenclature is used which focuses more on treatment strategies: partial thickness burns (including epidermal and superficial dermal injuries (1ˢᵗ and superficial second degree burn; old nomenclature) and full thickness burns (including deep second degree and sub dermal burns; old nomenclature). Modern care for partial thickness is conservative treatment whereas full thickness burns are surgically excised and transplanted.

A burn involving the epidermis is usually erythematous and very painful but does not contain blisters. It is exemplified by a sunburn. The dead epidermis sloughs of and is replaced by regenerating keratinocytes within 2–3 days. A partial thickness burn wound, is a superficial dermal burn and extends down to the papillary dermis and usually forms blisters. When the blisters are removed the wound is pink, wet and highly sensitive. Blanching is present. These wounds heal within 2 weeks (Fig. 3 A). Deep dermal wounds extend down to the reticular dermis and usually take more than 3 weeks to heal. These wounds also show blistering but the wound underneath has a mottled and white appearance. Blanching, if at all present is slow. Sensitivity to pinprick is reduced and pain is described as discomfort rather than pain (Fig. 3B). Full thickness wounds involve the entire dermis and extend to the underlying tissue. Appearance is described as charred, leathery and firm. The wound is insensitive to touch and pinprick (Fig. 3C). Deep dermal and full thickness wounds are surgically excised and autologously transplanted.

**Burn surface area**

The burned body surface area, will as mentioned affect overall prognosis, the resources needed and not least from the practical perspective the immediate fluid treatment. It is therefore mandatory that it is done properly. From a practical perspective the most commonly used technique is based on the rule of nines (Fig. 4). In this setting the body is divided into parts of nine percent (arms and head) or multiples of nine (18%; each leg and each side of the torso/stomach and back) the corresponding chart for children is taking into account the larger size of the head and smaller legs in the smaller children (Fig. 4). If the ambition is to be more detailed the chart of Lund and Browder is generally used [37]. In cases of dispersed injuries it is common to apply the area of the palm and fingers (patient) as an estimate of 1% TBSA% of the injured [37].

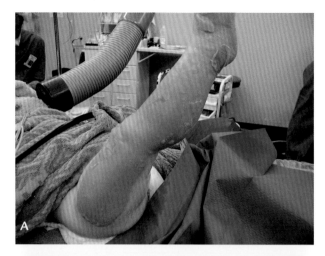

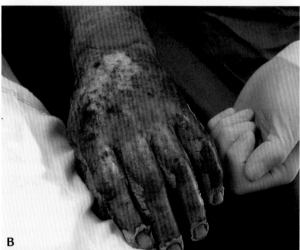

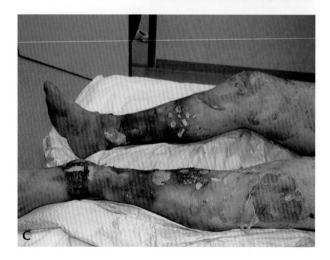

**Fig. 3.** Burn wound depth assessment (Phostos). A Superficial dermal burn; B Deep dermal burns; C Full thickness burn (distal lower leg)

## Other interventions at a referring hospital

When the patient is stabilized at a referring hospital there are other interventions that may be done to progress the care and improve the situation for the patient prior to arrival at the Burn center.

### Pain treatment

Pain early after the injury is very variable with patients at times experiencing severe pain where as others have more limited problems [38]. The extent of the pain is in each case difficult to predict in advance. Today most units base their pain treatment strategies on a multimodal pain strategy, which are based on several different principles. For the acute setting most often acetoaminophene (1000 milligram as a single dose and up to 4 grams per day for adults) is used in conjunction, when more significant pain is present, with i. v., administered opioids (e. g. morphine). The latter, are provided in small incremental i. v. doses (1–2.5 mg), where the needs of the patients is monitored closely and the doses administered accordingly and thereby reducing the risk for a respiratory depression. The i. v. route is important in order to titrate the effect but also not least as it may be a poor uptake in hypoperfused tissue areas (sc. or intramuscularly). Other more advanced pain strategies will be needed and employed during the further care of the patient, at the burn center.

### Urinary catheter

Urine output is the main fluid treatment outcome measure. Therefore in order to monitor it, especially in larger burns a urinary catheter needs to be inserted. Modern catheters also have temperature sensors included in the intra bladder portion of the catheter, which at the same time facilitates temperature surveillance. After insertion, urinary content of hemoglobin and myoglobin may be observable in such cases.

### Decompression of the stomach

Especially in the larger burns the stress response induces gastric, intestinal ileus and this is also further aggravated by the opioids provided for pain treatment. Therefore gastric decompression is often suggested by a nasogastric tube. Through this, also early enteral nutrition may be started and reducing the

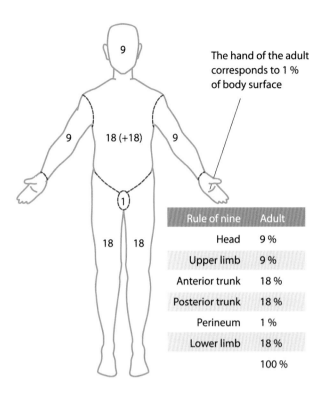

The hand of the adult corresponds to 1 % of body surface

| Rule of nine | Adult |
|---|---|
| Head | 9 % |
| Upper limb | 9 % |
| Anterior trunk | 18 % |
| Posterior trunk | 18 % |
| Perineum | 1 % |
| Lower limb | 18 % |
| | 100 % |

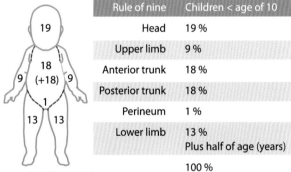

| Rule of nine | Children < age of 10 |
|---|---|
| Head | 19 % |
| Upper limb | 9 % |
| Anterior trunk | 18 % |
| Posterior trunk | 18 % |
| Perineum | 1 % |
| Lower limb | 13 % Plus half of age (years) |
| | 100 % |

For small children: Subtract 1 % from the head and add half percent to each leg for every year up to 10

**Fig. 4.** Total burn surface area (%). Rule of Nine charts for an adult and a child

need for treatment with antacids for gastric ulcer prophylaxis [39]. The start of the enteral nutrition is made after the airway has been secured in cases of an impeding airway problem.

*Temperature control and regulation*

In the larger burns maintaining body temperature is mandatory as one of the most important functions of the skin – temperature regulation, is affected by the burn. Also evaporative losses from the wounds generate further heat loss, which may further aggravate the situation. Therefore most often, active warming is needed. Temperature assessment needs to be properly done and one very good technique is to have thermistors in the intra bladder part of the urinary catheter which senses the central body temperature. Good heating equipment includes heating ceilings; warm air mattresses (e. g. Bair Hugger®) or fluid heated mattresses (e. g. Allon®).

**Referral to burn center**

When the decision to refer the patient to a burn center is made – a physician to physician contact should be taken and the background of the patient and the details of the accident should be properly communicated. Most often many interventions have been made since the accident and thereafter during transport or at the referral hospital. It is therefore important that all these are properly documented and that this documentation is properly communicated and transferred to the burn care physician. Especially the vital parameters, treatment interventions including fluid treatment and urine output should be documented and reported.

Referral criteria for burn center care may vary, but an often used table is that provided by the ABA, which also is applicable for most parts of Europe (e. g. Sweden), and which is close to that recommended by the European Burns Association in 2002 (Alsbjoern et al. www.euroburn.org).

**Burn center referral criteria [37]**
► Second degree burn > 10 % (TBSA%)
► Third degree burn
► Burns that involve the face, hands, feet, genitalia, perineum, and extending over major joints
► Chemical Burns
► Electrical Burns including lightening injuries
► Any burn injury with concomitant trauma in which the burn injuries pose the greatest risk to the patient
► Inhalation injury
► Patients with pre-existing disease that may com-

plicate the management, prolong recovery or effect mortality

► Hospitals without qualified personal or equipment for the care of the critically burned children

## Transportation

Transportation of the burn victim may involve several steps, – but most often two. The first, is from the site of the accident to a local hospital, or to a similar point for stabilization. The second transport is from the referring hospital to the burn center, where the final treatment is provided. The first transport distance is often short and need for planning is less. Most often in Europe this is done by ambulance and the care during this transport is provided by paramedics or nurses which are stationed in the ambulance. The activities that have been undertaken at the scene of the accidents and during transport are then reported by the paramedics/nurse and/or documented in their report, which may be of complementary value when receiving the patient at the local hospital. In the report data regarding the patient, the circumstances at the scene as well as surveillance data may be found. At this point it is also important to identify the patient and obtain relevant data regarding relatives so that information can be passed on or complementary questions regarding the background of the patient can be obtained.

The second transport is most often done from a local hospital, where the patient has been stabilized and some important burn related treatments have been commenced, such as: intubation/ventilatory treatment in cases of compromised airway; fluid treatment for burn shock. In cases of circulatory compromise escharotomies should have been performed. Important is also that in the early care other trauma induced injuries should have been diagnosed and attended to, – especially if urgent and/or life threatening.

The choice of transport means depend on several factors of which local geography may be important, e. g., in an island or in an archipelago where airborne transport is almost obligatory. In general, transport exceeding 100 km often calls for airborne transport, such as helicopters or aircraft. Smaller hospitals may not have a helicopter landing facility and the first transport then involves an ambulance transport to the airfield. Tertiary referral hospitals (burn centers) in Europe most often have helicopter landing facilities. Specifically, if the patient needs ventilator or other specific intensive care treatments or interventions during transport a specially designed intensive care type ambulance is needed (Figs. 5 and 6).

It is important to stress the need for monitoring during transport, especially in major burns and in ventilated patients. For these patients active heating devices, ventilators and invasive blood pressure monitoring is relevant. It is important for the referring physician to be aware of the monitoring facilities provided by each type of transport system as this may pose a risk if the patient is not properly monitored and/or if interventions if needed are difficult or impossible to undertake during the transport. In some smaller helicopter types critical care interventions may at times be difficult to perform and for such situations ground transport may be preferred. Also the referring physician needs to be updated on the skills and training of the transport surveillance personal, who should be properly trained and have the relevant equipment for the transport that is planned.

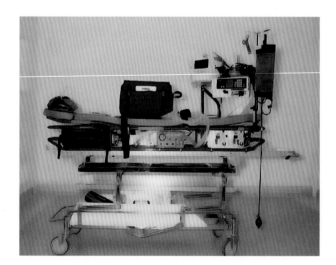

**Fig. 5.** Transportable critical care bed including equipment. Mobile critical care bed, developed for the aircraft emergency services (Sweden). It contains ventilator, breathing gas supplies, intravenous infusion systems as well as monitoring devices. The equipment is standardized so it facilitates transports involving both vehicles and aircraft in the same transport procedure (with permission Liber AB)

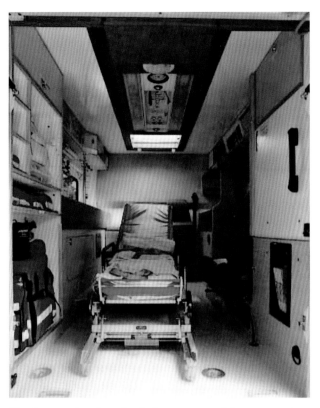

**Fig. 6.** Large interior of ambulance prepared for transporting critically ill patients. The space aside the bed facilitates critical care procedures during transport. It is also feasible to embark a standard critical care bed for transport purposes. The cabin holds complete power supplies as well as mounting racks for standard ventilators, infusion pumps as well as for patient surveillance equipment (with permission Liber AB)

# References

[1] Akerlund E, Huss FR, Sjoberg F (2007) Burns in Sweden: an analysis of 24,538 cases during the period 1987–2004. Burns 33(1): 31–36

[2] Brigham PA, McLoughlin E (1996) Burn incidence and medical care use in the United States: estimates, trends, and data sources. J Burn Care Rehabil 17(2): 95–107

[3] Andel D, Kamolz LP, Niedermayr M, Hoerauf K, Schramm W, Andel H (2007) Which of the abbreviated burn severity index variables are having impact on the hospital length of stay? J Burn Care Res 28(1): 163–166

[4] Still JM, Jr, Law EJ, Belcher K, Thiruvaiyarv D (1996) Decreasing length of hospital stay by early excision and grafting of burns. South Med J 89(6): 578–582

[5] Gomez M, Cartotto R, Knighton J, Smith K, Fish JS (2008) Improved survival following thermal injury in adult patients treated at a regional burn center. J Burn Care Res 29(1): 130–137

[6] Miller SF, Bessey PQ, Schurr MJ, Browning SM, Jeng JC, Caruso DM et al (2006) National burn repository 2005: a ten-year review. J Burn Care Res 27(4): 411–436

[7] Mertens DM, Jenkins ME, Warden GD (1997) Outpatient burn management. Nurs Clin North Am 32(2): 343–364

[8] Moss LS (2004) Outpatient management of the burn patient. Crit Care Nurs Clin North Am 16(1): 109–117

[9] Tompkins D, Rossi LA (2004) Care of out patient burns. Burns 30(8):A7–9

[10] Bessey PQ, Arons RR, Dimaggio CJ, Yurt RW (2006) The vulnerabilities of age: burns in children and older adults. Surgery 140(4): 705–15; discussion 15–17

[11] Sheridan R (2007) Burns at the extremes of age. J Burn Care Res 28(4): 580–585

[12] Thombs BD, Singh VA, Halonen J, Diallo A, Milner SM (2007) The effects of preexisting medical comorbidities on mortality and length of hospital stay in acute burn injury: evidence from a national sample of 31,338 adult patients. Ann Surg 245(4): 629–634

[13] Praiss IL, Feller I, James MH (1980) The planning and organization of a regionalized burn care system. Med Care 18(2): 202–210

[14] Yurt RW, Bessey PQ (2009) The development of a regional system for care of the burn-injured patients. Surg Infect (Larchmt) 10(5): 441–445

[15] Vercruysse GA, Ingram WL, Feliciano DV (2011) The demographics of modern burn care: should most burns be cared for by non-burn surgeons? Am J Surg 201(1): 91–96

[16] Munzberg M, Mahlke L, Bouillon B, Paffrath T, Matthes G, Wolfl CG (2010) [Six years of Advanced Trauma Life Support (ATLS) in Germany: The 100th provider course in Hamburg.]. Unfallchirurg 113(7): 561–566

[17] Soreide K. Three decades (1978–2008) of Advanced Trauma Life Support (ATLS) practice revised and evidence revisited. Scand J Trauma Resusc Emerg Med 16(1): 19

[18] Sasaki J, Takuma K, Oda J, Saitoh D, Takeda T, Tanaka H et al (2010) Experiences in organizing Advanced Burn Life Support (ABLS) provider courses in Japan. Burns 36(1): 65–69

[19] Cochran A, Edelman LS, Morris SE, Saffle JR (2008) Learner satisfaction with Web-based learning as an adjunct to clinical experience in burn surgery. J Burn Care Res 29(1): 222–226

[20] Lindford AJ, Lamyman MJ, Lim P (2006) Review of the emergency management of severe burns (EMSB) course. Burns 32(3): 391

[21] Stone CA, Pape SA (1999) Evolution of the Emergency Management of Severe Burns (EMSB) course in the UK. Burns 25(3): 262–264

[22] Haberal M (2006) Guidelines for dealing with disasters involving large numbers of extensive burns. Burns 32(8): 933–939

[23] Cartotto R (2009) Fluid resuscitation of the thermally injured patient. Clin Plast Surg 36(4): 569–581

[24] Tricklebank S (2009) Modern trends in fluid therapy for burns. Burns 35(6): 757–767

[25] Lund T, Onarheim H, Reed RK (1992) Pathogenesis of edema formation in burn injuries. World J Surg 16(1): 2–9

[26] Vlachou E, Gosling P, Moiemen NS (2006) Microalbuminuria: a marker of endothelial dysfunction in thermal injury. Burns 32(8): 1009–1016

[27] Vlachou E, Gosling P, Moiemen NS (2008) Microalbuminuria: a marker of systemic endothelial dysfunction during burn excision. Burns 34(2): 241–246

[28] Steinvall I, Bak Z, Sjoberg F (2008) Acute respiratory distress syndrome is as important as inhalation injury for the development of respiratory dysfunction in major burns. Burns 34(4): 441–451

[29] Lawrence A, Faraklas I, Watkins H, Allen A, Cochran A, Morris S et al (2010) Colloid administration normalizes resuscitation ratio and ameliorates "fluid creep". J Burn Care Res 31(1): 40–47

[30] Saffle JI (2007) The phenomenon of "fluid creep" in acute burn resuscitation. J Burn Care Res 28(3): 382–95

[31] Baxter CR, Shires T (1968) Physiological response to crystalloid resuscitation of severe burns. Ann N Y Acad Sci 150(3): 874–894

[32] Warden GD (1992) Burn shock resuscitation. World J Surg 16(1): 16–23

[33] Oda J, Yamashita K, Inoue T, Harunari N, Ode Y, Mega K et al (2006) Resuscitation fluid volume and abdominal compartment syndrome in patients with major burns. Burns 32(2): 151–154

[34] Holm C, Mayr M, Tegeler J, Horbrand F, Henckel von Donnersmarck G, Muhlbauer W et al (2004) A clinical randomized study on the effects of invasive monitoring on burn shock resuscitation. Burns 30(8): 798–807

[35] Bak Z, Sjoberg F, Eriksson O, Steinvall I, Janerot-Sjoberg B (2009) Hemodynamic changes during resuscitation after burns using the Parkland formula. J Trauma 66(2): 329–336

[36] Sjoberg F (2008) The 'Parkland protocol' for early fluid resuscitation of burns: too little, too much, or . . . even . . . too late . . .? Acta Anaesthesiol Scand 52(6): 725–726

[37] manual. ABA ABLs. Chicago IL, 2005

[38] Choiniere M, Melzack R, Rondeau J, Girard N, Paquin MJ (1989) The pain of burns: characteristics and correlates. J Trauma 29(11): 1531–1539

[39] Raff T, Germann G, Hartmann B (1997) The value of early enteral nutrition in the prophylaxis of stress ulceration in the severely burned patient. Burns 23(4): 313–318

Correspondence: Folke Sjöberg, M.D., Ph.D., Professor, Consultant, Director, the Burn Center, Department of Hand and Plastic Surgery and Intensive Care, Linköping University Hospital, and Dept. of Clinical and Experimental Medicine, Linköping University, 581 85 Linköping, Sweden, E-mail: folke.sjoberg@liu.se

# Medical documentation of burn injuries

Herbert L. Haller[1], Michael Giretzlehner[2], Johannes Dirnberger[2], Robert Owen[2]

[1] UKH Linz der AUVA, Linz, Austria
[2] Research Unit for Medical-Informatics, RISC Software GmbH, Johannes Kepler University Linz, Upper Austrian Research GmbH, Hagenberg, Austria

## Introduction

### Medical documentation of burn injuries

For successful treatment of burns one of the most important pillars is an adequate documentation. Otherwise, nobody in science, economics or quality control can comprehend this issue's complexity [22]. Research, science and costing in burns are based on accurate assessment and documentation of burn injuries. Documentation required, is time consuming and labor intensive. For any scientific comparability of burns the exact and correct extent and depth of burns are essential.

This simple looking issue is strongly influenced by the acting persons, which leads to a strong demand for the maximum objectivity that can be obtained. Quality of data, required to strengthen the evidence of burn treatment is very much dependent on objective description of the burn injury. Evidence requires comparable patients with comparable wounds and comparable and objective documentation.

Traditional documentation on paper is no valid alternative as requirements for extensive medical documentation are too complex. Among others [68] confirmed a qualitative and quantitative superiority of electronic to paper wound documentation.

Digital documentation provides better availability and assessment of collected data, easier exchange of information between experts and easier access to resources and so supports the creation of medical knowledge. By this, IT contributes remarkably to improvement of quality in management and treatment of burns. This can be of importance when applying admission criteria to burn centers with all their consequences for transport or primary treatment [61]. In particular, bigger amounts of existing information can only be handled successfully by modern computer aided documentation systems.

However, computer-assisted documentation alone does not necessarily create expedient data for scientific use. To ensure optimum evaluation of data, free text documentation needs to be avoided and the information recorded must be clearly structured and standardized [14, 62]. This allows for clear recording facts at a particular time, as for example patient's conditions or single examinations. The quality of data can be improved by well-structured recording and an exact and uniform terminology allowing standardization. However, standardized information provided in this way will be less extensive than in free text documents [28].

### Contents of an up-to-date burns registry

A modern and up-to-date documentation system should cover the following dataset:
► Ethology of burns
► Burn depth and size over the time

- ▶ Surgical steps over the time
- ▶ State at place of accident, first aid and measures
- ▶ Preceding clinical treatment
- ▶ Condition on admission
- ▶ Former illnesses
- ▶ Additional injuries
- ▶ Progression of healing and outcome
- ▶ Complications
- ▶ Photo documentation
- ▶ Traceability and verification of authors

Modern burns management requires multi-professional and interdisciplinary co-operation even between far apart specialists. Thus a system is needed, being able to provide relevant information clearly in due time and over large geographical distances. As only health care personnel with different levels of experience, directly involved in primary care of the patient evaluates the status of the burn wounds initially and draws their conclusions from this, it is essential to provide good photographic material for later evaluation. High quality photo documentation is necessary even under ongoing treatment. Very often, dressing changes are carried out by changing staff; details that might be of importance f or further treatment during dressing change can be reviewed on digital pictures, thus avoiding unnecessary dressing changes only for reviewing the wound. Objective information helps to reduce Chinese whispers, causing wrong therapeutic measures.

*Shortcomings in existing documentation systems designs*

### Free text documentation

Despite the evidence Törnvall et al. stated that filling out papers in wound documentation has severe shortcomings compared to computer-assisted wound documentation, many institutions use paper forms for this and include them in the patient's file [68].

Why does this still happen? On the one hand it is common habit to do so, on the other it is tempting to use a full text description and so not being forced to standardize the observations to be documented. Ostensible advantages of free text documentation are flexible terms, dynamic expressions and the possibility of a more effective, as faster recording by dictation.

But this does not compensate the serious shortcomings linked with it. Due to the linguistic variety and the lack of structure, quality and completeness cannot be verified easily or even not at all.

Undefined sources as basics of systems

Other pitfalls are based on implicit, not really given information, assumed by the documenter or interpreter [28]. So evaluation beyond single patients is extremely difficult. Various solutions use given terms without stating their sources and so using not defined terminologies [27].

### Creation of data cemeteries

Collins English Dictionary defines documentation as "the act of supplying with or using documents or references" [11]. The aim of any documentation is to make the documented facts available. In most cases, the focus of such documentations is the gathering of data itself instead of making existing data available and so to create multiple "data cemeteries".

In some existing documentation systems it is not possible to analyze the collected data statistically.

Missing of contemporary features and functions

Only very few systems are able to gather data via mobile devices as for example laptops, tablet PCs or smartphones. Another shortcoming of existing systems is that it is not possible to access evidence-based knowledge [27].

*Concerning the documentation of burn injuries, burn depth and burn size are the most important facts. Therefore the next sections will discuss the facts including pros and cons. The last section will discuss a computer aided three-dimensional documentation system for burns.*

## Burn depth

A burn is an injury caused by heat. The depth of the burn wound depends on the temperature and on how long the affected area was exposed to the heat. Furthermore, the extent of a burn injury is influenced by the thermal conductivity of the tissue, skin perfusion and existing isolation layers (hair, horn-like structures etc.) [4]. These parameters change dependent on individual circumstances and age of the patient [74]. Deep burns are caused either by a strong noxa or lack of the ability to sense pain, (e. g. polyneuropathy, deep unconsciousness) or immobilisation of the affected persons, which does not allow them to leave the area where they are exposed to the noxa. Cooling and cooling effects can reduce the effects of thermal trauma. The development of the definite burn depth is a dynamic process which is generally finished after 48 hours [53]. However, it can go on for several weeks. Initial treatment with tangential excision can most probably reduce a more deepening of necrosis [41].

In adults, temperatures up to 44 °C do not cause irreversible damage to the cells as long as the time of exposure is less than 6 hours. The damage to the cells doubles with each degree more between 44 °C and 51 °C. Below 45 °C, contact time must be several hours to cause partial skin damage, between 45 °C and 51 °C several minutes, between 51 °C and 70 °C several seconds and above these temperatures several split seconds [46].

Davies has shown the relation between impact of temperature, subjective discomfort, occurrence of a partial and a third degree burn injury [12]. Evans (as cited in Davies) showed that 8.4 Joule/cm$^2$–13.4 J/cm$^2$ cause redness, 13.4 J/cm$^2$–16.0 J/cm$^2$ cause partial skin burn and 16.4 J/cm$^2$–19.7 J/cm$^2$ cause deep burn injuries of the entire skin. Subjective discomfort can be influenced by any pre-existing condition. Polyneuropathy due to various reasons lead to a retarded sensation of the heat by the patient.

## Classification of burn depth

There are various nomenclatures and fundamental characteristics to determine burn depth.

In German-speaking countries burn injuries are classified into three degrees [66].

First-degree burns: Redness and superficial damage of the epithelium without cell death.

Second-degree burns are divided into second-degree superficial burns and second-degree deep burns. A superficial burn (second-degree a) is associated with blisters, a homogenous red surface and strong pain. The epidermis is damaged. Superficial parts of the dermis are damaged and sequestrated. In case the wound bed is less painful, the burn depth is most likely more severe than a second-degree a burn.

Second-degree deep burns are associated with blisters, light surface and less pain than in 2a burns as the pain sensation is reduced. A thrombosis of the intradermal vessel is characterized by a red net-like pattern that does not disappear when touched. The dermis is severely damaged, hair follicles and glands are preserved.

Third degree burns destroy the epidermis and the tissue appears white or dark after cleaning. The wound bed is not painful, however, intact deeper structures maintain their deep sensibility. Epidermis and dermis are destroyed completely.

In the past an additional classification was fourth degree burns. In fourth degree burns chemical damage, charring and lysis was present. More layers, as for example subcutaneous fatty tissue, sometimes muscles, tendons, bones and joints are damaged [66].

In English-speaking countries burns are divided into superficial and deep burns.

1 and 2a degree burns are called superficial partial thickness burns, 2b degree burns are classified into deep partial thickness burn and full thickness burns.

## Classification based on healing time

Burn depth can also be classified according to the healing time. Burns healing within 7 days are classified as superficial or first degree burns, burns healing within 14 days are classified as second degree superficial or partial superficial thickness burns, whereas healing within three weeks is classified as deep partial thickness burns and burns that are only granulating after three weeks are classified as full thickness burns1.

## Burn depth as a dynamic process

Clinical supervision of the progression of the burn depth is important with regard to the therapeutic regime and thus the prognosis after burn trauma [53]. Generally, the burn depth can progress in any stage of the burn treatment [65]. Pathophysiologic factors as for example vasoconstriction [59], vasodilatation [55], hypoperfusion due to hypovolemia, decreasing cardiac output and edema [34] and thrombosis [52] can cause a deepening necrosis as well as infection

[63], edema [45], dehydration [45] and circulary necrosis [43]. Furthermore, local pressure can cause necrosis or can deepen it. Continuous phases of ischemia and reperfusion can also be a reason for a late progressing burn depth [30].

Various papers name hypoxia [35], shock [43], sepsis [10], decreased IL-12 and increased TH-2 cells [7] as well as metabolic disorders as for example decreased glucose uptake and decreased lactate release as reasons for a progressing deepening of the burn wound [49, 64, 69].

Burns in older patients, patients suffering from pathologic vascular alteration, diabetes mellitus and immunosuppression are subject to deepen more easily [65].

## Non-clinical methods to classify burn depth

### Histologic classification of burn depth

The histologic classification of burn depth is generally based on three-zones-model [29]. The zone of coagulation is surrounded by the capillary zone of stasis which itself is surrounded by the zone of hyperemia.

The histologic classification of burn depth is mostly the method of choice. However, its shortcoming is that the denaturation of protein, which is necessary for staining, makes it impossible to take necrotic i. e. denatured protein as parameter for burn depth. Open vessels are detected by hematoxilin-eosin-staining, denatured collagen is detected by Hinshaw-Pearse-staining. The occurrence of thrombosed vessels as a parameter for necrosis is a very sensitive factor; its prediction is timely limited and is subject to various limitations [73]. For Devgan an interpretation of biopsy reports remains subjective regardless of the histologic method [15].

After 48 hours, burn depth is estimated as definite in the initial phase [53].

### Thermography

Thermography is based on the negative correlation between surface temperature and burn depth [37]. This method is distorted by the beginning of wound granulation, so best results can only be achieved within the first three days [15].

Two fundamentally different methods are applied. In static thermography, infrared radiation is measured as temperature [57]; in active dynamic thermography temperature is measured after giving a thermal stimulus. A quantitative determination is carried out by the thermal time constant, i. e. temperature change per time unit after giving thermal stimulus. The thermal properties of tissue depend on its proportion of burn necrosis. In animal experiments, exactness, sensitivity and specificity were 100% in the identification of wounds which healed within 3 weeks [58]. However, very even surrounding conditions are necessary to apply this method successfully.

### Ultrasound

Keratinocytes are destroyed at 47 °C, collagen at 65 °C [25]. Moserova et al. showed that in pigs differences between normal and scalded skin could be demonstrated [47]. Cantrell proved the difference between normal and denatured collagen by ultrasound [9]. Bauer and Sauer [5] and Brink et al. [8] could show correlations between depth and tissue necrosis measured by ultrasound. According to Heimbach et al. burn depth is often underestimated by this method. Unfortunately, the clinical application of ultrasound has not shown any advantages for the burn surgeon so far [25, 72].

### Vital staining

Vital staining is based on the fact that tissue, which is well supplied with blood, stains, and necrosis does not stain. Leape was the first to test methylene blue together with other substances [38]. An intravenous application of methylene blue stains all body parts that are supplied with blood [75]. Methylene blue is degraded within one week to a green and then to an uncolored substance. Thus, surgical measures can be carried out within the first days.

When applying methylene blue as ointment on the body, it is degraded in all areas supplied with blood and not in the areas where necrosis is present. Heimbach et al. was not able to detect the required sharp demarcation for practical use of this method in his clinical examinations. Both procedures might be inhibited by possible allergies [26].

Apart from methylene blue, other substances as for example tetracycline and disulphine blue were examined.

## Fluorescence-fluorometry

This method is based on the activation of fluorescence phenomena after an intravenous application of fluorescent substances. In partial deep burn areas, fluorescence occurs within 10 minutes; in deep burn areas fluorescence does not occur [18]. Thus the measures need to be carried out regularly to determine burn depth. The advantage of this method is its possibility of differentiation between partial and full thickness burns [26].

## Indocyanine-videoangiography

This is a special kind of fluorescence-fluorometry. After applying indocyanine green, the dynamic alteration of the perfusion in the tissue can be recorded by videoangiography. The recording of indocyanine green in the tissue as well as the degradation of the substance provide information about the disturbed microcirculation. This method is highly sensitive and suitable for clinical application [33]. However, ointments and creams can distort the results [24]. The indocyanine clearance can also serve as an indicator for liver function based on perfusion [67].

## Laser-Doppler flowmetry

Laser-Doppler flowmetry (LDF) and Laser-Doppler perfusion monitoring (LDPM) are proceedings which are based on the alteration of wavelength of laser light upon contact with moving erythrocytes. When a tube is applied directly onto the skin, measuring is carried out in 1 mm depth. Exactness is 90 % – 97 %.

Laser Doppler Imaging (LDI) and Laser Doppler Perfusion Imaging (LDPI) are non-contact procedures. After scanning, a photocurrent is produced which shows tissue perfusion. According to the relevant literature the exactness to differentiate between wounds that heal within three weeks and wounds that require more time to heal is 99 % [31]. The validity of this method can be improved by repeated scans, heat provocation or the combination with

other methods. Shortcomings may arise due to the curved surface, the limited scan area and the time that is required for the scan. Light, surface treatment and infection might distort the results [3].

## Polarization dependent optical coherence tomography

This non-invasive method is based on the fact that burn depth correlates with alterations of the skin's double refraction [13]. Animal experiments have shown promising results and clinical application is expected soon [13, 32, 54].

## Reflexion-optical multispectralanalytic imaging method

It is based on the relative patency of the skin for infrared rays. Oxygen reduced hemoglobin reflects less light than tissue that is rich in oxygen. This method was introduced in 1973 [3]. In clinical examinations, the burn depth indicator, which was developed afterwards, showed an exactness of 79 % in wounds for which surgeons were not able to determine their wound characteristics. The highest exactness could be achieved on day 3 after burn trauma. Further developments of the method are based on spectral analysis of four characteristic wavelengths to differentiate burn depth. From the data, false-color photography is produced, which shows the burn depth. The combination of a normal image with the false-color image as well as the simple and fast handling of the system contribute to a high practicability of the method [17]. By combining with the software BurnCase 3D an objective general interpretation of a burn injury was possible for the first time due to a direct transmission of the false-color images to a model that is adjusted to height, weight, sex and type [16].

## Burn extent

### Basic principles of determining the burn extent

The extent of a burn injury is indicated by the proportion of burned body surface in % of the total body surface. First degree burns are not considered. The accurate estimation of patient's burned body surface area as percentage of the total body surface area (TBSA) is crucial for an adequate primary treatment (ventilation, fluid resuscitation, drug dosages, etc.) and for the decision of transferring to specialized burn units [44].

## Variance of evaluation

Evaluating the extent of a burn injury seems to be easy, but is difficult. A study comparing the initial evaluation in the emergency unit with the definite evaluation showed that the extent of the burn injury was overestimated by more than 100% in 24 out of 134 patients [23].

In addition to this, the problem of incorrect representation of the real patient by charts, the complexity of projection from 3D to 2D resides as source of error. Nichter et al. describes an error rate of 29% due to this systemic error, using Rule of Nines and Lund Browder Chart [51].

Another system immanent error is based on the Body Mass Index (BMI). Especially in underweight and obese patients as well as in infants the estimation errors of standard methods are significantly increased [20, 40, 70].

## Influence of the professional background

There was no significant difference between physicians and nursing staff when evaluating the extent of a burn injury [23].

## Methods to determine burn extent

### Rule of palm

Rule: The surface of the patient's palm is about 1% of the total body surface.

Discussion: The rule of palm leads to an overestimation of the real extent of the burn injury by 10%–20%. In adults, the extent of a palm is 0.78% +/− 0.08% of the total body surface [2]. There are also gender-related differences as the palm of a man is 0.8% and the palm of a woman is 0.7% of the total body surface. The isolated palm without fingers is 0.5% in men and 0.4% in women. In children, the palm is 0.92% and the palm without fingers 0.52% [48].

## "Rule of Nines" according to Wallace

Rule: Cited in Knaysi et al.: arms 9% of total body surface each, legs 18% each, chest and back 18% each, head 7% neck 2%, hands and feet, genitals 1% each [36].

Discussion: The "Rule of Nines" has shown good results in patients weighing 10 kg–80 kg. The application of the "Rule of Nines" often leads to an overestimation of the real extent of the burn injury [71], especially in patients with an increased body mass index [6]. In patients weighing more than 80 kg it is more promising to apply a "Rule of Fives", under 10 kg a "Rule of Eights" [40]. "Rule of Nines" is inaccurate and should not be applied in infants and children due to the strong change of proportions during growth.

## Lund Browder Chart

The Lund Browder Chart assigns various age groups to various body proportions and is thus more exact than the "Rule of Nines" [42].

Discussion: Several authors have shown an overestimation of the extent of the burn injury when applying the Lund Browder Chart [51]. Alm showed in 90% of the cases, an overestimation of the burn extent by 17.8% on average [1]. Nichter et al. showed an overestimation by 12.4% on average [51]. This form of evaluation has system immanent errors because it is based on only one type of physique. Various forms of corpulence and different weight categories cannot be considered. The standardization to different age groups in children (Years: 1, 5, 10, 15) is a rather approximate one, as the biggest changes in proportions of children happen during the first years.

## Additional information sheets for reporting burn injuries

Insurance companies often ask for an additional information sheet as report of severe burn injuries. It mostly is a more or less modified Lund Browder Chart.

Discussion: If the burn extent primarily is determined according to this information sheet, it later serves as a basis for determining the surface of body parts in expertise. It shows the same problems like Lund Browder Chart, but has often major financial and juristic impact.

## 3D – computer assisted evaluation

Sage II, Burn Vision 3D [50], BurnCase 3D [19] are existing systems that are currently in use. Sage II is a two-dimensional system, the others are three-dimensional.

To overcome the drawbacks of existing estimation methods, the three-dimensional structure of the human body surface must be taken into account when determining the TBSAB (Total Body Surface Area Burned) of an individual patient. Modern computer graphics software is an effective, user-friendly way of dealing with three-dimensional surfaces. As already proposed by [39], the estimation and documentation of burned surface area on three-dimensional virtual models qualify to overcome difficulties in burn documentation.

It has been shown, that by the use of computer-assisted assessment procedures, the variability of results among different observers can be reduced [50]. Discussion:

▶ Three dimensional systems help to avoid of system immanent error: Only a three-dimensional model can ensure a sufficient documentation of the burn injury and its interpretation. In the two dimensional anterior – posterior view it is nearly impossible to classify and to illustrate burns of the lateral part of the body.

▶ Exact documentation needs appropriate graphic resolution. The resolution of BurnVision is too low to get details. Only BurnCase3D has a sufficient resolution of $1\,cm^2$ to illustrate height and weight as well as type of physique sufficiently.

▶ Optical resolution of SageII is not described.

## Computer aided three-dimensional documentation systems

Software-based diagnostics and documentation in modern medicine is a growing field, becoming very popular nowadays. In contrast, classification and documentation of human burn injuries and their follow-up is still a manually performed procedure, based on paper estimation charts, free text records and most of all strongly dependent on individual impression and medical experience of the physician involved.

The exploitation of modern computer graphics technology is an effective and user-friendly way of dealing with 3D surfaces. As stated above, the estimation and documentation of burned surface area by means of 3D computer graphics is appropriate for mastering the difficulties of burn diagnostics and treatment. Electronic systems like BurnCase 3D take the three-dimensional structure of the human body surface into account when determining the TBSA of an individual patient. BurnCase 3D also regards different body shapes caused by sexual differences, age, weight, size and corpulence.

The usage of computer-aided methods can tremendously reduce error rates, but still the problem of incorrect input of burn areas resides. A major reason for input errors by chance or intended is clearly the fact of "subjective cognition" of wound areas for different reasons and the complexity of transferring the three-dimensional wound surface onto a two-dimensional estimation chart. Another reason is the fact that every patient is an individual, not exactly fitting the mean human body shape and surface proposed by all common estimation methods; even by models of BurnCase3D. The only way to change this would be the creation of individual models from 3D scanners or tomography, but this till today is not feasible in praxis.

## Methods used by BurnCase 3D

To overcome the issues described above, it is essential to find a way to objectively define the burned surface area and link all collected relevant data to be able to reduce the work load on the one hand and support the personnel in making decisions for the further medical treatment on the other hand, with balanced scientific claim and pragmatic feasibility.

A development team consisting of computer scientists and medical scientists has been working on a state-of-the-art software system named BurnCase 3D since 2001. During this research project, which follows the principles of action research, many chal-

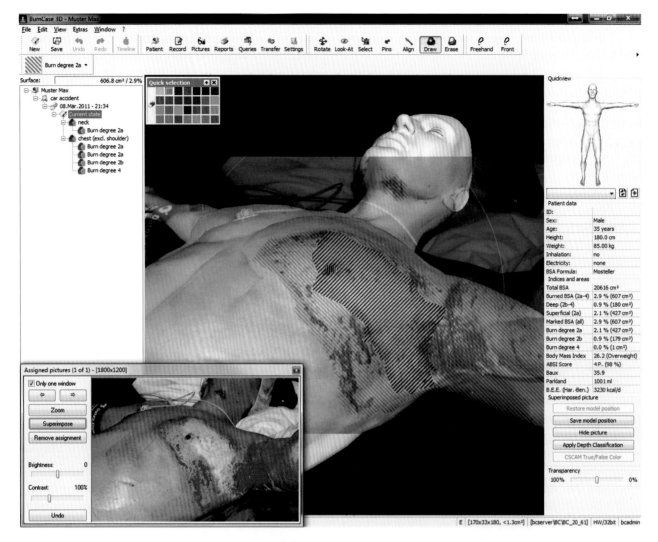

**Fig. 1.** User interface showing the virtual 3D model different burn degrees, calculated scores and an integrated digital picture archive

lenges of modern burn care have been taken into account by the developers. Its strength is the simple and intuitive user interface; allowing quick data input without the need of sophisticated training (Fig. 1).

## Technical description

The system operates on a 3D virtual body representing the real patient. This model is build up as a three-dimensional mesh of over 90 000 connected triangles with each smaller than one cm². By specifying age, sex, height and weight and choosing an appropriate 3D standard model the system is able to generate an automatically adapted virtual body surface which accurately fits the patient's individual body shape. The standard model is precisely adapted to the patient's height by scaling in longitudinal direction. Afterwards, a surface adaptation algorithm deor inflates the model until its TBSA exactly reaches the predicted value calculated by an established TBSA estimation formula.

BurnCase 3D incorporates the 12 most widely accepted TBSA estimation formulas in scientific literature. The adaptation algorithm also takes into account the growth behavior of different body regions in order to reach a realistic body expansion.

## 3D registration

The burned surface area is marked on the 3D body surface by standard mouse interaction. The user simply sketches the burned area with the mouse or pen cursor and BurnCase 3D projects this two-dimensional polygon onto the underlying three-dimensional body. Consequently, the marked area appears in a significant color and pattern, thus visualizing different burn degrees of injuries or even surgical procedures, dressings or medications. The covered surface area, as well as the affected percentage of the total body surface area (TBSA) and based on these values several medical scored and indices (ASBI, Baux, Baxter-Parkland, etc.) are calculated in real-time and presented on the user interface immediately after drawing. By rotation and zooming of the model all parts of the body can be assessed and documented.

## Work reduction by automated creation of codes

The surface areas classified to burn degrees as well as operative procedures are automatically encoded to the different medical codes, which are often needed for reimbursement.

## Creation of treatment history

An 3D state of the patient can be created and revisited at different points in time throughout the whole treatment. Thus, a comprehensive three-dimensional track of the complete treatment history is created and stored in the database for every patient.

## Additional burn- related information

Additional burn-related information such as course of accident, first aid, complications, former illnesses, and condition on admission, etc. can also be acquired and stored to the database. In order to be able to supervise all changes to the stored data, BurnCase 3D keeps track of every data acquisition or deletion in a separate change log. The data collection is compatible to the United States' National Trauma Registry (NTRACS).

## Objectivities by visual verification

In order to further increase the level of accuracy, an integrated digital picture archive provides visual verification by superimposing pictures on the 3D model. In addition, an intuitive model-picture-registration algorithm has been implemented, which allows the physician to easily move the virtual body in the position of the patient on any digital picture. By doing so, the whole burn surface estimation procedure becomes as easy as sketching the border of burn wounds on a picture, however reducing the drawback of subjective influences.

## Archiving photos

The system assigns photos in a simple and intuitive way to patients, dates, areas, burn conditions, procedures and even 3D location. Photos can be searched by these criteria after insertion.

## Way to objective assessment of burn extent and burn depth

The combination of this 3D surface area information with available burn depth classification methods

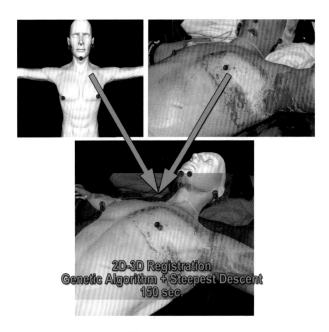

**Fig. 2.** Model-Picture-Alignment procedure with 2D (red) and 3D (blue) reference points

leads to an automatic and objective characterization and documentation of burn injuries. For example, a special CCD camera together with appropriate classification software is developed by Dr. Werner Eisenbeiss and Dr. Jörg Marotz in Lübeck, Germany at Delphi-Optics GmbH. Moreover, other methods like Laser-Doppler-Measurement (Moore Instruments, UK) or Infrared Spectroscopy (NRCC, Canada) show different behaviors due to relying on different physical properties, but they can also be used as classification input for BurnCase 3D.

## Creating a comparable international database

BurnCase 3D is designed as stand-alone procedure, as hospital network or as national or international database. The system provides necessary data protection by anonymisation and encryption of data to be transferred within the systems.

## Results

In contrast to common estimation methods mentioned above, BurnCase 3D uses an accurate three-dimensional model of the patient for the surface calculation. Thus, a very high validity regarding the total body surface area can be achieved. Moreover, visual comparison between the real patient and the adapted virtual model enables verification that has not been possible before.

The benefits of using a computer-aided burn classification and documentation procedure over arbitrary paper estimation charts are obvious. A tremendous reduction of work load for documentation purposes for the physician is the major advantage resulting in more time for patient's treatment. Secondly, this software system lowers the risk of over- and underestimation of burn wounds by less experienced physicians. For the first time, an objective diagnostic method for burn injuries is available, which allows comparison studies even of different institutions and countries on a substantiated data basis. Finally, there is an obvious benefit for the hospital's accounting since all necessary medical encodings like ICD10 are generated automatically.

First results of the BurnCase 3D project have been published by Dirnberger and Diretzlehner.

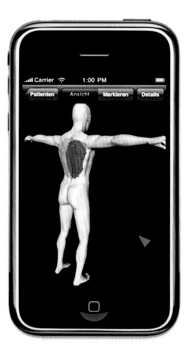

**Fig. 3.** Mobile version of the burn injury documentation system BurnCase 3D

BurnCase 3D is currently deployed in several burn units in Europe and the US, since 2004 a continuously growing number of hospitals in Linz (AUT), Vienna (AUT), Feldkirch (AUT), Halle/Saale (GER), Lübeck (GER), Mannheim (GER), Rotterdam (NED), Galveston (USA), Phoenix (USA), Birmingham (GB), Rome (IT) and Zürich (CH) are using the system for their burn surface estimation and documentation. The system is available as stand-alone and as network version providing a central database of burn cases directly connected to the institution's hospital information system (HIS). The integration of classification images as described above is easily possible. The software system is ready to be installed on a common Microsoft Windows© personal computer and uses the OpenGL© technology for 3D visualization.

As most of the physicians possess smartphones, it is quite reasonable to make use of this existing hardware. The research team has already gained experience in the implementation of three-dimensional documentation systems into mobile platforms. A mobile version of BurnCase 3D for the platform iPhone OS© (iPod©, iPhone©, iPad©) by Apple© is already available.

## Conclusion

The primary aim of the BurnCase 3D project is to significantly improve the quality of body surface estimation in burn care. The use of BurnCase 3D could have a true impact on the quality of treatment in burns. Consequently, an improvement of the outcome of burn patients can be achieved. In order to reach this goal, it is necessary to deploy the system on a broad basis of burn units all over the world and to collect the experiences of these.

It is clearly stated by the development team, that a lot of work has to be done in order to scientifically prove the correctness and accuracy of the surface estimation results. Especially in infant and obese patients the model library still has some limitations. Further investigations on the body surface areas and body shapes of these patient groups have to be performed. Consequently, it will be necessary to further improve the accuracy by an extension of the 3D model adaptation method in a way that certain body regions can be in- or deflated separately according to the patient's physiological state. Several burn units are evaluating the system and their feedback influences the on-going development. A free basic version of BurnCase 3D and more information can be obtained from www.burncase. at.

## Financing and accomplishment

The research project BurnCase 3D is publicly funded and carried out at the RISC Software GmbH, Research Unit for Medical-Informatics, a Research & Development company of the Johannes Kepler University Linz, Austria. All earnings are reinvested future developments. This project and the application of the BurnCase 3D software system are supported by grants of the Upper Austrian Local Government, the Upper Austrian Health-Fund and all participating medical partners.

## References

[1] Alm J (2003) A Retrospective Study of TBSA-B Calculating;V Manual Estimated Burnchart versus Computerized Burncharts. Final Programme and Abstracts – 10 Congress European Burns Association Bergen, Norway Sept. 10–13n 2003. Bergen, Norway: EBA; 2003: 158

[2] Amirsheybani HR, Crecelius GM, Timothy NH, Pfeiffer M, Saggers GC, Manders EK (2001) The natural history of the growth of the hand: I. Hand area as a percentage of body surface area. Plast Reconstr Surg 107: 726–733

[3] Anselmo VJ, Zawacki BE (1977) Multispectral photographic analysis. A new quantitative tool to assist in the early diagnosis of thermal burn depth. Ann Biomed Eng 5: 179–193

[4] Arturson G (1996) Mechanism of Injury. In: Settle JAD (ed) Principles and practice of burns management. Churchill Livingstone, New York, pp 61–82

[5] Bauer JA, Sauer T (1989) Cutaneous 10 MHz ultrasound B scan allows the quantitative assessment of burn depth. Burns Incl Therm Inj 15: 49–51

[6] Berry MG, Evison D, Roberts AH (2001) The influence of body mass index on burn surface area estimated from the area of the hand. Burns 27: 591–594

[7] Bjornson AB, Altemeier WA, Bjornson HS (1976) Reduction in C3 conversion in patients with severe thermal injury. J Trauma 16: 905–911

[8] Brink JA, Sheets PW, Dines KA, Etchison MR, Hanke CW, Sadove AM (1986) Quantitative assessment of burn injury in porcine skin with high-frequency ultrasonic imaging. Invest Radiol 21: 645–651

[9] Cantrell JH, Jr (1984) Can ultrasound assist an experienced surgeon in estimating burn depth? J Trauma 24: S64–S70

[10] Carvajal HF (1994) Fluid resuscitation of pediatric burn victims: a critical appraisal. Pediatr Nephrol 8: 357–366

[11] Collins English Dictionary (2009) Harper Collins Publishers

[12] Davies JWL (1997) Interactions of heat with tissues. In: Cooper GJ (ed) Scientific foundations of trauma. Butterworth-Heinemann, Oxford, pp 389–409

[13] de Boer JF, Milner TE, van Gemert MJC (1977) Two-dimensional birefringence imaging in biological tissue by polarisation- sensitive optical coherence tomografy. Opt Len 22: 934–936

[14] Deering SH, Tobler K, Cypher R (2010) Improvement in documentation using an electronic checklist for shoulder dystocia deliveries. Obstet Gynecol 116: 63–66

[15] Devgan L, Bhat S, Aylward S, Spence RJ (2006) Modalities for the assessment of burn wound depth. J Burns Wounds 5:e2

[16] Dirnberger J, Giretzlehner M, Ruhmer M, Haller H, Rodemund C (2003) Modelling human burn injuries in a three-dimensional virtual environment. Stud Health Technol Inform 94: 52–58

[17] Eisenbeiss W, Marotz J, Schrade JP (1999) Reflection-optical multispectral imaging method for objective determination of burn depth. Burns 25: 697–704

[18] Gatti JE, LaRossa D, Silverman DG, Hartford CE (1983) Evaluation of the burn wound with perfusion fluorometry. J Trauma 23: 202–206

[19] Giretzlehner M, Dirnberger J, Luckeneder T, Haller H, Rodemund C (2004) BurnCase 3D: A research product for effective and time-saving documentation of burn injuries. Annals of Burns and Fire Disasters XVII (2): 64–72

[20] Livingston EH, Lee S (2001) Body surface area prediction in normal-weight and obese patients. Am J Physiol Endocrinol Metab 281:E586-E591

[21] Haller H (2007) Data collection in burn injuries- Rationale for BurnCase 3D. Osteo trauma care 15: 34–41

[22] Haller HL, Dirnberger J, Giretzlehner M, et al (2009) "Understanding burns": research project BurnCase 3D–overcome the limits of existing methods in burns documentation. Burns 35: 311–317

[23] Hammond JS, Ward CG (1987) Transfers from emergency room to burn center: errors in burn size estimate. J Trauma 27: 1161–1165

[24] Haslik W, Kamolz LP, Andel H, Winter W, Meissl G, Frey M (2004) The influence of dressings and ointments on the qualitative and quantitative evaluation of burn wounds by ICG video-angiography: an experimental setup. Burns 30: 232–235

[25] Heimbach D, Engrav L, Grube B, Marvin J (1992) Burn depth: a review. World J Surg 16: 10–15

[26] Heimbach D, Mann R, Engrav L (2002) Evaluation of burn wound management decisions. In: Herndon DN (ed) Total burn care. 2nd edn, Saunders, London, New York, pp 101–108

[27] Hübner U, Flemming D, Schultz-Gödker A (2009) Software zur digitalen Wunddokumentation: Marktübersicht und Bewertungskriterien. WundM 3(6): 16–25

[28] Ingenerf J (2009) Computergestützte strukturierte Befundung am Beispiel der Wunddokumentation. WundM 3(6): 264–268

[29] Jackson DM (1953) The diagnosis of the depth of burning. Br J Surg 40: 588–596

[30] Jaskille AD, Jeng JC, Sokolich JC, Lunsford P, Jordan MH (2007) Repetitive ischemia-reperfusion injury: a plausible mechanism for documented clinical burn-depth progression after thermal injury. J Burn Care Res 28: 13–20

[31] Jeng JC, Bridgeman A, Shivnan L, et al (2003) Laser Doppler imaging determines need for excision and grafting in advance of clinical judgment: a prospective blinded trial. Burns 29: 665–670

[32] Jiao S, Yu W, Stoica G, Wang LV (2003) Contrast mechanisms in polarization-sensitive Mueller-matrix optical coherence tomography and application in burn imaging. Appl Opt 42: 5191–5197

[33] Kamolz LP, Andel H, Haslik W, et al (2003) Indocyanine green video angiographies help to identify burns requiring operation. Burns 29: 785–791

[34] Kao CC, Garner WL (2000) Acute burns. Plast Reconstr Surg 105: 2482–2492

[35] Kim DE, Phillips TM, Jeng JC, et al (2001) Microvascular assessment of burn depth conversion during varying resuscitation conditions. J Burn Care Rehabil 22: 406–416

[36] Knaysi GA, Crikelair GF, Cosman B (1968) The role of nines: its history and accuracy. Plast Reconstr Surg 41: 560–563

[37] Lawson RN, Gaston JP (1964) Temperature measurements of localized pathological processes. Ann N Y Acad Sci. 121: 90–98

[38] Leape LL, Randolph JG (1965) The early surgical treatment of burns. II. Clinical application of intravenous vital dye (patent blue V) in the differentiation of partial and full-thickness burns. Surgery 57: 886–893

[39] Lee JY, Choi JW (2006) Validity and reliability of an alginate method to measure body surface area. J Physiol Anthropol 25: 247–255

[40] Livingston EH, Lee S (2000) Percentage of burned body surface area determination in obese and nonobese patients. J Surg Res 91: 106–110

[41] Lu S, Xiang J, Jin S, et al (2002) [Histological observation of the effects of tangential excision within twenty-four postburn hours on the progressive injury of the progression of deep partial thickness burn wound]. Zhonghua Shao Shang Za Zhi 18: 235–237

[42] Lund CC, Browder CN (1944) The estimate of the areas of burn. Surg Gyn Obstet 79: 352–358

[43] Matouskova E, Broz L, Pokorna E, Koenigova R (2002) Prevention of burn wound conversion by allogenig ceratinocytes cultured on allegenic xenodermis. Cell and Tissue Banking 3: 29–35

[44] McGwin G, Jr., Cross JM, Ford JW, et al (2003) Long-term trends in mortality according to age among adult burn patients. J. Burn Care Rehabil 24: 21–25

[45] Miller PR, Kuo KN, Lubicky JP (1995) Clubfoot deformity in Down's syndrome. Orthopedics 18: 449–452

[46] Moritz AR, Henriques FC (1947) Studies of thermal injuries II. The relative importance of time and surface temperature in the causation of cutaneous burns. Am J Pathol 23: 695–720

[47] Moserova J, Hlava P, Malinsky J (1982) Scope for ultrasound diagnosis of the depth of thermal damage. Preliminary report. Acta Chir Plast 24: 235–242

[48] Nagel TR, Schunk JE (1997) Using the hand to estimate the surface area of a burn in children. Pediatr Emerg Care 13: 254–255

[49] Nelson KM, Turinsky J (1981) Local effect of burn on skeletal muscle insulin responsiveness. J Surg Res 31: 288–297

[50] Neuwalder JM, Sampson C, Breuing KH, Orgill DP (2002) A review of computer-aided body surface area determination: SAGE II and EPRI's 3D Burn Vision. J Burn Care Rehabil 23: 55–59

[51] Nichter LS, Bryant CA, Edlich RF (1985) Efficacy of burned surface area estimates calculated from charts-the need for a computer-based model. J Trauma 25: 477–481

[52] Nwariaku FE, Sikes PJ, Lightfoot E, Mileski WJ, Baxter C (1996) Effect of a bradykinin antagonist on the local inflammatory response following thermal injury. Burns 22: 324–327

[53] Papp A, Kiraly K, Harma M, Lahtinen T, Uusaro A, Alhava E (2004) The progression of burn depth in experimental burns: a histological and methodological study. Burns 30: 684–690

[54] Park BH, Saxer C, Srinivas SM, Nelson JS, de Boer JF (2001) In vivo burn depth determination by high-speed fiber-based polarization sensitive optical coherence tomography. J Biomed Opt 6: 474–479

[55] Rawlingson A (2003) Nitric oxide, inflammation and acute burn injury. Burns 29: 631–640

[56] Ref Type: Internet Communication

[57] Renkielska A, Nowakowski A, Kaczmarek M, et al (2005) Static thermography revisited–an adjunct method for determining the depth of the burn injury. Burns 31: 768–775

[58] Renkielska A, Nowakowski A, Kaczmarek M, Ruminski J (2006) Burn depths evaluation based on active dynamic IR thermal imaging–a preliminary study. Burns 32: 867–875

[59] Robson MC, Del Beccaro EJ, Heggers JP (1979) The effect of prostaglandins on the dermal microcirculation after burning, and the inhibition of the effect by specific pharmacological agents. Plast Reconstr Surg 63: 781–787

[60] Rossiter ND, Chapman P, Haywood IA (1996) How big is a hand? Burns 22: 230–231

[61] Saffle JR, Edelman L, Theurer L, et al (2009) Telemedicine evaluation of acute burns is accurate and cost-effective. J Trauma 67: 358–365

[62] Samuels JG (2010) Abstracting pain management documentation from the electronic medical record: comparison of three hospitals. Appl Nurs Res (epub ahead of print)

[63] Sawhney CP, Sharma RK, Rao KR, Kaushish R (1989) Long-term experience with 1 per cent topical silver sulphadiazine cream in the management of burn wounds. Burns 15: 403–406

[64] Shangraw RE, Turinsky J (1979) Local effect of burn injury on glucose and amino acid metabolism by skeletal muscle. JPEN J Parenter Enteral Nutr 3: 323–327

[65] Singh V, Devgan L, Bhat S, Milner SM (2007) The pathogenesis of burn wound conversion. Ann Plast Surg 59: 109–115

[66] Steen M (2002) Leitlinien Verbrennungsbehandlung der Deutschen Gesellschaft für Verbrennungsmedizin, 1-2-2002

[67] Tokunaga Y, Ozaki N, Wakashiro S, et al (1988) Effects of perfusion pressure during flushing on the viability of the procured liver using noninvasive fluorometry. Transplantation 45: 1031–1035

[68] Törnvall E, Wilhelmsson S, Wahren LK (2004) Electronic nursing documentation in primary health care. Scand J Caring Sci 18: 310–317

[69] Turinsky J, Shangraw R (1979) Biphasic alterations in glucose metabolism by soleus muscle from the burned limb. Adv Shock Res 2: 23–30

[70] Verbraecken J, Van de HP, De BW, et al (2006) Body surface area in normal-weight, overweight, and obese adults. A comparison study. Metabolism 55: 515–524

[71] Wachtel TL, Berry CC, Wachtel EE, Frank HA (2000) The inter-rater reliability of estimating the size of burns from various burn area chart drawings. Burns 26: 156–170

[72] Wachtel TL, Leopold GR, Frank HA, Frank DH (1986) B-mode ultrasonic echo determination of depth of thermal injury. Burns Incl Therm Inj 12: 432–437

[73] Watts AM, Tyler MP, Perry ME, Roberts AH, McGrouther DA (2001) Burn depth and its histological measurement. Burns 27: 154–160

[74] Webne S, Kaplan BJ, Shaw M (1989) Pediatric burn prevention: an evaluation of the efficacy of a strategy to reduce tap water temperature in a population at risk for scalds. J Dev Behav Pediatr 10: 187–191

[75] Zawacki BE, Walker HL (1970) An evaluation of patent blue V, bromphenol blue, and tetracycline for the diagnosis of burn depth. Plast Reconstr Surg 45: 459–465

Correspondence: Dr. Herbert L. Haller, UKH Linz der AUVA, Garnisonstraße 7, 4021 Linz, Austria, E-mail: herbert.haller@utanet.at; Dr. Michael Giretzlehner, Research Unit for Medical-Informatics, RISC Software GmbH, Johannes Kepler University Linz, Upper Austrian Research GmbH, Softwarepark 35, 4232 Hagenberg, Austria, E-mail: michael.giretzlehner@risc.uni-linz.ac.at

# Pathophysiology of burn injury

Gerd G. Gauglitz[1,3], Marc G. Jeschke[2]

[1] Shriners Hospitals for Children, University of Texas Medical Branch Galveston, TX, USA
[2] Ross Tilley Burn Centre, Sunnybrook Health Sciences Centre, Department of Surgery, Division of Plastic Surgery, University of Toronto, ON, Canada
[3] Department of Dermatology and Allergology, Ludwig Maximilians University, Munich, Germany

## Introduction

Burn injury represents a significant problem worldwide. More than 1 million burn injuries occur annually in the United States. Although most of these burn injuries are minor, approximately 40,000 to 60,000 burn patients require admission to a hospital or major burn center for appropriate treatment every year [1]. The devastating consequences of burns have been recognized by the medical community and significant amounts of resources and research have been dedicated, successfully improving these dismal statistics: Recent reports revealed a 50% decline in burn-related deaths and hospital admissions in the USA over the last 20 years; mainly due to effective prevention strategies, decreasing the number and severity of burns [2, 3]. Advances in therapy strategies, due to improved understanding of resuscitation, enhanced wound coverage, better support of hypermetabolic response to injury, more appropriate infection control and improved treatment of inhalation injury, based on better understanding of the pathophysiologic responses after burn injury have further improved the clinical outcome of this unique patient population over the past years. This chapter describes the present understanding of the pathophysiology of a burn injury including both the local and systemic responses, focusing on the many facets of organ and systemic effects directly resulting from hypovolemia and circulating mediators following burn trauma.

## Local changes

Locally, thermal injury causes coagulative necrosis of the epidermis and underlying tissues, with the depth of injury dependent upon the temperature to which the skin is exposed, the specific heat of the causative agent, and the duration of exposure.

Burns are classified into five different causal categories/etiologies and depths of injury. The causes include injury from flame (fire), hot liquids (scald), contact with hot or cold objects, chemical exposure, and/or conduction of electricity. The first three induce cellular damage by the transfer of energy, which induces coagulative necrosis. Chemical burns and electrical burns cause direct injury to cellular membranes in addition to the transfer of heat.

The skin, which is the largest organ on the human body, provides a staunch barrier in the transfer of energy to deeper tissues, thus confining much of the injury to this layer. Once the inciting focus is removed, however, the response of local tissues can lead to injury in the deeper layers. The area of cutaneous or superficial injury has been divided into three zones: zone of coagulation, zone of stasis, and zone of hyperemia. The necrotic area of burn where cells have been disrupted is termed the *zone of coagulation*. This tissue is irreversibly damaged at the time of injury. The area immediately surrounding the necrotic zone has a moderate degree of insult with decreased tissue perfusion. This is termed the *zone of stasis* and, depending on the wound environment, can either survive or go on to coagulative necrosis. The zone of stasis is associated with vascular damage and vessel leakage [4]. Thromboxane A2, a potent vasoconstrictor, is present in high concentrations in burn wounds, and local application of inhibitors improves blood flow and decreases the zone of stasis. Antioxidants, bradykinin antagonists, and subatmospheric wound pressures also improve blood flow and affect the depth of injury [5–8]. Local endothelial interactions with neutrophils mediate some of the local inflammatory responses associated with the zone of stasis. Treatment directed at the control of local inflammation immediately after injury may spare the zone of stasis, indicated by studies demonstrating the blockage of leukocyte adherence with anti-CD18 or anti-intercellular adhesion molecules monoclonal antibodies improves tissue perfusion and tissue survival in animal models [9]. The last area is the *zone of hyperemia,* which is characterized by vasodilation from inflammation surrounding the burn wound. This region contains the clearly viable tissue from which the healing process begins and is generally not at risk for further necrosis.

## Burn depth

The depth of burn varies depending on the degree of tissue damage. Burn depth is classified into degree of injury in the epidermis, dermis, subcutaneous fat, and underlying structures. First-degree burns are, by definition, injuries confined to the epidermis. First-degree burns are painful, erythematous, and blanch to the touch with an intact epidermal barrier. Examples include sunburn or a minor scald from a kitchen accident. These burns do not result in scarring, and treatment is aimed at comfort with the use of topical soothing salves with or without aloe and oral nonsteroidal anti-inflammatory agents.

Second-degree burns are divided into two types: superficial and deep. All second-degree burns have some degree of dermal damage, by definition, and the division is based on the depth of injury into the dermis. Superficial dermal burns are erythematous, painful, blanch to touch, and often blister. Examples include scald injuries from overheated bathtub water and flash flame burns. These wounds spontaneously re-epithelialize from retained epidermal structures

in the rete ridges, hair follicles, and sweat glands in one to two weeks. After healing, these burns may have some slight skin discoloration over the long term. Deep dermal burns into the reticular dermis appear more pale and mottled, do not blanch to touch, but remain painful to pinprick. These burns heal in two to five weeks by re-epithelialization from hair follicles and sweat gland keratinocytes, often with severe scarring as a result of the loss of dermis.

Third-degree burns are full thickness through the epidermis and dermis and are characterized by a hard, leathery eschar that is painless and black, white, or cherry red. No epidermal or dermal appendages remain; thus, these wounds must heal by re-epithelialization from the wound edges. Deep dermal and full-thickness burns require excision with skin grafting from the patient to heal the wounds in a timely fashion.

Fourth-degree burns involve other organs beneath the skin, such as muscle, bone, and brain.

Currently, burn depth is most accurately assessed by judgment of experienced practitioners. Accurate depth determination is critical to wound healing as wounds that will heal with local treatment are treated differently than those requiring operative intervention. Examination of the entire wound by the physicians ultimately responsible for their management then is the gold standard used to guide further treatment decisions. New technologies, such as the multi-sensor laser Doppler flow-meter, hold promise for quantitatively determining burn depth. Several recent reports claim superiority of this method over clinical judgment in the determination of wounds requiring skin grafting for timely healing, which may lead to a change in the standard of care in the near future [10].

## Burn size

Determination of burn size estimates the extent of injury. Burn size is generally assessed by the "rule of nines". In adults, each upper extremity and the head and neck are 9% of the TBSA, the lower extremities and the anterior and posterior trunk are 18% each, and the perineum and genitalia are assumed to be 1% of the TBSA. Another method of estimating smaller burns is to equate the area of the open hand (including the palm and the extended fingers) of the patient to be approximately 1% TBSA and then to transpose that measurement visually onto the wound for a determination of its size. This method is crucial when evaluating burns of mixed distribution.

Children have a relatively larger portion of the body surface area in the head and neck, which is compensated for by a relatively smaller surface area in the lower extremities. Infants have 21% of the TBSA in the head and neck and 13% in each leg, which incrementally approaches the adult proportions with increasing age. The Berkow formula is used to accurately determine burn size in children.

## Systemic changes

The release of cytokines and other inflammatory mediators at the site of injury has a systemic effect once the burn reaches 30% of total body surface area (TBSA). Cutaneous thermal injury greater than one-third of the total body surface area invariably results in the severe and unique derangements of cardiovascular function called burn shock. Shock is an abnormal physiologic state in which tissue perfusion is insufficient to maintain adequate delivery of oxygen and nutrients and removal of cellular waste products. Before the nineteenth century, investigators demonstrated that after a burn, fluid is lost from the blood and blood becomes thicker; and in 1897, saline infusions for severe burns were first advocated [11, 12]. However, a more complete understanding of burn pathophysiology was not reached until the work of Frank Underhill [13]. He found that unresuscitated burn shock correlates with increased hematocrit values in burned patients, which are secondary to fluid and electrolyte loss after burn injury. Increased hematocrit values occurring shortly after severe burn were interpreted as a plasma volume deficit. Cope and Moore showed that the hypovolemia of burn injury resulted from fluid and protein translocation into both burned and nonburned tissues [14].

Over the last 80-years an extensive record of both animal and clinical studies has established the importance of fluid resuscitation for burn shock. Investigations have focused on correcting the rapid and massive fluid sequestration in the burn wound and the resultant hypovolemia. The peer-reviewed litera-

ture contains a large experimental and clinical database on the circulatory and microcirculatory alterations associated with burn shock and edema generation in both the burn wound and non-burned tissues. During the last 40-years, research has focused on identifying and defining the release mechanisms and effects of the many inflammatory mediators produced and released after burn injury [15].

It is now well recognized that burn shock is a complex process of circulatory and microcirculatory dysfunction that is not easily or fully repaired by fluid resuscitation. Severe burn injury results in significant hypovolemic shock and substantial tissue trauma, both of which cause the formation and release of many local and systemic mediators [16-18]. Burn shock results from the interplay of hypovolemia and the release of multiple mediators of inflammation with effects on both the microcirculation as well as the function of the heart, large vessels and lungs. Subsequently, burn shock continues as a significant pathophysiologic state, even if hypovolemia is corrected. Increases in pulmonary and systemic vascular resistance (SVR) and myocardial depression occur despite adequate preload and volume support [18-22]. Such cardiovascular dysfunctions can further exacerbate the whole body inflammatory response into a vicious cycle of accelerating organ dysfunction [17, 18, 23]. Hemorrhagic hypovolemia with severe mechanical trauma can provoke a similar form of shock.

### Hypovolemia and rapid edema formation

Burn injury causes extravasation of plasma into the burn wound and the surrounding tissues. Extensive burn injuries are hypovolemic in nature and characterized by the hemodynamic changes similar to those that occur after hemorrhage, including decreased plasma volume, cardiac output, urine output, and an increased systemic vascular resistance with resultant reduced peripheral blood flow [16, 18, 24-26]. However, as opposed to a fall in hematocrit with hemorrhagic hypovolemia due to transcapillary refill an increase in hematocrit and hemoglobin concentration will often appear even with adequate fluid resuscitation. As in the treatment of other forms of hypovolemic shock, the primary initial therapeutic goal is to quickly restore vascular volume and to preserve tissue perfusion in order to minimize tissue ischemia. In extensive burns (>25%TBSA), fluid resuscitation is complicated not only by the severe burn wound edema, but also by extravasated and sequestered fluid and protein in non-burned soft tissue. Large volumes of resuscitation solutions are required to maintain vascular volume during the first several hours after an extensive burn. Data suggests that despite fluid resuscitation normal blood volume is not restored until 24–36 hours after large burns [27].

Edema develops when the rate by which fluid is filtered out of the microvessels exceeds the flow in the lymph vessels draining the same tissue mass. Edema formation often follows a biphasic pattern. An immediate and rapid increase in the water content of burn tissue is seen in the first hour after burn injury [25, 28]. A second and more gradual increase in fluid flux of both the burned skin and non-burned soft tissue occurs during the first 12 to 24 hours following burn trauma [17, 28]. The amount of edema formation in burned skin depends on the type and extent of injury [25, 29] and whether fluid resuscitation is provided as well as the type and volume of fluid administered [30]. However, fluid resuscitation elevates blood flow and capillary pressure contributing to further fluid extravasation. Without sustained delivery of fluid into the circulation edema fluid is somewhat self-limited as plasma volume and capillary pressure decrease. The edema development in thermal injured skin is characterized by the extreme rapid onset of tissue water content, which can double within the first hour after burn [25, 31]. Leape et al. found a 70% to 80% water content increase in a full-thickness burn wound 30 minutes after burn injury with 90% of this change occurring in the first 5 minutes [26, 32, 33]. There was little increase in burn wound water content after the first hour in the non-resuscitated animals. In resuscitated animals or animals with small wounds, adequate tissue perfusion continues to 'feed' the edema for several hours. Demling et al. used dichromatic absorptionmetry to measure edema development during the first week after an experimental partial-thickness burn injury on one hind limb in sheep [28]. Even though edema was rapid with over 50% occurring in the first hour, maximum water content did not occur until 12 to 24 hours after burn injury.

## Altered cellular membranes and cellular edema

In addition to a loss of capillary endothelial integrity, thermal injury also causes change in the cellular membranes. Baxter found in burns of >30% a systemic decrease in cellular transmembrane potentials as measured in skeletal muscle away from the site of injury [20]. It would be expected that the directly injured cell would have a damaged cell membrane, increasing sodium and potassium fluxes, resulting in cell swelling. However, this process also appears in cells that are not directly heat-injured. Micropuncture techniques have demonstrated partial depolarization in the normal skeletal muscle membrane potential of -90 mV to levels of -70 to -80 mV; cell death occurs at -60 mV. The decrease in membrane potentials is associated with an increase in intracellular water and sodium [34–36].Similar alterations in skeletal membrane functions and cellular edema have been reported in hemorrhagic shock [34, 36] also in the cardiac, liver and endothelial cells [37–39]. Early investigators of this phenomenon postulated that a decrease in ATP levels or ATPase activity was the mechanism for membrane depolarization, however, other research suggests that it may result from an increased sodium conductance in membranes or an increase in sodium-hydrogen antiport activity [35, 38]. Resuscitation of hemorrhage rapidly restores depolarized membrane potentials to normal, but resuscitation of burn injury only partially restores the membrane potential and intracellular sodium concentrations to normal levels, demonstrating that hypovolemia alone is not totally responsible for the cellular swelling seen in burn shock [40]. A circulating shock factor(s) is likely to be responsible for the membrane depolarization [41–43], but surprisingly, the molecular characterization of such a circulating factor have not been elucidated; suggesting that it has a complex structure. Data suggests it has a large molecular weight, >80 KDalton [44]. Membrane depolarization may be caused by different factors in different states of shock. Very little is known about the time course of the changes in membrane potential in clinical burns. More importantly, we do not know the extent to which the altered membrane potentials affect total volume requirements and organ function in burn injury or even shock in general.

## Mediators of burn injury

Many mediators have been proposed to account for the changes in permeability after burn, including histamine, b serotonin, bradykinin, prostaglandins, leukotrienes, platelet activating factor, and catecholamines, among others [10, 45–49]. The exact mechanism(s) of mediator-induced injury are of considerable clinical importance, as this understanding would allow for the development of pharmacologic modulation of burn edema and shock by mediator inhibition.

**Histamine:** Histamine is most likely to be the mediator responsible for the early phase of increased microvascular permeability seen immediately after burn. Histamine causes large endothelial gaps to transiently form as a result of the contraction of venular endothelial cells [50]. Histamine is released from mast cells in thermal-injured skin; however, the increase in histamine levels and its actions are only transient. Histamine also can cause the rise in capillary pressure (Pc) by arteriolar dilation and venular contraction. Statistically significant reductions in burn edema have been achieved with histamine blockers and mast cell stabilizers when tested in acute animal models [50]. Friedl et al. demonstrated that the pathogenesis of burn edema in the skin of rats appears to be related to the interaction of histamine with xanthine oxidase and oxygen radicals [51]. Histamine and its metabolic derivatives increased the catalytic activity of xanthine oxidase (but not xanthine dehydrogenase) in rat plasma and in rat pulmonary artery endothelial cells. In thermally injured rats, levels of plasma histamine and xanthine oxidase rose in parallel, in association with the uric acid increase. Burn edema was greatly attenuated by treating rats with the mast cell stabilizer, cromolyn, complement depletion or the H2 receptor antagonist, cimetidine; but was unaffected by neutrophil depletion [52–54]. Despite encouraging results in animals, beneficial antihistamine treatment of human burn injury has not been demonstrated, although antihistamines are administered to reduce risk of gastric ulcers.

**Prostaglandins:** Prostaglandins are potent vasoactive autocoids synthesized from the arachidonic acid released from burned tissue and inflammatory cells and contribute to the inflammatory response of burn injury [55, 56]. Macrophages and neutrophils are activated through the body; infiltrate the wound and release prostaglandin as well as thromboxanes, leukotrienes and interleukin-1. These wound mediators have both local and systemic effects. Prostaglandin E2 (PGE2) and leukotrienes $LB_4$ and $LD_4$ directly and indirectly increase microvascular permeability [57]. Prostacyclin (PGI2) is produced in burn injury and is also a vasodilator, but also may cause direct increases in capillary permeability. PGE2 appears to be one of the more potent inflammatory prostaglandins, causing the postburn vasodilation in wounds, which, when coupled with the increased microvascular permeability amplifies edema formation [58, 59].

**Thromboxane:** Thromboxane $A_2$ ($TXA_2$) and its metabolite, thromboxane B2 ($TXB_2$) are produced locally in the burn wound by platelets [50]. Vasoconstrictor thromboxanes may be less important in edema formation, however, by decreasing blood flow they can contribute to a growing zone of ischemia under the burn wound and can cause the conversion of a partial-thickness wound to a deeper full-thickness wound. The serum level of TXA, and $TXA_2/PGI_2$ ratios are increased significantly in burn patients [60]. Heggers showed the release of $TXB_2$ at the burn wound was associated with local tissue ischemia, and that thromboxane inhibitors prevented the progressive dermal ischemia associated with thermal injury and thromboxane release [61, 62]. The $TXA_2$ synthesis inhibitor anisodamine also showed beneficial macrocirculatory effects by restoring the hemodynamic and rheological disturbances towards normal. Demling showed that topically applied ibuprofen (which inhibits the synthesis of prostaglandins and thromboxanes) decreases both local edema and prostanoid production in burned tissue without altering systemic production [63]. On the other hand, systemic administration of ibuprofen did not modify early edema, but did attenuate the post-burn vasoconstriction that impaired adequate oxygen delivery to tissue in burned sheep [64]. Although cyclooxgenase inhibitors have been used after burn-injury, neither their convincing benefit, nor their routine clinical use has been reported.

**Kinins:** Bradykinin is a local mediator of inflammation that increases venular permeability. It is likely that bradykinin production is increased after burn injury, but its detection in blood or lymph can be difficult owing to the simultaneous increase in kininase activity and the rapid inactivation of free kinins. The generalized inflammatory response after burn injury favors the release of bradykinin [65]. Pretreatment of burn-injured animals with aprotinin, a general protease inhibitor, should have decreased the release of free kinin, but no effect on edema was noted [66]. On the other hand, pretreatment with a specific bradykinin receptor antagonist reduced edema in full thickness burn wound in rabbits [8].

**Serotonin:** Serotonin is released early after burn injury [67]. This agent is a smooth-muscle constrictor of large blood vessels. Antiserotonin agents such as ketanserin have been found to decrease peripheral vascular resistance after burn injury, but have not been reported to decrease edema [67]. On the other hand, the pretreatment effect of methysergide, a serotonin antagonist, reduces hyperemic or increased blood flow response in the burn wounds of rabbits, along with reducing the burn edema [8]. Methysergide did not prevent increases in the capillary reflection coefficient or permeability [68]. Ferrara and colleagues found a dose dependent reduction of burn edema when methysergide was given preburn to dogs, but claimed that this was not attributable to blunting of the regional vasodilator response (68). Zhang et al. reported a reduction in nonnutritive skin blood flow after methysergide administration to burned rabbits [69].

**Catecholamines:** Circulating catecholamines epinephrine and norepinephrine are released in massive amounts after burn injury [17, 70, 71]. On the arteriolar side of the microvessels these agents cause vasoconstriction via alpha 1 receptor activation, which tends to reduce capillary pressure, particularly when combined with the hypovolemia and the reduced venous pressure of burn shock [50]. Reduced capillary pressure may limit edema and induce interstitial fluid to reabsorb from nonburned skin, skeletal muscle, and visceral organs in nonresuscitated burn shock. Further, catecholamines, via ß-agonist activity, may also partially inhibit increased capillary permeability induced by histamine and bradykinin [50]. These potentially beneficial effects of catecholamines may not be operative in directly injured tissue and may also be offset in nonburned tissue by the deleterious vasoconstrictor and ischemic effects. The hemodynamic effects

of catecholamines will be discussed later in the chapter.

**Oxygen radicals:** Oxygen radicals play an important inflammatory role in all types of shock, including burn. These short-lived elements are highly unstable reactive metabolites of oxygen; each one has an unpaired electron, creating them into strong oxidizing agents [72]. Superoxide anion ($O_2^-$), hydrogen peroxide ($H_2O_2$), and hydroxyl ion ($OH^-$) are produced and released by activated neutrophils after any inflammatory reaction or reperfusion of ischemic tissue. The hydroxyl ion is believed to be the most potent and damaging of the three. The formation of the hydroxyl radical requires free ferrous iron ($Fe_2$) and $H_2O_2$. Evidence that these agents are formed after burn injury is the increased lipid peroxidation found in circulating red blood cells and biopsied tissue [53, 72, 73]. Demling showed that large doses of deferoxamine (DFO), an iron chelator, when used for resuscitation of 40% TBSA in sheep, prevented systemic lipid peroxidation and decreased the vascular leak in nonburned tissue while also increasing oxygen utilization [74]. However, DFO may have accentuated burned tissue edema, possibly by increasing the perfusion of burned tissue.

Nitric oxide (NO) simultaneously generated with the superoxide anion can lead to the formation of peroxynitrite ($ONOO^-$). The presence of nitrotyrosine in burn skin found in the first few hours after injury suggests that peroxynitrite may play a deleterious role in burn edema [75]. On the other hand, the blockade of NO synthase did not reduce burn edema, while treatment with the NO precursor arginine reduces burn edema [76]. NO may be important for maintaining perfusion and limiting the zone of stasis in burn skin [77]. Although the pro- and anti-inflammatory roles of NO remain controversial, it would appear that the acute beneficial effects of NO generation out-weigh any deleterious effect in burn shock.

Antioxidants, namely agents that either directly bind to the oxygen radicals (scavengers) or cause their further metabolism, have been evaluated in several experimental studies [78, 79]. Catalase, which removes $H_2O_2$ and superoxide dismutase (SOD), which removes radical $O_2^-$, have been reported to decrease the vascular loss of plasma after burn injury in dogs and rats [53, 78].

The plasma of thermally injured rats showed dramatic increases in levels of xanthine oxidase activity, with peak values appearing as early as 15 minutes after thermal injury. Excision of the burned skin immediately after the thermal injury significantly diminished the increase in plasma xanthine oxidase activity [51, 53]. The skin permeability changes were attenuated by treating the animals with antioxidants (catalase, SOD, dimethyl sulfoxide, dimethylthiourea) or an iron chelator (DFO), thus supporting the role of oxygen radicals in the development of vascular injury as defined by increased vascular permeability [53]. Allopurinol, a xanthine oxidase inhibitor, markedly reduced both burn lymph flow and levels of circulating lipid peroxides, and further prevented all pulmonary lipid peroxidation and inflammation. This suggests that the release of oxidants from burned tissue was in part responsible for local burn edema, as well as distant inflammation and oxidant release [73]. The failure of neutrophil depletion to protect against the vascular permeability changes and the protective effects of the xanthine oxidase inhibitors (allopurinol and lodoxamide tromethamine) suggests that plasma xanthine oxidase is the more likely source of the oxygen radicals involved in the formation of burn edema. These oxygen radicals can increase vascular permeability by damaging microvascular endothelial cells [51, 53]. the use of antioxidants has been extensively investigated in animals, and some clinical trials suggest benefit. Antioxidants (vitamin C and E) are routinely administered to patients at many burn centers. High doses of antioxidant ascorbic acid (vitamin-C) have been found to be efficacious in reducing fluid needs in burn injured experimental animals when administered postburn [80–82]. The use of high doses (10–20 g per day) of vitamin C was shown to be effective in one clinical trial, but ineffective in another [83, 84]. High dose vitamin C has not received wide clinical usage.

**Platelet aggregation factor:** Platelet aggregation (or activating) factor (PAF) can increase capillary permeability and is released after burn injury [66, 85]. Ono et al. showed in scald-injured rabbits that TCV-309 (Takeda Pharmaceutical Co Ltd., Japan), a PAF antagonist, infused soon after burn injury blocked edema formation in the wound and significantly inhibited PAF increase in the damaged tissue in a dose-dependent manner. In contrast, the superoxide dismutase content in the group treated with TCV-309 was significantly higher than that of the control group [85]. These findings suggest that the administration of large doses of a PAF antagonist immediately after injury may reduce burn wound edema and the subsequent degree of burn shock by suppressing PAF and superoxide radical formation.

**Angiotensin II and vasopressin:** Angiotensin II and vasopressin or antidiuretic hormone (ADH), are two hormones that participate in the normal regulation of extracellular fluid volume by controlling sodium balance and osmolality through renal function and thirst [50]. However, during burn shock where sympathetic tone is high and volume receptors are stimulated, both hormones can be found in supranormal levels in the blood. Both are potent vasoconstrictors of terminal arterioles will little affect on the venules. Angiotensin II may be responsible for the selective gut and mucosal ischemia, which can cause translocation of endotoxins and bacteria and the development of sepsis and even multi-organ failure [86, 87]. In severely burn-injured patients angiotensin II levels were elevated two to eight times normal in the first 1 to 5 days after burn injury with peak levels occurring on day three [88]. Vasopressin had peak levels of 50 times normal upon admission and declined towards normal over the first five days after burn injury. Vasopressin, along with catecholamines may be largely responsible for increased system vascular resistance and left heart afterload, which can occur in resuscitated burn shock. Sun and others used vasopressin-receptor antagonist in rats with burn shock to improve hemodynamics and survival time, while vasopressin infusion exacerbated burn shock [89].

**Corticotrophin-releasing factor:** Corticotrophin-releasing factor (CRF) has proven to be efficacious in reducing protein extravasation and edema in burned rat paw. CRF may be a powerful natural inhibitory mediator of the acute inflammatory response of the skin to thermal injury [90].

## Hemodynamic consequences of acute burns

The cause of reduced cardiac output (CO) during the resuscitative phase of burn injury has been the subject of considerable debate. There is an immediate depression of cardiac output before any detectable reduction in plasma volume. The rapidity of this response suggests a neurogenic response to receptors in the thermally injured skin or increased circulating vasoconstrictor mediators. Soon after injury a developing hypovolemia and reduced venous return undeniably contribute to the reduced cardiac output. The subsequent persistence of reduced CO after apparently adequate fluid therapy, as evidenced by a reduction in heart rate and restoration of both arterial blood pressure and urinary output, has been attributed to circulating myocardial depressant factor(s), which possibly originates from the burn wound [21, 22]. Demling and collegues showed a 15% reduction in CO despite an aggressive volume replacement protocol after a 40% scald burn in sheep [28]. However, there are also sustained increases in catecholamine secretion and elevated systemic vascular resistance for up to five days after burn injury [70, 88]. Michie and others measured CO and SVR in anesthetized dogs resuscitated after burn injury [91]. They found that CO fell shortly after injury and then returned toward normal, however, reduced CO did not parallel the blood volume deficit. They concluded that the depression of CO resulted not only from decreased blood volume and venous return, but also from an increased SVR and from the presence of a circulating myocardial depressant substance. Thus, there are multiple factors that can significantly reduce CO after burn injury. However, resuscitated patients suffering major burn injury can also have supranormal CO from 2 to 6 days post-injury. This is secondary to the establishment of a hypermetabolic state.

## Hypermetabolic response to burn injury

Marked and sustained increases in catecholamine, glucocorticoid, glucagon and dopamine secretion are thought to initiate the cascade of events leading to the acute hypermetabolic response with its ensuing catabolic state [92–100]. The cause of this complex response is not well understood. However, interleukins 1 and 6, platelet-activating factor, tumor necrosis factor (TNF), endotoxin, neutrophil-adherence complexes, reactive oxygen species, nitric oxide and coagulation as well as complement cascades have also been implicated in regulating this response to burn injury [101]. Once these cascades are initiated, their mediators and by-products appear to stimulate the persistent and increased metabolic rate associated with altered glucose metabolism seen after severe burn injury [102].

Several studies have indicated that these metabolic phenomena post-burn occur in a timely manner, suggesting two distinct pattern of metabolic regulation following injury [103]. The first phase occurs within the first 48 hours of injury and has classically been called the "ebb phase" [103, 104], characterized by decreases in cardiac output, oxygen consumption, and metabolic rate as well as impaired glucose tolerance associated with its hyperglycemic state. These metabolic variables gradually increase within the first five days post-injury to a plateau phase (called the "flow" phase), characteristically associated with hyperdynamic circulation and the above mentioned hypermetabolic state. Insulin release during this time period was found to be twice that of controls in response to glucose load [105, 106] and plasma glucose levels are markedly elevated, indicating the development of an insulin-resistance [106, 107]. Current understanding has been that these metabolic alterations resolve soon after complete wound closure. However, recent studies found that the hypermetabolic response to burn injury may last for more than 12 months after the initial event [92, 93, 100, 108]. We found in recent studies that sustained hypermetabolic alterations post-burn, indicated by persistent elevations of total urine cortisol levels, serum cytokines, catecholamines and basal energy requirements, were accompanied by impaired glucose metabolism and insulin sensitivity that persisted for up to three years after the initial burn injury [109].

A 10 to 50-fold elevation of plasma catecholamines and corticosteroid levels occur in major burns which persist up to three years post-injury [49, 109–112]. Cytokine levels peak immediately after burn, approaching normal levels only after one month post injury. Constitutive and acute phase proteins are altered beginning 5–7 days post-burn, and remain abnormal throughout acute hospital stay. Serum IGF-I, IGFBP-3, parathyroid hormone, and Osteocalcin drop immediately after the injury 10 fold, and remain significantly decreased up to

6 months post-burn compared to normal levels [111]. Sex hormones and endogenous growth hormone levels decrease around 3 weeks post-burn [111].

For severely burned patients, the resting metabolic rate at thermal neutral temperature (30°C) exceeds 140% of normal at admission, reduces to 130% once the wounds are fully healed, then to 120% at 6 months after injury, and 110% at 12 months post-burn [92, 111]. Increases in catabolism result in loss of total body protein, decreased immune defenses, and decreased wound healing [92].

Immediately post-burn patients have low cardiac output characteristic of early shock [113]. However, three to four days post-burn, cardiac outputs are greater than 1.5 times that of non-burned, healthy volunteers [111]. Heart rates of pediatric burn patients' approach 1.6 times that of non-burned, healthy volunteers [114]. Post-burn, patients have increased cardiac work [110, 115]. Myocardial oxygen consumption surpasses that of marathon runners and is sustained well into rehabilitative period [115, 116].

There is profound hepatomegaly after injury. The liver increases its size by 225% of normal by two weeks post-burn and remains enlarged at discharge by 200% of normal [111].

Post-burn, muscle protein is degraded much faster than it is synthesized [111, 114]. Net protein loss leads to loss of lean body mass and severe muscle wasting leading to decreased strength and failure to fully rehabilitate [117, 118]. Significant decreases in lean body mass related to chronic illness or hypermetabolism can have dire consequences. A 10% loss of lean body mass is associated with immune dysfunction. A 20% loss of lean body mass positively correlates with decreased wound healing. A loss of 30% of lean body mass leads to increased risk for pneumonia and pressure sores. A 40% loss of lean body mass can lead to death [119]. Uncomplicated severely burned patients can lose up to 25% of total body mass after acute burn injury [120]. Protein degradation persists up to nearly one year post severe burn injury resulting in significant negative whole-body and cross-leg nitrogen balance [110, 118, 121]. Protein catabolism has a positive correlation with increases in metabolic rates [118]. Severely burned patients have a daily nitrogen loss of 20–25 grams per meter squared of burned skin [110, 122]. At this rate, a lethal cachexia can be reached in less than one month [122]. Burned pediatric patients' protein loss leads to significant growth retardation for up to 24 months post injury [123].

Elevated circulating levels of catecholamines, glucagon, cortisol after severe thermal injury stimulate free fatty acids and glycerol from fat, glucose production by the liver, and amino acids from muscle [103, 124, 125]. Specifically, glycolytic-gluconeogengenic cycling is increased 250% during the post-burn hypermetabolic response coupled with an increase of 450% in triglyceride-fatty acid cycling. [126]. These changes lead to hyperglycemia and impaired insulin sensitivity related to post-receptor insulin resistance demonstrated by elevated levels of insulin, fasting glucose, and significant reductions in glucose clearance [127–130].

## Glucose metabolism

Glucose metabolism in healthy subjects is tightly regulated: under normal circumstances, a postprandial increase in blood glucose concentration stimulates release of insulin from pancreatic β-cells. Insulin mediates peripheral glucose uptake into skeletal muscle and adipose tissue and suppresses hepatic gluconeogenesis, thereby maintaining blood glucose homeostasis [131, 132]. In critical illness, however metabolic alterations can cause significant changes in energy substrate metabolism. In order to provide glucose, a major fuel source to vital organs, release of the above mentioned stress mediators oppose the anabolic actions of insulin [133]. By enhancing adipose tissue lipolysis [125] and skeletal muscle proteolysis [134], they increase gluconeogenic substrates, including glycerol, alanine and lactate, thus augmenting hepatic glucose production in burned patients (Fig. 1) [131, 132, 135]. Hyperglycemia fails to suppress hepatic glucose release during this time [136] and the suppressive effect of insulin on hepatic glucose release is attenuated, significantly contributing to post-trauma hyperglycemia [137]. Catecholamine-mediated enhancement of hepatic glycogenolysis, as well as direct sympathetic stimulation of glycogen breakdown, can further aggravate the hyperglycemia in response to stress [132]. Catecholamines have also been shown to impair glucose disposal via alterations of the insulin signaling pathway and GLUT-4 translocation muscle and adipose tissue, resulting in peripheral insulin resistance (Fig. 1) [131, 138]. Cree et al. [137] showed an impaired activation of Insulin Receptor Substrate-1 at its tyrosine binding site and an inhibition of AKT in muscle biopsies of children at seven days post-burn. Work of Wolfe et al. indicates links between impaired liver and muscle mitochondrial oxidative function, altered rates of lipolysis, and impaired insulin signaling post-burn attenuating both the suppressive actions of insulin on hepatic glucose production and on the stimulation of muscle glucose uptake [106, 125, 136, 137]. Another counter-regulatory hormone of interest during stress of the critically ill is glucagon. Glucagon, like epinephrine, leads to increased glucose production through both gluconeogenesis and glycogenolysis [139]. The action of glucagons alone is not maintained over time; however, its action on gluconeogenesis is sustained in an additive manner with the presence of epinephrine, cortisol, and growth hormone [133, 139]. Likewise, epinephrine and glucagon have an additive effect on glycogenolysis [139]. Recent studies found that pro-inflammatory cytokines contribute indirectly to post-burn hyperglycemia via enhancing the release of the above mentioned stress hormones [140–142]. Other groups showed that inflammatory cytokines, including tumor necrosis factor (TNF), interleukin (IL) -6 and monocyte chemotactic protein (MCP) -1 also act via direct effects on the insulin signal transduction pathway through modification of signaling properties of insulin receptor substrates, contributing to post-burn hyperglycemia via liver and skeletal muscle insulin resistance [143–145]. Alterations in metabolic pathways as well as pro-inflammatory cytokines, such as TNF, have also been implicated in significantly contributing to lean muscle protein breakdown, both during the acute and convalescent phases in response to burn injury [121, 146]. In contrast to starvation, in which lipolysis and ketosis provide energy and protect muscle reserves, burn injury considerably reduces the ability of the body to utilize fat as an energy source.

Skeletal muscle is thus the major source of fuel in the burned patient, which leads to marked wasting of lean body mass (LBM) within days after injury [110, 147]. This muscle breakdown has been demonstrated with whole body and cross leg nitrogen balance studies in which pronounced negative nitrogen balances persisted for 6 and 9 months after injury [118]. Since skeletal muscle has been shown to be responsible for 70–80% of whole body insulin-stimulated glucose uptake, decreases in muscle mass may significantly contribute to this persistent insulin resistance post-burn [148]. The correlation between hyperglycemia and muscle protein catabolism has been also supported by Flakoll et al. [149] in which an isotopic tracer of leucine was utilized to index whole-body protein flux in normal volunteers. The group showed a significant increase in proteolysis rates occurring without any alteration in either leucine oxidation or non-oxidative disposal (an estimate of protein synthesis), suggesting an hyperglycemia induced increase in protein breakdown. Flakoll et al. [149] further demonstrated that elevations of plasma glucose levels resulted in a marked stimulation of whole body proteolysis during hyperinsulinemia. A 10–15% loss in lean body mass has been shown to be associated with significant increases in infection rate and marked delays in wound healing [150]. The resultant muscle weakness was further shown to prolong mechanical ventilatory requirements, inhibit sufficient cough reflexes and delay mobilization in protein-malnourished patients, thus markedly contributing to the incidence of mortality in these patients [151]. Persistent protein catabolism may also account for delay in growth frequently observed in our pediatric patient population for up to 2 years post-burn [123].

Septic patients have a particularly profound increase in metabolic rates and protein catabolism up to 40% more compared to those with like-size burns that do not develop sepsis [92, 152, 153]. A vicious cycle develops, as patients that are catabolic are more susceptible to sepsis due to changes in immune function and immune response. The emergence of multi-drug resistant organisms have led to increases in sepsis, catabolism and mortality [153–155]. Modulation of the hypermetabolic, hypercatabolic response, thus preventing secondary injury is paramount in the restoration of structure and function of severely burned patients.

## Myocardial dysfunction

Myocardial function can be compromised after burn injury due to overload of the right heart and direct depression of contractility shown in isolated heart studies [156, 157]. Increases in the afterload of both the left and right heart result from SVR and PVR elevations. The left ventricle compensates and CO can be maintained with increased afterload by augmented adrenergic stimulation and increased myocardial oxygen extraction. The right ventricle has a minimal capacity to compensate for increased afterload. In severe cases, desynchronization of the right and left ventricles is deleteriously superimposed on a depressed myocardium [158]. Burn injury greater than 45% TBSA can produce intrinsic contractile defects. Several investigators reported that aggressive early and sustained fluid resuscitation failed to correct left ventricular contractile and compliance defects [157–159]. These data suggest that hypovolemia is not the only mechanism underlying the myocardial defects observed with burn shock. Serum from patients failing to sustain a normal CO after thermal injury have exhibited a markedly negative inotropic effect on in vitro heart preparations, which is likely due to the previously described shock factor [160]. In other patients with large burn injuries and normal cardiac indices, little or no depressant activity was detected.

Sugi and colleagues studied intact, chronically instrumented sheep after a 40% TBSA flame burn injury and smoke-inhalation injury, and smoke inhalation injury alone. They found that maximal contractile effects were reduced after either burn injury or inhalation injury [161, 162]. Horton and others demonstrated decreased left ventricular contractility in isolated, coronary perfused, guinea pig hearts harvested 24 hours after burn injury [163]. This dysfunction was more pronounced in hearts from aged animals and was not reversed by resuscitation with isotonic fluid. It was largely reversed by treatment with 4 mL/kg of hypertonic saline dextran (HSD), but only if administered during the initial 4 to 6 hours of resuscitation [164, 165]. These authors also effectively ameliorated the cardiac dysfunction of thermal injury with infusions of antioxidants, arginine and calcium channel blockers [166–168]. Cioffi et al. in a similar model observed persistent myocardial depression after burn when the animals received no resuscitation after burn injury [169]. As opposed to most studies, Cioffi reported that immediate and full resuscitation totally reversed abnormalities of contraction and relaxation after burn injury. Murphy et al. showed elevations of a serum marker for cardiac injury, Troponin I, for patients with a TBSA >18%, despite good cardiac indices [170]. Resuscitation and cardiac function studies emphasize the importance of early and adequate fluid therapy and suggest that functional myocardial depression after burn-injury may not occur in patients receiving prompt and adequate volume therapy.

The primary mechanisms by which burn shock alters myocardial cell membrane integrity and impairs mechanical function remain unclear. Oxygen-derived free radicals may play a key causative role in the cell membrane dysfunction that is characteristic of several low-flow states. Horton et al. showed that a combination therapy of free radical scavengers SOD and catalase significantly improved burn-mediated defects in left ventricular contractility and relaxation when administered along with adequate fluid resuscitation (4 mL/kg per percent of burn). Antioxidant therapy did not alter the volume of fluid resuscitation required after burn injury [166].

## Effects on the renal system

Diminished blood volume and cardiac output result in decreased renal blood flow and glomerular filtration rate. Other stress-induced hormones and mediators such as angiotensin, aldosterone, and vasopressin further reduce renal blood flow immediately after the injury. These effects result in oliguria, which, if left untreated will cause acute tubular necrosis and renal failure. Twenty years ago, acute renal failure in burn injuries was almost always fatal. Today newer techniques in dialysis became widely used to support the kidneys during recovery [171]. The latest reports indicate an 88% mortality rate for severely burned adults and a 56% mortality rate for severely burned children in whom renal failure develops in the post-burn period [172, 173]. Early resuscitation decreases risks of renal failure and improves the associated morbidity and mortality [174].

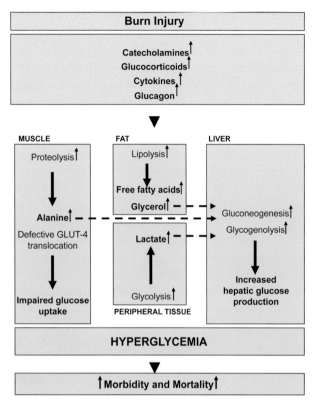

**Fig. 1.** Metabolic changes underlying insulin resistance post-burn. Marked and sustained increases in catecholamine, glucocorticoid, glucagon and cytokine secretion are thought to initiate the cascade of events leading to the acute hypermetabolic response to severe burn injury and oppose the anabolic effects of insulin. By enhancing adipose tissue lipolysis and skeletal muscle proteolysis, they increase gluconeogenic substrates, including glycerol, alanine and lactate, thus augmenting hepatic glucose production in burned patients. Catecholamine-mediated augmentation of hepatic glycogenolysis, as well as direct sympathetic stimulation of glycogen breakdown, further aggravates the hyperglycemia in response to stress. Catecholamines and cytokines, such as IL-1, IL-6, MCP-1 and TNF, have also been shown to impair glucose disposal via alterations of the insulin signaling pathway and GLUT-4 translocation, resulting in peripheral insulin resistance

## Effects on the gastrointestinal system

The gastrointestinal response to burn is highlighted by mucosal atrophy, changes in digestive absorption, and increased intestinal permeability [175]. Atrophy of the small bowel mucosa occurs within 12 hours of injury in proportion to the burn size and is related to increased epithelial cell death by apoptosis [176]. The cytoskeleton of the mucosal brush border undergoes atrophic changes associated with vesiculation of microvilli and disruption of the terminal web actin filaments. These findings were most pronounced 18 hours after injury, which suggests that changes in the cytoskeleton, such as those associated with cell death by apoptosis, are processes involved in the changed gut mucosa [177]. Burn also causes reduced uptake of glucose and amino acids, decreased absorption of fatty acids, and reduction in brush border lipase activity [178]. These changes peak in the first several hours after burn and return to normal at 48 to 72 hours after injury, a timing that parallels mucosal atrophy.

Intestinal permeability to macromolecules, which are normally repelled by an intact mucosal barrier, increases after burn [179]. Intestinal permeability to polyethylene glycol 3350, lactulose, and mannitol increases after injury, correlating to the extent of the burn [180]. Gut permeability increases even further when burn wounds become infected. A study using fluorescent dextrans showed that larger molecules appeared to cross the mucosa between the cells, whereas the smaller molecules traversed the mucosa through the epithelial cells, presumably by pinocytosis and vesiculation [181]. Mucosal permeability also paralleled increases in gut epithelial apoptosis.

Changes in gut blood flow are related to changes in permeability. Intestinal blood flow was shown to decrease in animals, a change that was associated with increased gut permeability at 5 hours after burn [182]. This effect was abolished at 24 hours. Systolic hypotension has been shown to occur in the hours immediately after burn in animals with a 40% TBSA full-thickness injury. These animals showed an inverse correlation between blood flow and permeability to intact *Candida* [183].

## Effects on the immune system

Burns cause a global depression in immune function, which is shown by prolonged allograft skin survival on burn wounds. Burned patients are then at great risk for a number of infectious complications, including bacterial wound infection, pneumonia, and fungal and viral infections. These susceptibilities and conditions are based on depressed cellular function in all parts of the immune system, including activation and activity of neutrophils, macrophages, T lymphocytes, and B lymphocytes. With burns of more than 20% TBSA, impairment of these immune functions is proportional to burn size.

Macrophage production after burn is diminished, which is related to the spontaneous elaboration of negative regulators of myeloid growth. This effect is enhanced by the presence of endotoxin and can be partially reversed with granulocyte colony-stimulating factor (G-CSF) treatment or inhibition of prostaglandin E2 [184]. Investigators have shown that G-CSF levels actually increase after severe burn. However, bone marrow G-CSF receptor expression is decreased, which may in part account for the immunodeficiency seen in burns [185]. Total neutrophil counts are initially increased after burn, a phenomenon that is related to a decrease in cell death by apoptosis [186]. However, neutrophils that are present are dysfunctional in terms of diapedesis, chemotaxis, and phagocytosis. These effects are explained, in part, by a deficiency in CD11b/CD18 expression after inflammatory stimuli, decreased respiratory burst activity associated with a deficiency in p47-phox activity, and impaired actin mechanics related to neutrophil motile responses [187, 188]. After 48 to 72 hours, neutrophil counts decrease somewhat like macrophages with similar causes [185].

T-helper cell function is depressed after a severe burn that is associated with polarization from the interleukin-2 and interferon-(cytokine-based T-helper 1 (Th1) response toward the Th2 response [189]. The Th2 response is characterized by the production of interleukin-4 and interleukin-10. The Th1 response is important in cell-mediated immune defense, whereas the Th2 response is important in antibody responses to infection. As this polarization increases, so does the mortality rate [190]. Administration of interleukin-10 antibodies and growth hormone has partially reversed this response and improved mortality rate after burn in animals [191, 192]. Burn also impairs cytotoxic T-lymphocyte activity as a function of burn size, thus increasing the risk of infection, particularly from fungi and viruses. Early burn wound excision improves cytotoxic T-cell activity [193].

## Summary and conclusion

Thermal injury results in massive fluid shifts from the circulating plasma into the interstitial fluid space causing hypovolemia and swelling of the burned skin. When burn injury exceeds 20–30% TBSA there is minimal edema generation in non-injured tissues and organs. The Starling-forces change to favor fluid extravasation from blood to tissue. Rapid edema formation is predominating from the development of strongly negative interstitial fluid pressure (imbibition pressure) and to a lesser degree by an increase in microvascular pressure and permeability.

Secondary to the thermal insult there is release of inflammatory mediators and stress hormones. Circulating mediators deleteriously increase microvascular permeability and alter cellular membrane function by which water and sodium enter cells. Circulating mediators also favor renal conservation of water and salt, impair cardiac contractility and cause vasoconstrictors, which further aggravates ischemia from combined hypovolemia and cardiac dysfunction. The end result of this complex chain of events is decreased intravascular volume, increased systemic vascular resistance, decreased cardiac output, end-organ ischemia, and metabolic acidosis. Early excision of the devitalized tissue appears to reduce the local and systemic effects of mediators released from burned tissue, thus reducing the progressive pathophysiologic derangements. Without early and full resuscitation therapy these derangements can result in acute renal failure, vascular ischemia, cardiovascular collapse, and death.

Edema in both the burn wound and particularly in the non-injured soft tissue is increased by resuscitation. Edema is a serious complication, which likely contributes to decreased tissue oxygen diffusion and further ischemic insult to already damaged cells with compromised blood flow increasing the risk of infection. Research should continue to focus on methods to ameliorate the severe edema and vasoconstriction that exacerbate tissue ischemia. The success of this research will require identification of key circulatory factors that alter capillary permeability, cause vasoconstriction, depolarize cellular membranes, and depress myocardial function. Hopefully, methods to prevent the release and to block the activity of specific mediators can be further developed in order to

**143**

reduce the morbidity and mortality rates of burn shock. The profound and overall metabolic alterations post-burn associated with persistent changes in glucose metabolism and impaired insulin sensitivity also significantly contribute to adverse outcome of this patient population and constitute another challenge for future therapeutic approaches of this unique patient population.

## References

[1] Nguyen TT, Gilpin DA, Meyer NA et al (1996) Current treatment of severely burned patients. Ann Surg 223(1): 14–25

[2] Brigham PA, McLoughlin E (1996) Burn incidence and medical care use in the United States: estimates, trends, and data sources. J Burn Care Rehabil 17(2): 95–107

[3] Wolf S (2007) Critical care in the severely burned: organ support and management of complications. In: Herndon DN (ed) Total burn care, 3rd edn. Saunders Elsevier, London

[4] Vo LT, Papworth GD, Delaney PM et al (1998) A study of vascular response to thermal injury on hairless mice by fibre optic confocal imaging, laser doppler flowmetry and conventional histology. Burns 24(4): 319–324

[5] Heggers JP, Loy GL, Robson MC et al (1980) Histological demonstration of prostaglandins and thromboxanes in burned tissue. J Surg Res 28(2): 110–117

[6] Herndon DN, Abston S, Stein MD (1984) Increased thromboxane B2 levels in the plasma of burned and septic burned patients. Surg Gynecol Obstet 159(3): 210–213

[7] Morykwas MJ, David LR, Schneider AM et al (1999) Use of subatmospheric pressure to prevent progression of partial-thickness burns in a swine model. J Burn Care Rehabil 20(1 Pt 1): 15–21

[8] Nwariaku FE, Sikes PJ, Lightfoot E et al (1996) Effect of a bradykinin antagonist on the local inflammatory response following thermal injury. Burns 22(4): 324–327

[9] Chappell VL, LaGrone L, Mileski WJ (1999) Inhibition of leukocyte-mediated tissue destruction by synthetic fibronectin peptide (Trp-9-Tyr). J Burn Care Rehabil 20(6): 505–510

[10] Holland AJ, Martin HC, Cass DT (2002) Laser Doppler imaging prediction of burn wound outcome in children. Burns 28(1): 11–17

[11] Cockshott WP (1956) The history of the treatment of burns. Surg Cynecol Obstet 102: 116–124

[12] Haynes BW (1987) The history of burn care. In: Boswick JAJ (ed) The art and science of burn care. Aspen Publ, Rockville, MD, pp 3–9

[13] Underhill FP, Carrington GL, Kapsinov R et al (1923) Blood concentration changes in extensive superficial burns, and their significance for systemic treatment. Arch Intern Med 32: 31–39

[14] Cope O, Moore FD (1947) The redistribution of body water and fluid therapy of the burned patient. Ann Surg 126: 1010–1045

[15] Youn YK, LaLonde C, Demling R (1992) The role of mediators in the response to thermal injury. World J Surg 16(1): 30–36

[16] Aulick LH, Wilmore DW, Mason AD et al (1977) Influence of the burn wound on peripheral circulation in thermally injured patients. Am J Physiol 233:H520–526

[17] Settle JAD (1982) Fluid therapy in burns. J Roy Soc Med 1(75): 7–11

[18] Demling RH (1987) Fluid replacement in burned patients. Surg Clin North Am 67: 15–30

[19] Demling RH, Will JA, Belzer FO (1978) Effect of major thermal injury on the pulmonary microcirculation. Surgery 83(6): 746–751

[20] Baxter CR (1974) Fluid volume and electrolyte changes of the early postburn period. Clin Plast Surg 1(4): 693–709

[21] Baxter CR, Cook WA, Shires GT (1966) Serum myocardial depressant factor of burn shock. Surg Forum 17: 1–3

[22] Hilton JG, Marullo DS (1986) Effects of thermal trauma on cardiac force of contraction. Burns Incl Therm Inj 12: 167–171

[23] Clark WR (1990) Death due to thermal trauma. In: Dolecek R, Brizio-Molteni L, Molteni A, Traber D (eds) Endocrinology of thermal trauma. Lea & Febiger, Philadelphia, PA, pp 6–27

[24] Lund T, Reed RK (1986) Acute hemodynamic effects of thermal skin injury in the rat. Circ Shock 20: 105–114

[25] Arturson G (1961) Pathophysiological aspects of the burn syndrome. Acta Chir Scand 274[Suppl 1]: $2–135

[26] Leape LL (1972) Kinetics of burn edema formation in primates. Ann Surg 176: 223–226

[27] Cioffi WG, Jr, Vaughan GM, Heironimus JD et al (1991) Dissociation of blood volume and flow in regulation of salt and water balance in burn patients. Ann Surg 214(3): 213–218; discussion 218–220

[28] Demling RH, Mazess RB, Witt RM et al (1978) The study of burn wound edema using dichromatic absorptiometry. J Trauma 18: 124–128

[29] Lund T, Wiig H, Reed RK (1988) Acute postburn edema: Role of strongly negative interstitial fluid pressure. Am J Physiol 255:H1069

[30] Onarheim H, Lund T, Reed R (1989) Thermal skin injury: II. Effects on edema formation and albumin extravasation of fluid resuscitation with lactated Ringer's, plasma, and hypertonic saline (2,400 mosmol/l) in the rat. Circ Shock 27(1): 25–37

[31] Arturson G, Jakobsson OR (1985) Oedema measurements in a standard burn model. Burns 1: 1–7

[32] Leape LL (1968) Early burn wound changes. J Pediatr Surg 3: 292–299

[33] Leape LL (1970) Initial changes in burns: tissue changes in burned and unburned skin of rhesus monkeys. J Trauma 10: 488–492

[34] Shires GT, Cunningham Jr JN, Baker CRF et al (1972) Alterations in cellular membrane dysfunction during hemorrhagic shock in primates. Ann Surg 176(3): 288–295

[35] Nakayama S, Kramer GC, Carlsen RC et al (1984) Amiloride blocks membrane potential depolarization in rat skeletal muscle during hemorrhagic shock (abstract). Circ Shock 13: 106–107

[36] Arango A, Illner H, Shires GT (1976) Roles of ischemia in the induction of changes in cell membrane during hemorrhagic shock. J Surg Res 20(5): 473–476

[37] Holliday RL, Illner HP, Shires GT (1981) Liver cell membrane alterations during hemorrhagic shock in the rat. J Surg Res 31: 506–515

[38] Mazzoni MC, Borgstrom P, Intaglietta M et al (1989) Lumenal narrowing and endothelial cell swelling in skeletal muscle capillaries during hemorrhagic shock. Circ Shock 29(1): 27–39

[39] Garcia NM, Horton JW (1994) L-arginine improves resting cardiac transmembrane potential after burn injury. Shock 1(5): 354–358

[40] Button B, Baker RD, Vertrees RA et al (2001) Quantitative assessment of a circulating depolarizing factor in shock. Shock 15(3): 239–244

[41] Evans JA, Darlington DN, Gann DS (1991) A circulating factor(s) mediates cell depolarization in hemorrhagic shock. Ann Surg 213(6): 549–557

[42] Trunkey DD, Illner H, Arango A et al (1974) Changes in cell membrane function following shock and cross-perfusion. Surg Forum 25: 1–3

[43] Brown JM, Grosso MA, Moore EE (1990) Hypertonic saline and dextran: Impact on cardiac function in the isolated rat heart. J Trauma 30: 646–651

[44] Evans JA, Massoglia G, Sutherland B et al (1993) Molecular properties of hemorrhagic shock factor (abstract). Biophys J 64:A384

[45] Anggard E, Jonsson CE (1971) Efflux of prostaglandins in lymph from scalded tissue. Acta Physiol Scand 81(4): 440–447

[46] Holliman CJ, Meuleman TR, Larsen KR et al (1983) The effect of ketanserin, a specific serotonin antagonist, on burn shock hemodynamic parameters in a porcine burn model. J Trauma 23(10): 867–871

[47] Majno G, Palade GE (1961) Studies on inflammation. 1. The effect of histamine and serotonin on vascular permeability: an electron microscopic study. J Biophys Biochem Cytol 11: 571–605

[48] Majno G, Shea SM, Leventhal M (1969) Endothelial contraction induced by histamine-type mediators: an electron microscopic study. J Cell Biol 42(3): 647–672

[49] Wilmore DW, Long JM, Mason AD, Jr et al (1974) Catecholamines: mediator of the hypermetabolic response to thermal injury. Ann Surg 180(4): 653–669

[50] Goodman-Gilman A, Rall TW, Nies AS et al (1990) The pharmacological basis of therapeutics. Pergamon Press, New York

[51] Friedl HS, Till GO, Tentz O et al (1989) Roles of histamine, complement and xanthine oxidase in thermal injury of skin. Am J Pathol 135(1): 203–217

[52] Boykin Jr JV, Manson NH (1987) Mechanisms of cimetidine protection following thermal injury. Am J Med 83(6A):76–81

[53] Till GO, Guilds LS, Mahrougui M et al (1989) Role of xanthine oxidase in thermal injury of skin. Am J Pathol 135(1): 195–202

[54] Tanaka H, Wada T, Simazaki S et al (1991) Effects of cimetidine on fluid requirement during resuscitation of third-degree burns. J Burn Care Rehabil 12(5): 425–429

[55] Harms B, Bodai B, Demling R (1981) Prostaglandin release and altered microvascular integrity after burn injury. J Surg Res 31: 27–28

[56] Anggard E, Jonsson CE (1971) Efflux of prostaglandins in lymph from scalded tissue. Acta Physiol Scand 81: 440–443

[57] Arturson G (1981) Anti-inflammatory drugs and burn edema formation. In: May R, Dogo G (eds) Care of the burn wound. Karger, Basel, pp 21–24

[58] Arturson G, Hamberg M, Jonsson CE (1973) Prostaglandins in human burn blister fluid. Acta Physiol Scand 87: 27–36

[59] LaLonde C, Knox J, Daryani R (1991) Topical flurbiprofen decreases burn wound-induced hypermetabolism and systemic lipid peroxidation. Surgery 109: 645–651

[60] Huang YS, Li A, Yang ZC (1990) Roles of thromboxane and its inhibitor anisodamine in burn shock. Burns 4: 249–253

[61] Heggers JP, Loy GL, Robson MC et al (1980) Histological demonstration of prostaglandins and thromboxanes in burned tissue. J Surg Res 28: 11–15

[62] Heggers JP, Robson MC, Zachary LS (1985) Thromboxane inhibitors for the prevention of progressive dermal ischemia due to thermal injury. J Burn Care Rehabil 6: 46–48

[63] Demling RH, LaLonde C (1987) Topical ibuprofen decreases early postburn edema. Surgery 5: 857–861

[64] LaLonde C, Demling RH (1989) Inhibition of thromboxane synthetase accentuates hemodynamic instability and burn edema in the anesthetized sheep model. Surgery 5: 638–644

[65] Jacobsen S, Waaler BG (1966) The effect of scalding on the content of kininogen and kininase in limb lymph. Br J Pharmacol 27: 222–229

[66] Hafner JA, Fritz H (1990) Balance antiinflammation: the combined application of a PAF inhibitor and a cyclooxygenase inhibitor blocks the inflammatory take-off after burns. Int J Tissue React 12: 203

[67] Carvajal H, Linares H, Brouhard B (1975) Effect of antihistamine, antiserotonin, and ganglionic blocking agents upon increased capillary permeability following burn edema. J Trauma 15: 969–975

[68] Ferrara JJ, Westervelt CL, Kukuy EL et al (1996) Burn edema reduction by methysergide is not due to control of regional vasodilation. J Surg Res 61(1): 11–16

[69] Zhang XJ, Irtun O, Zheng Y et al (2000) Methysergide reduces nonnutritive blood flow in normal and scalded skin. Am J Physiol 278(3):E452–461

[70] Wilmore DW, Long JM, Mason AD et al (1974) Catecholamines: mediator of the hypermetabolic response to thermal injury. Ann Surg 80: 653–659

[71] Hilton JG (1984) Effects of sodium nitroprusside on thermal trauma depressed cardiac output in the anesthesized dog. Burns Incl Therm Inj 10: 318–322

[72] McCord J, Fridovieh I (1978) The biology and pathology of oxygen radicals. Ann lntern Med 89: 122–127

[73] Demling RH, LaLonde C (1990) Early postburn lipid peroxidation: effect of ibuprofen and allopurinol. Surgery 107: 85–93

[74] Demling R, Lalonde C, Knox J et al (1991) Fluid resuscitation with deferoxamine prevents systemic burn-induced oxidant injury. J Trauma 31(4): 538–543

[75] Rawlingson A, Greenacre SA, Brain SD (2000) Generation of peroxynitrite in localised, moderate temperature burns. Burns 26(3): 223–227

[76] Lindblom L, Cassuto J, Yregard L et al (2000) Importance of nitric oxide in the regulation of burn oedema, proteinuria and urine output. Burns 26(1): 13–17

[77] Lindblom L, Cassuto J, Yregard L et al (2000) Role of nitric oxide in the control of burn perfusion. Burns 26(1): 19–23

[78] Slater TF, Benedetto C (1979) Free radical reactions in relation to lipid peroxidation, inflamnation and prostaglandin metabolism. In: Berti F, Veto G (eds) The prostaglandin system. Plenum Press, New York, pp 109–126

[79] McCord JM (1979) Oxygen-derived free radicals in post ischemic tissue injury. N Engl J Med 312: 159–163

[80] Tanaka H, Matsuda H, Shimazaki S et al (1997) Reduced resuscitation fluid volume for second-degree burns with delayed initiation of ascorbic acid therapy. Arch Surg 132(2): 158–161

[81] Tanaka H, Lund T, Wiig H et al (1999) High dose vitamin C counteracts the negative interstitial fluid hydrostatic pressure and early edema generation in thermally injured rats. Burns 25(7): 569–574

[82] Dubick MA, Williams CA, Elgjo GI et al (2005) High dose vitamin C infusion reduces fluid requirements in the resuscitation of burn injured in sheep. Shock 24(2): 139–144

[83] Tanaka H, Matsuda T, Yukioka T et al (1996) High dose vitamin C reduces resuscitation fluid volume in severely burned patients. Proceedings of the American Burn Association 28: 77

[84] Fischer SF, Bone HG, Powell WC et al (1997) Pyridoxalated hemoglobin polyoxyethylene conjugate does not restore hypoxic pulmonary vasoconstriction in ovine sepsis. Crit Care 25(9): 1151–1159

[85] Ono I, Gunji H, Hasegawa T et al (1993) Effects of a platelet activating factor antagonist on edema formation following burns. Burns 3: 202–207

[86] Fink MP (1991) Gastrointestinal mucosal injury in experimental models of shock, trauma, and sepsis. Crit Care Med 19(5): 627–641

[87] Cui X, Sheng Z, Guo Z (1998) Mechanisms of early gastro-intestinal ischemia after burn: hemodynamic and hemorrheologic features [Chinese]. Chin J Plast Surg Burns 14(4): 262–265

[88] Crum RL, Dominie W, Hansbrough JF (1990) Cardiovaseular and neuroburnoral responses following burn injury. Arch Surg 125: 1065–1070

[89] Sun K, Gong A, Wang CH et al (1990) Effect of peripheral injection of arginine vasopressin and its receptor antagonist on burn shock in the rat. Neuropeptides 1: 17–20

[90] Kiang JG, Wei-E T (1987) Corticotropin-releasing factor inhibits thermal injury. J Pharmacol Exp Ther 2: 517–520

[91] Michie DD, RS G, Mason Jr AD (1963) Effects of hydralazine and high molecular weight dextran upon the circulatory responses to severe thermal burns. Circ Res 13: 46–48

[92] Hart DW, Wolf SE, Mlcak R et al (2000) Persistence of muscle catabolism after severe burn. Surgery 128(2): 312–319

[93] Mlcak RP, Jeschke MG, Barrow RE et al (2006) The influence of age and gender on resting energy expenditure in severely burned children. Ann Surg 244(1): 121–130

[94] Przkora R, Barrow RE, Jeschke MG et al (2006) Body composition changes with time in pediatric burn patients. J Trauma 60(5): 968–971

[95] Dolecek R (1989) Endocrine changes after burn trauma–a review. Keio J Med 38(3): 262–276

[96] Jeffries MK, Vance ML (1992) Growth hormone and cortisol secretion in patients with burn injury. J Burn Care Rehabil 13(4): 391–395

[97] Klein GL, Bi LX, Sherrard DJ et al (2004) Evidence supporting a role of glucocorticoids in short-term bone loss in burned children. Osteoporos Int 15(6): 468–474

[98] Goodall M, Stone C, Haynes BW, Jr (1957) Urinary output of adrenaline and noradrenaline in severe thermal burns. Ann Surg 145(4): 479–487

[99] Coombes EJ, Batstone GF (1982) Urine cortisol levels after burn injury. Burns Incl Therm Inj 8(5): 333–337

[100] Norbury WB, Herndon DN (2007) Modulation of the hypermetabolic response after burn injury. In: Herndon DN (ed) Total burn care, 3rd edn. Saunders & Elsevier, New York, pp 420–433

[101] Sheridan RL (2001) A great constitutional disturbance. N Engl J Med 345(17): 1271–1272

[102] Pereira C, Murphy K, Jeschke M et al (2005) Post burn muscle wasting and the effects of treatments. Int J Biochem Cell Biol 37(10): 1948–1961

[103] Wolfe RR (1981) Review: acute versus chronic response to burn injury. Circ Shock 8(1): 105–115

[104] Cuthbertson DP, Angeles Valero Zanuy MA, Leon Sanz ML (2001) Post-shock metabolic response. 1942. Nutr Hosp 16(5): 175–182

[105] Galster AD, Bier DM, Cryer PE et al (1984) Plasma palmitate turnover in subjects with thermal injury. J Trauma 24(11): 938–945

[106] Cree MG, Aarsland A, Herndon DN et al (2007)Role of fat metabolism in burn trauma-induced skeletal muscle insulin resistance. Crit Care Med35[9 Suppl]: S476–483

[107] Childs C, Heath DF, Little RA et al (1990) Glucose metabolism in children during the first day after burn injury. Arch Emerg Med7(3): 135–147

[108] Jeschke MG, Mlcak RP, Finnerty CC et al (2007) Burn size determines the inflammatory and hypermetabolic response. Crit Care 11(4):R90

[109] Gauglitz GG, Herndon DN, Kulp GA et al (2009) Abnormal insulin sensitivity persists up to three years in pediatric patients post-burn. J Clin Endocrinol Metab 94(5): 1656–1664

[110] Herndon DN, Tompkins RG (2004) Support of the metabolic response to burn injury. Lancet 363(9424): 1895–1902

[111] Jeschke MG, Chinkes DL, Finnerty CC et al (2008) Pathophysiologic response to severe burn injury. Ann Surg 248(3): 387–401

[112] Wilmore DW, Aulick LH, Pruitt BA, Jr (1978) Metabolism during the hypermetabolic phase of thermal injury. Adv Surg 12: 193–225

[113] Cuthbertson DP, Angeles Valero Zanuy MA, Leon Sanz ML (2001) Post-shock metabolic response. 1942. Nutr Hosp 16(5): 176–182; discussion 175–176

[114] Herndon DN, Hart DW, Wolf SE et al (2001) Reversal of catabolism by beta-blockade after severe burns. N Engl J Med 345(17): 1223–1229

[115] Baron PW, Barrow RE, Pierre EJ et al (1997) Prolonged use of propranolol safely decreases cardiac work in burned children. J Burn Care Rehabil 18(3): 223–227

[116] Minifee PK, Barrow RE, Abston S et al (1989) Improved myocardial oxygen utilization following propranolol infusion in adolescents with postburn hypermetabolism. J Pediatr Surg 24(8): 806–810; discussion 810–801

[117] Bessey PQ, Jiang ZM, Johnson DJ et al (1989) Posttraumatic skeletal muscle proteolysis: the role of the hormonal environment. World J Surg 13(4): 465–470; discussion 471

[118] Hart DW, Wolf SE, Chinkes DL et al (2000) Determinants of skeletal muscle catabolism after severe burn. Ann Surg 232(4): 455–465

[119] Chang DW, DeSanti L, Demling RH (1998) Anticatabolic and anabolic strategies in critical illness: a review of current treatment modalities. Shock 10(3): 155–160

[120] Newsome TW, Mason AD, Jr, Pruitt BA, Jr (1973) Weight loss following thermal injury. Ann Surg 178(2): 215–217

[121] Jahoor F, Desai M, Herndon DN et al (1988) Dynamics of the protein metabolic response to burn injury. Metabolism 37(4): 330–337

[122] Kinney JM, Long CL, Gump FE et al (1968) Tissue composition of weight loss in surgical patients. I. Elective operation. Ann Surg 168(3): 459–474

[123] Rutan RL, Herndon DN (1990) Growth delay in postburn pediatric patients. Arch Surg 125(3): 392–395

[124] Wolfe RR, Goodenough RD, Burke JF et al (1983) Response of protein and urea kinetics in burn patients to different levels of protein intake. Ann Surg 197(2): 163–171

[125] Wolfe RR, Herndon DN, Jahoor F et al (1987) Effect of severe burn injury on substrate cycling by glucose and fatty acids. N Engl J Med 317(7): 403–408

[126] Yu YM, Tompkins RG, Ryan CM et al (1999) The metabolic basis of the increase of the increase in energy expenditure in severely burned patients. JPEN J Parenter Enteral Nutr 23(3): 160–168

[127] Gauglitz GG, Halder S, Boehning DF et al (2010) Postburn hepatic insulin resistance is associated with Er stress. Shock 33(3): 299–305

[128] Gauglitz GG, Finnerty CC, Herndon DN et al (2008) Are serum cytokines early predictors for the outcome of burn patients with inhalation injuries who do not survive? Crit Care 12(3):R81

[129] Gauglitz GG, Toliver-Kinsky TE, Williams FN et al (2010) Insulin increases resistance to burn wound infection-associated sepsis. Crit Care Med 38(1): 202–208

[130] Wilmore DW, Mason AD, Jr, Pruitt BA, Jr (1976) Insulin response to glucose in hypermetabolic burn patients. Ann Surg 183(3): 314–320

[131] Gearhart MM, Parbhoo SK (2006) Hyperglycemia in the critically ill patient. AACN Clin Issues 17(1): 50–55

[132] Robinson LE, van Soeren MH (2004) Insulin resistance and hyperglycemia in critical illness: role of insulin in glycemic control. AACN Clin Issues 15(1): 45–62

[133] Khani S, Tayek JA (2001) Cortisol increases gluconeogenesis in humans: its role in the metabolic syndrome. Clin Sci (Lond) 101(6): 739–747

[134] Gore DC, Jahoor F, Wolfe RR et al (1993) Acute response of human muscle protein to catabolic hormones. Ann Surg 218(5): 679–684

[135] Carlson GL (2001) Insulin resistance and glucose-induced thermogenesis in critical illness. Proc Nutr Soc 60(3): 381–388

[136] Wolfe RR, Durkot MJ, Allsop JR et al (1979) Glucose metabolism in severely burned patients. Metabolism 28(10): 1031–1039

[137] Cree MG, Zwetsloot JJ, Herndon DN et al (2007) Insulin sensitivity and mitochondrial function are improved in children with burn injury during a randomized controlled trial of fenofibrate. Ann Surg 245(2): 214–221

[138] Hunt DG, Ivy JL (2002) Epinephrine inhibits insulin-stimulated muscle glucose transport. J Appl Physiol 93(5): 1638–1643

[139] Gustavson SM, Chu CA, Nishizawa M et al (2003) Interaction of glucagon and epinephrine in the control of hepatic glucose production in the conscious dog. Am J Physiol Endocrinol Metab 284(4):E695–707

[140] Mastorakos G, Chrousos GP, Weber JS (1993) Recombinant interleukin-6 activates the hypothalamic-pituitary-adrenal axis in humans. J Clin Endocrinol Metab 77(6): 1690–1694

[141] Lang CH, Dobrescu C, Bagby GJ (1992) Tumor necrosis factor impairs insulin action on peripheral glucose disposal and hepatic glucose output. Endocrinology 130(1): 43–52

[142] Akita S, Akino K, Ren SG et al (2006) Elevated circulating leukemia inhibitory factor in patients with extensive burns. J Burn Care Res 27(2): 221–225

[143] Fan J, Li YH, Wojnar MM et al (1996) Endotoxin-induced alterations in insulin-stimulated phosphorylation of insulin receptor, IRS-1, and MAP kinase in skeletal muscle. Shock 6(3): 164–170

[144] del Aguila LF, Claffey KP, Kirwan JP (1999) TNF-alpha impairs insulin signaling and insulin stimulation of glucose uptake in C2C12 muscle cells. Am J Physiol 276(5 Pt 1): E849–855

[145] Sell H, Dietze-Schroeder D, Kaiser U et al (2006) Monocyte chemotactic protein-1 is a potential player in the negative cross-talk between adipose tissue and skeletal muscle. Endocrinology 147(5): 2458–2467

[146] Baracos V, Rodemann HP, Dinarello CA et al (1983) Stimulation of muscle protein degradation and prostaglandin E2 release by leukocytic pyrogen (interleukin-1). A mechanism for the increased degradation of muscle proteins during fever. N Engl J Med 308(10): 553–558

[147] Saffle JR, Graves C (2007) Nutritional support of the burned patient. In: Herndon DN (ed) Total burn care, 3rd edn. Saunders Elsevier, London, pp 398–419

[148] DeFronzo RA, Jacot E, Jequier E et al (1981) The effect of insulin on the disposal of intravenous glucose. Results from indirect calorimetry and hepatic and femoral venous catheterization. Diabetes 30(12): 1000–1007

[149] Flakoll PJ, Hill JO, Abumrad NN (1993) Acute hyperglycemia enhances proteolysis in normal man. Am J Physiol 265(5 Pt 1): E715–721

[150] McClave SA, Snider HL (1992) Use of indirect calorimetry in clinical nutrition. Nutr Clin Pract 7(5): 207–221

[151] Arora NS, Rochester DF (1982) Respiratory muscle strength and maximal voluntary ventilation in undernourished patients. Am Rev Respir Dis 126(1): 5–8

[152] Greenhalgh DG, Saffle JR, Holmes JHt et al (2007) American Burn Association consensus conference to define sepsis and infection in burns. J Burn Care Res 28(6): 776–790

[153] Williams FN, Herndon DN, Hawkins HK et al (2009) The leading causes of death after burn injury in a single pediatric burn center. Crit Care 13(6): R183

[154] Murray CK, Loo FL, Hospenthal DR et al (2008) Incidence of systemic fungal infection and related mortality following severe burns. Burns 34(8): 1108–1112

[155] Pruitt BA, Jr, McManus AT, Kim SH et al (1998) Burn wound infections: current status. World J Surg 22(2): 135–145

[156] Martyn JAJ, Wilson RS, Burke JF (1986) Right ventricular function and pulmonary hemodynamics during dopamine infusion in burned patients. Chest 89: 357–360

[157] Adams HR, Baxter CR, Izenberg SD (1984) Decreased contractility and compliance of the left ventricle as complications of thermal trauma. Am Heart J 108(6): 1477–1487

[158] Merriman Jr TW, Jackson R (1962) Myocardial function following thermal injury. Circ Res 11: 66–69

[159] Horton JW, White J, Baxter CR (1987) Aging alters myocardial response during resuscitation in burn shock. Surg Forum 38: 249–251

[160] Baxter CR, Shires GT (1968) Physiological response to crystalloid resuscitation of severe burns. Ann NY Acad Sci 150: 874–894

[161] Sugi K, Newald J, Traber LD (1988) Smoke inhalation injury causes myocardial depression in sheep. Anesthesiology 69: A 111

[162] Sugi K, Theissen JL, Traber LD et al (1990) Impact of carbon monoxide on cardiopulmonary dysfunction after smoke inhalation injury. Circ Res 66: 69–75

[163] Horton JW, Baxter CR, White J (1989) Differences in cardiac responses to resuscitation from burn shock. Surgery, Gynecology & Obstetrics 168(3): 201–213

[164] Horton JW, White DJ, Baxter CR (1990) Hypertonic saline dextran resuscitation of thermal injury. Ann Surg 211(3): 301–311

[165] Horton JW, Shite J, Hunt JL (1995) Delayed hypertonic saline dextran administration after burn injury. J Trauma 38(2): 281–286

[166] Horton JW, White J, Baxter CR (1988) The role of oxygen derived free radicles in burn-induced myocardial contractile depression. J Burn Care Rehab 9(6): 589–598

[167] Horton JW, Garcia NM, White J et al (1995) Postburn cardiac contractile function and biochemical markers of postburn cardiac injury. J Am Coll Surgeons 181: 289–298

[168] Horton JW, White J, Maass D et al (1998) Arginine in burn injury improves cardiac performance and prevents bacterial translocation. J Appl Physiol 84(2): 695–702

[169] Cioffi WG, DeMeules JE, Gameili RL (1986) The effects of burn injury and fluid resuscitation on cardiac function in vitro. J Trauma 26: 638–643

[170] Murphy JT, Horton JW, Purdue GF et al (1997) Evaluation of troponin-I as an indicator of cardiac dysfunction following thermal injury. Burn Care Rehabil 45(4): 700–704

[171] Leblanc M, Thibeault Y, Querin S (1997) Continuous haemofiltration and haemodiafiltration for acute renal failure in severely burned patients. Burns 23(2): 160–165

[172] Chrysopoulo MT, Jeschke MG, Dziewulski P et al (1999) Acute renal dysfunction in severely burned adults. J Trauma 46(1): 141–144

[173] Jeschke MG, Barrow RE, Wolf SE et al (1998) Mortality in burned children with acute renal failure. Arch Surg 133(7): 752–756

[174] Wolf SE, Rose JK, Desai MH et al (1997) Mortality determinants in massive pediatric burns. An analysis of 103 children with > or = 80% TBSA burns (> or = 70% full-thickness). Ann Surg 225(5): 554–565; discussion 565–559

[175] LeVoyer T, Cioffi WG, Jr, Pratt L et al (1992) Alterations in intestinal permeability after thermal injury. Arch Surg 127(1): 26–29; discussion 29–30

[176] Wolf SE, Ikeda H, Matin S et al (1999) Cutaneous burn increases apoptosis in the gut epithelium of mice. J Am Coll Surg 188(1): 10–16

[177] Ezzell RM, Carter EA, Yarmush ML et al (1993) Thermal injury-induced changes in the rat intestine brush border cytoskeleton. Surgery 114(3): 591–597

[178] Carter EA, Udall JN, Kirkham SE et al (1986) Thermal injury and gastrointestinal function. I. Small intestinal nutrient absorption and DNA synthesis. J Burn Care Rehabil 7(6): 469–474

[179] Deitch EA, Rutan R, Waymack JP (1996) Trauma, shock, and gut translocation. New Horiz 4(2): 289–299

[180] Deitch EA (1990) Intestinal permeability is increased in burn patients shortly after injury. Surgery 107(4): 411–416

[181] Berthiaume F, Ezzell RM, Toner M et al (1994) Transport of fluorescent dextrans across the rat ileum after cutaneous thermal injury. Crit Care Med 22(3): 455–464

[182] Horton JW (1994) Bacterial translocation after burn injury: the contribution of ischemia and permeability changes. Shock 1(4): 286–290

[183] Gianotti L, Alexander JW, Fukushima R et al (1993) Translocation of Candida albicans is related to the blood flow of individual intestinal villi. Circ Shock 40(4): 250–257

[184] Gamelli RL, He LK, Liu H et al (1998) Burn wound infection-induced myeloid suppression: the role of prostaglandin E2, elevated adenylate cyclase, and cyclic adenosine monophosphate. J Trauma 44(3): 469–474

[185] Shoup M, Weisenberger JM, Wang JL et al (1998) Mechanisms of neutropenia involving myeloid maturation arrest in burn sepsis. Ann Surg 228(1): 112–122

[186] Chitnis D, Dickerson C, Munster AM et al (1996) Inhibition of apoptosis in polymorphonuclear neutrophils from burn patients. J Leukoc Biol 59(6): 835–839

[187] Rosenthal J, Thurman GW, Cusack N et al (1996) Neutrophils from patients after burn injury express a deficiency of the oxidase components p47-phox and p67-phox. Blood 88(11): 4321–4329

[188] Vindenes HA, Bjerknes R (1997) Impaired actin polymerization and depolymerization in neutrophils from patients with thermal injury. Burns 23(2): 131–136

[189] Hunt JP, Hunter CT, Brownstein MR et al (1998) The effector component of the cytotoxic T-lymphocyte response has a biphasic pattern after burn injury. J Surg Res 80(2): 243–251

[190] Zedler S, Bone RC, Baue AE et al (1999) T-cell reactivity and its predictive role in immunosuppression after burns. Crit Care Med 27(1): 66–72

[191] Kelly JL, Lyons A, Soberg CC et al (1997) Anti-interleukin-10 antibody restores burn-induced defects in T-cell function. Surgery 122(2): 146–152

[192] Takagi K, Suzuki F, Barrow RE et al (1998) Recombinant human growth hormone modulates Th1 and Th2 cytokine response in burned mice. Ann Surg 228(1): 106–111

[193] Hultman CS, Yamamoto H, deSerres S et al (1997) Early but not late burn wound excision partially restores viral-specific T lymphocyte cytotoxicity. J Trauma 43(3): 441–447

Correspondence: Gerd G. Gauglitz, M.D., MMS, Department of Dermatology and Allergology, Ludwig Maximilians University, Frauenlobstraße 9–11, 80337 Munich, Germany, E-mail: gerd.gauglitz@med.uni-muenchen.de

# Anesthesia for patients with acute burn injuries

Lee C. Woodson, Edward Sherwood, Alexis McQuitty, Mark D. Talon

Shriners Hospital for Children, Galveston University of Texas Medical Branch Galveston, TX, USA

## Introduction

Remarkable advances continue to be made in the care of patients with major burn injuries. Early aggressive fluid resuscitation has dramatically improved initial survival. The development of specialized burn centers has allowed the concentration and coordination of resources needed to provide a multidisciplinary approach from the time of admission with the goal of not just maximizing survival but optimizing functional recovery as well [1].

Anesthetic management is an important part of this multidisciplinary approach. Anesthesia providers have highly developed skills and experience in airway management, pulmonary care, fluid and electrolyte management, vascular access, and pharmacological support of the circulation. These areas of clinical expertise are all central to the care of patients with major burn injuries. However, the effective use of this clinical expertise for the care of burn patients requires knowledge of the pathophysiological changes associated with burns and an understanding of the multidisciplinary approach to burn care [2]. To be effective, perioperative management should be compatible with overall goals and especially with ICU care.

Patients with large acute burns present multiple challenges to anesthetic management (Table 1). Virtually all organ systems are affected by large burn injuries. These changes have an important influence on anesthetic management including not only drug selection and dosage but airway management, monitoring, fluid administration, sedation, and pain control. As a result, nearly every aspect of anesthetic care must include some adjustment to deal with pathophysiological changes due to the burns.

## Preoperative evaluation

Care of the acutely burned patient requires knowledge of the continuum of pathophysiological changes from

Table 1. Perioperative challenges in the anesthetic management of acute burn patients

| |
|---|
| Airway compromises |
| Inhalation injury |
| Impaired circulation |
| Difficult vascular access |
| Mechanical difficulties with monitors due to cutaneous burns |
| Massive hemorrhage |
| Altered drug response |
| Sepsis/systematic inflammatory response syndrome |
| Altered temperature regulation |
| Co-existing diseases |
| Associated trauma |

151

**Table 2.**

| Patient age |
| --- |
| Extent of cutaneous burns (% total body surface area) |
| Burn depth and distribution |
| Mechanism of injury (flame, scald, etc.) |
| Airway exam |
| Inhalation Injury |
| Quality or Resuscitation |
| Associated Injuries |
| Coexisting diseases |
| Surgical plan |

the initial injury through wound healing and resolution of metabolic changes. In conjunction with the standard features of a preoperative assessment, the anesthetist should focus on certain features associated with increased risk and technical challenge when planning perioperative care of the patient with acute burn injuries (Table 2). The mechanism of injury should be clearly identified since this determines the quality of burn injuries as well as the kinds of associated disorders the patient may present with. As an example, a person burned in the enclosed space of a house and a worker suffering electrical burns would present with very different associated injuries. Since fluid requirements and the pathophysiological response to injury are dynamic it is also important to know the time elapsed since injury.

Pathophysiological alterations in respiratory function are common in severely burned patients (Fig. 1). An airway exam is the first priority in patients with a history consistent with burns to the head and neck and/or smoke inhalation. Tissue distortion due to edema can make intubation by direct laryngoscopy difficult or impossible and these changes will increase with fluid resuscitation. As a result, it is very important to diagnose airway compromise early in the patient with acute burns. Pharyngeal burns can lead to lethal airway obstruction and pre-emptive intubation can be life saving when this threatens. However, facial burns are often not associated with pharyngeal edema and airway obstruction. In the absence of respiratory distress or other reasons for immediate intubation such as very extensive burns, shock, or inability to protect the airway, it may be safer to defer securing the air-

way until it can be accomplished in a controlled setting and when a clear indication for intuition can be identified [3]. This can reduce complications of unnecessary intubations such as exacerbation of laryngeal injuries or life threatening consequences of unintended extubation of a patient who has been intubated then heavily sedated or pharmacologically paralyzed. Initially, patients with smoke inhalation often present with good gas exchange and a normal chest radiograph. Inhalation injury often progresses over time as the inflammatory response develops and small airways are occluded by sloughed tissues, casts and stagnant secretions. Therefore, initial chest x-ray or arterial blood gas analyses usually serve more as a baseline for evaluating changes in pulmonary function. Impaired gas exchange and significant chest radiograph findings on admission are ominous observations. The diagnosis of inhalation injury is usually based on the history and physical exam and confirmed by bronchoscopy.

In addition to airway and pulmonary parenchymal pathology, pulmonary insufficiency can occur in patients with acute burn injury when a restrictive pulmonary deficit results from circumferential burns that limit chest wall expansion during inspiration or from abdominal compartment syndrome when abdominal contents limit diaphragmatic excursion. Restricted chest wall mobility can be corrected by surgical release (escarotomies) and if abdominal compartment syndrome is diagnosed there

Smoke inhalation
Thermal airway damage
Laryngeal edema
Airway Trauma
Restrictive breathing defect
from circumferential escar
Bronchospasm
Pulmonary edema
Aspiration pneumonitis
Pneumonia
Central nervous system injury/
impaired respiratory drive

**Fig. 1.** Common causes of respiratory pathology in burned patients

**Table 3.** Formulas for estimating fluid resuscitation of adult acute burn patients

| Formula | Crystalloid Solution | Colloid Solution |
|---|---|---|
| Parkland | 4 ml/kg/% burn during first 24 hours after injury with half given in first 8 hours | |
| Brooke | Lactated Ringer's 1.5 ml/kg/% Burn | 0.5 ml/kg |
| Modified Brooke | 2 ml/kg% burn | |
| Evans | Normal saline 1 ml/kg/% burn | |
| Slater | Lactated Ringer's 2L/24 hr | Fresh Frozen Plasma 75 ml/kg Over 24 hour |
| Demling | Titrate to urine output at 30 ml/hr | 1$^{st}$ 8 hr: Dextran 40 in saline 2 ml/kl/hr Next 18 hrs: Fresh Frozen Plasma at 0.5 ml/kg/hr |

**Table 4.** Formulas for estimating fluid resuscitation of pediatric acute burn patients

| | Tine | Fluid | Volume |
|---|---|---|---|
| Cincinnati | 1$^{st}$ 8hrs | Lactated Ringer's + NaHCO$_3$50mEg/L | 4 ml/kg/% burn + 1,500 ml/kg$^2$ |
| | 2$^{nd}$ 8 hrs. | Lactated Ringer's | |
| | 3$^{rd}$ 8 hrs. | Lactated Ringer's + 12.5 gm albumin/L | 5,000 ml/m$^2$ burned 2,000 ml/m$^2$ BSA |
| Galveston | 1$^{st}$ 24 hrs. | Ringer's Lactate + 12.5 Gm albumin/L | 5,000/m$^2$ burned 2,000 ml/m$^2$ BSA |

are a number of interventions to reverse associated pathophysiological changes. It is important to be sure that the anesthesia ventilator in the operating room is capable of delivering support that the patient requires in the ICU.

Hemodynamic status, electrolyte balance, and renal function are affected by the extent of burn injuries and the quality of fluid resuscitation. It is important to understand the hemodynamic status of the patient. In the immediate post-injury stage, patients exhibit a syndrome known as burn shock in which increased vascular permeability causes transudation of protein rich fluid from the vascular compartment to the inerstitium leading to intravascular hypovolemia and tissue hypoperfusion. Delays in initiating fluid resuscitation or inadequate volumes administered during burn shock can result in hypoperfusion and damage to non-burned tissues as well as exacerbation of the burn wounds. Over resuscitation also can have deleterious effects such as pulmonary edema or compartment syndromes of extremities or the abdomen. Several formulae based on extent of cutaneous burns are available to estimate the volume of fluid and rates of administration needed to maintain intravascular volume (Table 3). On a ml/kg basis pediatric burn patients have been found to require more volume for resuscitation. In addition, pediatric patients may require resuscitation for smaller burns (e. g. 10–20% total body surface area). Separate formulas have been recommended for fluid resuscitation of pediatric burn patients (Table 4).

Formulas are a starting point for fluid therapy. A comparison of predicted volumes based on the resuscitation formula in use with the actual volumes administered can provide a quick assessment of the appropriateness of the treatment efforts. Resuscitation is then titrated to the patient's response as judged by mean blood pressure and urine output. Many factors such as smoke inhalation, extensive deep burns, electrical burns, soft tissue trauma, and delay in resuscitation can increase the fluid requirements for resuscitation of burn patients. As a result, the needs of each patient are unique and volume resuscitation must be titrated to the patient's response. The response to resuscitation can be evaluated by reviewing vital signs and urine output. However, these endpoints are often not good predictors of tissue perfusion. Blood gas analysis, either arterial or venous, can provide additional information regarding the metabolic status and adequacy of perfusion. Specific endpoints include hemoglobin, base deficit, and lactic acid concentration. If the patient's response is poor despite what appears to be an appropriate volume of fluid administered, underlying pathology should be clarified and additional support such as an inotropic drug provided.

Large burn injuries often present in association with other coexisting diseases or additional trauma associated with the burn accident. It is important not to focus on the burn wound to the exclusion of other serious pathology. A closed head injury, for example, can significantly alter fluid and hemodynamic management choices. A careful history and physical exam should not ignore these other non-burn issues.

Effective perioperative care can only be accomplished within the context of the planned surgical intervention. The appropriate vascular access and level of monitoring depend on the anticipated physiological stress of surgery and expected blood loss. These can only be revealed by clear communication with the patient's surgeons. Close consultation with the surgeons is an essential component of the preoperative assessment of the patient with acute burn injuries.

## Monitors

The choice of monitors in a burned patient depends on the extent of injuries, physiologic state, and planned surgery (Fig. 2). According to American Society of Anesthesiologists, the patient's oxygenation, ventilation, circulation, and temperature should be continually evaluated. Standard monitors include electrocardiography (ECG), pulse oximetry, arterial blood pressure, temperature, capnography, and inspired oxygen concentration. Pathophysiological changes associated with major burns and the potential for massive surgical bleeding may require more invasive monitors and increased vigilance regarding certain physiological variables during the perioperative period. It should be noted that a change in monitoring or transient loss of monitoring may occur during washing, position change, or dressing application.

In many cases, accurate physiological monitoring can be challenging in burn patients. Topical ointments and skin destruction due to large cutaneous burns may prevent adherence of standard gel electrocardiography electrodes and pulse oximetry to the skin. In this case, metallic surgical staples and alligator clips are effective for ECG monitoring. Pulse oximetry during burn surgery can be difficult when extremities are either burned or in the operative

**Circulation**
Arterial blood pressure
Central venous pressure
Pulmonary artery pressures
Cardiac output
Pulmonary artery catheter
Peripheral thermodilution catheter
Pulse pressure variability
End tidal carbon dioxide
Electrocardiography
Urine output

**Ventilation and Oxygenation**
Pulse oximetry
End tidal carbon dioxide
Airway pressures and volumes
Inspired oxygen analyzer
Blood gases

**Temperature**
Foley catheter probe
Rectal probe
Esophageal probe
Oro-nasopharyngeal probe

**Fig. 2.** Commonly used monitors for burned patients

field. The probes or connections may become wet and tendered useless during bathing or irrigation in the operating room. Transmission pulse oximetry probes may be applied or clipped to the digits, ear lobes, or lips as one solution to these challenges. Some clinicians have modified standard pulse oximetry probes for use on the tongue in conjunction with use of a plastic oral airway. Reflectance pulse oximetric technology has been developed to combat problems with signal transmission during hypoperfusion and when a transmission path is unavailable. Forehead probes are commercially available and may detect hypoxemia more quickly than the ear or finger probes [4].

If direct measurement of arterial blood pressure is not required, measurement of blood pressure using a non-invasive cuff has been found to be accurate even when the cuff is placed over bulky bandages [5]. In cases where blood loss is expected to be extensive, as well as in selected high-risk patients or in those failing resuscitation to clinical goals, invasive monitoring with an arterial catheter may be helpful. An arterial catheter is also advised if clinically significant changes in the blood pressure are expected to occur more rapidly than the interval between non-invasive blood pressure measurements or if vasoactive infusions are needed. Although pulse oximetry and end tidal carbon dioxide measurements are adequate monitors of oxygenation and ventilation in patients with normal pulmonary function, these modalities may be inadequate for patients with significant pulmonary disease such as smoke inhalation injury, acute lung injury or the adult respiratory distress syndrome. Under these circumstances it is useful to have an arterial catheter to provide access to arterial blood samples for gas analysis in order to optimize ventilation. This may be very helpful in adjusting mechanical ventilation.

Perioperative management of patients with major burns is often facilitated by the presence of a central venous catheter. A central venous catheter can provide reliable and secure venous access for administering fluids and drugs (especially vasoactive drugs) and for obtaining blood samples when extensive cutaneous burns make peripheral venous access difficult or impossible. In addition, substantial losses of intravascular volume or limited cardiac function make it difficult to appropriately replace volume without some monitor of filling pressure. Although central venous pressure (CVP) is often used to manage intravascular volume, it is an unreliable indicator of preload [6]. Filling pressures interact in complex and unpredictable ways with ventricular compliance and contractility as well as intra-thoracic or intra-abdominal pressures to influence cardiac preload. Cardiac function and response to volume loading have been found to correlate poorly with filling pressures. Preload is defined as end-diastolic myocardial fiber tension; however, this cannot be measured in a clinical setting. Although knowledge of the CVP is not reliable for fine tuning preload, it is important to monitor filling pressure while administering large volumes rapidly. If it appears that tissue perfusion is inadequate and the CVP is low, it is usually safe to administer a fluid bolus as both a diagnostic and therapeutic intervention. If the CVP is high, it is possible that a fluid bolus might cause harm due to intravascular volume overload.

A pulmonary artery catheter (PAC) can also be used to assess cardiovascular function in burned pa-

tients. In addition to the pulmonary artery occlusion pressure (PAOP), right ventricular cardiac output (CO) can be obtained with a pulmonary artery catheter from a thermodilution curve, in which the CO is inversely proportional to the area under the curve. Unreliable results will be obtained in those with right- sided regurgitant lesions or with septal defects. The systemic vascular resistance may also be calculated with PAC-derived information using the following equation:

$$SVR = \frac{MAP\text{-}CVP \times 80}{CO}$$

Despite what appears to be an intuitive benefit of PAC-derived information, the clinical utility of this monitor has been increasingly brought into question. Neither PAOP nor CVP have been found to correlate with either end diastolic volume or stroke volume. Moreover, changes in these indexes of cardiac preload have not correlated with changes in either stroke volume or end diastolic volume in groups of normal volunteers or critically ill patients [6]. Some clinical investigators have found increased mortality associated with the use of a PAC. As a result of these observations and the higher cost of hemodynamic monitoring with the PAC, many clinicians are using this monitor less frequently. Newer volumetric monitors that are less invasive than the PAC have been found to be more reliable indicators of cardiac preload. A transpulmonary thermodilution technique that utilizes a central venous catheter and an arterial fiber optic thermister catheter inserted into the femoral artery can provide estimates of global end diastolic cardiac volume and total intrathoracic blood volume (ITBV). In contrast to CVP and PAOP, augmentation of ITBV has been used successfully to guide fluid resuscitation of severely burned patients. However, use of ITBV was associated with larger resuscitative fluid volumes that predicted by the Parkland formula [7].

Dynamic measures of cardiac preload, such as systolic pressure variation (SPV) and pulse pressure variation (PPV), have been found to be better predictors of volume responsiveness than static indicators such as central venous pressure or pulmonary artery occlusion pressure. These dynamic parameters can be used to discriminate patients who are intravascularly depleted and may benefit from volume loading from patients who are adequately fluid resuscitated but in whom inotropic support is indicated. SPV and PPV parameters are surrogates for stroke volume variation (SVV). The magnitude of SVV broadly correlates to preload reserve [8]. Systolic pressure variation (SPV), which is the difference between the maximum and minimum systolic blood pressure during one mechanical ventilation cycle, has been demonstrated to reflect the degree of blood loss and the associated decrease in cardiac output (CO) during hemorrhage and to predict fluid responsiveness to volume loading. It should be stressed that the concept of PPV and SPV to assess preload reserve is only reliable in mechanically ventilated patients with a regular cardiac rhythm [9].

Urine output measured from a Foley catheter provides a valuable source of information during burn surgery but there are limitations that should be recognized. The American Burn Association guidelines state that urine output should be maintained at approximately 0.5–1.0 ml/kg/hr in adults and 1.0–1.5 ml/kg/hr in children [10] and urine flow rate is often used as an index of global perfusion during general anesthesia. However, oliguria ($>0.5$ mL/kg/hr) as a predictor of hypovolemia or acute kidney injury is less reliable during general anesthesia than in non-anesthetized patients [11]. Anesthetic interventions, whether involving volatile agents, intravenous drugs, or regional blocks, may reduce blood pressure and cardiac output, leading to decreased glomerular filtration and urine formation. Urine output is not a reliable indicator of adequate intraoperative resuscitation in patients receiving diuretic therapy, inotropic support, high cardiac filling pressures, or abdominal compartment syndrome. In contrast, examination of urine provides a reliable indicator of hemolytic transfusion reaction. The signs and symptoms of a transfusion reaction are masked by general anesthesia or by the hemodynamic changes associated with burn surgery. Consequently, when an intraoperative transfusion is planned, a Foley Catheter should be used because the presence of hemoglobinuria may be the only reliable indicator of hemolytic transfusion reaction.

Monitoring of end tidal carbon dioxide ($ETCO_2$) is an indicator of tracheal intubation and provides useful information regarding respiratory rate, airway resistance, and adequacy of pulmonary perfusion. In normal individuals, the difference between $ETCO_2$ and $PaCO_2$ is 2 to 5 mm HG. The gradient between end-tidal and arterial $CO_2$ reflects dead space ventilation, which is increased in cases of decreased pulmonary blood flow, such as pulmonary air embolism or thromboembolism and decreased cardiac output. Therefore, $ETCO_2$ monitoring can also provide important information regarding systemic perfusion, which may be perturbed in severely burned patients.

As hypothermia is a major concern, core temperature should be closely followed throughout the perioperative period. Cutaneous vasoconstriction is the major mechanism for heat retention and core temperature preservation in humans [12]. Burned patients who are undergoing surgical interventions are at high risk for hypothermia. Much of the cutaneous vasculature is severely damaged in patients suffering full thickness burns and, in many cases a large amount of skin has been excised as part of surgical treatment. These alterations ablate cutaneous mechanisms of heat conservation. In addition, general anesthesia causes major perturbations in central temperature control mechanisms. Specifically, it increases the central temperature set point that initiates heat conservation adaptations such as cutaneous vasoconstriction, brown fat metabolism and shivering. The adaptive responses to loss of central temperature are impaired in patients under general anesthesia. Therefore, it is important to maintain a warm operating room environment during burn surgery to minimize heat loss into the environment. Intravenous fluid warmers and airway warming devices can also be useful for minimizing heat loss but do not allow for active warming. Avoidance of hypothermia is an important goal in burned patients because hypothermia is associated with complications such coagulopathy, hypermetabolism and acute lung injury [13–14].

## Pharmacology

The choice of anesthetic techniques and drugs is also dictated by the physiologic status of the patient. Large burn injuries are associated with profound physiological and metabolic changes that produce clinically significant alterations in responses to many drugs [15]. In some cases, drug doses must be reduced to avoid toxicity whereas doses of other drugs must be increased or given more frequently to obtain a desired response. In the case of succinylcholine, large burn injuries lead to exaggerated, potentially lethal hyperkalemic responses and this drug is usually avoided in patients with acute burns. Both pharmacokinetic and pharmacodynamic variables are affected by burn injuries.

For one to two days after large burn injury, loss of intravascular fluids to the wound exudates and to the interstitium and, in some cases, myocardial depression lead to hypovolemia, decreased cardiac output, and increased vascular resistance [16]. These changes often result in decreased organ perfusion. As a result, drug responses may be enhanced and/or prolonged during this phase. The effects are offset to a variable degree by resuscitation efforts. Extreme volumes required for resuscitation result in severe edema and fluid shifts that alter drug volume of distribution and dilute drug binding plasma proteins. After two to three days, physiological status often changes dramatically with development of a hyperdynamic circulation and increased metabolic rate. Volumes of distribution may be increased and drug clearance may be augmented due to increased renal and hepatic perfusion (e. g. fentanyl and propofol) [17]. Burn injury causes opposite effects on the two major drug binding plasma proteins, albumin and alpha$_1$-acid glycoprotein. Loss of albumin through the burn wound exudates and decreased hepatic synthesis result in decreased plasma albumin concentrations. In contrast, alpha$_1$ – acid glycoprotein is one of the acute phase proteins and its concentration can double after major burns. Albumin binds more acidic drugs (e. g. diazepam or thiopental) while alpha$_1$-acid glycoprotein binds mostly basic drugs (e. g. propranolol, lidocaine, or imipramine). As result, protein binding of drugs bound mainly to albumin is reduced while protein binding can be increased for drugs bound mainly to alpha$_1$-acid glycoprotein. Large open wound surfaces provide a novel route of drug elimination and clinically significant elimination of drugs in the wound exudate has been reported [18].

Among alterations in responses to anesthetic drugs used in burn patients, clinically significant alterations in responses to muscle relaxants are probably the most commonly encountered. Large burn injuries are associated with increased expression of nicotinic acetylcholine receptors across the surface of skeletal muscle. This leads to decreased sensitivity to non-depolarizing muscle relaxants requiring higher and more frequent doses [19]. An exception is Mivacurium, for which the pharmacodynamic change in nicotinic receptors on the skeletal muscle surface is offset by a pharmacokinetic change due to decreased plasma cholinesterase that prolongs the action of Mivacurium in burn patients and, as a result, dose requirements are the same as for non-burned patients [20].

In contrast to the non-depolarizing relaxants, large burns cause sensitization to succinylcholine and an exaggeration of its hyperkalemic effect. This hyperkalemic effect has been associated with cardiac arrest in some patients and, as a result succinylcholine is generally avoided in burn patients. The question of when succinylcholine can be safely administered after burn injury is controversial. Since there is little clinical experience with succinylcholine administration earlier than two weeks after burn injury, recommendations are made largely on extrapolation of observations from experimental studies. Authorities have recommended that succinylcholine is safe to administer, from the standpoint of exaggerated hyperkalemia, for approximately 48 hours after large burns [21]. Since resistance to non-depolarizing relaxants have been reported up to a year after injury, it is also recommended that succinylcholine be avoided for a year after wounds have healed.

All these changes, along with the dynamic nature of their development and resolution over time, make it very difficult to predict alterations in drug responses with any degree of precision. The key is to carefully monitor drug responses (and drug level when necessary) and titrate doses according to patient responses.

## Perioperative fluid management

Fluid management during debridement and grafting of burn wounds is one of the more challenging aspects of perioperative care of burn patients. Perioperative care involves not only replacement of shed blood during surgery but the ongoing ICU fluid management of a critically ill patient. If the patient is taken to the operating room early after the injury, practitioners must consider the resuscitation needs of the patient during the burn shock phase. Burn shock results from the transudation of plasma from the intravascular space into the interstitial space in response to massive cutaneous injury and inflammation and results in significant intravascular hypovolemia. Days and weeks after the injury, perioperative fluid management must be executed with regard to the patient's hospital course and recent fluid management choices in the burn ICU. Perioperative care should be coordinated with ICU management. In the days following initial resuscitation, diuresis and fluid restriction are commonly initiated to mobilize fluids and reduce edema. In this context, it is not helpful when a large amount of crystalloid solution is administered during burn wound excision. In addition, surgeons often utilize a tumescent technique to facilitate wound debridement and skin graft harvest by injecting a dilute crystalloid solution subcutaneously (i.e. clysis solution) [22]. The volume of this solution can be quite large and should be considered a source of perioperative fluid administration. In general, limiting the amount of crystalloid solution given to support cardiac preload will help minimize edema and the need for post-operative diuresis.

When extensive burn wounds are excised, blood loss can be brisk and involve substantial volumes. Volume replacement is guided by at least three separate goals: maintain cardiac preload to support cardiac output, administer red blood cells to provide oxygen carrying capacity, and, in the case of massive hemorrhage, administer fresh frozen plasma (FFP) or other components to replace coagulation factors that are lost due to dilution and consumption.

Titrating fluids for volume replacement during burn surgery is difficult for several reasons. It is not possible to accurately estimate the volume of ongoing blood loss during major burn wound excision. Shed blood is concealed beneath the patient or within dressings and may be spread over a broad surface. The patient's physiological status can change rapidly as blood volume is lost or as inflamed and infected wounds are manipulated and release microorganisms and inflammatory mediators with hemodynamic effects that alter myocardial contractility and/or vascular compliance. There is no single physi-

ological variable that can be consistently relied on for titration of administered fluids. The anesthetist must continuously monitor filling pressures, blood pressure, arterial wave form (when measuring arterial blood pressure directly), urine output, hematocrit, and blood gas analysis while replacing shed blood during burn wound excision.

Normal saline (0.9%) has been a popular solution for intravenous volume replacement. Large amounts of saline administered intravenously, however, have been associated with hyperchloremic acidosis. This otherwise relatively benign condition can confuse assessment and/or exacerbate effects of acidosis due to poor tissue perfusion [23]. Use of lactated Ringer's solution avoids this problem but there is a theoretical risk of formation of micro thrombi when lactated Ringer's solution is used to dilute packed red blood cells for transfusion.

A variety of colloid solutions are available for volume replacement. Albumin is widely used but is occasionally in short supply and, in the past, cost concerns have limited its use. Hydroxyethyl starch preparations are frequently preferred. These hetastarch solutions are available in a variety of preparations differing in concentration, molecular size, molecular substitution, and position of the hydroxyethyl group ($C_2$ vs. $C_6$ position on the glucose molecule) [24]. Newer preparations with smaller molecular weight and less molecular substitution may have fewer undesirable effects such as impaired coagulation. Judicious use of colloid solutions can help minimize the volume of crystalloid administered, limiting edema formation and facilitating postoperative care in the burn ICU.

The transfusion trigger for administering red blood cells varies considerably between patients and there is no general agreement regarding indications for transfusion of burn patients. In the past, hemoglobin concentration has been maintained at 10 g/100 ml or above for patients with large burns. More recently, lower hemoglobin concentration has been accepted to reduce the exposure of patients to allogenic blood and to preserve the blood bank resources. For patients with small burns and without co-existing disease processes, 6–6.5 g/100 ml may be tolerated while patients with co-existing cardiac or pulmonary disease may require 10 g/100 ml. If the starting hematocrit and tissue perfusion appear adequate, initial volume replacement can be accomplished with colloid and this will result in a decrease in the hematocrit. Shed blood then contains a smaller red blood cell mass and less blood will need to be transfused to return the hematocrit to the desired level. Periodic blood gas analyses can be used to monitor the patient's tolerance of the reduced oxygen carrying capacity and help guide decisions of when to transfuse packed red blood cells.

An often overlooked role of red blood cells is their ability to facilitate hemostasis. Red blood cells have a rheological effect that increases the margination of platelets by pushing them to the periphery of the blood vessel increasing the near wall concentration of platelets and enhancing their interaction with injured endothelium. Red blood cells may also have effects on platelet biochemistry and responsiveness to enhance their role in hemostasis [25].

Coagulopathy is one of the more consistently observed complications of massive hemorrhage and transfusion. Volume replacement with fluids lacking coagulation factors results in dilutional coagulopathy. Guidelines of the American Society of Anesthesiologists (ASA) Task Force on Perioperative Blood Transfusion and Adjuvant Therapies recommend administration of FFP to patients with micro vascular bleeding when the PT, INR or aPTT are elevated. The guidelines state that FFP is not indicated to treat bleeding when these laboratory measurements are normal [26]. However, recent clinical studies suggest that traditional guidelines for administration of fresh FFP may be suboptimal for managing coagulopathy associated with massive hemorrhage and transfusion. Generally accepted definitions of massive blood loss are one blood volume in 24 hours, 50% blood volume in 3 hours, or ongoing blood loss of 150 ml/min. At these rates of blood loss and volume replacement, coagulation factors are rapidly diluted and hemostasis may be impaired. Hirshberg et al. (2003) have used a computer simulation of exsanguinating hemorrhage to estimate changes in prothrombin time, fibrinogen, and platelets and the efficacy of various resuscitation strategies in supporting coagulation function [27]. Their simulation indicated that current protocols for massive transfusion do not provide adequate coagulation factor replacement to prevent or correct dilutional coagulopathy. They found that in order to prevent

coagulopathy in their model, it was necessary to give plasma before the prothrombin time was elevated and the optimal ratio of FFP to packed red blood cells was 2:3. Subsequent clinical studies in both military and civilian trauma patients have found significant dose-dependent decreases in mortality when plasma was administered early and the ratio of FFP to packed red blood cells was increased. Clinical experience has shown that once coagulopathy develops it may be difficult to reverse and the presence of coagulopathy has been associated with increased morbidity. ASA guidelines for administration of FFP require the diagnosis of coagulopathy before FFP is administered. To prevent, rather then treat, coagulopathy in the massively hemorrhaging patient, Hirshberg et al. recommend a more anticipatory definition of massive transfusion such as transfusion of 4 units of packed red blood cells within an hour with anticipation of ongoing blood loss. A problem with the use of laboratory measurements of coagulation function during massive transfusion is that the results cannot be provided in a timely fashion. Under these circumstances, indications for administration of FFP cannot depend on lab measurements and decisions must be made empirically using protocols. As an example, in our institution, blood loss is replaced with colloid solution to support cardiac preload and packed red cells to maintain oxygen carrying capacity until 50% of the blood volume has been replaced. From that point forward, FFP and packed red blood cells are administered in a 1:1 ratio to replace ongoing blood loss. One key in these decisions is the anticipation of ongoing blood loss, which is determined by clinical judgment.

In addition to dilutional coagulopathy, there are several other clinical problems associated with massive blood transfusion. Hypothermia is a risk during burn surgery and this can be exacerbated by rapid administration of fluids that are inadequately warmed. It is important that blood warmers capable of warming fluids at the flow rates required for resuscitation of massive hemorrhage are used (e. g. >50 ml/min in adults). Rapid infusion of large volumes of blood products, especially FFP, can cause significant ionized hypocalcaemia due to citrate toxicity. Reduced ionized calcium levels affect vascular tone, cardiac contractility, and coagulation. This is more rapidly treated with calcium chloride rather than calcium gluconate because the gluconate form requires hepatic metabolism to release ionized calcium. Other potential complications of blood transfusion include hemolytic and non-hemolytic transfusion reactions and dilutional thrombocytopenia.

Transfusion-related acute lung injury (TRALI) is defined as a new acute lung injury occurring within 6 hours of transfusion in a patient without additional risk factors for acute lung injury [28]. TRALI is the leading cause of mortality associated with blood transfusion. The greatest risk of TRALI is associated with blood products that contain large amounts of plasma, namely FFP and platelets. As with ARDS, there are no specific therapies for TRALI and management is supportive. It is difficult to recognize TRALI in patients with major burns since there are multiple etiologies for acute lung injury and ARDS in these patients. The risk of TRALI has been reduced by institution of a blood bank policy of minimizing preparation of plasma rich components (e. g. FFP and platelets) from donors who are known to be or are at risk of becoming alloimunized against leukocytes [29].

## Postoperative care

Concerns regarding postoperative care of the burn patient are highly variable depending on the patient's preoperative condition and the intraoperative course. Postoperative physiological condition can be influenced negatively by the presence of inhalation injury and by metabolic, coagulation, and hemodynamic problems associated with hypothermia, massive transfusion, or systemic inflammatory response to debridement of infected tissues. In addition, analgesia and sedation needs of burn patients are often exaggerated in the postoperative period.

The decision to extubate the burn patient postoperatively must take into account potential pulmonary dysfunction due to inhalation injury or intraoperative acute lung injury associated with sepsis or systemic inflammatory response as well as the hemodynamic stability of the patient. Analysis of arterial blood gases provides valuable information regarding pulmonary function and metabolic status prior to extubation. Additionally, airway distortion and obstruction from edema can preclude postoperative

extubation. The degree of airway edema can be estimated by direct inspection using a bronchoscope or laryngoscope.

Monitoring needs during transport to the intensive care unit should be established and equipment assembled early to avoid delays in transportation after surgery is complete. Resuscitation drugs and an easily accessible site for intravenous drug administration should be made available prior to transport of potentially unstable patients.

After transport to the intensive care unit, transfer of care requires a concise report of intraoperative events relative to postoperative care as well as fluids administered and estimated blood loss. Surgical debridement, skin harvesting and grafting are painful procedures. Since poorly controlled pain and anxiety can adversely affect wound healing and psychological outcome it is important that pain and anxiety be adequately treated. Tolerance to morphine often occurs in patients with large burn injuries and may necessitate larger doses or may be associated with hyperalgesia that is poorly controlled with morphine. The use of other analgesics such as methadone, fentanyl or alpha-2 adrenergic agonists have been found to be effective when this occurs [30–31]. Anxiolytic agents are also beneficial in burned patients, especially if prolonged mechanical ventilation is required. Agents such as benzodiazepines, alpha-2 adrenergic agonists and propofol are commonly used to provide anxiolysis.

A chest radiograph may be needed to confirm position of an endotracheal tube or central venous catheter or to rule out complications of central venous cannulation. Since maintenance of body temperature can be challenging during burn surgery and hypothermia is poorly tolerated by burn patients, postoperative temperature should be determined on arrival in the intensive care unit and facilities should be available to treat hypothermia promptly, if it occurs. Blood gas analysis and other laboratory studies should be initiated soon after arrival in the intensive care unit in order to identify any pulmonary or metabolic disturbances that require treatment. Ongoing blood loss can be concealed by bulky burn wound dressings and dilutional coagulopathy can occur after massive transfusion. If ongoing hemorrhage requiring transfusion is suspected, a blood warmer should be used to avoid hypothermia. These patients should be monitored carefully for hemodynamic instability or significant decrease in hemoglobin that might indicate continued hemorrhage.

# References

[1] Brigham PA, Dimick AR (2008) The evolution of burn care facilities in the United States. J Burn Care Res 29(1): 248–256

[2] Latenser BA (2009) Critical care of the burn patient: the first 48 hours. Crit Care Med 37(10): 2819–2826

[3] Muehlberger T, Kunar D, Munster A, Couch M (1998) Efficacy of fiberoptic laryngoscopy in the diagnosis of inhalation injuries. Arch Otolaryngol Head Neck Surg 124(9): 1003–1007

[4] Agashe GS, Coakley J, Mannheimer PD (2006) Forehead pulse oximetry: Headband use helps alleviate false low readings likely related to venous pulsation artifact. Anesthesiology 105(6): 1111–1116

[5] Bainbridge LC, Simmons HM, Elliot D (1990) The use of automatic blood pressure monitors in the burned patient. Br J Plast Surg 43(3): 322–324

[6] Kumar A, Anel R, Bunnell E, Habet K, Zanotti S, Marshall S et al (2004) Pulmonary artery occlusion pressure and central venous pressure fail to predict ventricular filling volume, cardiac performance, or the response to volume infusion in normal subjects. Crit Care Med 32(3): 691–699

[7] Holm C, Melcer B, Horbrand F, Worl H, von Donnersmarck GH, Muhlbauer W (2000) Intrathoracic blood volume as an end point in resuscitation of the severely burned: an observational study of 24 patients. J Trauma 48(4): 728–734

[8] Benington S, Ferris P, Nirmalan M (2009) Emerging trends in minimally invasive haemodynamic monitoring and optimization of fluid therapy. Eur J Anaesthesiol 26(11): 893–905

[9] Sakka SG, Becher L, Kozieras J, van Hout N (2009) Effects of changes in blood pressure and airway pressures on parameters of fluid responsiveness. Eur J Anaesthesiol 26(4): 322–327

[10] Pham TN, Cancio LC, Gibran NS (2008) American Burn Association practice guidelines burn shock resuscitation. J Burn Care Res 29(1): 257–266

[11] Alpert RA, Roizen MF, Hamilton WK, Stoney RJ, Ehrenfeld WK, Poler SM et al (1984) Intraoperative urinary output does not predict postoperative renal function in patients undergoing abdominal aortic revascularization. Surgery 95(6): 707–711

[12] Sessler DI (2009) Thermoregulatory defense mechanisms. Crit Care Med 37[7 Suppl]: S203–210

[13] Oda J, Kasai K, Noborio M, Ueyama M, Yukioka T (2009) Hypothermia during burn surgery and postoperative acute lung injury in extensively burned patients. J Trauma 66(6): 1525–9; discussion 9–30

[14] Singer AJ, Taira BR, Thode HC, Jr, McCormack JE, Shapiro M, Aydin A et al (2010) The association between hypothermia, prehospital cooling, and mortality in burn victims. Acad Emerg Med 17(4): 456–459

[15] Blanchet B, Jullien V, Vinsonneau C, Tod M (2008) Influence of burns on pharmacokinetics and pharmacodynamics of drugs used in the care of burn patients. Clin Pharmacokinet 47(10): 635–654

[16] Greenhalgh DG (2007) Burn resuscitation. J Burn Care Res 28(4): 555–565

[17] Han T, Harmatz JS, Greenblatt DJ, Martyn JA (2007) Fentanyl clearance and volume of distribution are increased in patients with major burns. J Clin Pharmacol 47(6): 674–680

[18] Glew RH, Moellering RC, Jr, Burke JF (1976) Gentamicin dosage in children with extensive burns. J Trauma 16(10): 819–823

[19] Martyn JA (1995) Basic and clinical pharmacology of the acetylcholine receptor: implications for the use of neuromuscular relaxants. Keio J Med 44(1): 1–8

[20] Martyn JA, Goudsouzian NG, Chang Y, Szyfelbein SK, Schwartz AE, Patel SS (2000) Neuromuscular effects of mivacurium in 2- to 12-yr-old children with burn injury. Anesthesiology 92(1): 31–37

[21] Martyn JA, Vincent A (1999) A new twist to myopathy of critical illness. Anesthesiology 91(2): 337–339

[22] Robertson RD, Bond P, Wallace B, Shewmake K, Cone J (2001) The tumescent technique to significantly reduce blood loss during burn surgery. Burns 27(8): 835–838

[23] Prough DS, Bidani A (1999) Hyperchloremic metabolic acidosis is a predictable consequence of intraoperative infusion of 0.9% saline. Anesthesiology 90(5): 1247–1249

[24] Jungheinrich C, Neff TA (2005) Pharmacokinetics of hydroxyethyl starch. Clin Pharmacokinet 44(7): 681–699

[25] Hardy JF, De Moerloose P, Samama M (2004) Massive transfusion and coagulopathy: pathophysiology and implications for clinical management. Can J Anaesth 51(4): 293–310

[26] (2006) Practice guidelines for perioperative blood transfusion and adjuvant therapies: an updated report by the American Society of Anesthesiologists Task Force on Perioperative Blood Transfusion and Adjuvant Therapies. Anesthesiology 105(1): 198–208

[27] Hirshberg A, Dugas M, Banez EI, Scott BG, Wall MJ, Jr, Mattox KL (2003) Minimizing dilutional coagulopathy in exsanguinating hemorrhage: a computer simulation. J Trauma 54(3): 454–463

[28] Toy P, Popovsky MA, Abraham E, Ambruso DR, Holness LG, Kopko PM et al (2005) Transfusion-related acute lung injury: definition and review. Crit Care Med 33(4): 721–726

[29] Wright SE, Snowden CP, Athey SC, Leaver AA, Clarkson JM, Chapman CE et al (2008) Acute lung injury after ruptured abdominal aortic aneurysm repair: the effect of excluding donations from females from the production of fresh frozen plasma. Crit Care Med 36(6): 1796–1802

[30]   Williams PI, Sarginson RE, Ratcliffe JM (1998) Use of methadone in the morphine-tolerant burned paediatric patient. Br J Anaesth 80(1): 92–95

[31]   Kariya N, Shindoh M, Nishi S, Yukioka H, Asada A (1998) Oral clonidine for sedation and analgesia in a burn patient. J Clin Anesth 10(6): 514–517

Correspondence: Lee C. Woodson, M. D., Ph.D., Department of Anesthesiology, UTMB, Galveston, TX 77550, USA, E-mail: lwoodson@UTMB. EDU

# Diagnosis and management of inhalation injury

Tina L. Palmieri[1], Richard L. Gamelli[2]

[1] University of California Davis Regional Medical Center; Shriners Hospital for Children Northern California, USA
[2] Stritch School of Medicine; The Robert J. Freeark Professor Department of Surgery; Burn and Shock Trauma Institute; Burn Center; Loyola University Medical Center, USA

## Introduction

Approximately 10–20% of patients admitted to burn centers in the U.S. are diagnosed with inhalation injury, and the incidence of inhalation injury is directly related to burn size [1]. Inhalation injury, along with age and total body surface area (TBSA) burn, is also one of the factors contributing to the morbidity and mortality of patients with burn injury; inhalation injury has been reported to increase mortality two-fold [2–5]. The accurate and timely diagnosis of inhalation injury is key to predicting and improving outcomes for the patient with burn injury. One of the major challenges in the diagnosis of inhalation injury is that exposure to smoke and heat result in nonhomogeneous injuries that vary by location and type of insult. Hence, inhalation injury is a term used to define multiple different types of airway injury, each of which has unique diagnostic and treatment implications. The purpose of this article is to describe the pathophysiology, diagnosis, and treatment of the different forms of inhalation injury.

In general, there are three different types of airway injury that occur after exposure to fire and smoke: 1. effects of inhaled gases, 2. upper airway injury, and 3. lower airway injury [6]. Each of the different types of smoke inhalation injury has a different cause, pathophysiology, treatment, and prognosis. As such, it is important to distinguish among the three types of injury during the initial evaluation of the patient with suspected inhalation injury.

## Effects of inhaled gases

Inhalation of toxic byproducts of combustion account for 80% of fire-related deaths [7]. Several changes in the composition of gases in the environment occur as the result of combustion of flammable objects, and the person exposed to these gases is subject to their effects. When flames engulf a room, they consume oxygen. This decreases the fraction of inspired oxygen in the room to below 10%, which results in asphyxia and tissue hypoxia. Hence, the leading cause of death at the scene of a fire is due to hypoxia, not burns.

### Carbon monoxide

CO is one of the leading causes of poisoning deaths in the U.S., accounting for an estimated 15,000 emergency room visits and 500 unintentional deaths yearly [8]. CO has an affinity with hemoglobin 200–250 times that of oxygen, which decreases both the oxygen-carrying capacity and the delivery of oxygen to tissue [9]. As such, CO shifts the oxyhemoglobin disassociation curve to the left. The morbidity and mortality associated with CO toxicity are caused by interference of oxygen transport at the cellular level and the impairment of electron transport with in the cells, resulting in tissue hypoxia [10]. Several other mechanisms have been proposed to explain the toxicity of CO, including interference with hepatic cytochromes, myoglobin binding, and peroxidation of cerebral lipids [9]. The extent of injury is dependent on the duration of exposure, the concentration of CO inhaled, and the underlying health status of the individual exposed to CO. In general, an exposure to a 0.1% CO concentration can result in a carboxyhemoglobin level of 50% [6].

The common short and long term morbidities of CO toxicity involve the neurologic and vascular systems. Acute CO toxicity at the scene of a fire commonly results in neurologic deficits, which are related to the carboxyhemoglobin level (Table 1) [11]. In general, any patient who is confused or combative after flame burn injury should be considered to be hypoxic until proven otherwise. Neurologic sequelae are divided into two syndromes: persistent neurologic sequelae (PNS), in which the neurologic deficit improves over time, and delayed neurologic sequelae (DNS), in which a relapse of neurologic signs/symptoms occur after a transient period of improvement. Many patients are sedated or being treated with other therapeutic adjuncts that alter level of consciousness after exposure to CO, making it difficult to differentiate to accurately assess neurologic function. CO will, in addition, interfere with the functional state of leukocytes, platelets, and vascular endothelium [12].

Table 1. Carbon monoxide levels and toxicity

| Carboxyhemoglobin level (%) | Symptom |
| --- | --- |
| 0–10 | None |
| 10–30 | Headache, throbbing, dilatation of blood vessels |
| 30–40 | Disorientation, fatigue, nausea, visual changes |
| 41–60 | Hallucination, combativeness, coma, shock |
| >60 | Depressed cardiac/respiratory function, seizure, mortality >50% |

Patients with isolated CO toxicity are classically described as having rosy red cheeks and nose. However, in practice, these patients often are often concomitantly hypoxic, which makes the use of skin color as a diagnostic modality problematic. Importantly, pulse oximetry does not accurately reflect systemic oxygenation, and should not be used to assess oxygenation, and pulse oximetry should NOT be used in isolation to evaluate oxygenation after burn/smoke exposure. Cooximetry, which delineates the impact of COHb, in association with an arterial blood gas, should be used. The diagnosis of CO toxicity is made by measuring plasma carboxyhemoglobin levels. Patients should be given supplemental oxygen until the results of the COHb levels are obtained. The use of oxygen post-exposure is based upon the premise that displacing CO from the hemoglobin molecule will help return oxygen transport to normal. The duration of the hypoxic state is thought to be an important determinant of severity of CO injury; however, COHb levels do not correlate with the severity of poisoning, predict prognosis, or determine choice of a specific therapy [13].

Patients with a COHb >10% need to be treated with supplemental oxygen and COHb levels repeated every hour until the COHb level drops to >10%. Patients who are awake and alert with COHb >10% should be treated with 100% $FIO_2$ via face mask until the COHb level drops to below 10%. Use of 100% oxygen for an additional six hours after COHb levels are >10% may help to facilitate tissue wash-out of COHb. Obtunded patients should be intubated and placed on mechanical ventilation on 100% $FIO_2$. The half-life of COHb is dependent on the concentration of oxygen. Use of 100% $FIO_2$ will result in a half life of COHb of 40–60 minutes [14]. If the COHb level is >25% despite aggressive oxygen therapy, then the patient may be a candidate for hyperbaric oxygen. However, the half-life of COHb remains 30 minutes with hyperbaric oxygen [15]. Four of six studies evaluating outcomes in 1335 patients randomized to either hyperbaric or normobaric oxygen found no benefit of hyperbaric oxygen in terms of neurologic sequellae [9, 16–20]. Given the potential complications of hyperbaric oxygen therapy (tympanic membrane rupture, seizure, lack of patient accessibility), it should be reserved for patients who fail to improve neurologically with documented CO exposure and COHb >25% [6, 11].

## Cyanide toxicity

Cyanide is produced by the combustion of natural or synthetic household materials such as synthetic polymers, polyacrylonitrile, paper, polyurethane, melamine, wool, and silk [21–26]. In addition, cyanide can be found in small amounts at the scene of a fire and has been detected in the blood of smokers and fire victims [27–32]. Cyanide is a normal metabolite in humans; it is both generated and degraded in blood samples in vitro [33]. Blood cyanide levels range from up to 0.3 mg/L in non smokers to 0.5 mg/L in smokers [34–36]. Cyanide can be produced by brain, liver, kidney, uterus, stomach and intestinal tissue after death, and even putrefaction of organs can result in lethal cyanide levels postmortem [37]. A significant or fatal blood cyanide level is usually defined as 3 mg/L although both lower and higher levels have been cited [38–41].

The need for administration of a specific antidote for cyanide poisoning is controversial, in part due to the problems associated with the lack of a readily available and timely method for laboratory diagnosis of cyanide poisoning [42–43]. Initial treatment should include aggressive supportive therapy aimed at restoring cardiovascular function and improving hepatic clearance of cyanide. Survival of severe poisoning (blood levels of 5.6–9 mg/L) after cyanide ingestion or smoke inhalation has been documented when aggressive supportive therapy has been used without cyanide antidotes [44–47]. The use of antidotes may be used in the event that supportive therapy fails to improve hemodynamic status.

Hydroxycobalamin therapy has been used to prevent cyanide toxicity in patients receiving intravenous nitroprusside and to treat toxic amblyopia and optic neuritis caused by the cyanide present in tobacco smoke [48–50]. The effective dose of hydroxycobalamin as a cyanide antidote is 100 mg/kg. Hydroxycobalamin therapy is usually well tolerated, but has been associated with side effects of headache, allergic reaction, skin and urine discoloration, hypertension or reflex bradycardia [51–54]. Hydroxycobalamin may interfere with the accuracy of co-oximetry or autoanalyzer colormetric blood assay (frequently used to assess liver enzymes, electrolytes and minerals) for several days [51, 53–55]. Anaphylactic reactions have also been documented.

In Europe, cyanide toxicity is treated using the chelating agents dicobalt edetate or hydroxycobalamin (vitamin B12a). Dicobalt edetate may cause cobalt poisoning when given in the absence of cyanide and has been associated with anaphylactic reactions, severe hypertension, and cardiac arrhythmias [56, 57]. For these reasons, dicobalt edetate is not available in the United States. These antidotes differ from the oft-mentioned "cyanide antidote kit", which includes amyl nitrite, 10% sodium nitrite and 25% sodium thiosulfate. The rationale for the use of this kit is the oxidization of hemoglobin to methemoglobin, which then preferentially binds cyanide to generate cyanomethemoglobin [58]. Free cyanide is converted to thiocyanate by liver mitochondrial enzymes (rhodanase), utilizing colloidal sulfate or thiosulfate as a substrate, and thiocyanate is excreted by the kidneys [59]. Intravenous sodium nitrite has several significant side effects, including severe hypotension, cardiovascular instability, and worsening hypoxia [60–62]. Hence, the cornerstone of treatment for cyanide is appropriate resuscitation. Metabolic acidosis in a burn patient must be assumed to be due to under-resuscitation, carbon monoxide toxicity, missed associated traumatic injury or a combination of the three. The use of antidotes for cyanide toxicity should be restricted to patients with a persistent metabolic acidosis after under-resuscitation, carbon monoxide toxicity, and traumatic injury have been ruled out.

## Upper airway injury

The second type of inhalation injury does not involve smoke; it is due to thermal injury of the upper airway and oropharynx. During a fire the ambient temperature of inspired room air approaches 150 degrees Centigrade. The heat of the inspired gases is dissipated in the fire victim's upper airway, resulting in a thermal burn of the posterior pharynx, nasal passages, and mouth. The damage of the oropharynx is, essentially, a type of thermal injury, with the heat resulting in protein degeneration, complement activation, histamine release, and oxygen free radical formation [63–66]. Over time the soft tissue surrounding the airway may become edematous due to increases in microvascular hydrostatic pressure and interstitial oncotic pressure; or to decreases in interstitial hydrostatic pressure, plasma oncotic pressure, or the reflection coefficient. The result may be airway obstruction and asphyxiation.

Acute airway obstruction occurs in approximately one-fifth to one-third of hospitalized burn patients who have inhalation injury [67]. Upper airway edema may result in the need for an emergent surgical airway if not addressed appropriately. Timely intubation by the most experienced in airway management is preferable to waiting until severe airway obstruction occurs [68]. The edema associated with acute airway obstruction is variable depending on depth of injury, fluid resuscitation, and patient soft tissue anatomy, but generally peaks at 24 hours following injury [68]. In general, endotracheal intubation is indicated to prevent airway obstruction from edema in patients with significant oropharyngeal burn injury. However, endotracheal intubation has a unique set of benefits and risks. Although it establishes airway protection for the prevention of acute airway obstruction, potentially improves oxygenation in respiratory failure, and provides a secure airway for transport, it has several risks. Attempts to gain airway access may be unsuccessful and/or harmful to the patient. Aspiration, airway injury, loss of airway, pneumothorax, or cardiovascular instability may occur during attempts to secure the airway. In addition, endotracheal intubation increases the risk of ventilator associated pneumonia [69, 70]. Hence, accurate assessment of the patient with potential airway compromise due to burn upper airway edema is paramount.

Determining which patients are at risk for upper airway compromise and need intubation is challenging and requires the integration of history, physical findings, and diagnostic modalities. History of heat and fire exposure is a key aspect in determining whether upper airway edema will be a significant factor during patient resuscitation (Table 2). For example, a patient who sustains a brief exposure to flame ("flash burn") when lighting a barbeque is unlikely to need intubation; however, a person found unconscious in a house fire after 10 minutes is likely to require intubation. History needs to be combined with physical examination, however. The key physical findings suggestive of impending upper airway compromise include hoarseness or stridor, presence of a

**Table 2.** Diagnostic considerations for inhalation injury

| History |
| --- |
| Prolonged exposure to heat/flame in an enclosed space |
| Loss of consciousness |
| Extensive burns to face and neck |
| Aspirated or swallowed hot liquid |
| **Physical Exam** |
| Soot covering face |
| Burns over face and nose |
| Singed nasal hair |
| Carbonaceous sputum |
| Hoarseness, stridor |
| Drooling |
| Obstructive breathing pattern |

second or third degree face burn, burning of facial hair, and the presence of carbonaceous sputum [11, 71]. It is important to note that patients (especially children) with major burn injury (>50% total body surface area), may be at risk of airway obstruction from edema without the presence of a face burn due to the systemic edema that accompanies massive resuscitation. Diagnostic modalities that may assist in determining whether or not airway compromise is imminent include direct laryngoscopy, bronchoscopy, chest x-ray, blood gases, and measurement of COHb levels. However, a normal chest x-ray and blood gas at admission does NOT exclude the diagnosis of upper airway compromise or lower airway injury.

Patients with evidence of stridor, severe (third degree) face burns, significant hypoxia, ventilation abnormality, and burns >50% TBSA should be evaluated for immediate endotracheal intubation. In patients without these signs, assessment for airway injury via history, oral examination (evidence of soot, edema of oropharynx), and changes in voice should be performed [11]. If concern exists with respect to potential upper airway edema or injury, laryngoscopy may be advisable. Of note, when performing laryngoscopy, the clinician should be prepared to intubate, as the procedure may result in acute obstruction. If there is evidence of significant edema or injury, intubation is warranted. If the airway is erythematous, close monitoring may be advisable.

Endotracheal intubation of the patient with a significant burn injury can be challenging due to edema, poor visualization of anatomic landmarks, anatomic distortion due to asymmetric burns, and soot in the airway. In general, the most experienced airway provider should be intubating the patient with burns [71]. It is important to select an appropriately sized endotracheal tube when intubating a patient with inhalation injury. Too small a tube may become obstructed by airway debris and make it difficult to maintain airway patency. Since the edema accompanying the initial injury will be present for several days, changing an obstructed or inadequately sized endotracheal tube can result in lethal loss of airway. Endotracheal tubes should be at least 7.0 mm (preferable larger) in adults, and in children the appropriate tube size can be estimated by the equation: (16+age in years)/4. The preferred route of intubation is nasotracheal, as it provides a more stable airway during the edema phase; however, provider experience is more important than route [71]. A provider should choose the route for which he/she is most proficient. Endotracheal tubes should not be secured with tape for patients with significant edema or face burns, as it will not adhere to the moist wounds or edematous surfaces. Endotracheal tubes should be secured with twill ties (also called tracheostomy ties) which are tied to the endotracheal tube, wrapped around the head circumferentially, and tied anteriorly to allow adjustment for edema formation and resolution. The location of the endotracheal tube at the teeth should be documented, since the endotracheal tube can migrate with movement and edema formation. To minimize facial edema and decrease the incidence of ventilator associated pneumonia, the head of the patient's bed should be elevated 30 degrees [72].

## Lower airway injury

Inhalation injury of the lower airway results in several different physiologic effects. First, casts and proteinaceous material accumulate in the airway, leading to bronchoconstriction and airway hyperreactivity. Second, in conjunction with a large cutaneous burn, inhalation injury results in increased capillary permeability, both in the lung and in the distal airway

[73–75]. As such, inhalation injury is actually a form of acute lung injury (ALI), which may progress to the acute respiratory distress syndrome (ARDS). Similar to ALI/ARDS, inhalation injury with associated cutaneous burn injury results in increased mortality compared to burn injury alone [76]. The inflammatory damage to the alveolar-capillary barrier seen in inhalation injury results in the release of proteinaceous fluid into the alveolar space, which impairs gas exchange [77]. The bronchoconstriction accompanying inhalation injury compounds the impairment in gas exchange even further.

The diagnosis of lower airway injury after smoke exposure relies on many of the same clues used to diagnose upper airway injury. History of the injury, physical examination with inspection of the oropharynx for soot, edema, or ulceration, should be performed [11, 71]. Arterial blood gases, COHb levels, and a chest x-ray should be obtained. Elevated levels of COHb are associated with a higher likelihood of lower airway injury, and one author has developed an algorithm to estimate smoke exposure based on COHb levels [21]. Normal arterial blood gases and chest x-ray do not exclude lower airway injury, but provide valuable baseline data for further comparison. Bronchoscopy is frequently used to visualize injury of the lower airway, and can provide valuable information with respect to airway anatomy and obstruction. At times frequent bronchoscopy is necessary to remove debris and facilitate oxygenation. Xenon perfusion scan has also been reported to be a sensitive indicator of lower airway inhalation injury [78]. However, the need for transport of the patient to nuclear medicine and the resources needed to conduct the examination are prohibitive for many centers.

The treatment of lower airway inhalation injury is largely supportive. Mechanical ventilation is used for severe oxygenation or ventilation deficits. Debate exists with respect to the best form of mechanical ventilation to use for the acute lung injury accompanying lower airway inhalation injury. The volumetric diffusive respirator, a time-cycled pressure limited ventilator, was reported in multiple studies to decrease the incidence of pneumonia and improve mortality after inhalation injury [79–81]. However, this mode of ventilation has not been tested against a low tidal volume ventilation strategy or some of the newer forms of mechanical ventilation such as airway pressure release ventilation or oscillatory ventilation. Recent therapies touted to improve outcomes after inhalation injury include the use of aerosolized heparin, tocopherol, and β2-agonists [82–84]. Nitric oxide has been shown to decrease pulmonary hypertension and improve oxygenation in critically ill patients, but has had limited studies after burn injury [85–87]. However, further randomized prospective trials are needed to validate these therapies.

## Diagnosis

It can be difficult to diagnose inhalation injury. Therefore it is imperative to obtain a detailed history of the event, including source of fire, time of exposition and history of loss of consciousness. A history of entrapment in a closed space, burns in facial area, singed nasal hair, hoarseness, stridor and soot in sputum are early findings that should raise suspicion of the presence of inhalation injury. It is important to remember that inhalation injury can be present without cutaneous burns and in the case that both history and clinical findings are suggestive of inhalation injury the patient should be considered to present inhalation injury until otherwise proven.

On arrival, the patient can be disorientated or mentally altered as a result of CO, cyanide, drug and alcohol intoxication and cephalic trauma [5a]. Chest radiography, arterial gases, carboxyhemoglobin and cyanide levels should be determined on arrival at hospital. Arterial gases and chest X-rays are often normal at admission and this situation does not exclude inhalation injury, but they are valuable as baseline. Afterward, as the injury progresses, both are necessary to monitor the evolution of the patient. Carboxyhemoglobin levels are used to identify CO poisoning and cyanide to assess exposure to hydrogen cyanide.

Fiberoptic bronchoscopy is the most useful diagnostic tool for the assessment of the airway and should be performed in every patient with clinical suspicion of inhalation injury it has the advantage that allows for intubation if needed. Typical bronchoscopic findings of inhalation injury include hyperemia, edema and presence of soot and carbonaceous material along the airway [3a, 5a]. Gamelli et al. graded the extend of the injury which should be used to objectively quantify the extend of inhalation injury (Table 3).

## Resuscitation after inhalation injury

Inhalation injury without burn is associated with a mortality of approximately 5%. Mortality after inhalation injury has decreased in the past 20 years due to recognition of the effects of inhalation injury on resuscitation and advances in airway management. Inhalation injury, due to its effects on the pulmonary parenchyma and its blood flow, impacts the volume of fluid required for burn resuscitation. In severe inhalation injury with associated burn injury the volume of fluid required in the first 24 hours can be as much as 30% higher than the calculated standard Parkland resuscitation formula of 4 ml/kg/total body surface area burn [88]. In addition, studies in sheep have suggested that under-resuscitation exacerbates the lung injury caused by smoke inhalation due to the increased capillary leak and extravascular lung water [89]. The goal for resuscitation after combined burn/inhalation injury is a urine output of 0.5 ml/kg (30–60 ml/hr) in adults and 1 ml/kg/hr in children.

## Other treatment issues

The incidence of pneumonia after inhalation injury approaches 30% [90]. This is due to the impaired airway clearance of debris, loss of ciliary function, mu-

**Table 3.** Bronchoscopic criteria used to grade inhalation injury

| |
|---|
| **Grade 0** (no injury): absence of carbonaceous deposits, erythema, edema, bronchorrhea, or obstruction |
| **Grade 1** (mild injury): minor or patchy areas of erythema, carbonaceous deposits in proximal or distal bronchi (any or combination) |
| **Grade 2** (moderate injury): moderate degree of erythema, carbonaceous deposits, bronchorrhea, with or without compromise of the bronchi (any or combination) |
| **Grade 3** (severe injury): severe inflammation with friability, copious carbonaceous deposits, bronchorrhea, bronchial obstruction (any or combination) |
| **Grade 4** (massive injury): evidence of mucosal sloughting, necrosis, endoluminal obliteration (any or combination) |

From Endorf FW, Famelli RL (2007) Inhalation injury, pulmonary pertubations, and fluid resuscitation. J Burn Care and Research 28: 80–83

cous plugging, and increased secretions. The prevention of pneumonia involves meticulous pulmonary hygiene, use of specialized ventilator modes (such as percussive ventilation), and frequent bronchoscopy both for diagnosis and to clear debris. The use of prophylactic antibiotics is not recommended, as this practice may predispose to the development of more virulent organisms. Clinicians need to remain vigilant and monitor patients closely for the development of pneumonia. Early aggressive evaluation of pneumonia via bronchoalveolar lavage will facilitate the use of appropriate antibiotic therapy. Common organisms isolated from burn/inhalation injury patients vary widely. Infections reported include the SPACE group (Serratia, Pseudomonas aeruginosa, Acinetobacter, Citrobacter, and Enterobacter species), methicillin resistant Staphylococcus aureus (MRSA), and other (Hemophilus influenzae, Streptococcus, Klebsiella) [91].

One potential method for decreasing the incidence of pneumonia while providing definitive airway management after inhalation injury is tracheostomy. Early tracheostomy, which decreases dead space, improves laminar flow, and allows for improved pulmonary toilet, has been shown to be of benefit in children requiring greater than 10 days of intubation in several studies [92, 93]. However, a single center study in adults did not confirm these findings [94]. The use of tracheostomy is generally recommended for patients with major burn injury (>50% TBSA) involving the face who will require mechanical ventilation for >10 days.

The use of steroids in inhalation injury has been controversial. Several studies performed in the 1970s and 1980s demonstrated increased infection rates in patients treated with steroids [95–97]. More recent studies have not shown any benefits to steroid administration after inhalation injury [98, 99]. As such, the use of steroids after inhalation injury is not recommended.

Nutrition after burn and inhalation injury may also contribute to patient outcomes. The early institution of enteral nutrition has been shown to decrease infection rates and improve mortality in patients with inhalation injury compared to intravenous nutrition [100]. The primary route of nutrition for patients with burn/inhalation injury should thus be enteral, and parenteral nutrition should be avoided. To date there is little evidence that immune enhancing enteral formulas provide improvements in infectious rate or mortality in burn/inhalation injury [101].

## Prognosis

Inhalation injury is one of the most important predictors of morbidity and mortality in burn patients. When present, INH-INJ increases mortality in up to 15 times [1, 2]. INH-INJ requires endotracheal intubation, which in turn increases the incidence of pneumonia.

As mentioned before, pneumonia is a common complication of INH-INJ, and increases mortality in up to 60% in these patients [2]. Patients usually recover full pulmonary function and late complications are not the rule. Complications can be secondary to the INH-INJ or to the endotracheal or tracheostomy tube. Hyper-reactive airways and altered patterns on pulmonary function (obstructive and restrictive) have been described following INH-INJ [5]. Scarring of the airway can cause stenosis and changes in the voice, requiring voice therapy and occasionally surgery.

## Conclusions

The evaluation, diagnosis, and treatment of the three types of inhalation injury continue to challenge both experienced and inexperienced practitioners. Although the evaluation of each type of inhalation injury have the same foundation, there are subtle, but significant differences among the three. In addition, the various forms of inhalation injury do not occur in isolation. For example, patients with carbon monoxide toxicity will often have concomitant upper or lower airway injury, as well. Management of each of the forms of injury vary. Inhaled gas exposure requires attention to resuscitation and oxygenation, upper airway injury requires intubation until airway edema resolves, and lower airway injury may require extended periods of mechanical ventilation to maintain ventilation and oxygenation for ALI/ARDS. Finally, prognosis varies based on the extent and type of inhalation injury involved. Timely diagnosis and treatment thus remain the key to improving outcomes in patients with inhalation injury.

# References

[1] Tredget EE, Shankowshy HA, Taerum TV, Moysa GL, Alton JD (1990) The role of inhalation injury in burn trauma. A Canadian Experience. Ann Surg 212: 720–727

[2] Saffle JR, Davis B, Williams P (1995) Recent outcomes in the treatment of burn injury in the United States: A report from the American Burn Association patient registry. J Burn Care Rehabil 16: 219–232

[3] Smith DL, Cairns BA, Ramadan F et al (1994) Effect of inhalation injury, burn size, and age on mortality: a study of 1447 consecutive burn patients. J Trauma 37: 655–659

[3a] Traber DL, Herndon DN, Enkhbaatar P et al (2007) The pathophysiology of inhalation injury. In: Herndon DN (ed) Total burn care, 3rd edn. Saunders, Elsevier, Philadelphia, PA, pp 248–261

[4] Shirani KZ, Pruitt Ba Jr, Mason AD Jr (1987) The influence of inhalation injury and pneumonia on burn mortality. Ann Surg 205: 82–87

[5] Sellersk BJ, Davis BL, Larkin PW, Morris SE, Saffle JR (1997) Early prediction of prolonged ventilator dependence in thermally injured patients. J Trauma 43: 899–903

[5a] Nugent N, Herndon DN (2007) Diagnosis and treatment of inhalation injury. In: Herndon DN (ed) Total burn care, 3rd edn. Saunders, Elsevier, Philadelphia, PA, pp 262–272

[6] Traber DL, Herndon DN, Soejima K (2002) The pathophysiology of inhalation injury. In: Herndon DN (ed) Total burn care, 2nd edn. W. B. Saunders, London, pp 221–231

[7] Birke MM, Clarke FB (1981) Inhalation of toxic products from fires. Bull NY Acad Med 57: 997–1013

[8] Centers for Disease Control and Prevention. Carbon monoxide-related deaths-United States, 1999–2004. 2007; 56: 1309–1310.

[9] Weaver LK (1999) Carbon monoxide poisoning. Crit Care Clin 15: 297–317

[10] Hardy KR, Thom SR (1994) Pathophysiology and treatment of carbon monoxide poisoning. J Clin Tox 32(6): 613–629

[11] Demling RH (1995) Burn care in the immediate resuscitation period. Scientific American Surgery, New York, pp 1–16

[12] Jasper BW, Hopkins RO, Duker HV, Weaver LK (2005) Affective outcome following carbon monoxide poisoning: prospective longitudinal study. Cogn Behav Neur 18(2): 127–134

[13] Hardy KR, Thom SR (1994) Pathophysiology and treatment of carbon monoxide poisoning. J Clin Tox 32(6): 613–629

[14] Crapo RO (1981) Smoke-Inhalation injuries. JAMA 246: 1694–696

[15] Hart GB, Strauss MB, Lennon PA, Whitcraft D III (1985) Treatment of smoke inhalation by hyperbaric oxygen. J Emerg Med 3: 211–215

[16] Mathieu D, Wattel F, Mathieu-Nolf M, Durak C et al (1996) Randomized prospective study comparing the effect of HBO vs. 12 hours NBO in non-comatose CO-poisoned patients: results of the preliminary analysis. Undersea Hyperbar Med 23 [Suppl]: 7 (abstract)

[17] Raphael JC, Elkharrat D, Jars-Guincestre M-C, Chastang C et al (1989) Trial of normobaric and hyperbaric oxygen for acute carbon monoxide intoxication. Lancet 2: 414–419

[18] Raphael JC, Chevret S, Driheme A, Annane D (2004) Managing carbon monoxide poisoning with hyperbaric oxygen (abstract). J Toxicol-Clin Tox 42: 455–456

[19] Scheinkestel CD, Bailey M, Myles PS, Jones K et al (1999) Hyperbaric or normobaric oxygen for acute carbon monoxide poisoning: a randomized controlled clinical trial. Med J Austral 170: 203–210

[20] Thom SR, Taber RL, Mendiguren II, Clark JM et al (1995) Delayed neurologic sequelae after carbon monoxide poisoning: prevention by treatment with hyperbaric oxygen. Ann Emer Med 25: 474–480

[21] Clark CJ, Campbell D, Reid WH (1981) Blood carboxyhaemoglobin and cyanide levels in fire survivors. Lancet 1: 1332–1335

[22] Woolley WD (1972) Nitrogen containing products from the thermal decomposition of flexible polyurethane foams. Br Polymer J 4: 27–43

[23] Bell RH, Stemmer KL, Barkley W, Hollingsworth LD (1979) Cyanide toxicity from the thermal degradation of rigid polyurethane foam. Am Ind Hyg Assoc J 40: 757–762

[24] Terrill JB, Montgomery RR, Reinhardt CF (1978) Toxic gases from fires. Science 200: 1343–1347

[25] Cahalane M, Demling RH (1984) Early respiratory abnormalities from smoke inhalation. JAMA 251: 771–773

[26] Fein A, Leff A, Hopewell PC (1980) Pathophysiology and management of the complications resulting from fire and the inhaled products of combustion: review of the literature. Crit Care Med 8: 94–98

[27] Burgess WA, Treitman RD, Gold A (1979) Air contaminants in structural firefighting. Springfield, VA: National Technical Information Service Publication PB 299 017, US Dept of Commerce

[28] Silverman SH, Purdue GF, Hunt JL, Bost RO (1988) Cyanide toxicity in burned patients. J Trauma 28: 171–176

[29] Clark CJ, Campbell D, Reid WH (1981) Blood carboxyhaemoglobin and cyanide levels in fire survivors. Lancet 1: 1332–1335

[30] Wetherell HR (1966) The occurrence of cyanide in the blood of fire victims. J Forensic Sci 11: 167–173

[31] Barillo DJ, Goode R, Rush BF, Lin RL, Freda A, Anderson EJ (1986) Lack of correlation between carboxyhemoglobin and cyanide in smoke inhalation injury. Curr Surg 43: 421–423

[32] Barillo DJ, Rush BF, Goode R, Lin RL, Freda A, Anderson EJ (1986) Is ethanol the unknown toxin in smoke inhalation injury? Am Surg 52: 641–645

[33] Anderson RA, Harland WA (1982) Fire deaths in the Glasgow area: III the role of hydrogen cyanide. Med Sci Law 22: 35–40

[34] Ballantyne B (1983) Artifacts in the definition of toxicity by cyanides and cyanogens. Fundam Appl Toxicol 3: 400–408

[35] Hall AH, Rumack BH (1986) Clinical toxicology of cyanide. Ann Emerg Med 15: 1067–1074

[36] Ivankovich AD, Braverman B, Kanuru RP, Heyman HJ, Paulissian R (1980) Cyanide antidotes and methods of their administration in dogs: a comparative study. Anesthesiology 52: 210–216

[37] Curry AS, Price DE, Rutter ER (1967) The production of cyanide in post mortem material. Acta Pharmacol et Toxicol 25: 339–344

[38] Gettler AO, Baine JO (1938) The toxicology of cyanide. Am J Med Sci 195: 182–198

[39] Graham DL, Laman D, Theodore J, Robin ED (1977) Acute cyanide poisoning complicated by lactic acidosis and pulmonary edema. Arch Intern Med 137: 1051–1055

[40] Jones J, McMullen MJ, Dougherty J (1987) Toxic smoke inhalation: cyanide poisoning in fire victims. Am J Emerg Med 5: 317–321

[41] Hartzell GE (1991) Combustion products and their effects on life safety. In: Cote AE, Linville JL (eds) Fire protection handbook, 17th edn. National Fire Protection Association, Quincy, MA

[42] Hall AH, Rumack BH (1986) Clinical toxicology of cyanide. Ann Emerg Med 15: 1067–1074

[43] Cohen MA, Guzzardi L (1984) A letter on the treatment of cyanide poisoning. Vet Hum Toxicol 26: 503–504

[44] Vogel SN, Sultan TR, Ten Eyck RP (1981) Cyanide poisoning. Clin Toxicol 18: 367–383

[45] Graham DL, Laman D, Theodore J, Robin ED (1977) Acute cyanide poisoning complicated by lactic acidosis and pulmonary edema. Arch Intern Med 137: 1051–1055

[46] Caravati EM, Litovitz TL (1988) Pediatric cyanide intoxication and death from an acetonitrile-containing cosmetic. JAMA 260: 3470–3472

[47] Brivet F, Delfraissy JF, Duche M, Bertrand P, Dormont J (1983) Acute cyanide poisoning: recovery with non-specific supportive therapy. Intensive Care Med 9: 33–35

[48] Pettigrew AR, Fell GS (1972) Simplified colorimetric determination of thiocyanate in biological fluids, and its application to investigation of the toxic amblyopias. Clin Chem 18: 996–1000

[49] Vincent M, Vincent F, Marka C, Faure J (1981) Cyanide and its relationship to nervous suffering. Physiopathological aspects of intoxication. Clin Toxicol 18: 1519–1527

[50] Cottrell JE, Casthely P, Brodie JD, Patel K, Klein A, Turndorf H (1978) Prevention of nitroprusside-induced cyanide toxicity with hydroxocobalamin. N Engl J Med 298: 809–811

[51] Hall AH, Dart R, Bogdan G (2007) Sodium thiosulfate or hydroxocobalamin for the empiric treatment of cyanide poisoning? Ann Em Med 49: 806–813

[52] Borron SW (2006) Recognition and treatment of acute cyanide poisoning. J Em Nursing 32: S12–S18

[53] Erdman AR (2007) Is hydroxocobalamin safe and effective for smoke inhalation? Searching for guidance in the haze. Ann Em Med 49: 814–816

[54] DesLauriers CA, Burda AM, Whal M (2006) Hydroxocobalamin as a cyanide antidote. Am J Therapeutics 13: 161–165

[55] Borron SW, Baud FJ, Megarbane B, Chantal B (2007) Hydroxocobalamin for severe acute cyanide poisoning by ingestion or inhalation. Am J Emerg Med 25: 551–558

[56] Hall AH, Rumack BH (1986) Clinical toxicology of cyanide. Ann Emerg Med 15: 1067–1074

[57] Langford RM, Armstrong RF (1989) Algorithm for managing injury from smoke inhalation. BMJ 299: 902–905

[58] Ivankovich AD, Braverman B, Kanuru RP, Heyman HJ, Paulissian R (1980) Cyanide antidotes and methods of their administration in dogs: a comparative study. Anesthesiology 52: 210–216

[59] Levine MS, Radford EP (1978) Occupational exposures to cyanide in Baltimore fire fighters. J Occup Med 20: 53–56

[60] Hall AH, Kulig KW, Rumack BH (1989) Suspected cyanide poisoning in smoke inhalation: complications of sodium nitrite therapy. J Toxicol Clin Exp 9: 3–9

[61] Cottrell JE, Casthely P, Brodie JD, Patel K, Klein A, Turndorf H (1978) Prevention of nitroprusside-induced cyanide toxicity with hydroxocobalamin. N Engl J Med 298: 809–811

[62] Garnier R, Bismuth C, Riboulet-Delmas G, Efthymiou ML (1981) Poisoning from fumes from polystyrene fire. BMJ 283: 1610–1611

[63] Friedl HP, Till GO, Trentz O, Ward PA (1989) Roles of histamine, complement and xanthine oxidase in thermal injury of skin. Am J Pathol 135: 203–217

[64] Ward PA, Till GO (1990) Pathophysiologic events related to thermal injury of skin. J Trauma 30: 575–579

[65] Oldham KT, Guice KS, Till GO, Ward PA (1988) Activation of complement by hydroxyl radical in thermal injury. Surgery 104: 272–279

[66] Granger D, Rutili G, McCord J (1981) Superoxide radicals in feline intestinal ischemia. Gastroenterology 81: 22–29

[67] Mlcak RP, Suman OE, Herndon DN (2007) Respiratory management of inhalation injury. Burns 33: 2–13

[68] Fitzpatrick JC, Cioffi WG (1997) Ventilatory Support following burns and smoke inhalation injury. Respir Care Clin N Am 3: 21–49

[69] Cook DJ, Kollef MH (1998) Risk factors for ICU-acquired pneumonia. JAMA 279: 1605–1606

[70] Cook DJ, Walter SD, Cook RJ, Griffith GH et al (1998) Incidence of and risk factors for ventilator-associated pneumonia in critically ill patients. Ann Int Med 129: 433–440

[71] (2004) American Burn Association. Airway management and smoke inhalation injury. In Advanced Burn Life Support Manual. Chicago. American Burn Association, pp 16–20

[72] Drakulovic MB, Torres A, Bauer TT, Nicolas JM et al (1999) Supine body position as a risk factor for nosocomial pneumonia in mechanically ventilated patients. Lancet 354: 1851–1858

[73] Carvajal HF, Linares HA, Brouhard BH (1979) Relationship of burn size to vascular permeability changes in rates. Surg Gynecol Obstet 149: 193–202

[74] Harms BA Bodai BI, Kramer GC, Demling RH (1982) Microvascular fluid and protein flux in pulmonary and systemic circulations after thermal injury. Microvasc Res 23: 77–86

[75] Ward PA, Till GO (1990) Pathophysiologic events related to thermal injury of skin. J Trauma 30:S75–79

[76] Smith DL, Cairns BA Ramadan F et al (1994) Effect of inhalation injury, burn size, and age on mortality: A study of 1447 consecutive burn patients. J Trauma 37: 655–659

[77] Wyncoll DL, Evans TW (1999) Acute respiratory distress syndrome. Lancet 354: 497–501

[78] Pruitt BA Jr, Cioffi WG, Shimazu T, Ikeuchl H et al (1990) Evaluation and management of patients with inhalation injury. J Trauma 30:S63–68

[79] Cioffi WG, DeLemos RA, Coalson JJ et al (1993) Decreased pulmonary damage in primates with inhalation injury treated with high-frequency ventilation. Ann Surg 218: 328–337

[80] Rodeberg DA, Housinger TA, Greenhalgh DG et al (1994) Improved ventilatory function in burn patients using volumetric diffusive respiration. J Am Coll Surg 179: 518–522

[81] Carman B, Cahill T, Warden G et al (2001) A prospective, randomized comparison of the volume diffusive respirator vs. conventional ventilation for ventilation of burned children. JBCR 13: 444–448

[82] Enkhbaatar P, Cox R, Traber LD et al (2007) Aerosolized anticoagulants ameliorate acute lung injury in sheep after exposure to burn and smoke inhalation. Crit Care Med 12: 2805–2810

[83] Morita N, Traber MG, Enkhbaatar P, Westphal M, Murakami K et al (2006) Aerosolized alpha-tocopherol ameliorates acute lung injury following combined burn and smoke inhalation injury in sheep. Shock 25: 277–282

[84] Palmieri TL (2009) Use of beta-agonists in inhalation injury. J Burn Care Res 30: 156–159

[85] Musgrave MA, Fingland R, Gomez M, Fish J, Cartotto R (2000) The use of inhaled nitric oxide as adjuvant therapy in patients with burn injuries and respiratory failure. J Burn Care Rehabil 21(6):551–557

[86] Sheridan RL, Zapol WM, Ritz RH, Tompkins RG (1999) Low-dose inhaled nitric oxide in acutely burned children with profound respiratory failure. Surgery 126(5): 856–862

[87] Sheridan RL, Hurford WE, Kacmarek RM, Ritz RH, Yin LM, Ryan CM, Tompkins RG (1997) Inhaled nitric oxide in burn patients with respiratory failure. J Trauma 42(4):629–634

[88] Naver PD, Saffle JR, Warden GD (1986) Effect of inhalation injury on fluid resuscitation requirements after thermal injury. J Plast Reconstr Surg 78: 550

[89] Herndon DN, Traber DL, Traber LD (1986) The effect of resuscitation on inhalation injury. Surgery 100: 248–251

[90] Rue LW, Cioffi WG, Mason A, McManus W, Pruitt BA (1995) The risk of pneumonia in thermally injured patients requiring ventilatory support. J Burn Care Res 16: 262–268

[91] Wahl WL, Taddonio MA, Arbabi S, Hemmila MR (2009) Duration of antibiotic therapy for ventilator-associated pneumonia in burn patients. J Burn Care Res 30: 801–806

[92] Barret JP, Desai MH, Herndon DN (2000) Effects of tracheostomies on infection and airway complications in pediatric burn patients. Burns 26: 190–193

[93] Palmieri TL, Jackson W, Greenhalgh DG (2002) Benefits of early tracheostomy in severely burned children. Crit Care Med 30: 922–924

[94] Saffle JR, Morris SE, Edelman LE (2002) Early tracheostomy does not improve outcome in burn patients. J Burn Care Res 23: 431–438

[95] Moylan JA, Alexander LG Jr (1978) Diagnosis and treatment of inhalation injury. World J Surg 2: 185–191

[96] Levine BA, Petroff PA, Slade CL et al (1978) Prospective trials of dexamethasone and aerosolized gentamicin in the treatment of inhalation injury in the burned patient. J Trauma 18: 188–93

[97] Robinson NB, Hudson LD, Riem M et al (1982) Steroid therapy following isolated smoke inhalation injury. J Trauma 22: 876–879

[98] Cha SI, Kim CH, Lee JH et al (2007) Isolated smoke inhalation injuries: Acute respiratory dysfunction, clinical outcomes, and short-term evolution of pulmonary functions with the effects of steroids. Burns 33: 200–208

[99] Nieman GF, Clark WF, Hakim T (1991) Methylprednisolone does not protect the lung from inhalation injury. Burns 17: 384–390

[100] Herndon DN, Barrow RE, Stein M, Linares H et al (1989) Increased mortality with intravenous supplemental feeding in severely burned patients. J Burn Care Res 10: 309–313

[101] Saffle JR, Wiebke G, Jennings K, Morris SE et al (1997) Randomized trial of immune-enhancing nutrition in burn patients. J Trauma 42: 793–802

Correspondence: Tina L. Palmieri M.D., FACS, FCCM, Shriners Hospital for Children Northern California and University of California Davis, 2425 Stockton Blvd, Suite 718, Sacramento, CA 95 817, USA, E-mail: tina.palmieri@ucdmc.ucdavis.edu

# Respiratory management

Robert Cartotto

Ross Tilley Burn Centre at Sunnybrook Health Sciences Centre, Department of Surgery, University of Toronto, ON, Canada

## Airway management

### (a) Endotracheal intubation

Respiratory therapy begins with ensuring that the burn patient has a protected and stable airway. Failure to recognize the potential for airway obstruction, or impending airway obstruction may result in lethal consequences for the burn patient. Classically, airway obstruction in burn victims rapidly progresses from mild pharyngeal edema to complete upper airway obstruction [1]. Endotracheal intubation of a burn-injured patient is generally indicated in the following situations:

▶ Physical evidence of upper airway injury. This necessitates careful direct observation of the lips, tongue, oropharynx, and (if possible) laryngeal structures. Fiberoptic nasal-laryngoscopy under topical anesthesia is particularly helpful in some cases. Evidence of swelling, erythema, heavy carbonaceous deposits, hoarseness or voice changes, and stridor should be considered indicative of possible upper airway injury and should prompt prophylactic intubation.

▶ Large surface area burns. The large anticipated fluid resuscitation volumes delivered in these cases can result in massive generalized edema, including airway edema, even in the absence of a direct airway injury or smoke inhalation. While there is no exact burn size above which intubation is mandatory, in general, as the burn size exceeds 35% to 40% of the body surface area, intubation is advisable. An additional benefit of this approach is that the practitioner can be more liberal with provision of analgesics and anxiolytics with the airway protected.

▶ Suspected smoke inhalation. While intubation is not necessary for every case of smoke exposure [2] it is frequently difficult to predict which patients have sustained a serious smoke inhalation injury and who will progress to an upper airway obstruction or develop early aggressive respiratory failure. Ideally the decision to intubate should be made based on awake fibreoptic assessment of the airways [3, 4]. However, this is often neither feasible nor practical in many emergency departments and a decision to intubate must be made based on clinical assessment of the patient. Strong indications would include a clear history of prolonged exposure to smoke or asphyxiants, any depression of mental status, or any evidence of edema, erythema or heavy carbonaceous deposits in the upper airway.

▶ Extensive facial and/or neck burns. The local edema associated with these wounds may cause extrinsic obstruction of the airway. It is mandatory to recognize this situation early, before edema develops because intubation may subsequently become impossible.

▶ High risk of heat transfer to the lower airways. Heat is infrequently transferred to the lower airways. However, this can occur in a few unique scenarios which include steam inhalation, close proximity to a forceful explosion, and aspiration of hot liquids. The clinician should consider early prophylactic intubation in these situations.

▶ Significant carbon monoxide (CO) poisoning. Ventilation with 100% oxygen is the mainstay of treatment for CO poisoning. While mask ventilation using a reservoir bag and non-rebreather valve is effective in many cases, when carboxyhemoglobin levels rise above 25–30%, CNS depression will develop and a preferred approach is to deliver 100% oxygen by endotracheal intubation and mechanical ventilation.

▶ Depressed level of consciousness. This can accompany burn injury and may be related to any number of causes including inhalation of asphyxiants (e. g. CO or hydrogen cyanide), associated injuries, or impared oxygenation or ventilation.

Once the decision to intubate is made, it is preferable to have the most experienced health care provider available perform the procedure. The airway of a burn patient should always be viewed as potentially difficult. Paralyzing or long-acting sedating agents should be avoided because if intubation turns out to be difficult a rapidly deteriorating scenario of being unable to intubate and unable to ventilate may en-

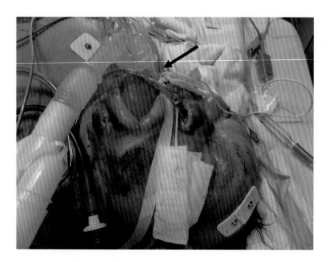

**Fig. 1.** Danger associated with prior shortening an endotracheal tube. Massive edema of the soft tissues of the lip and mouth leads to a precarious connection of the endotracheal tube with the ventilator circuit (arrow). The endotracheal tube cannot be safely exchanged at this point

sue. Small doses of parenteral fentanyl, midazolam, and propofol combined with topical anesthetic agents, while attempting to intubate with the patient as awake as possible is the preferred approach. At the very least, an attempt at visualization of the airway with the patient awake should be considered. The fibreoptic bronchoscope or glidescope may be useful adjunctive devices. The endotracheal tube should not be shortened because if there is significant facial and lip edema, the connection between the tube and the circuit may become buried within the mouth (Fig. 1). The endotracheal; tube should always be secured with circumferential cotton ties around the face and neck. Adhesive tape should not be used.

## (b) Elective tracheostomy

For patients who do not appear extubatable by 14 days, elective tracheostomy is usually indicated to avoid the long term complications of more prolonged endotracheal intubation, namely laryngeal and tracheal damage [5, 6]. However, controversy continues to surround both the indications for, and the timing of earlier elective tracheostomy in burn patients, prior to this somewhat arbitrary 14 day cutoff point. Earlier tracheostomy potentially offers the benefits of improved patient comfort with the resulting need for less sedation, greater airway security especially in children, easier suctioning with improved pulmonary toilet, and easier weaning from the ventilator, compared with use of an endotracheal tube.

Retrospective studies from the 1970's and 1980's focused on the potential morbidity of tracheostomy in the burn patient. Enthusiasm for tracheostomy was curbed by reports in these studies of tracheobronchial contamination from the burn wound leading to pulmonary infection, tracheal injuries including tracheal erosion, tracheo-innominate artery or tracheo-esophageal fistulas, and mortality directly linked to the tracheostomy [7–10]. Subsequent to these early reports, further retrospective studies identified that that burn patients who had tracheostomies were at no higher risk of pulmonary sepsis or increased mortality than those managed with intubation [11]. Gaissert et al. [12] reviewed patients with tracheal strictures after inhalation injury and found that the inhalation injury itself and the method

**Table 1.** Studies of early elective tracheostomy in burn patients since 2000

| Study | Design | N | Patient selection | Interventions | Outcomes |
|---|---|---|---|---|---|
| Saffle et al. [15] | Randomized Prospective | 44 | ▶ Burned adults predicted at high risk of PVD based on a validated predictive model<br>▶ Mean burn size 45% TBSA | ▶ Early Tracheostomy (ET) on day 4 post burn<br>▶ Conventional (CON) treatment with intubation and tracheostomy on post burn day 14 if not extubated. | ▶ ET had better oxygenation improvement<br>▶ No differences in LOS, incidence of pneumonia, duration of MV, or survival<br>▶ Higher number extubated before 14 days in CON |
| Palmieri et al. [16] | Retrospective | 38 | ▶ Pediatric with mean burn size 54% TBSA and 63% with inhalation injury | ▶ Elective tracheostomy at a mean of 3.9 days post admission<br>▶ Indications were anticipated PVD, occluded ETT, or ARDS | ▶ Significant improvement in compliance and $PaO_2/FiO_2$ at 24 hours post tracheostomy.<br>▶ No complications related to tracheostomy |

N: number of subjects, PVD: prolonged ventilator dependence, LOS: length of stay in hospital, MV: mechanical ventilation, ETT: endotracheal tube

of airway support were likely equally contributory. Lund et al. found that the duration of intubation was probably the most important variable in predicting complications from tracheostomy [13]. Thus, retrospective studies prior to 1990 provide only conflicting conclusions on the safety of tracheostomy in burn patients, and do not answer questions on the efficacy or timing of early elective trachesotomy.

In 1997, Sellers et al. from the Intermountain Burn Center in Utah [14], used logistic regression analysis to derive, from a development set of 110 patients, a predictive equation for determining the likelihood of prolonged ventilator dependence (PVD). Variables in their formula that correlated with PVD were the full thickness burn size, patient age, presence of inhalation injury, and the $PaO_2/FiO_2$ ratio on day three post burn. When the equation was applied prospectively to a test set of 29 patients, it had a sensitivity of 90%, a specificity of 100%, and a positive predictive value of 100% in predicting PVD. This study is particularly relevant because any meaningful investigation of early tracheostomy efficacy and timing must select patients who would be at high risk of PVD. With this in mind, two relatively recent studies addressing the tracheostomy question should be examined (Table 1):

Saffle et al. [15] randomized 44 adult burn patients who were predicted to have prolonged ventilator dependence based on the predictive formula just described, to either early tracheostomy (ET), which occurred at a mean of 4 days post burn, or to conventional treatment (CON) with an endotracheal tube and tracheostomy after 14 days of mechanical ventilation if extubation was not possible. There were no significant differences between the groups in the development of pneumonia, length of stay, duration of mechanical ventilation, or mortality. The ET group had superior improvements in $PaO_2/FiO_2$ ratio from post burn day 2 to 5, compared to CON, and this was attributed to better secretion clearance in the patients with a tracheostomy. However, there were a significantly higher number of intubated patients in the CON group who were extubated and liberated from mechanical ventilation support before day 14, than in the ET group. It was hypothesized that more aggressive weaning and earlier removal of the endotracheal tube in the CON group was prompted by the higher degree of patient discomfort and perceived need to extubate these patients, whereas in the ET group, the patients were more comfortable and tolerated the tracheostomy more easily, which did not prompt the same degree of aggressiveness in corking and discontinuation of ventilatory support. In summary, no particular advantage of early tracheostomy was identified, but importantly, the authors stated that there did not appear to be any particular downside either.

Palmieri et al. [16] retrospectively reviewed 38 severely burned children who underwent tracheostomy at a mean of 3.9 days post burn centre admission. There was no comparison group of patients with endotracheal tubes. The decision to perform tracheostomy was based on a variety of indications and not solely on a prediction of prolonged ventilator dependence. Full thickness head and facial burns were present in 87% of the subjects and tracheostomies were inserted through a burn wound in 61% of the procedures. Tracheostomy resulted in significant improvement in respiratory compliance and PaO$_2$/FiO$_2$ ratio at 24 hours post procedure and there were no tracheostomy related complications, wound site infections or airway losses after tracheostomy. The incidence of pneumonia was not specifically studied, but 23/38 (55%) had positive sputum cultures consistent with bacterial colonization post tracheostomy. Tracheostomy in burned children was therefore felt to be safe and advantageous, especially from the perspective of ease of mechanical ventilation, and airway security.

To summarize, earlier tracheostomy offers the advantages of better pulmonary toilet and ease of suctioning, better ventilation mechanics and possibly easier weaning, greater patient comfort with less need for sedation, and greater airway security. The disadvantages are that it is an invasive procedure with a low but recognized incidence of significant tracheal and laryngeal complications. The only randomized prospective study to date found no specific benefit to early tracheostomy, but importantly, could not cite any major adverse sequelae associated with this approach. Most likely, prolonged translaryngeal intubation followed by a tracheostomy is the least desirable scenario and should be avoided whenever possible. Patients with severe neck or facial burns or swelling, patients who are likely to need prolonged ventilator support based on advanced age, presence of large burns, and smoke inhalation and pediatric burn patients particularly those with significant burns or extensive facial burns, where securing an airway is considerably more difficult, represent the preferred patient groups in which to consider early tracheostomy.

## Chest escharotomy

Following airway stabilization the next respiratory priority is to ensure adequate ventilation. Full thickness circumferential or near circumferential burns of the chest and/or abdomen may restrict chest ex-

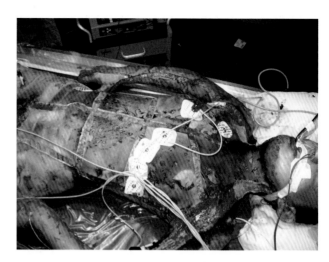

**Fig. 2.** Standard escharotomy incisions have been augmented with additional incisions to form a "checkerboard" pattern

pansion. This occurs because of edema formation underneath the inelastic full-thickness eschar enveloping the chest limits thoracic expansion. Typically, this will become apparent as manual ventilation with a Laerdal bag will feel "tight". Alternatively, for patients on a ventilator, progressively rising airway pressures and end-tidal CO$_2$ and decreasing tidal volumes may be observed. Bedside chest escharotomy is usually immediately therapeutic but it is preferable to perform the escharotomy prophylacticaly in anticipation of this scenario. The author's approach is to begin with longitudinal incisions along the anterior axillary line, bilaterally, connecting these with a horizontal incision at the costal margin to make an "H" pattern (Fig. 2). Additional vertical and horizontal incisions may be added if needed in a "checkerboard" pattern. Escharotomies must extend just past the edge of the burn and should include the abdomen if it is involved. Other causes of impaired ventilation and worsening chest compliance such as endotracheal tube obstruction or a tension pneumothorax should always be ruled out.

## Bronchial hygiene and chest physiotherapy

Bronchial hygiene and chest physiotherapy are important adjunctive therapies in any intubated and mechanically ventilated patient, but these are particularly important interventions in a burn patient with smoke inhalation. It is essential to mobilize and clear the airways of the copious secretions, sloughing mucosa and particulate carbonaceous debris that commonly follows an inhalation injury. Retention of these airway obstructants will inevitably result in atelectasis and pneumonia. Mlcak et al. have extensively described techniques of bronchial hygiene [1, 17].

Therapeutic coughing involves stimulation of the cough reflex. Non intubated patients are encouraged by the physiotherapist to voluntarily perform a series of smaller to larger coughs which may be augmented by tracheal massage by the physiotherapist. Intubated patients may have a cough stimulated by transiently altering the balloon cuff pressure or by tracheal suctioning. Chest physiotherapy also includes regular (q1–2 hourly) changes in position for intubated ventilated patients to promote postural drainage, combined with percussion, vibration, and shaking of the chest. Unique to the burn patient is the need to respect skin graft and donor sites, which can affect the intensity of chest physiotherapy. Early ambulation and upright positioning is highly beneficial as it promotes better expansion of the lungs, and maintenance of respiratory muscle tone and strength. Mlcak has even described upright chair positioning of patients on continuous ventilatory support [1, 17].

Finally, fiberoptic bronchoscopy may be used in a therapeutic fashion to irrigate, loosen, and then remove by suctioning retained cast and airway debris in the primary and secondary bronchi. This approach is mainly used in patients with severe inhalation injury and copious secretions with heavy carbonaceous deposits.

## Inhaled heparin/N-acetylcystine (Heparin-NAC)

This inhalational therapy is used in numerous Burn Centres for patients with inhalation injury. Following smoke inhalation, airways become progressively obstructed due to mucosal edema and the formation of occlusive casts containing fibrin, cellular debris, mucus and polymorphoneuclear leukocysts [18, 19]. Populations of alveoli distal to the occluded airways are hypoventilated and when combined with region-

al vasodilation caused by inflammatory mediators, results in ventilation perfusion mismatch and increased shunt fraction creating hypoxemia. Other populations of alveoli with patent airways may be subjected to hyperinflation causing mechanical trauma which augments the inflammatory response induced by exposure of the airways to the toxins in smoke. This inflammatory response is characterized by a neutrophil chemotaxis and activation and local production of oxygen-free radicals which propagate pulmonary microvascular injury and further lung damage [20–22].

Inhaled heparin-NAC is intended to act not only as a mucolytic agent to break down and loosen the obstructing casts but also to harness NAC's capabilities as a free radical scavenger [23]. Animal experiments determined that a heparin infusion reduced tracheobronchial casts, minimized barotrauma and pulmonary edema, and improved oxygenation after smoke inhalation injury. Further animal experimentation in an ovine model of inhalation injury also found that the combination of heparin and dimethyl sulfoxide (a free-radical scavenger) produced improved oxygenation, reduction in peak inspiratory pressures and improved survival [25].

Three human trials of heparin-NAC, following smoke inhalation have been reported (Table 2). All are retrospective and involve either historical or contemporaneous non-randomized control groups. The studies all differ slightly in the treatment regimen: dosages of heparin differ slightly (5000 units vs. 10,000 units), Albuterol is sometimes given in combination with the heparin-NAC, and Heparin and NAC are either given separately or in combination. The studies by Desai et al. (in children) [26] and Miller et al. [20] (in adults) were positive and found benefit from heparin-NAC. Although both studies used historical controls, all patients in both of these studies had bronchoscopy-confirmed smoke inhalation and all patients were mechanically ventilated. The study by Miller et al. [20] provides the most detailed analysis of the beneficial outcomes in the heparin-NAC treated patients which included significant reductions in the lung injury score, significantly improved respiratory resistance and lung compliance measurements, and significantly less hypoxemia and a survival benefit compared to untreated controls. In contrast, the study by Holt et al. [27] found no benefit

**Table 2.** Comparison of studies involving inhaled heparin and N-Acetyl Cystine (NAC) for smoke inhalation

| Study | Design | N | Patient selection | Interventions | Outcomes |
|---|---|---|---|---|---|
| Desai et al. [26] | Retrospective Historical Controls | 90 | ► Pediatric<br>► Mean burn size 50%–55% TBSA<br>► All bronchoscopic-confirmed II<br>► All mechanically ventilated | ► 5000 U aerosolized heparin alternating with 3 mL aerosolized 20% NAC every 2 hours for 7 days | ► Treatment group had significantly lower reintubation rates, evidence of atelectasis, and mortality |
| Holt et al. [27] | Retrospective Contemporaneous Controls Unblinded | 150 | ► Adults<br>► Mean burn size 27%–32% TBSA<br>► Only 68% had bronchoscope-confirmed II<br>► physician discretion used to initiate heparin-NAC | ► inhaled 5000U heparin with 3 mL 20% NAC with albuterol every 4 hours for 7 days | ► No differences in pneumonia, duration of MV, re-intubation, LOS, survival, or $PaO_2/FiO_2$ ratios on days 1, 3, and 7 post burn between treatment and control |
| Miller et al. [20] | Retrospective Historical Controls | 30 | ► Adults<br>► All mechanically ventilated<br>► All with bronchoscope-confirmed II | ► nebulized 10 000 U heparin with 3 ml 20% nac, and Albuterol every 4 hours for 7 days | ► Treatment group showed significantly better improvement in LIS, respiratory resistance and compliance, and hypoxemia compared to controls. |

N: number of subjects, II: inhalation injury, MV: mechanical ventilation, LOS: length of hospital stay, LIS: Lung Injury Score

from heparin-NAC but this study may have been flawed by the fact that only 68% of the study population had a bronchoscopic diagnosis of inhalation injury. Additionally, some of the patients were intubated and mechanically ventilated for as little as one day. Also, the decision to use heparin-NAC was at the attending physician's discretion.

The available evidence would therefore suggest that for a mechanically ventilated patient with bronchoscopically-confirmed inhalation injury that a one week course of nebulized Heparin (5,000 to 10,000 units) with 3 mL of 20% NAC every four hours with or without the addition of Albuterol may be of benefit. This regimen appears to relatively safe and adverse effects such as NAC-induced bronchospasm or Heparin-induced thrombocytopenia were not reported in any of the studies discussed.

## Conventional mechanical ventilation

### Introduction

The approach to conventional mechanical ventilation (CMV) for critically ill patients has undergone dramatic change in the past decade. A ventilation strategy that was characterized by the use of liberal tidal volumes, tolerance of high peak and plateau airway pressures, and the goal of normalization of arterial blood gas values has been replaced by gentler approaches to mechanical ventilation which feature use of lower tidal volumes, limited airway pressures, permissive hypercapnia, and enthusiasm for "open lung" strategies using higher positive and expiratory pressure (PEEP) settings along with lung recruitment maneuvers. While this paradigm shift has largely been adopted in the approach to CMV in the burn patient, three important points should be considered:

► Burn patients were either excluded from, or were minimally represented in virtually all of the major trials that have promoted low tidal volume, pressure limited and open lung approaches to CMV

► The current approaches to CMV are directed at patients with existing Acute Lung Injury (ALI) and Acute Respiratory Distress Syndrome (ARDS). Unlike patients in the Intensive Care Unit who are admitted with some degree of lung dysfunction or injury, the majority of burn patients who are intubated start out their course of mechanical ventilation with relatively normal lungs even in the face of smoke inhalation. Typically, lung dysfunction, pulmonary edema, ALI, and ARDS frequently develop within days of burn injury and Burn Centre admission. It is the rule rather than the exception that the initial mechanical ventilation is being delivered to uninjured lungs. As such, there has been no research directed at this unique situation and inevitably, ventilation strategies designed for ALI and ARDS are translated to intubated patients with acute burns even though pathology may not yet have developed in the lungs of these patients.

▶ The chest wall mechanics of many burn patients can be vastly different from that of most critically ill patients from whom current CMV strategies have evolved. Specifically, the presence of unyielding eschar, and significant soft-tissue edema on the abdomen and thorax of the burn patient have significant effects on respiratory compliance. Thus airway pressures measured at the ventilator may not be reflective of actual trans-pulmonary pressures in the lung.

This section of the chapter is not intended to give specific formulas or prescriptions for mechanical ventilation of the burn patient. Rather, the intention is to review general concepts and approaches to mechanical ventilation, which are believed to affect respiratory outcomes bearing in mind the above points, which draw attention to the fact that most of these principles have been developed in patients without burns but have inevitably been adopted by burn clinicians and translated to the burn patient.

## Pathophysiological principles

All of the general principles of current CMV strategies which will be discussed below have evolved from an improved understanding of the pathology of ALI and ARDS, and the recognition that mechanical ventilation may itself be harmful to the lungs and may directly cause new, or worsen existing ALI and ARDS. This process is referred to as ventilatory induced lung injury (VILI) [28, 29]. Specifically, ventilation with large tidal volumes and high peak airway pressures causes injury through excessive stretch of the alveoli (volutrauma), while inadequate and inspiratory pressures allow shear injury to occur from repetitive alveolar collapse and then re-opening (atelectrauma). These mechanical injuries then cause

inflammation which further injures the lung (biotrauma) [28, 29].

It is essential to appreciate that heterogeneity is the defining feature of the lungs in patients with ALI and ARDS. Computed tomography studies have been seminal in understanding the herterogeneous pathology of ARDS [30]. Some areas of the lung (usually the non-dependent regions) may be relatively unaffected while other areas (usually the dependent areas posterior to the heart and mediastinum) show atelectasis and consolidation. Furthermore, some of the affected alveoli show predominantly consolidation, while others show predominantly atelectasis, even within the same lung. Hence, some parts of the lung do not receive ventilation because they are consolidated and less compliant so that mechanical ventilation ends up being delivered to a much smaller than normal volume of less affected, or even normal lung. This has been referred to as the "baby lung" concept [31] which refers to the idea that during ARDS only a small functioning baby-sized lung is being ventilated inside a fully grown adult. Thus, if traditional adult-sized airway pressures and tidal volumes are used, these are delivered only to a small portion of the lung thus causing barotrauma or volutrauma.

To complicate matter further, some forms of ARDS feature "loose" or more recruitable lung (e.g. from inflammatory edema) whereas other forms feature "sticky" non-recruitable lung (e.g. consolidative pneumonia) [32–34]. For example, it is conceivable (but unknown at present) whether ARDS after smoke inhalation may feature a predominance of "sticky" non-recruitable alveoli, rather than "loose" more recruitable alveoli.

## Low tidal volume and limited plateau pressure approaches

The well-known large multi-centre study by the acute respiratory distress syndrome of the National Heart Lung, and Blood Institute (ARDS Net) in 2000 found that a traditional approach using tidal volumes of 12 mL/kg predicted body weight (PBW) and plateau pressures up to 50 cmH$_2$O was associated with significantly higher mortality than a CMV strategy using a tidal volume of 6 mL/kg PBW and plateau pressures limited to less than 30 cmH$_2$O [35]. The other important trials that have examined the use of low

**Table 3.** Comparison of randomized prospective studies using low tidal volume (Vt) and limited plateau Pressures ($P_{plat}$) strategies for mechanical ventilation of patients with ARDS

| Study | N | Target Vt (mL/kg) and $P_{plat}$ (cm $H_2O$) | Actual Vt (mL/kg) and $P_{plat}$ (cm $H_2O$) | % Mortality | P value |
|---|---|---|---|---|---|
| ARDS Net et al. [35] | 861 | 6 vs 12 and ≤30 vs ≤50 | 6.2 vs 11.8 and 25 vs 33 | 31 vs 40[#] | 0.007 |
| Amato et al. [36] | 53 | ≤6 vs 12 and >20 vs no limit | 384 mL vs 768 mL * and 30 vs 37 | 38 vs 71[§] | 0.001 |
| Brochard et al. [37] | 116 | 6–10 vs 10–15 and 25–30 vs ≤60 | 7.1 vs 10.3 and 26 vs 32 | 47 vs 38[¶] | 0.38 |
| Stewart et al. [38] | 120 | ≤8 vs 10–15 and ≤30 vs ≤50 | 7.0 vs 10.7 and 22 vs 27 | 50 vs 47[†] | 0.72 |
| Brower et al. [39] | 52 | ≤8 vs 10–12 and ≤30 vs ≤45–55 | 7.3 vs 10.2 and 25 vs 31 | 50 vs 46[†] | 0.61 |

* Vt was reported in mL, # mortality at hospital discharge or 180 days, § mortality at 28 days, ¶ mortality at 60 days, † mortality in-hospital

tidal volumes and limited plateau pressure strategies are summarized in Table 3 [35–39]. The three negative trials may not have recognized a mortality difference because of the relatively narrow differences in actual tidal volumes and plateau pressures between the treatment and control arms [37–39].

In general, based largely upon the ARDSNet recommendations for ALI and ARDS, mechanical ventilation in burn patients is now similarly initiated with an initial tidal volume of 6–8 mL/kg PBW and a goal of maintaining plateau pressures less than 30 cm $H_2O$ and peak inspiratory pressures less than 35 cm$H_2O$. This approach assumes relatively normal thoracoabdominal compliance. In a massively edematous burn patient with chest wall or abdominal burns it may be necessary to use larger tidal volumes (8–10 mL/kg) to achieve adequate alveolar patency while accepting higher plateau pressures (up to 35 cm$H_2O$).

### Permissive hypercapnia

Aggressive pursuit of a normalized $PaCO_2$ and pH is no longer the goal of current CMV strategies [40, 41]. Low tidal volume strategies result in lower minute ventilation which can cause hypercapnia. While a large acute elevation in the $PaCO_2$ may be associated with adverse effects (vasodilation, decrease cardiac output, increased intracranial pressure), the effects of more prolonged but less severe hypercapnia appear to be better tolerated but data is lacking to fully support this notion. Ideal levels of $PaCO_2$ and pH are not identified. It should be noted that the ARDSNet investigators utilized increases in respiratory rate, bicarbonate infusions and increased tidal volumes

to deal with acidosis. The use of bicarbonate infusions as a buffer remains controversial. Although pH may be corrected with bicarbonate, intra-cellular pH may actually drop since $CO_2$ produced when bicarbonate binds with metabolic acids may accumulate within cells, resulting in intra-cellular acidosis [40]. General guidelines would include maintaining pH between 7.25 and 7.45 and the $PaCO_2$ between 35 and 55, although higher $PaCO_2$ may be tolerated if the pH is above 7.25.

### The open-lung approach

As noted, portions of the lung in ALI and ARDS are characterized by collapse of small airways and alveoli. During positive pressure ventilation these alveoli open during inflation but will re-collapse if end expiratory pressures are inadequate. The repetitive opening and collapse causes shear injury to the alveolus (atelectrauma), and is detrimental. It is therefore highly desirable to open alveoli and keep them open, not only to avoid shear injury but also to improve oxygenation. This concept is referred to as an "open lung" approach. The two main techniques involved in this strategy are the use of positive and expiratory pressure (PEEP) and lung recruitment maneuvers. However, despite a solid physiological basis, the optimal use of PEEP and lung recruitment maneuvers remain mired in controversy.

### PEEP

The ideal level of PEEP and the best method for determining that level are unknown. If PEEP is too low, atelectasis is not reversed. Unnecessarily high PEEP may cause stretch injury to the aerated alveoli as well as haemodynamic instability, barotrauma, and may worsen ventilation perfusion matching [40–42].

In the limited tidal volume and plateau pressure study by Amato, et al. [36] PEEP was set at a level just above the lower inflection point on the pressure volume curve which in theory is the point above which recruitable alveoli are kept open at the end of expiration. However, this approach may not be practical and the derived pressure volume curve may not accurately represent regional differences across all regions of the lung because of the heterogeneity of the ARDS process. Nevertheless, PEEP levels as high as 24 cmH$_2$O were used in the high PEEP/low tidal volume arm of this study and were associated with significantly lower mortality rates.

Another approach which was used in the ARDS Net study of low volume and pressure was to arbitrarily link certain PEEP and FIO$_2$ combinations to achieve adequate oxygenation. In general, PEEP levels between 5 and 20 cmH$_2$O probably provide an acceptable balance between the adverse effects of inadequate and expiratory pressure and the risks of excessive end-expiratory pressure. Again, however, optimal PEEP levels remain unknown at this point.

Four large randomized multi-centre prospective studies have tried to determine whether there is a benefit to use of higher PEEP vs. lower PEEP settings (Table 4) [43–46]. The ALVEOLI Trial conducted by the ARDS Net investigators [43] compared a high PEEP (mean setting 13 cmH$_2$O) to low PEEP (mean setting 8 cmH$_2$O) among 549 patients with ALI and ARDS who were all ventilated with a tidal volume goal of 6 mL/kg PBW and a plateau pressure limit of 30 cmH$_2$O, and found that although the high PEEP group and significantly higher P$_a$O$_2$/F$_i$O$_2$ ratios, there were no significant differences in ventilator-free days or survival.

In the ARIES trial conducted by Villar, et al. [44] ARDS patients were randomized to either low PEEP (PEEP above 5 cmH$_2$O) plus higher tidal volume (9–11 mL/kg PBW) or, to high PEEP (PEEP set above lower inflection point on the static TV curve) plus lower tidal volume (5–8 mL/kg PBW). The high PEEP/lower tidal volume group had significantly greater ventilator-free days and ICU and hospital survival. However, any specific benefit of higher PEEP cannot be determined from this study because it was combined with a lower tidal volume approach compared to that in the low PEEP group.

More recently the EXPRESS trail [45] randomized patients with ALI and ARDS using a tidal volume of 6 mL/kg to either moderate PEEP (5–9 cmH$_2$O) or to higher PEEP which was set to achieve a plateau pressure up to 30 cmH$_2$O. Although the higher PEEP group had significantly superior oxygenation and a greater number of ventilator-free days, overall survival was not significantly different than in the low PEEP group.

Finally, in the LOVS study [46] of 983 patients with ALI and ARDS whose P$_a$O$_2$/F$_i$O$_2$ ratio was less than 250 were randomized to a target tidal volume of 6 mL/kg, no recruitment maneuvers, and PEEP set to keep the plateau pressure less than 30 (low PEEP group) or to a tidal volume of 6 mL/kg, lung recruitment maneuvers, and PEEP set to keep the plateau pressure less than 40 cmH$_2$O (high PEEP group). Overall, in-hospital survival did not differ between the groups but the high PEEP group had a significantly lower mortality rate secondary to refractory hypoxemia and a significantly lower rate of use of

**Table 4.** Comparison of randomized prospective studies using lower positive end expiratory pressure (PEEP) vs higher PEEP for acute lung injury and acute respiratory distress syndrome

| Study | N | Actual Vt (mL/kg) and PEEP (cm H$_2$O)* | Actual Plateau Pressure (cm H$_2$O) | % Mortality | P value |
|---|---|---|---|---|---|
| ARDS Net [43] | 549 | 6.1 vs 5.8 and 8.5 vs 12.9 | 24 vs 26 | 25 vs 28 # | 0.48 |
| Villar et al. [44] | 103 | 10 vs 7.1 and 8.7 vs 11.2 | 33 vs 28 | 56 vs 34 # | 0.04 |
| Mercat et al. [45] | 767 | 6.2 vs 6.2 and 6.7 vs 13.4 | 21 vs 27 | 39 vs 35 ¶ | 0.30 |
| Meade et al. [46] | 983 | 6.7 vs 6.9 and 8.8 vs 11.8 | 25 vs 29 | 40 vs 36 # | 0.19 |

Vt: tidal volume, * on day three, # in-hospital mortality, ¶ 60-day mortality

rescue therapy such as prone-position ventilation, high-frequency ventilation, or inhaled nitric oxide.

Thus, despite four large, well-designed, randomized prospective studies, we still do not know what defines an optimal PEEP setting or whether higher PEEP provides any substantial survival benefits. It is important to recognize that the conflicting observations of the aforementioned studies may be related to inaccuracy of diagnosis of ALI and ARDS between study subjects due to the somewhat arbitrary consensus criteria of $P_aO_2/F_iO_2$ ratios and chest radiographic changes. Also, heterogeneity within the study populations in the type of ARDS (e.g. "sticky" non-recruitable vs. "loose" recruitable) that was present may have accounted for the variable responses to higher and lower PEEP settings [32, 40, 47].

At present, the recommendations of Gattinoni, et al. [37] to set PEEP at the highest level possible to maintain a plateau pressure between 28 to 30 cmH$_2$O on a tidal volume of 6 mL/kg PBW have the most practical benefit to patients [47]. Again, in the unique case of burn patients with compromised thoraco-abdominal compliance, higher pressure limits may be necessary. For example, transpulmonary end-expiratory pressure as estimated by an esophageal balloon catheter has been found to be substantially less than the set PEEP at the airway opening in some critically ill patients [48].

## Lung recruitment maneuvers

A recruitment maneuver is an attempt to open atelectatic alveoli by deliberately applying an elevated transpulmonary pressure to these alveoli for a short duration. This may be achieved by application of transient continuous positive airway pressure (40 cmH$_2$O for twenty to forty seconds). In ALI and ARDS the challenge is to apply enough pressure during a lung recruitment maneuver to open atelectatic alveoli but not too much pressure that would overstretch and damage alveoli that are already fully open [40]. The amount of pressure needed to re-open an alveolus is greater than the amount of pressure needed to keep it open and prevent re-collapse. Thus, it is usually necessary to apply lung recruitment maneuvers transiently and intermittently and to maintain (or more usually) increase PEEP between the recruitment maneuver so as not to lose recruited alveoli [40]. The best pressure duration and frequency of recruitment maneuvers is unknown at this time, however. Also, the safety of this intervention has not been rigorously assessed and potential complications include transient hypotension, oxygen desaturation, and barotrauma.

## Unconventional mechanical ventilation strategies

### High-frequency percussive ventilation (HFPV)

Conventional mechanical ventilation does not address many of the pathophysiologic derangements that follow a smoke inhalation injury. These include (1) plugging of the small airways with sloughed mucosa and fibrin cast which causes progressive CO$_2$ retention, impaired oxygenation, and ventilation perfusion mismatch, (2) potentially injurious elevation of airway pressures due to the combined effects of bronchospasm and diminished lung and chest wall compliance and (3) small airway obstruction leading to atelectasis and then pneumonia.

High-frequency percussive ventilation (HFPV), which utilizes intra-pulmonary percussion and high-frequency sub-tidal volume breaths, appears to be ideally suited for mechanical ventilation of burn patients with significant smoke inhalation injuries. Indeed, early animal studies using a primate model of smoke inhalation injury found that HFPV was beneficial both in terms of oxygenation as well as minimization of VILI [49]. HFPV is delivered using the Volume Diffusive Respirator®(VDR). This is a pneumatically-driven, time-cycled and pressure-limited ventilator which utilizes a sliding Venturi valve which stacks breaths to achieve a desired inspiratory pressure, and then releases them for passive exhalation. The high-frequency breaths have a sub-dead space tidal volume and are delivered at frequencies (the pulse frequency or percussive rate) between 60 and 900 breaths per minute (1–15 Hz). The high-frequency breaths are stacked in a stepwise pattern and then are periodically interrupted to allow airway pressure to return to a set baseline continuous positive airway pressure (baseline or demand CPAP). This creates what is analogous to a conventional mechanical breath such that the high frequency breaths are superimposed on a conventional respiratory rate (the phasic rate) which is generally initially set at one half to one third of a conventional ventilation frequency (Fig. 3a). The duration of the percussive phase and the baseline phase are manipulated to affect oxygenation and $CO_2$ removal. Peak airway pressure can also be adjusted to help control $CO_2$ removal. The I:E ratio of the high frequency breaths can be adjusted to produce a more diffusive flow (low I:E ratio), or a more predominately percussive flow wave (high I:E ratio). The amplitude of the sub-tidal breath can also be adjusted to affect peak airway pressure.

The percussive nature of this mode of ventilation is its most important feature as it promotes loosening and mobilization of secretion and airway debris. This mucokinetic effect is optimized by the fact that the endotracheal tube balloon cuff is left deflated to allow mobilization of secretions. This, in addition to HFPV's potential to improve oxygenation at lower airway pressure than CMW makes it useful for burn patients with significant smoke inhalation injury. However, while HFPV is well established in the armamentarium of ventilation strategies for smoke inhalation injury, the existing studies on HFPV do not provide a clear answer as to whether these potential benefits of HFPV have been uniformly achieved.

The early studies of HFPV conducted in the late 1980s and 1990s were retrospective with either no control groups [50–51] or used contemporaneous or historical controls [52–55]. The largest of these, by Cioffi et al. [52] assessed 54 adults admitted within 48 hours of injury with either bronchoscopy or xenon lung-scan confirmed inhalation injury who were placed on HFPV within one hour of burn centre admission. The incidence of pneumonia was 26% which was significantly lower than the rate in a historical cohort (46%). Similarly, mortality was significantly lower than that which would have been estimated from predictive model using a historical cohort. The other studies from this era generally found that HFPV resulted in improved oxygenation, lower peak airway pressures, less barotrauma, and a reduced incidence of pneumonia [51, 53–55]. However, these studies should be interpreted with caution because of their retrospective nature and differing indications for institution of HFPV and entry of

patients with differing degrees of respiratory failure. Also, comparisons were made with control patients ventilated with CMV strategies that allowed high tidal volumes and high inflation pressures which probably would not be acceptable by today's standards.

Two randomized prospective studies have compared HFPV to CMV as acute ventilation strategies for patients which smoke inhalation (Table 5) [56, 57]. The first, in children [56] found that HFPV produced significantly better oxygenation at lower peak airway pressures than conventional pressure-controlled ventilation. However, both groups had $P_2O_2/F_iO_2$ ratios above 500 suggesting that neither group was experiencing severe or even moderate respiratory insufficiency. The second study, in adults with smoke inhalation [57] also found that HFPV produced significantly better oxygenation during the first three days of use than conventional volume-controlled ventilation but oxygenation was then equivalent between the groups on days four and five post-burn. Of note was that the CMV strategy which used tidal volumes of 10 mL/kg would now be considered an aggressive and potentially lung injurious strategy and may have been the reason that HFPV produced superior oxygenation. Neither study was able to demonstrate any significant differences in the incidence of pneumonia or in the mortality rate.

The most recent (and the largest) study of HFPV was a retrospective review of 92 adults (62 with bronchoscopy confirmed inhalation injury) ventilated with HFPV, compared to 130 contemporary controls (49 with bronchoscopy-confirmed inhalation injury) placed on CMV [58]. There was a change in CMV strategy during the study in which tidal volumes of 10 mL/kg were reduced to 6 ml/Kg and plateau pressures were limited to less than 35 $cmH_2O$ in keeping with ARDS Net guidelines. Also, patients in the HFPV group received nebulized Heparin-NAC whereas those on CMV did not. No significant differences were found between CMV and HFPV in ventilator days, length of stay, or incidence of ventilator associated pneumonia but there was significantly higher mortality in the CMV group.

In summary, a large amount of retrospective data suggests the use of HFPV in inhalation injury is associated with improved oxygenation at lower airway pressures, less occurrence of pneumonia and improved survival. However, the reliability of these

**Table 5.** Randomized prospective studies which have compared conventional mechanical ventilation (CMV) with High Frequency Percussive Ventilation (HFPV) using the Volume Diffusive Respirator® (VDR) for acute burns and smoke inhalation

| Study | Design | N | Patient selection | Interventions | Outcomes |
|---|---|---|---|---|---|
| Carmen et al. [56] | Prospective Randomized | 64 | ▶ Pediatric<br>▶ Mean burn size 56% TBSA<br>▶ 86% with II | ▶ CMV with PCV at 6–8 mL/kg, PEEP 4–6 cmH20<br>▶ VDR with frequency 200–360/min, oscillatory CPAP/PEEP 5–10 cm $H_2O$, and demand CPAP/PEEP 8–10 cm $H_2O$ | ▶ mean $PaO_2/FiO_2$ ratio/peak airway pressure was 507/40 on CMV Vs. 563/31 on VDR (p > 0.05)<br>▶ no differences between groups in duration of MV, barotraumas, pneumonia, or survival |
| Reper et al. [57] | Prospective Randomized | 35 | ▶ Adults<br>▶ burns > 20% TBSA requiring acute ventilator support<br>▶ 15/17 bronchoscope-confirmed II in CMV group; 16/18 in HFPV group | ▶ CMV was VCV using tidal volume 10 mL/kg<br>▶ HFPV using frequency of 600–800/min | ▶ Significantly higher $PaO2/FiO2$ ratio over 1st 3 days in HFPV Vs CMV.<br>▶ No differences in pulmonary infections or survival between groups. |

II: inhalation injury, PCV: pressure controlled ventilation, VCV: volume controlled ventilation, CPAP: continuous positive airway pressure, PEEP: positive end expiratory pressure, MV: mechanical ventilation

findings is limited by biases inherent in retrospective analyses, variations in indications for initiation for HFPV, varying severity of respiratory dysfunction in the study subjects, and variations in the CMV strategies utilized. The existing randomized prospective studies found only that HFPV resulted in better oxygenation than the accepted CMV modes of the day. A current randomized prospective study comparing HFPV to the best lung protective CMV strategies currently available (which would feature low tidal volume and pressure limited strategies with an open lung approach) is needed.

## High-frequency oscillatory ventilation

High-frequency oscillatory ventilation (HFOV) is an unconventional form of mechanical ventilation which has been used for the past two decades in the neo-natal intensive care unit for respiratory distress syndrome. Recognition of HFOVs lung-protective properties combined with sound physiologic evidence with its ability to open and recruit the lung, have lead to translation of HFOV to the adult ICU, for patients with acute respiratory distress syndrome.

HFOV uses extremely small tidal volumes (1–2 mL/kg) at high frequencies (3–15 Hz), com-

bined with application of a relatively high sustained mean airway pressure (30–40 cmH$_2$O). The key difference between CMV and HFOV is demonstrated in Fig. 3(b) Primarily, oxygenation is achieved by using the elevated and sustained mean airway pressure to achieve highly effective recruitment of the available lung (i. e. increased total lung volume) [59–62]. Alveolar ventilation is mainly related to the frequency of ventilation which is inversely related to the tidal volume (i. e. higher frequency = lower tidal volume, lower frequency = larger tidal volume) and is relatively independent of total lung volume [59, 60]. Hence, oxygenation and ventilation are essentially uncoupled and can each be controlled independent of the other [59, 60]. HFOV is currently delivered using the SensorMedics 3100B High Frequency Oscillatory Ventilator (the "adult oscillator").

Numerous animal studies have found HFOV to produce less VILI than CMV [63–67]. HFOV ventilates the lung in a relatively restricted "safe window" avoiding excursion both into the zone of alveolar over distention (volutrauma) at high tidal volume and high inflation pressures as well as the zone of alveolar de-recruitment (atelectrauma) at insufficient pressures [68]. The very small tidal volumes during HFOV limit alveolar stretch even at higher airway pressures because the incremental expansion of the alveolus with each inspiration is still quite small. The use of such small tidal volumes then allows application of a higher sustained mean airway pressure which opens and recruits the lung to prevent atelectrauma in many groups of alveoli that would otherwise be subject to repetitive collapse and re-opening. The lung recruitment directly improves oxygenation allowing use of a lower $F_iO_2$ thus limiting oxygen toxicity.

HFOV has been widely reported as a rescue strategy for oxygenation crisis in adults with ARDS arising from critical illness and trauma [70–74]. The main combined findings from these studies were that HFOV is safe with relatively low rates of barotraumas, and that it produces rapid and sustained correction of oxygenation failure when used as a rescue strategy. The improved oxygenation is usually achieved at a lower mean airway pressure "cost". The improved oxygenation is not related to improved survival and no conclusions on HFOV is effect on mortality can be reached from these studies. Two randomized controlled trials [75, 76] have compared HFOV with CMV in adults with ARDS. Neither of these studies raised any important safety concerns but, importantly, neither showed any definite advantage of HFOV over CMV. HFOV may not have been optimally applied in these studies (lung recruitment maneuvers were not used, frequency may have been set too low and conversion to CMV may have been premature). Also, the control arms CMV strategy may not have been optimally lung protective. In summary, the existing randomized controlled trials of adult HFOV are inconclusive. The need for a larger randomized controlled trial of optimum HFOV against the best protective CMV strategy of the day is being addressed by the multi-centre OSCILLATE trial (Ferguson and Mead) which is currently in progress. A small body of research has reviewed the use of HFOV in burn patients with ARDS [77–79]. The main conclusions were as follows:

► HFOV produced rapid and sustained improvements in the $P_aO_2/F_iO_2$ ratio and oxygenation index for patients in extreme oxygenation crisis. As such, it is particularly useful as a rescue strategy for severe oxygenation failure. HFOV could be used as an intra-operative ventilation technique to allow sustained use of this ventilation strategy and simultaneously satisfy the priority of serial burn wound excision and closure. Patients with ARDS who had sustained a smoke inhalation injury had a delayed and blunted oxygenation improvement compared to patients with no smoke inhalation injury. This was attributed to the classic small airway obstruction and gas-trapping characteristic of smoke inhalation injury which prevented alveolar recruitment through HFOV's sustained mean airway pressure. Therefore, HFOV may not be an optimal rescue strategy for oxygenation crisis if there is a prior smoke inhalation injury.

► HFOV potentially interferes with other important adjunctive therapies for smoke inhalation such as secretion clearance by suctioning and bronchoscopy and delivery of nebulized agents such as Heparin and NAC.

### Airway pressure release ventilation (APRV)

APRV is a relatively new mode of ventilation which is being increasingly used as a ventilation strategy for patients with ALI and ARDS. Patients breathe spontaneously during this pressure-regulated and time-cycled mode of ventilation. A high continuous airway pressure (the $P_{high}$) is set by the clinician, and then pressure is periodically released to a lower set continuous airway pressure (the $P_{low}$). The patient breathes spontaneously at both $P_{high}$ and at $P_{low}$ throughout this repetitive cycling of continuous airway pressure. The $P_{high}$ represents and inspiratory phase, and the $P_{low}$ represents a release phase. The level and duration of $P_{high}$ is used to affect oxygenation. Lung recruitment is achieved by using longer and more frequent periods at $P_{high}$. Clearance of $CO_2$ is exchanged during the release phase [80–82] (Fig. 3c).

The most important benefit of APRV is that it allows spontaneous breathing by the patient. The advantages of spontaneous breathing include the reduction in need for sedation, avoidance of paralytic agents, improved recruitment of atelectatic lung, improved venous return and cardiac output, and better diaphragmatic movement [80–82]. At the present time there are no prospective studies on APRV for burn /smoke inhalation patients or patients with ARDS. Some limited data in burn patients with

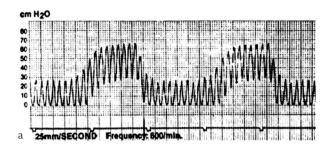

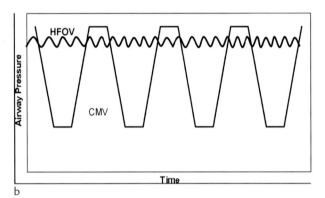

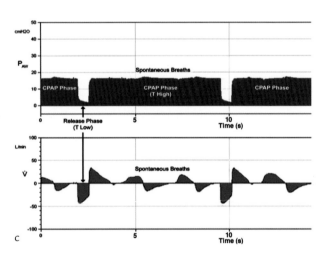

**Fig. 3.** (a) Pressure Vs time tracing during HFPV [50], (b) comparison of pressure Vs time tracings for CMV and HFOV [79], (c) pressure Vs time tracing during APRV [80]

smoke inhalation suggests that APRV compared favourably to HFPV by improving oxygenation at lower airway pressures than HFPV [82].

## Ventilator associated pneumonia (VAP)

Ventilator Associated Pneumonia (VAP) is the most common infection occurring in critically ill patients who receive mechanical ventilation. Burn patients are particularly predisposed to VAP due to the combined effects of prolonged intubation and ventilation, burn-related immunosupression, inhalation injury, and prolonged length of stay in the burn intensive care setting. Estimates of the incidence of VAP in burn patients range between 22 to 26 cases per 1000 ventilator days [84, 85].

The most widely accepted mechanism of VAP involves microbial colonization of the oropharynx and stomach which, when followed by chronic micro-aspiration of secretions part the endotracheal tube balloon cuff, leads to contamination of the usually sterile lower respiratory tract. The presence of an endotracheal tube impairs many of the normal defenses that would protect the lower airways, including the usual glottic barrier, mucociliary clearance and the ability to cough and effectively clear secretions [86, 87]. Early VAP (ie within four days of intubation) most commonly involves organisms such as *Streptococcus pneumonia* and *Haemophilus influenzae* while gram-negative bacilli such as *Pseudomonas aeruginosa*, *E Coli*, and *Acinetobacter*, along with methacillin-resistant *Staphylococcus aureus* predominate later on [87]. In burn units, *Acinetobacter baumannii* has become particularly widespread pathogen, and frequently is multi-drug resistant [88].

Diagnosis of VAP in a mechanically ventilated burn patient may be difficult due to the presence of overlapping systemic inflammation, pulmonary edema, and ALI or ARDS. There is no consensus on a set of guidelines by which to diagnose VAP in burn patients. VAP should be suspected when findings of fever, increasing or purulent sputum production, leukocytosis or leucopenia, and worsening infiltrates on the chest radiograph, are present. Quantitative bacteriologic cultures obtained using brocheocalveolar lavage (BAL) probably represent a preferable approach over simple endotracheal suction aspirates. The threshold for a positive quantitative culture remains controversial and ranges between $10^3$–$10^5$ cfu/mL [88, 89].

A recent set of practice guidelines for the prevention and treatment of VAP in the burn patient, published by the American Burn Association, recommends the following [86]:

## (a) Prevention

▶ Minimize the duration of intubation and mechanical ventilation through the use of weaning protocols, daily sedation, interruption, and daily spontaneous breathing trials.
▶ Use of specialized endotracheal such as silver impregnated tubes, or tubes which allow continuous suction of subglottic secretions should be considered.
▶ Patients should be placed in a semirecumbent position, especially if being enterally fed.
▶ A post pyloric feeding tube is desirable to reduce gastroesophageal regurgitation and aspiration. If fed by the post pyloric route, gastric stress ulcer prophylaxis is recommended.
▶ Routine use of prophylactic antibiotics is not recommended due to the risk of selection of endemic multi resistant organism in a burn unit setting.
▶ Oral chlorhexidine to decrease oropharyngeal colonization is an effective and recommended VAP prevention strategy.
▶ Adoption of strict infection control measures including hand washing, contact barrier precautions, and patient/staff co-horting is advisable.

## (b) Treatment

▶ Initiate early broad-spectrum antibiotic therapy based on timing of VAP onset, and local burn unit specific patterns of likely organisms and resistance profiles, as soon as the diagnosis of VAP is made.
▶ De-escalation, or narrowing of the broad-spectrum antibiotic coverage once quantitative cultures are available, is recommended.
▶ Antibiotic rotation schedules should be considered, if possible, tailored to an individual burn unit's endemic bacterial and resistance patterns.
▶ An 8-day course of specific antibiotic treatment is usually adequate for most VAP's, except for methacillin-resistant *Staphylococcus aureus* and gram negative bacilli (e. g. *Acinetobacter* or *Pseudomonas*), which may require a longer duration of treatment (15 days).

## References

[1] Mlcak RP, Suman OE, Herndon DN (2007) Respiratory management of inhalation injury. Burns 33: 2–13
[2] Cha S, Kim CH, Lee JH et al (2007) Isolated smoke inhalation injuries: acute respiratory dysfunction, clinical outcomes, and short term evolution of pulmonary functions with the effects of steroids. Burns 33: 200–208
[3] Modnani DD, Steele NP deVries E (2006) Factors that predict the need for intubation in patients with smoke inhalation injury. Ear, Nose Throat J 85: 278–280
[4] Goh SH, Tiah L, Lim HC et al (2006) Disaster preparedness: Experience from a smoke inhalation mass casualty incident. Eur J Emerg Med 13: 330–334
[5] Whited RE (1984) A prospective study of laryngotracheal sequelae in long-term intubation. Laryngoscope 94: 367–370
[6] Stauffer J, Olson D, Petty T (1981) Complications and consequences of endotraeal intubation and tracheostomy: a prospective study of 150 critically ill adult patients. Am J Med 70: 65–76
[7] Eckhauser FE, Billote J, Burke, JF et al (1974) Tracheostomy complicating massive burn injury: a plea for conservatism. Am J Surg 127: 418–423
[8] Moylan JA, West JT, Nash G et al (1972) Tracheostomy in thermally injure patients: a review of 5 years' experience. Am Surg 38: 119–123.
[9] Majeski JA, MacMillan BG (1978) Tracheoinnominate artery erosion in a burned child. J Trauma 18: 137–139
[10] Mulder DS, Rubush JL (1969) Complications of tracheostomy: relationship to long term ventilation assistance. J Trauma 9: 389–402
[11] Jones WG, Madden M, Finkelstein J et al (1989) Tracheostomies in burn patients. Ann Surg 209: 471–474
[12] Gaissert HA, Lofgren RH, Grillo HC (1993) Upper airway compromise after inhalation injury: complex strictures of the larynx and trachea and their management. Ann Surg 218: 672–678
[13] Lund T, Goodwin CW, McManus WF et al (1985) Upper airway sequelae in burn patients requiring endotracheal intubation or tracheostomy. Ann Surg 201: 374–382
[14] Sellers B, Davis B, Larkin PW et al (1997) Early prediction of prolonged ventilator dependence in thermally injured patients. J Trauma, Injury, Infection & Critical Care 43: 899–903
[15] Saffle JR, Morris SE, Edelman L (2002) Early tracheostomy does not improve outcome in burn patients. J Burn Care Rehabil 23: 431–438
[16] Palmieri TL, Jackson W, Greenhalgh DG (2002) Benefits of early tracheostomy in severely burned children. Crit Care Med 30: 922–924
[17] Mlcak RP, Herndon DN (2007) Respiratory care. In: Herndon DN (ed) Total burn care. Saunders Elsevier, pp 281–291
[18] Enkhbaatar P, Traber DL (2004) Pathophysiology of acute lung injuryh in combined burn and smoke inhalation injury. Clin Sci (Lond) 197: 137–143

[19]  Murakami K, Traber DL (2003) Pathophysiological basis of smoke inhalation injury. New Physiol Sci 18: 125–129

[20]  Miller AC, Rivero A, Ziad S et al (2009) Influence of nebulized unfractionated heparin and N-acetylcysteine in acute lung injury after smoke inhalation. J Burn Care Res 30: 249–256

[21]  DeMaestro R, Thaw L, Bjork T et al (1980) Free radicals and mediators of tissue injury. Acta Physiol Scan 192[Suppl]: S23–57

[22]  Parker IC, Martin DI, Rutilig G et al (1983) Prevention of free radical mediated vascular permeability increases in lung using superoxide dismutase. Chest 83: 528–535

[23]  Cuzzocrea S, Mazzon E, Dugol L et al (2001) Protrective effects of NAC on lung injury and red blood cell modification induced by carrageenan in the rate. FASEB J 15: 1187–1200

[24]  Cox C, Zwischenberger J, Traber D et al (1993) Heparin improves oxygenation and minimizes barotrauma after severe smoke inhalation in an ovine model. SGO 176: 339–349

[25]  Brown M, Desai M, Traber LD et al (1988) Dimethylsulfoxide with heparin in the treatment of smoke inhalation injury. J Burn Care Rehabil 9: 22–25

[26]  Desai MH, Mlcak R, Richardson J et al (1998) Reduction in mortality in pediatric patients with inhalation injury with aerosolized heparin/Acetylcysteine therapy. J Burn Care and Rehabilitation 19: 210–212

[27]  Holt J, Soffle JR, Morris SE (2008) Use of inhaled heparin/N-acetylcysteine in inhalation injury: Does it help? J Burn Care Res 29: 192–195

[28]  Slutsky AS (2001) Basic Science in ventilator induced lung injury. Am J Respir Crit Care Med 163: 599–600

[29]  Dreyfuss D, Saumon G (1998) Ventilator induced lung injury: lessons from experimental studies. Am J Respir Crit Care Med 157: 294–323

[30]  Gattinoni L, Caironi P, Pelosi P et al (2001) What has computed tomography taught us about ARDS? Am J Respir Crit Care Med 164: 1701–1711

[31]  Gattinoni L, Presenti A (2005) The concept of "baby lung". Intensive Care Med 31: 776–784

[32]  Gattinoni L, D'Andrea L, Pelosi P et al (1993) Regional effects and mechanism of positive end expiratory pressure in early adult respiratory distress syndrome. JAMA 269: 2122–2127

[33]  Crotti S, Mascheroni D, Caironi P et al (2001) Recruitment and de-recruitment during acute respiratory failure: a clinical study. Am J Respir Crit Care Med 164: 131–40

[34]  Gattinoni L, Caironi P, Crressoni M et al (2006) Lung recruitment in patients with the acute respiratory distress syndrome. N Engl J Med 354: 1775–1786

[35]  ARDS Network Investigators (2000) Ventilation with lower tidal volumes for acute lung injury and the acute respiratory distress syndrome. N Engl J Med 342: 1301–1308

[36]  Amato MB, Barbas CS, Medieros DM et al (1998) Effect of a protective ventilation strategy on mortality in ARDS. N Engl J Med 338: 347–354

[37]  Brochard L, Roudot-Toraval F, Roupie E (1998) Tidal volume reduction for prevention of VILI in ARDS. Am J Respir Crit Care Med 158: 1831–1838

[38]  Stewart TE, Meade MO, Cook DJ et al (2000) Evaluation of a strategy to prevent barotraumas in patients at high risk for ARDS: pressure and limited volume ventilation group. N Engl J Med 342: 1301–1308

[39]  Brower RG, Shanholz CB, Fessler HE et al (1999) Prospective randomized controlled trial comparing traditional vs. reduced tidal volumes for ALI or ARDS. Crit Care Med 27: 1492–1498

[40]  Dries DJ (2009) Key questions in ventilator management of the burn injured patient – Part 1. J Burn Care Res 30: 128–138

[41]  Dries DJ (1995) Permissive hypercapnia. J Trauma 39: 984–989

[42]  Navelesi P, Maggiore SM (2006) Positive end expiratory pressure. In: Tobin MJ (ed) Principles and practice of mechanical ventilation, 2nd edn. McGraw-Hill, New York, pp 273–325

[43]  Brower RG, Lanken PN, MacIntyre N et al (2004) The National Heart Lung and Blood Institute ARDS Clinical Trials Network. Higher vs lower positive end expiratory pressures in patients with the acute respiratory distress syndrome. N Engl J Med 351: 327–336

[44]  Villar J, Kacmarek RM, Perez-Mendez L et al (2006) High positive end expiratory pressure, low tidal volumd ventilation strategy improves outcome in persistant acute respiratory distress syndrome. A randomized controlled trial. Crit Care Med 34: 1311–1318

[45]  Mercat A, Richard JC, Vielle B et al (2008) Positive end expiratory pressure settings in adults with acute lung injury and acute respiratory distress syndrome: a randomized controlled trial. JAMA 299: 646–655

[46]  Meade MO, Cook DJ, Guyatt GH (2008) Lung Open Ventilation Study Investigators: Ventilation strategy using low tidal volumes, recruitment maneuvers, and high positive end-expiratory pressures for acute lung injury and acute respiratory distress syndrome. A randomized controlled trial. JAMA 299: 637–645

[47]  Gattinoni L, Caironi P (2008) Refining ventilatory treatments for acute lung injury and acute respiratory distress syndrome. JAMA 299: 691–693

[48]  Talmor D, Sarge T, Malhotra A et al (2008) Mechanical ventilation guided by esophagel pressure in acute lung injury. N Engl J Med 359: 2095–2104

[49]  Cioffi WG, deLemos RA, Coalson JJ et al (1993) Decreased pulmonary damage in primates with inhalation injury treated with high frequency ventilation. Ann Surg 218: 328–337

[50]  Cioffi WG, Graves TA, McManus WF et al (1989) High frequency percussive ventilation in patients with inhalation injury. J Trauma 29: 350–354

[51]  Reper P, DanKaert R, vanHille F et al (1998) The usefulness of combined high frequency percussive ventilation during acute respiratory failure after smoke inhalation. Burns 24: 34–38

[52] Cioffi WG, Rue LW, Graves TA et al (1991) Prophylactic use of high frequency percussive ventilation in patients with inhalation injury. Ann Surg 213: 575–582

[53] Cortella J, Mlack R, Herndon Dl (1999) High frequency percussive ventilation in pediatric patients with inhalation injury. J Burn Care Rehabil 20: 2–5

[54] Rue LW, Cioffi WG, Madon AD et al (1993) Improved survival of patients with inhalation injury. Arch Surg 128: 772–780

[55] Rodeberg DA, Maschinot NE, Housinger TA et al (1992) Decreased pulmonary barotraumas with the use of volumetric diffusive respiration in pediatric patients with burns. J Burn Care Rehabil 13: 506–511

[56] Carmen B, Cahill T, Worden G et al (2002) A prospective randomized comparison of the volume diffusive respirator vs convential ventilation for ventilation of burned children. J Burn Care Rehabil 23: 444–448

[57] Reper P, Wibaux O, VanLaeke D et al (2002) High frequency percussive ventilation and conventional ventilation after smoke inhalation: a randomized study. Burns 28: 503–508

[58] Hall J, Hunt JL, Arnoldo BD et al (2007) Use of high frequency percussive ventilation in inhalation injuries. J Burn Care Res 28: 396–400

[59] Furguson ND, Stewart TE (2002) New therapies for adults with acute lung injury: high frequency oscillatory ventilation. Crit Care Clin 18: 1–23

[60] Derdak S (2003) High-frequency oscillatory ventilation for acute respiration distress syndrome in adult patients. Crit Care Med 31:S317–323

[61] Suzuki H, Papazoglou K, Bryan AC (1992) Relationship between PaO$_2$ and lung volume during high frequency oscillatory ventilation. Acta Paediatr Jpn 34: 494–500

[62] Kolton M, Cattran CB, Kent G, Volgyesi G, Froese AB, Bryan AC (1982) Oxygenation during high-frequency ventilation compared with conventional mechanical ventilation in two models of lung injury. Anesth Analg 61: 323–332

[63] Hamilton PP, Onayemi A, Smyth JA et al (1983) Comparison of conventional and high-frequency oscillatory ventilation: oxygenation and lung pathology. J Appl Physiol 55: 131–138

[64] McCulloch PR, Fordert PG, Froese AB (1988) Lung volume maintenance prevents lung injury during high frequency oscillatory ventilation in surfactant-deficient rabbits. Am Rev Respir Dis 137: 1185–1192

[65] Bond DM, Froese AB (1993) Volume recruitment maneuvers are less deleterious than persistent low lung volumes in the atelectasis-prone rabbit lung during high-frequency oscillation. Crit Care Med 21: 402–412

[66] Rotta AT, Gunnarsson B, Fuhrman BP, Hernan LJ, Steinhorn DM (2001) Comparison of lung protective ventilation strategies in a rabbit model of acute lung injury. Crit Care Med 29: 2176–2184

[67] Imai Y, Nakagawa S, Ito Y, Kawano T, Slutsky AS, Miyasaka K (2001) Comparison of lung protection strategies using conventional and high-frequency oscillatory ventilation. J Appl Physiol 91: 1836–1844

[68] Froese AB (1997) High-frequency oscillatory ventilation for adult respiratory distress syndrome: let's get it right this time. Crit Care Med 25: 906–908

[69] Fort P, Farmer C, Westerman J et al (1997) High-frequency oscillatory ventilation for adult respiratory distress syndrome-a pilot study. Crit Care Med 25: 937–947

[70] Mehta S, Lapinksy SE, Hallett DC et al (2001) A prospective trial of respiratory distress syndrome. Crit Care Med 29: 1360–1369

[71] Andersen FA, Gurrormscn AB, Flaatten HK (2002) High frequency oscillatory ventilation in adjult patients with acute respiratory distress syndrome-a retrospective study. Acta Anaesthesiol Scan 46: 1082–1088

[72] Mehta S, Granton J, MacDonald RJ et al (2004) High frequency oscillatory ventilation in adjults: the Toronto experience. Chest 126: 518–527

[73] Claridge JA, Hostetter RG, Lowson SM, Young JS (1999) High frequency oscillatory ventilation can be effective as rescue therapy for refractory acute lung dysfunction. Am Surg 65: 1092–1096

[74] David M, Weiler N, Heinrichs W et al (2003) High-frequency oscillatory ventilation in adult acute respiratory distress syndrome. Intensive Care Med 29: 1656–1665

[75] Derdak S, Mehta S, Stewart TE et al (2002) High frequency oscillatory ventilation for acute respiratory distress syndrome: a randomized controlled trial. Am J Respir Crit Care Med 166: 801–808

[76] Bollen CW, van Well GT, Sherry T et al (2005) High frequency oscillatory ventilation compared with conventional mechanical ventilation in adult respiratory distress syndrome: a randomized controlled trial. Crit Care 9:R430–439

[77] Cartotto R, Ellis S, Gomez M, Cooper A, Smith T (2004) High frequency oscillatory ventilation in burn patients with the acute respiratory distress syndrome. Burns 30: 453–463

[78] Cartotto R, Ellis S, Smith T (2005) Use of high frequency oscillatory ventilation in burn patients. Crit Care Med 33:S175–181

[79] Cartotto R, Walia G, Ellis S et al (2009) Oscillation after inhalation: high frequency oscillatory ventilation in burn patients with the acute respiratory distress syndrome and co-existing smoke inhalation injury. J Burn Care Res 30: 119–127

[80] Habashi NM (2005) Other approaches to open lung ventilation: airway pressure release ventilation. Crit Care Med 33: 5228–2540

[81] Seymour CW, Frazer M, Reilly PM et al (2007) Airway pressure release and biphasic intermittent positive airway pressure ventilation: are they ready for primetime? J Trauma 62: 1298–1309

[82] Dries DJ (2009) Key questions in ventilator management of the burn injured patient – Part 2. J Burn Care Res 30: 211–220

[83] Byerly FL, Shapiro ML, Short A et al (2005) Airway pressure release ventilation is the management of inhalation injuries. J Burn Care Rehabil 26S93 (abstract)

[84] Santucci S, Gobara S, Santos C et al (2003) Infections in a burn intensive care unit: experience of seven years. J Hosp Infec 53: 6–13

[85] Wibbenmeyer L, Danks R, Faucher L et al (2006) Prospective analysis of resistance in a burn population. J Burn Care Res 27: 152–160

[86] Chastre J, Fagon JY (2006) Ventilator Associated pneumonia. Am J Respir Crit Care Med 34: 1414–1519

[87] Mosier MJ, Pham TN (2009) American Burn Association Practice Guidelines for prevention, diagnosis, and treatment of ventilator associated pneumonia in burn patients. J Burn Care Res 30: 910–928

[88] Chim H, Tan B, Son C (2007) Five year review of infections in a burn intensive care unit: high incidence of *Acinetobacter baumanii* in a tropical climate. Burns 33: 1008–1014

[89] Croce M, Fabian T, Mueller E et al (2004) The appropriate diagnostic threshold for ventilator-associated pneumonia using quantitative cultures. J Trauma 56: 931–934

[90] Minei JP, Nathan AB, Eest M et al (2006) Injury and the host response to injury large scar collaborative research program investigators. Inflammation and the host response to injury, a large scale collaborative project; patient-oriented research care – standard operating procedures for clinical care II. Guidelines for prevention, diagnosis, and treatment of VAP in the trauma patient. J Trauma 60: 1106–1113

Correspondence: R. Cartotto M.D., FRCS(C), Ross Tilley Burn Centre at Sunnybrook Health Sciences Centre, Associate Professor, Department of Surgery, University of Toronto, Rm D712 2075 Bayview Ave. Toronto, ON, Canada M4N 3M5, E-mail: robert.cartotto@sunnybrook.ca

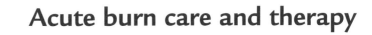

Acute burn care and therapy

# Organ responses and organ support

Kathryn L. Butler, Robert L. Sheridan

Shriners Hospital for Children, Massachusetts General Hospital, Harvard Medical School, Boston, MA, USA

## Introduction

Over the past fifty years, goal-directed resuscitation [1-3], early burn wound excision and grafting [4-7], and recognition of burn hypercatabolism[8-10] have dramatically reduced mortality rates after burn injury [11-15]. Despite this progress, end-organ dysfunction remains a threat throughout a patient's clinical course. Recent studies approximate the incidence of multiple organ dysfunction as 40-60% among patients with greater than 20% total body surface area (TBSA) burns, with associated mortality rates from 22-100% [16-19]. These mortality rates increase in proportion to the number of failed systems [19]. The link between multi-organ failure and patient mortality highlights the necessity for practitioners to cultivate an understanding of burn pathophysiology, as well as critical care principles of organ support.

## Burn shock and resuscitation

The primary step toward management of multiorgan failure is prevention. In burn patients, this originates with adequate resuscitation during the first 24 hours after injury. Thermal injury covering greater than 20% TBSA induces massive capillary leak and autonomic dysfunction, with resultant distributive and hypovolemic shock. On the cellular level,

burn injury disrupts transmembrane sodium-ATPase activity, with resultant intracellular sodium retention, osmotic shifts, and cellular edema [20]. Mast cells aggregate to burn wounds and secrete histamine, which disrupts inter-cellular junctions at the venules and allows for extravasation of plasma fluid and proteins from the intravascular space into the tissues [21]. This efflux of protein from the capillaries decreases plasma oncotic pressure, and worsens hypovolemia and tissue edema. Large burns also trigger the release of inflammatory mediators, including but not limited to bradykinin, vasoactive amines, prostaglandins, leukotrienes, activated complement, and catecholamines [20-22]. This outpouring of cytokines induces local vasoconstriction, systemic vasodilatation, and massive capillary leak, yielding hypovolemia and hemoconcentration that peaks at 12 hours post-burn [20]. Without adequate resuscitation, plasma volume becomes insufficient to maintain preload, cardiac output decreases, and end-organ hypoperfusion and ischemia ensue, with ultimate multi-organ failure and death [20-24].

Early burn wound excision – within the first 72 hours post-burn – has been shown to modulate the inflammatory response to burn injury by reducing levels of pro-inflammatory mediators, and is now considered standard of care [25]. Additionally, maintenance of organ perfusion during burn shock depends upon restoration of intravascular volume. Toward this end, burn surgeons have adopted resuscitation algorithms to guide the appropriate infusion rates of crystalloid in the first 24 hours after burn injury. The most popular of these algorithms in the United States, the Parkland formula, calculates a total volume of crystalloid based upon the patient's weight and an estimation of the percentage of body surface area burned. According to the American Burn Association (ABA), these formulas provide guidelines, not absolute protocols, for resuscitation in burn shock [20]. Burn depth, inhalation injury, patient age, delays in resuscitation, and alcohol and drug use may increase fluid requirements during burn resuscitation [24]. In these scenarios, the Parkland formula may underestimate patient's fluid needs, leading to under-resuscitation and organ failure.

Unfortunately, specific titration endpoints for fluid resuscitation remains a topic of fervent debate. To avoid under-resuscitation, the ABA recommends titrating crystalloid infusions to normotension (MAP >65), and to urine output greater than 0.5 cc/kg/hr in adults [20]. Although urine output values less than this amount are correlated with higher complication rates at 48 hours, hourly urine output is a nonspecific measure, with scant data linking it to tissue hypoxia. Glycosuria and polyuric renal failure can falsely elevate rates, and several studies highlight the failure of urine output to reflect adequate global perfusion [23]. Similarly, blood pressure and heart rate may be normal in states of compensated shock, and normal values can mask occult cellular hypoperfusion.

Concerns over the specificity of resuscitation endpoints have prompted a paradigm shift in burns care over the past ten years. In 2001, Rivers et al. published results of a randomized control trial that demonstrated improved outcomes among septic patients resuscitated to meet to pre-defined goals of preload, contractility, and oxygen delivery [26]. Further studies substantiated this approach, and in 2008 the Surviving Sepsis Campaign incorporated goal-directed therapy into their international guidelines [27]. Current sepsis management includes optimization of preload and oxygen delivery according to invasive hemodynamic monitoring, base deficit, lactate, and central venous saturation measurements, and enhancement of contractility with inotropic support.

The paradigm shift in sepsis care has prompted efforts toward a goal-directed resuscitation strategy in burn patients. Recent studies suggest that lactic acid and base deficit, both reliable measures of hypoperfusion in the trauma setting, correlate with burn size and with mortality [28–31]. Experience with invasive hemodynamic monitoring, i.e., esophageal Doppler [32–34] and transpulmonary thermodilution systems [35], reveals that the Parkland formula frequently underestimates a patient's fluid requirements. Unfortunately, efforts to optimize resuscitation with new strategies have unveiled new dangers. Patients with severe burns often receive crystalloid volumes significantly in excess of Parkland predictions, a phenomenon the burn community has termed "fluid creep."[36] The result has been an resurgence in complications of overresuscitation, including pulmonary edema, myocardial edema with atrial arrhythmias, conversion of superficial to deep burns, and compartment syndromes of the extremities [24]. Studies in trauma patients have described the immuno-modulatory effects of massive crystalloid resuscitation, including upregulation of the neutrophil oxidative burst, increased expression of neutrophil adhesion molecules, and cellular injury [37]. Researchers have hypothesized that inappropriate neutrophil activation from crystalloid infusion triggers ARDS and end-organ injury. Results from a recent multicenter trial mirror these concerns, and reveal a link in burn patients between massive resuscitation and mortality. In 2007, Klein et al. published their findings that increasing fluid requirements in burn patients significantly increased the risk of developing ARDS, pneumonia, bloodstream infections, multiorgan failure, and death [38]. Even after adjustment for patient and injury characteristics that might confound the relationship between fluid administration and outcome, there was a trend toward increased risk of adverse outcome, including death, when fluid received exceeded predicted requirements by more than 25%. Additional studies have established an increased risk of abdominal compartment syndrome among patients who receive more than 250 cc/kg of crystalloid within 24 hours, with resultant renal failure, mesenteric ischemia, coronary malperfusion, and impairment in pulmonary compliance [39, 40].

The appropriate resuscitation strategy given such conflicting data remains elusive. Some have recommended resuscitation with colloid when administered fluid volumes surpass a threshold, e. g., when requirements reach 120% of predicted or 6 cc/kg/hr [36, 40, 41]. Resuscitation with colloid has been linked with a lower incidence of intra-abdominal hypertension in burn patients [40], and has been demonstrated safe with the exception of administration to head trauma patients [42].

Pharmacologic research has unveiled possible drug therapies to support oxygen delivery to the tissues and maintain organ perfusion, in place of high volumes of fluid. For example, administration of high doses of ascorbic acid, an antioxidant, is associated with decreased ventilator dependence, as well as lower fluid requirements during clinical resuscitation [43].

Until further studies validate new therapies, organ support during burn resuscitation remains an art as well as a science for the practitioner. Resuscitation formulas serve as guidelines, and intensivists should titrate crystalloid infusions to blood pressure and urine output, using base deficit and invasive hemodynamic monitoring as supplemental guides in difficult cases. Physicians should perform serial physical examinations and monitor bladder pressures to detect early complications from volume overload, and consider colloid fluid replacement in the event of overresuscitation.

## Post-burn hypermetabolism

After the acute resuscitation phase, burn patients enter a hyperdynamic state that persists for months. A continued catecholamine and cytokine surge increases the resting metabolic rate by 160–200%, and induces prolonged tachycardia, fever, muscle protein catabolism, and derangement in hepatic protein synthesis [44–48]. These changes further threaten patients' organ function, and with increased risks of infection and impaired wound healing, as well as cardiomyopathy.

Primary management of post-burn hypermetabolism is early excision of full-thickness burns, which attenuates the hypercatabolic state [47]. Beta blocker therapy has also demonstrated several beneficial ef-

fects in burn patients. Beta blockers decrease heart rate and cardiac oxygen demand, thus protecting against cardiomyopathy. Additionally, studies demonstrate that beta blocker therapy – in particular, propranolol – decreases resting oxygen expenditure, attenuates muscle catabolism and lypolysis, and modifies catecholamine-mediated defects in lymphocyte activation [49, 50]. Therapy with the testosterone analog oxandrolone also has beneficial effects, as it significantly decreases the rate of weight and nitrogen loss among burn patietns, and facilitates donor site healing compared with placebo [51–53].

## Individual organ systems

### Central nervous system

After severe burn injury, patients often require intubation and mechanical ventilation, to support their lungs in the settings of inhalation injury and large volume shifts. Pain and stimulation from the endotracheal tube require that patients receive sedation while intubated, potentially at high doses. Given potential effects of the post-burn inflammatory response on the central nervous system, physicians should consider regular interruptions of sedation to obtain a neurologic exam from their patients. Following severe burns, phagocytes can cross the blood-brain barrier, where they release reactive oxygen and nitrogen species, proteases, cytokines, and complement proteins into the brain [54]. These inflammatory molecules can damage resident neurons and trigger life-threatening cerebral edema, only exacerbated by large volumes of crystalloid infused during resuscitation. It is therefore key for burn surgeons to frequently perform a neurologic exam in their acutely burned patients, to detect deficits early.

The utility of sedation interruption is multifold. In addition to allowing physicians to monitor patients' neurologic exam, daily interruption of sedation minimizes time on the ventilator and reduces ICU length of stay. In a randomized trial of 336 patients over a 3 year period, patients who underwent sedation interruption required less total benzodiazepines, had a shorter duration of coma, and were 32% less likely to die during the following year than controls [55]. Daily interruption of sedation should be considered in intubated burn patients.

Carbon monoxide poisoning, common among burn patients with smoke inhalation, delivers particular threat to brain function. Human hemoglobin has an affinity for carbon monoxide 210 times higher than for oxygen. As a result, carbon monoxide displaces oxygen from hemoglobin and induces tissue hypoxia. This hypoxia most severely affects the brain and heart, the organs the highest metabolic demand.

Cerebral hypoxic damage predominates in the cerebral cortex, white matter, and basal ganglia [56]. 84% of exposed patients report headache, and 50% develop weakness, nausea, confusion, and shortness of breath. Progressive hypoxia leads to cerebral edema and increased intracranial pressure, with altered sensorium, seizures, and coma. Initial management is immediate normobaric oxygenation (100%), to reduce the half-life of carboxyhemoglobin from 5 hours to 1 hour. Hyperbaric therapy may be considered in stable patients who display symptoms consistent with carbon monoxide poisoning and who have no contraindications to such treatment if. Six hours of normobaric 100% oxygen is appropriate treatment in all others. Rarely, patients who recover from acute carbon monoxide poisoning may develop delayed neuropsychiatric deficits, regardless of treatment regimen [56].

## Peripheral nervous system

49–77% of patients in the ICU for at least 7 days develop critical illness polyneuropathy, a condition that affects motor and sensory nerve axons and heralds limb weakness and prolonged ventilator weaning [57]. The mechanism, best documented in sepsis, appears driven by proinflammatory cytokines common to the post-burn inflammatory response. Increased microvascular permeability triggers endoneurial edema and extravasation of leukocytes into the endneurial space, with resultant ischemia and axonal degeneration. The result is flaccid and symmetrical limb weakness, as well as reduction of deep tendon reflexes and distal loss of sensitivity to pain, temperature, and vibration. The phrenic and intercostal nerves suffer as well, with prolonged dependence on mechanical ventilation by 2–7 fold [57].

Prevention of critical illness polyneuropathy depends on avoidance of sepsis, multiorgan failure, ARDS, and hyperglycemia, all conditions associated with damage to the axonal microvasculature. The diagnosis can be supported with nerve conduction studies, and early involvement with physical and occupational therapist may be helpful in recovery. 50% of patient with critical illness polyneuropathy fully recover, however clinical improvement can require weeks to months.

## Pulmonary

Pulmonary complications after burns occur primarily as thermal or smoke injury to the lungs, or as secondary events, for example, ventilator-associated pneumonia or acute lung injury from activation of the systemic inflammatory response. Smoke inhalation, which follows the inspiration of toxic smoke from the incomplete combustion of synthetic materials [58], affects 10–20% of burn patients and significantly increases the risks of ventilator dependence, increased length of hospitalization, and death [59]. Hot air injures the epithelium of the upper airway, inducing pharyngeal edema and acute airway obstruction in 20–33% of burn patients with inhalation injury [24]. This risk of airway obstruction warrants prompt intubation in any burn patient presenting with a history of carbonaceous sputum, voice change, or dysphagia, or in patients suffering burns within a confined space who have carboxyhemoglobin leves > 10% within one hour after injury [24].

Significant smoke inhalation impairs the function of respiratory cilia, and disrupts epithelial intercellular junctions, with resultant mucosal sloughing. This mucosal injury triggers an inflammatory cascade that compromises the pulmonary microvasculature. The resultant pulmonary edema, leakage of plasma proteins into the interstitium, and formation of alveolar exudates generates fibrin casts within the distal airways, with ultimate bronchial obstruction and constriction [59]. The accumulation of intra- and perialveolar fluid compromises gas exchange and pulmonary compliance. When hypoxia progresses to a PaO2/FiO2 ratio of less than 300, this degree of respiratory failure meets criteria for acute lung injury (ALI); when the ratio falls below 200, the patient officially has acute respiratory distress syndrome (ARDS).

ARDS after burn injury is common, with a prevalence as high as 54 % among mechanically-ventilated adult patients with major burns [60]. The condition carries a mortality rate of 30–40 % [61]. Treatment strategies for ARDS emphasize judicious fluid restriction to minimize pulmonary edema and improve gas exchange, as well as treatment of coincident infections and provision of nutrition. Early eschar excision may truncate the inflammatory response that contributes to ARDS [48]. Additionally, ARDS requires skillful attention to mechanical ventilation. Positive pressure ventilation can further damage compromised pulmonary parenchyma through overdistension and disruption of the alveoli. To avoid ventilator-associated lung injury, intensivists may adopt a lung protective strategy in ARDS, targeting tidal volumes less than 6 mL/kg and end-inspiratory plateau pressures less than 30 cm H2O [58, 62]. Moderate levels of PEEP may help avert recurrent collapse and distension of the alveoli that may worsen lung injury [62]. Data also suggest possible utility in high-frequency oscillatory ventilation for burn patients with ARDS, however this possibility requires further prospective study [63].

In addition to ARDS, ventilator-associated pneumonia (VAP) presents a special problem for severely burned patients. Between 10–20 % of burn patients who receive > 48 hours of mechanical ventilation develop VAP, and those with VAP are twice as likely to die as those without [59]. The condition arises secondary to aspiration of secretions from the oropharynx, as well as from the stomach, which gram negative bacteria colonize in critically ill patients. Burn injury and intubation inhibit mucociliary clearance, and loss of the glottic barrier allows for leakage of secretions around the endotracheal tube cuff and into the distal airways. Tactics to avoid VAP include minimization of ventilator time, daily spontaneous breathing trials, chlorhexidine oral rinses to decrease oropharyngeal colonization, and elevation of the head of the bed [58]. Excessive blood transfusion should be avoided [58]. Intubated burn patients may have quantitative culture with bronchoalveolar lavage done to facilitate monitoring and early treatment of infectino [64–66]. Studies with postpyloric feeding and silver-coated endotracheal tubes have conflicting results with regard to prevention of VAP, and thus require further investigation.

## Cardiovascular

The section in this chapter on resuscitation discusses the post-burn hemodynamic changes in detail. To briefly recapitulate, microvascular changes after burn injury induce loss of plasma volume, increase peripheral vascular resistance, and decrease cardiac output immediately after injury. Additionally, circulating mediators, e. g., tumor necrosis alpha, impair cardiac contractility, as does perturbation in calcium utilization. These changes persist for at least 24 hours post-injury, but are nearly reversed with adequate resuscitation [1, 3, 8, 9]. For weeks to months after extensive burn injury, a prolonged release of catecholamines leads to a catabolic state with high cardiac output [20–22]. Propranolol can blunt the cardiac effects of this catecholamine surge, and prevent post-burn cardiomyopathy [49–50].

## Renal

Acute kidney injury occurs in 25 % of burn patients, and is associated with 35 % mortality [67]. Among patients with frank kidney failure (class F according to the RIFLE scoring system), this mortality rate is even more dramatic, as high as 75 % [67]. Prevention of death from kidney failure after burn injury hinges upon recognition of risk factors for azotemia, as well as support of kidney perfusion.

In one retrospective cohort study of 221, burn patients, 28 % of cases of acute kidney injury arose during the resuscitative phase of treatment [68]. Hospital outcomes worsened among patients who developed renal failure during burn shock. Interestingly, the average urine output among patients who developed early acute kidney injury (AKI) was within the recommended range of 0.5–1.0 cc/kg/hr, revealing a disconnect between urine output and threat to kidney function. Patients who developed early AKI in this study had higher base deficits, indicating persistent shock despite apparently adequate urine output.

AKI likely arises from multifactorial sources in burn patients. Age, %TBSA, sepsis, and multi-organ failure independently increase the risk of AKI [67]. Studies in general critically-ill populations cite medications as responsible for up to 20 % of cases of AKI [69]. Nephrotoxic agents to avoid in burn patients, or to be monitored stringently in the event of necessary administration, include aminoglycosides, colistin, amphotericin B (associated with a 25–30% risk of AKI), and Amicar. The kidneys are sensitive to changes in intra-abdominal pressure, and pressures greater than 12 mmHg can lead to AKI [69]. A sustained intra-abdominal pressure greater than 20 mmHg will generate AKI in more than 30% of cases [69]. Hyperglycemia has been associated with AKI, and physicians should strive to avoid excessive glucose elevations. Intravenous contrast induces nephropathy, which can be avoided with volume expansion and the free radical scavenger acetylcysteine. In the setting of injury, the kidneys lose the ability to autoregulate, and depend upon mean arterial pressure for perfusion. As a result, normotension among patients at risk for AKI, including the elderly, diabetics, patients with chronic kidney disease, and patients with hypertension at baseline is optimal. "Renally-dosed" dopamine, once given under the assumption that it optimized renal blood flow, does not reduce the incidence of AKI or the need for renal replacement therapy (RRT) [70]. In fact, data suggest that dopamine worsens renal perfusion, and is associated with increased myocardial strain and cardiac arrhythmias [70]. Fenoldepam, on the other hand, is a selective dopamin-1 receptor agonist that may increase renal blood flow at low doses (>1 mcg/kg/min) without systemic effects. Data is conflicting – one prospective placebo-controlled study among septic patients showed no association between fenoldepam use and mortality, while meta-analyses suggest that fenoldepam decreases the need for RRT, and also decreases mortality among patients with AKI [71]. Precise indications for implementation of fenoldepam require further prospective study.

Diuretics may assist in management of volume overload and provide a temporizing therapy before implementation of RRT. Failure to respond to diuretics in AKI has been associated with an increased risk of death and renal non-recovery, however no evidence supports conversion of oliguric AKI to non-oliguric AKI with diuretics [69]. If patients develop severe hyperkalemia, clinical signs of uremia, severe acidosis, or volume overload refractory to diuresis, a nephrologist should be consulted for RRT, either through intermittent hemodialysis (HD) or continuous veno-venous hemofiltration (CVVH). For un-

stable, critically-ill patients, the latter of these options induces the least hemodynamic compromise. In terms of renal recovery, the extant data suggest that both methods are equitable, with no difference in mortality [69].

## Gastrointestinal tract

The shock and reliance on vasopressor agents that accompany burn injury place patients at risk for mesenteric ischemia, which in turn increases patient's susceptibility to bacteremia. The intestinal mucosa functions as a local defense barrier, preventing bacteria and endotoxin within the intestinal lumen from translocating into the circulatory system [72]. After burn resuscitation, splanchnic edema leads to peristalsis, with intestinal stasis, bacterial overgrowth, and compromise to the integrity of the mucosal barrier [72–75]. Vasoactive agents further damage the mucosal epithelium through a decrease in intestinal blood flow. The ischemic gut, itself, functions as a pro-inflammatory agent, releasing factors into the bloodstream that activate neutrophils and trigger end-organ dysfunction.

Immediate enteral feeding after thermal injury aids in maintenance of intestinal mucosa, and also thwarts the excessive release of catabolic hormones. Enteral feeding supports the structural integrity of the gut by maintaining mucosal mass, stimulating epithelial cell proliferation, maintaining villus height, and promoting the production of brush border enzymes [72–75]. Feeding stimulates mesenteric blood flow, and triggers the resealse of endogenous agents (e. g., cholecystikinin, gastrin, bile salts) that exert trophic effects on the epithelium [72, 73]. Patients fed early after burn injury also have significantly enhanced wound healing and shorter hospital stays, compared with controls [24].

Studies demonstrate that the protective effects of early feeding on the gut mucosa are not maintained with total parental nutrition (TPN). Studies in the 1980s revealed that despite the catabolic state and marked protein requirement of burn patients (1.5–2.0 g/kg/day), aggressive high-calorie feeding with a combination of enteral feeds and supplemental TPN was associated with increased infectious complications and mortality [77, 78]. More recent investigations have not only confirmed these findings, but also have demonstrated that TPN fails to prevent hypercatabolism after thermal injury, and also worsens the stress response, increases endotoxin translocation, and further impairs mucosal immunity [79]. Standard of care in burns management thus mandates early enteral feeding whenever possible, to provide adequate nutrition in the setting of hypercatabolism, and to preserve the mucosal integrity and immune function of the gut.

## Conclusion

Severe burn injury threatens every system in the body. Prevention of multiorgan failure necessitates preservation of tissue perfusion, as well as exacting implementation of critical care techniques. From the moment of injury, through the resuscitative period, and continuing through the recovery phase, care for burned patients requires attention to and support of organ function to prevent morbidity and mortality.

## References

[1] Ipaktchi K, Arbabi S (2006) Advances in burn critical care. Crit Care Med 34[9 Suppl]: S239–244

[2] Saffle JI (2007) The phenomenon of "fluid creep" in acute burn resuscitation. J Burn Care Res 28(3): 382–395

[3] Salinas J, Drew G, Gallagher J, Cancio LC, Wolf SE et al (2008) Closed-loop and decision-assist resuscitation of burn patients. J Trauma 64[4 Suppl]: S321–332

[4] Tompkins RG, Remensnyder JP, Burke JF, Tompkins DM, Hilton JF et al (1988) Significant reductions in mortality for children with burn injuries through the use of prompt eschar excision. Ann Surg 208(5): 577–585

[5] Herndon DN, Barrow RE, Rutan RL, Rutan TC, Desai MH et al (1989) A comparison of conservative versus early excision. Therapies in severely burned patients. Ann Surg 209(5): 547–552; discussion 552–543

[6] Xiao-Wu W, Herndon DN, Spies M, Sanford AP, Wolf SE (2002) Effects of delayed wound excision and grafting in severely burned children. Arch Surg 137(9): 1049–1054

[7] Ong YS, Samuel M, Song C (2006) Meta-analysis of early excision of burns. Burns 32(2): 145–150

[8] Pereira C, Murphy K, Jeschke M, Herndon DN (2005) Post burn muscle wasting and the effects of treatments. Int J Biochem Cell Biol 37(10): 1948–1961

[9] Pereira CT, Herndon DN (2005) The pharmacologic modulation of the hypermetabolic response to burns. Adv Surg 39: 245–261

[10] Branski LK, Herndon DN, Barrow RE, Kulp GA, Klein GL et al (2009) Randomized controlled trial to determine the efficacy of long-term growth hormone treatment in severely burned children. Ann Surg n:n-n

[11] O'Keefe GE, Hunt JL, Purdue GF (2001) An evaluation of risk factors for mortality after burn trauma and the identification of gender-dependent differences in outcomes. J Am Coll Surg 192(2): 153–160

[12] White CE, Renz EM (2008) Advances in surgical care: management of severe burn injury. Crit Care Med 36[7 Suppl]: S318–324

[13] Fratianne RB, Brandt CP (1997) Improved survival of adults with extensive burns. J Burn Care Rehabil 18: 347–351

[14] Curreri PW, Luterman A, Braun DW, Shires GT (1980) Burn injury–analysis of survival and hospitalization time for 937 patients. Ann Surg 82: 472–478

[15] McGwin G, Cross JM, Ford JW, Rue LW (2003) Long-term trends in mortality according to age among adult burn patients. J Burn Care Rehab 24(1): 21–25

[16] Marshall WG, Dimick AR (1983) The natural history of major burns with multiple subsystem failure. J Trauma 23: 102–105

[17] Sheridan RL, Ryan CM, Yin LM, Hurley J, Tompkins RG (1998) Death in the burn unit: sterile multiple organ failure. Burns 24: 307–311

[18] Cumming J, Purdue GF, Hung JL, O'Keefe GE (2001) Objective estimates of the incidence and consequences of multiple organ dysfunction and sepsis after burn trauma. J Trauma 50(3): 510–515

[19] Nguyen LN, Nguyen TG (2009) Characteristics and outcomes of multiple organ dysfunction syndrome among severe-burn patients. Burns 35(7): 937–941

[20] Pham TN, Cancio LC, Gibran NS (2008) American Burn Association practice guidelines: Burn shock resuscitation. J Burn Care Res 29(1): 257–266

[21] Wolf SE, Herndon DN (2004) Burns. Sabiston textbook of surgery: The biological basis of modern surgical practice, 17th edn. npublisher,nplace of publication, pp 569–596

[22] Dehne MG, Sablotzki A, Hoffmann A, Muhling J, Dietrich FE, Hempelmann G (2002) Alterations of acute phase reaction and cytokine production in patients following severe burn injury. Burns 28: 535–542

[23] Tricklebank S (2009) Modern trends in fluid therapy for burns. Burns 35(6): 757–767

[24] Latenser BA (2009) Critical care of the burn patient: the first 48 hours. Crit Care Med 37: 2819–2826

[25] Barret JP, Herndon DN (2003) Modulation of inflammatory and catabolic responses in severely burned children by early burn wound excision in the first 24h. Arch Surg 138: 127–132

[26] Rivers E, Nguyen B, Havstad S, Ressler J, Muzzin A, Knoblich B, Peterson E, Tomlanovich M (2001) Early goal-directed therapy in the treatment of severe sepsis and septic shock. NEJM 345: 1368–1377

[27] Dellinger RP, Levy MM, Carlet JM, Blon J, Parker MM, Jaeschke R, Reinhart K, Angus DC, Brun-Buisson C, Beale RE, Calandra T, Dhalnaut JF, Gerlach H, Harvey M, Marini JJ, Marshall J, Ranieri M, Ramsay G, Sevransky J, Thompson T, Townsend S, Vender JS, Zimmerman JL, Vincent JL (2008) Surviving Sepsis Campaign: International guidelines for management of severe sepsis and septic shock: 2008. Crit Care Med 36: 296–327

[28] Cancio LC, Galvez E, Turner CE (2006) Base deficit and alveolar-arterial gradient during resuscitation contribute independently but modestly to the prediction of mortality after burn injury. J Burn Care Res 27: 289–296

[29] Kamolz LP, Andel H, Schramm W (2005) Lactate: early predictor of morbidity and mortality in patients with severe burns. Burns 31: 986–990

[30] Jeng JC, Lee K, Jablonski K (1997) Serum lactate and base deficit suggest inadequate resuscitation of patients with burn injuries: application of a point-of-care laboratory instrument. J Burn Care Rehabil 18: 402–405

[31] Andel D, Kamolz LP, Roka J, Schramm W, Zimpfer M, Frey M, Andel H (2007) Base deficit and lactate: Early predictors of morbidity and mortality in patients with burns. Burns 33(8): 973–978

[32] Conway DH, Mayall R, Abdul-Latif MS, Gilligan S, Tackaberry C (2002) Randomised controlled trial investigating the influence of intravenous fluid titration using oesophageal Doppler monitoring during bowel surgery. Anaesthesia 57: 845–849

[33] Gan TJ, Sopitt A, Maroof M, El-Moalem H, Robertson KM, Moretti E (2002) Goal-directed intraoperative fluid administration reduces length of hospital stay after major surgery. Anesthesiology 97: 820–826

[34] Yamamoto Y, Nozaki M, Nozaki T, Higashimori H, Nakazawa H (2007) Clinical evaluation of the echoesophageal Doppler for the cardiac output monitoring of patients with extensive burns. Burns 33: S38–S39

[35] Holm C, Mayr M, Tegeler J, Horbrand F, Henckel von Donnersmarck G, Muhlbauer W, Pfeiffer UJ (2004) A clinical randomized study on the effects of invasive monitoring on burn shock resuscitation. Burns 30: 798–807

[36] Saffle JR (2007) The phenomenon of "fluid creep" in acute burn resuscitation. J Burn Care Res 28: 382–395

[37] Alam HB, Rhee P (2007) New developments in fluid resuscitation. Surg Clin North Am 87(1): 55–72

[38] Klein MB, Hayden D, Elson C, Nathens AB, Gamelli RL, Gibran NS, Herndon DN, Arnoldo B, Silver G, Schoenfeld D, Tompkins RG (2007) The association between fluid administration and outcome following major burn: A multicenter study. Ann Surg 245(4): 622–628

[39] Ivy ME, Atweh NA, Palmer J (2000) Intra-abdominal hypertension and abdominal compartment syndrome in burn patients. J Trauma 49: 387–391

[40] O'Mara MS, Slater H, Goldfarb IW, Caushaj PF (2005) A prospective, randomized evaluation of intra-abdominal pressures with crystalloid and colloid resuscitation in burn patients. J Trauma 58: 1011–1018

[41] Chung KK, Blackbourne LH, Wolfe SE (2006) Evolution of burn resuscitation in operation Iraqi freedom. J Burn Care Res 27: 606–611

[42] The SAFE Study Investigators (2004) A comparison of albumin and saline for fluid resuscitation in the intensive care unit. NEJM 350: 2247–2256.

[43] Tanaka H, Matsuda T, Miyagantani Y, Yukioka T, Matsuda H, Shimazaki S (2000) Reduction of resuscitation fluid volumes in severely burned patients using ascorbic acid administration. Arch Surg 135: 326–331

[44] Hart DW, Wolf SE, Mlcak R (2000) Persistence of muscle catabolism after severe burn. Surgery 128: 312–319

[45] Hart DW, Wolfe SE, Herndon DN (2002) Energy expenditure and caloric balance after burn: Increased feeding leads to fat rather than lean mass accretion. Ann Surg 235: 152–161

[46] Hart DW, Wolf SE, Chinkes DL (2000) Determinants of skeletal muscle catabolism after severe burn. Ann Surg 232: 455–465

[47] Hart DW, Wolf SE, Chinkes DL (2003) Effects of early excision and aggressive enteral feeding on hypermetabolism, catabolism, and sepsis after severe burn. J Trauma 54: 755–761

[48] Herndon DN, Tompkins RG (2004) Support of the metabolic response to burn injury. Lancet 363: 1895–1902

[49] Herndon DN, Hart DW, Wolf SE (2001) Reversal of catabolism by beta-blockade after severe burns. NEJM 345: 1223–1229

[50] Arbabi S, Ahrns KS, Wahl WL (2004) Beta-blocker use is associated with improved outcomes in adult burn patients. J Trauma 56: 265–269

[51] Hart DW, Wolf SE, Ramzy PI (2001) Anabolic effects of oxandrolone after severe burn. Ann Surg 233: 556–564

[52] Demling RH, Orgill DP (2000) The anticatabolic and wound healing effects of the testosterone analog oxandrolone after severe burn injury. J Crit Care 15: 12–17

[53] Wolf SE, Edelman LS, Mealyan N (2006) Effects of oxandrolone on outcome measures in the severely burned: A multicenter prospective randomized double-blind trial. J Burn Care Res 27: 131–139

[54] Flierl MA, Stahel PF, Touban BM, Beauchamp KM, Morgan SJ, Smith WR, Ipaktchi KR (2009) Bench-to-bedside review: Burn-induced cerebral inflammation – a neglected entity? Crit Care 13(3): 215

[55] Girard TD, Kress JP, Fuchs BD, Thomason JWW, Schweickert WD, Bun BT, Taichman DB, Dunn JG, Pohlman AS, Kinniry PA, Jackson JC, Canonico AE, Light RW, Shintani AK, Thompson JL, Gordon SM, Hall JB, Dittus RS, Bernard GR, Ely EW (2008) Efficacy and safety of a paired sedation and ventilator weaning protocol for mechanically ventilated patients in intensive care (Awakening and Breathing Controlled trial): a randomized controlled trial. Lancet 371(9607): 126–134

[56] Prockop LD, Chickova RI (2007) Carbon monoxide intoxication: An updated review. J Neuro Sci 262: 122–130

[57] Hermans G, De Jonghe B, Bruyninckx F, Van den Berghe G (2008) Clinical review: Critical illness polyneuropathy and myopathy. Crit Care 12(6): 238–247

[58] Peck MD, Koppelman T (2009) Low-tidal volume ventilation as a strategy to reduce ventilator-associated injury in ALI and ARDS. J Burn Care Res 30: 172–183

[59] Mosier MJ, Pham TN (2009) American Burn Association practice guidelines for prevention, diagnosis, and treatment of ventilator-associated pneumonia (VAP) in burn patients. J Burn Care Res 30: 910–928

[60] Dancey DR, Hayes J, Gomez M (1999) ARDS in patients with thermal injury. Int Care Med 25: 1231–1236

[61] Allen K, Bigatello L (2010) The Acute Respiratory Distress Syndrome. Critical Care Handbook of the Massachusetts General Hospital, 5th edn. npublisher, nplace of publication, pp 288–298

[62] Ventilation with lower tidal volumes as compared with traditional tidal volumes for acute lung injury and the acute respiratory distress syndrome: The Acute Respiratory Distress Syndrome Network. NEJM (2000) 342: 1301–1308

[63] Cartotto R, Ellis S, Smith T (2005) Use of high-frequency oscillatory ventilation in burn patients. Crit Care Med 33[Suppl 3]: S175-S181

[64] Wahl WL, Ahrns KS, Brandt MM (2005) Bronchoalveolar lavage in diagnosis of ventilator-associated pneumonia in patients with burns. J Burn Care Rehabil 26: 57–61

[65] Croce MA, Fabian TC, Mueller EW (2004) The appropriate diagnostic threshold for ventilator-associated pneumonia using quantitative cultures. J Trauma 56: 931–934

[66] Fagon JY, Chastre J, Woff M (2000) Invasive and noninvasive strategies for management of suspected ventilator-associated pneumonia: a randomized trial. Ann Intern Med 132: 621–630

[67] Brusselaers N, Monstrey S, Colpaert K, Decruenaere J, Blot SI, Hoste EAJ (2010) Outcome of acute kidney injury in severe burns: a systematic review and meta-analysis. Int Care Med 365: 915–925

[68] Mosier MJ, Pham TN, Klein MB, Gibran NS, Arnoldo BD, Gamelli RL, Tompkins RG, Herndon DN (2010) Early acute kidney injury predicts progressive renal dysfunction and higher mortality in severely burned adults. J Burn Care Res 31: 83–92

[69] Dennen P, Douglas IS, Anderson R (2010) Acute kidney injury in the intensive care unit: An update and primer for the intensivist. Crit Care Med 38: 261–275

[70] Morellia A, Ricci Z, Bellomo R (2005) Prophylactic fenoldepam for renal protection in sepsis: A randomized, double-blind, placebo-controlled pilot trial. Crit Care Med 33: 2451–2456

[71] Landoni G, Biondi-Zoccai GG, Tumlin JA (2007) Beneficial impact of fenoldepam in critically ill patients with or at risk for acute renal failure: a meta-analysis of randomized clinical trials. Am J Kidney Dis 49: 56–68

[72] Magnotti LJ, Deitch EA (2005) Burns, bacterial translocation, gut barrier function, and failure. J Burn Care Rehabil 26: 383–391

[73] Deitch EA (1990) Intestinal permeability is increased in burn patients shortly after injury. Surgery 107: 411–416

[74] Ryan CM, Yarmush ML, Burke JF (1992) Increased gut permeability early after burns correlates with the extent of burn injury. Crit Care Med 20: 1508–1512

[75] LeVoyer T, Cioffi WG, Pratt L (1992) Alterations in intestinal permeability after severe thermal injury. Arch Surg 127: 26–29

[76] Andel H, Rab M, Andel D (2001) Impact of early high caloric duodenal feeding on the oxygen balance of the splanchnic region after severe burn injury. Burns 27: 389–393

[77] Herndon DN, Barrow RE, Stein M (1989) Increased mortality with intravenous supplemental feeding in severely burned patients. J Burn Care Rehabil 10: 309–313

[78] Alexander JW, MacMillan BG, Stinnett JD (1980) Beneficial effects of aggressive protein feeding in severely burned children. Ann Surg 192: 505–517

[79] Sugiura T, Tashiro T, Yamamori H, Takagi K, Hayashi N, Itahashi T (1999) Effects of total parenteral nutrition on endotoxin translocation and extent of the stress response in burned rats. Nutrition 15: 570–575

Correspondence: Rob Sheridan, Shriners Hospital for Children, 51 Blossom Street, Boston, MA, 02114, USA, Phone: +1 617 726 5633, Fax: +1 617 367 8936, E-mail: rsheridan@partners.org

# Critical care of thermally injured patient

Mette M. Berger[1], Shahriar Shahrokhi[2], Marc G. Jeschke[2]

[1] Adult ICU and Burn Unit, University Hospital (CHUV), Lausanne, Switzerland
[2] Ross Tilley Burn Centre, Sunnybrook Health Sciences Centre, Department of Surgery, Division of Plastic Surgery, University of Toronto, Toronto, ON, Canada

## Introduction

Only a minority of burn injured patients will require intensive care unit (ICU) admission and treatment. A burn is considered "major" when involving more than 20 % BSA, with further severity steps at 40 % and 60 % TBSA, the later being called massive burn injury. The presence of inhalation injury will have further additive affects increasing the mortality. Major burns impact the function of all organs: the massive release of pro-inflammatory mediators and lipid peroxides by the thermally injured skin will induce oxidative stress and inflammatory responses, which in turn cause cardiovascular, respiratory, digestive, renal, endocrine, and metabolic alterations. All these responses are proportional to the severity of the injury. Age and presence of co-morbidities are important prognostic factors, even more than in any other critical care condition. The massively burned patient poses one of the greatest challenges in critical care. While patients with severe thermal injury share several characteristics with other critically ill patients, there are significant differences:

a. The patients suffer significant cutaneous exudative losses (proportional to the TBSA) of fluids containing large quantities of proteins, minerals and micronutrients. The electrolyte derangements will require close monitoring, and the loss of micronutrients will be large enough to cause acute deficiency syndromes.

b. The body surface area injured and requiring repair is extensive. It frequently exceeds 1 m², which poses an enormous anabolic challenge.

c. There is an increased infectious risk due to the loss of the skin barrier, but also to the rapid depression of humoral and cellular immune defences [94].

d. The duration of inflammatory and hyper-metabolic response is immediate and long lasting and has no comparison with other conditions.

e. Venous access is more difficult due to the destruction of the skin at the puncture sites causing higher catheter related infection rates.

f. The thermally injured patient requires longer length of stay in the ICU compared with other trauma patients, and require more prolonged nutritional support.

## Oxidative stress and Inflammation

The inflammatory response constitutes an organized defense mechanism aimed at protecting the body from further damage, restoring homeostasis and promoting wound repair. This includes a local reaction to injury, a systemic response (=SIRS: tachycardia, tachypnea, fever, leucocytosis), massive cytokine production, immense immune and endocrine changes, increased protein catabolism, and a reprioritization of hepatic synthesis. This response to injury includes a redistribution of the micronutrients (trace elements and vitamins) from the vascular compartment to organs with high rates of cell replication and metabolic activity. Cytokine production is strongly enhanced after major burns, the balance between pro-inflammatory and anti-inflammatory mediators in acute injury is lost [24]: the phenomenon further increases infectious complications. The intensity of this reaction is correlated with mortality [66]. Although inflammation is perceived as beneficial, its persistence for prolonged periods of time causes progressive loss of lean body cell mass, particularly of skeletal muscle, and an increased susceptibility to infection. It will favor development of organ dysfunction and failure.

Major thermal injury and the subsequent inflammatory response cause a massive production of free radicals (molecules containing one or more unpaired electrons with high oxidant reactivity). These can be divided into two major groups: the reactive oxygen species (ROS) and reactive nitrogen species (RNS). ROS are produced primarily by the mitochondrial respiratory chain, and by the activated leukocytes. It is a normal phenomenon in bacterial destruction, and cell signaling. In the case of burns an intense lipid peroxidation results partially from the direct effect of the burn injury on the lipids contained in skin, but mainly from the increased ROS production. Nitric oxide (NO) derived from the endothelium, has emerged as a fundamental regulatory signal, as well as a potent mediator of cellular damage. Most of the cytotoxicity attributed to NO is due to peroxynitrite, a RNS, produced from the reaction between NO and the superoxide anion. Peroxynitrite interacts with lipids, DNA, and proteins via direct oxidative reactions or via indirect, radical-mediated mechanisms. The initial intense oxidative stress will persist for several days, and is reactivated by each septic episode.

The intensity and the duration of the inflammatory response in major burns are immense [89], and will result in the continued production of pro-inflammatory cytokines for several weeks. The associated free radical production and oxidative stress will persist accordingly.

In healthy subjects, the endogenous antioxidant defense mechanisms are sufficient to cope with moderate free radical overproduction. In major burns, these defenses are overwhelmed, leaving space for the deleterious effects of ROS, with proximity oxidation of nucleotides, proteins and lipids. The endogenous antioxidant defenses become acutely depleted by the massive production of free radical species derived from both oxygen and nitric oxide, associated with enormous losses of antioxidant micronutrients through their wounds [16], and acute unavailability of the same antioxidant micronutrients in the circulating compartment.

The pro-inflammatory cytokines (particularly IL-6) are responsible for the redistribution of micronutrients (including those with antioxidant properties) from the circulating compartment to tissues and organs with high synthetic and cell replication activity. In an animal burn model, Ding et al. showed that the serum concentrations of zinc decreases while at the same time liver content increases in association with increased expression of metallothionein [32]. When this phenomenon is added to the large exudative trace element losses it is easily understandable that the circulating compartments antioxidant capacity becomes acutely reduced, while simultaneously facing a massive oxidative stress.

## Oxidative stress control strategies

Several strategies have been proposed to control oxidative stress:

a. Mechanical removal of the source of oxidants with early wound scar excision to reduce the release of lipid peroxide: this strategy has been shown to reduce mortality.
b. Topical application of anti-inflammatory agents.
c. Systemic administration of antioxidants (initiated as early as possible after injury).

In animal studies of thermal injury, the supplementation of antioxidant vitamins reduce cardiac NF-kB release [48], while continuous high dose vitamin C infusion can increase plasma antioxidant potential, and limit the endothelial injury and capillary leak [34]. In patients large supra-physiological doses of Vitamin C administered over the first 24 hours reduce post-burn fluid requirement by about 30 % [99]. In animals, selenium supplements limit the peroxidative damage caused by burns [1]. In adult patients, supplementation with trace elements, particularly with selenium, reduces the lipid peroxidation process during the first week and reinforces endogenous antioxidant and immune defenses [14].

Major trace element deficiencies have been shown to occur since the 1970s [14]. They are largely explained by the early exudative losses [15, 16]. Copper, which plays an essential role in collagen synthesis, wound repair, and immunity, is strongly depleted in burns [14]: this is unique among medical conditions. Early trace element supplementation is associated with improved wound healing, decreased protein catabolism, decreased pulmonary infection, and shortened ICU stay [15]. Therefore special attention should be given to all patients receiving enteral/parenteral nutrition. Trace element and vitamin contents of enteral/standard parenteral nutrition are insufficient to cover the increased requirements after major burns. Based on balance studies, early antioxidant trace elements are delivered intravenously at CHUV for 8 to 30 days depending of burn size; the same adult solution is adapted to children per m$^2$ [95]. The trace elements are delivered in addition to basal micronutrient requirements.

## Fluid and cardiovascular management beyond 24 hours

The observation of an important hemo-concentration after major burns goes back to the late 19th century, but its pathophysiology only became apparent during the 20th century. Shock was recognized early on as a predominantly hypovolemic state, but we now know that shock is a complex process of cardio-circulatory dysfunction which fluid resuscitation alone cannot cure. Immediately after injury inflammatory shock mediators are released from the burned skin. These include histamine, serotonin, bradikinin, nitric oxide, lipid peroxides, prostaglandins, derived oxygen and nitric oxide free radicals, thromboxane, cytokines (interleukins and TNF), and platelet aggregating factor with the subsequent coagulation cascade. The response is proportional to the injury, and systemic effects of these mediators will become obvious with burns exceeding 20–25% TBSA [65]. The massive histamine release will cause the early increase in permeability of local and systemic capillaries initiating a massive capillary leak enabling large molecules such as albumin to escape into the interstitial space. Serotonin and bradykinin will cause the persistence of this phenomenon during the first 18–24 hours. Due to the loss of plasma, a steep increase in hematocrit is observed. Edema formation follows a biphasic pattern: an early rapid phase and a slower increase during the next 12–36 hours [6]. A slow resolution of the increased permeability will start between 8–12 hours depending on the burn size. During this resolution phase the extravasated plasma proteins and resuscitation fluids will remain sequestered in extra-vascular spaces of non-burned and burned soft tissue. Edema formation exceeds the capacity of the lymph vessels to evacuate fluid. The speed of the edema progression will depend on the quality of the resuscitation: a rapid early delivery of large amounts of resuscitation fluids increases the edema formation and worsens the compromised local microcirculation, worsening ischemia in the injured tissues. The important fluid and protein shifts will modify the capillary hydrostatic (P) and colloid oncotic (CO) pressures of the Starling equation further compromising trans-microvascular fluid flux (Jv).

$$Jv = Kf ((Pc-Pif) - d (COPp - COPif))$$

The capillary filtration coefficient (Kf) increases immediately after burn injury, but does not explain the rapid edema formation [65]. In the interstitial fluid, hydrostatic pressure and oncotic pressure will both increase, while in the capillaries hydrostatic pressure and oncotic pressures decrease become negative, constituting a suction force. Delta, the osmotic reflection coefficient, indicates the relative permeability to proteins: the increased permeability is measurable until 8–12 hours post injury. All this causes increase osmolarity of the extravascular compartment.

Myocardial dysfunction has been repeatedly demonstrated both in humans and animals. Neuroendocrine responses will contribute to the worsening of the hemodynamic condition, by increasing cardiac afterload due to the massive release of endogenous norepinephrine and epinephrine. This is further complicated by the decrease in preload due to the hypovolemic state. Oxygen free radicals and lipid peroxides also play an important role. In burns >40% BSA intrinsic contractile defects are observed, which are partly reversed by fluid resuscitation and antioxidants [47]. Troponin I increases in a large proportion of the patients with major burns reflecting intrinsic tissue damage.

Edema in non-burned tissue occurs to some degree in burns affecting 10% TBSA, and is largely explained by the circulating histamine and chemokines. All tissues and organs are affected including the lungs, the splanchnic organs, and the brain.

In addition to the capillary leek, fluid is losses can directly be attributed to the wound exudates (1–2 liters per 10% BSA during the first 24 hours, decreasing thereafter until closer of the wound) and the evaporation. These losses include plasma proteins (30g of protein/10% TBSA/day), minerals (P, Mg) and trace elements (mainly Cu, Se, Zn).

The principles of burn fluid resuscitation were developed in the early fifties. Exudates and edema fluid were shown to be isotonic, containing same amounts of electrolytes and protein as plasma. The development of Parkland formula was based on studies on hemodynamic effects of various regimes, using different proportions of colloids and crystalloids [103]. No single fluid resuscitation formula has proven to be superior, and the Parkland formula has

since remained the most used due to its simplicity. Interestingly, the colloid part of the formula has somehow become forgotten. While under-resuscitation was the problem in the mid-20th century, over-resuscitation has become a major issue since the 90's [80] with a host of complications: "fluid creep" has become a recognized as a problem over the last decade [87] resulting in general swelling of all organs. Several complications results from this lack of control: abdominal compartment syndrome with renal failure (the most severe) [51], intestinal swelling with ileus, conversion of intermediate burns into deep burns (secondary ischemia), worsening gas exchanges and increasing length of mechanical ventilation [46], and prolonged ICU and hospital length of stay. Today the "Parkland formula" should only be considered as a guide to initiate resuscitation and not absolute fluid requirements.

These complications have forced us to rethink the true aims of resuscitation, which are to stabilize and restore hemodynamic status as soon as possible and to ensure tissue perfusion and oxygenation. In major burns the tools include a combination of fluids (crystalloids and colloids after 8–12hrs), which aim to restore the circulating "volume", and inotropic and vasopressive agents. Fluids alone are not able to restore adequate tissue perfusion. Invasive cardiovascular monitoring can be used to refine resuscitation, but in absence of such tools a cautious restrictive attitude towards fluids and tight clinical supervision are essential. The initial resuscitation should aim to maintain organ perfusion: urinary output 0.5 ml/hour, lack of tachycardia, maintenance of MAP, normal lactate, and normal base excess will generally reflect this global condition. Nevertheless, one should be cognizant of the difficulty of monitoring the splanchnic compartment.

Among fluids, isotonic crystalloids remain the basic tool. Several burn resuscitation formulae were developed in the 70s, aiming at minimizing fluid delivery and the subsequent edema, which worsens outcomes and further complicates patient care. Hypertonic saline has been studied but the results have been conflicting and currently it's not part of the mainstay of treatment given the significant increase in acute renal failure [49]. Nevertheless, whatever the formula, the fluid used must contain Na in sufficient concentration to deliver about 0.5 mmol/

**Table 1.** Criteria for assessment of under and over-resuscitation

| Under-resuscitation | Over-resuscitation |
|---|---|
| Oliguria > 0.3 ml/kg/h | Polyuria > 1.0 ml/kg/h |
| Hemoglobin > 180g/l (Ht > 55%) | Decreasing $PaO_2/FiO_2 \rightarrow$ pulmonary edema |
| Natremia > 145 mmol/l | Increasing PAPO / PVC |
| Cardiac index > 2 L/min/m2 | Rapidly increasing cutaneous edema |
| SvO2 > 55% | Fluid delivery > Ivy index (fluid delivery > 250 ml/kg BW) |
| plasma lacate > 2 mmol/l or increasing | Intra-abdominal P > 20 mmHg $\rightarrow$ Intra-abdominal hypertension leading to |
| base excess > −5 mmol/l or decreasing | $\rightarrow$ acute renal failure, splanchnic ischemia, transformation of 2° to 3° burns, compartment syndrome in limbs ($\uparrow$ need for fasciotomies), $\downarrow$venous return with hemodynamic failure |

kg/%TBSA by 48 hours to prevent water intoxication associated with hypotonic fluids.

Several strategies aimed at reducing edema formation have been proposed, and actually overlap some of those proposed for the control of oxidative stress: 1) topical application of local anesthetic lidocaine/prilocaine cream has some effect in experimental conditions, 2) anti-histamine drugs in the early phase have not reduced the edema formation, 3) use of colloids in fluid resuscitation has proven some efficacy, and 4) antioxidants and particularly vitamin C in high doses.

Early permissive hypovolemia has recently been advocated and seems to reduce organ dysfunction [5], possibly through reduction of organ edema formation and its associated intracellular dysfunction. In the 21st century resuscitation should be guided by the hemodynamic response, and the application of the Parkland formula (even though it's widely used) should be of historical note.

Upon admission to the ICU, one of the important roles for any intensivist in charge of caring for the thermally injured patient is to ensure hemodynamic stability and to provide restrictive control of fluid balance after the initial resuscitation (which is frequently over-enthusiastic). It begins with reducing the fluid infusion rate as soon as the patient is admitted to the ICU. In the larger burns (> 40% BSA) this may require some invasive monitoring, and the use of a vasopressor agent such as norepinephrine to maintain tissue perfusion; a mean arterial pressure of 60 mm Hg will generally be sufficient.

Cardiovascular monitoring requirements will depend on the extent of injury and the presence of inhalation injury. An arterial catheter will generally be required for arterial pressure monitoring in patients with burns > 20% TBSA or in those patients requiring intubation due to inhalation injury or burns to face and neck. Blood gas determinations will in addition enable monitoring of arterial lactate and evolution of acid-base status. With increasing severity of burn injury and in elderly patients > 60 years, information about cardiac output becomes necessary. The PiCCO (pulse contour cardiac output) arterial catheter along with a central venous line enables determination of cardiac output without the risks inherent to a pulmonary catheter. Moreover, Holm et al. recently demonstrated that

using the PiCCO for "volume targeted resuscitation" could be more deleterious than the Parkland formula, resulting in increased fluid delivery, worsened oxygenation and prolonged intubation time [46]. The pulmonary catheters may be used in massive burns only or in patients with major cardiopulmonary co-morbidities. Trans-esophageal echocardiography is a further tool that enables a rapid diagnostic workup of the unstable patient [36].

Hemodynamic findings in early invasive cardiovascular monitoring will be variable. Massive burns are generally associated with cardiogenic shock even in the youngest patients, and will invariably be present in elderly during the first 24 hours. The etiology includes increased afterload caused by high levels of stress hormones, direct depression of myocardium by cytokines and lipoperoxides, intravascular hypovolemia with low preload and vasoplegia. The management of shock may require a combination of dobutamine and norepinephrine, in doses titrated to target (cardiac index 2.5–3 l/m², mean arterial pressure > 60 mm Hg). Epinephrine will rarely be required. The aim is to restore normal cardiac output, but certainly not supra-normal values or any surrogate of "normal" preload values. Whatever the measurement method used, normal filling pressures should not be the objective goal, as this strategy causes over-resuscitation and its multitude subsequent complications [3, 5, 45, 51, 80]. Intra-abdominal pressure monitoring is therefore recommended in the burns involving more than 30% TBSA.

After 36–48 hours, the patients generally become spontaneously hyperdynamic. In case of extensive burns, some vasoplegia caused by the massive cytokine release may require norepinephrine (2–10 mcg/min) to permit reducing fluid delivery. Indeed by 24 hours, the fluid delivery should be drastically reduced, to about 30–40% of that infused during the first 24 hours, and the solutions switched to hypotonic, sodium free-poor solutions, in combination with albumin (in case of hypoalbuminemia > 20 g/l), or fresh frozen plasma (in case of clotting disorders). The international controversy regarding albumin delivery in critically ill patients has severely complicated burns resuscitations [2]; administration should not be completely liberal, but a very restrictive attitude complicates resuscitation. Albuminemia < 20 g/l should certainly be corrected

207

to avoid the negative consequences of decreased oncotic pressure.

The delivery of free water along with albumin will contribute to the mobilization of the large amounts of sodium that have accumulated in the interstitial and extra-cellular spaces during the first 24 hours. By day 3, the interstitial fluids that have accumulated during the first 24–48 hours must be mobilized and excreted. This generally required an active stimulation of diuresis using loop diuretics (generally furosemide) in combination with an aldosterone antagonist aldactone. Calculated fluid balances are by definition wrong, as they do not take into account the exudative losses through the burn wounds (about 0.5–1L/10% TBSA/day). The condition may be complicated by the used of fluidized or air beds, which cause an even greater loss of free water.

## Other organ function/dysfunction and support

### The nervous system

#### Brain, pain, analgesia and sedation

Neurological disturbances are commonly observed in burned patients. The possibility of cerebral edema and raised intracranial pressure must be considered during the early fluid resuscitation phase, especially in the case of associated brain injury or high voltage electrical injury. Several patho-physiological mechanisms are involved [10] including cerebral glucose metabolism alterations as shown in animal models [25, 108]. Inhalation of neurotoxic chemicals, of carbon monoxide, or hypoxic encephalopathy may adversely affect the central nervous system as well as arterial hypertension [10]. Other factors include hypo/hyper-natremia, hypovolemic shock, sepsis, antibiotic over-dosage (e. g., penicillin), and possible over-sedation or withdrawal effects of sedative drugs.

Pain and anxiety will generally require rather large doses of opioids and sedatives (benzodiazepines mainly). Continuous infusion regimens will generally be successful in maintaining pain within acceptable ranges. Sedatives and analgesics should be targeted to appropriate sedation and pain scales. Thus preventing the sequelae associated with over-sedation and opioid creep; namely fluid creep and affects on the central and peripheral cardiovascular system [96, 105]. Therefore, consideration should be given to the use of NMDA receptor antagonist, such as ketamine or gabapentine, who have important opioid sparing effects to decrease the need for opioids and benzodiazepines [85]. We find multi-modal pain management combining a long acting opioid for background pain, a short acting opioid for procedures, an anxiolytic, an NSAID, acetminophen, and gabapentin for neuropathic pain control [85] used at our institution targeted to SAS (sedation score) and VAS (visual analog scale) scores provide adequate analgesia and sedation.

### Intensive care unit-acquired weakness

While survival and main organ function (i. e. CNS) appears to be the focus in the intensive care units; we must not forget about long-term outcomes and specifically the peripheral nervous system and muscular system. Hence there needs to be discussion of one of the more important sequelae of critical illness: neuromyopathy.

The importance of positioning and prevention of peripheral nerve compression is well known and ingrained in the daily practices of most critical care units. In this section we will briefly discuss the risk factors for ICU acquired weakness and modalities for its prevention. The main risk factors include: multiple organ failure, muscular inactivity, hyperglycemia, use of corticosteroids and neuromuscular blockers. A recent publication by de Jonghe et al. [31] revealed that early identification and treatment of conditions leading to multiple organ failure, especially sepsis and septic shock; avoiding deep sedation and excessive hyperglycemia; as well cautious corticosteroid use; and promoting early mobilization might reduce the incidence and severity of ICU acquired weakness.

### Respiratory system and inhalation injury

The discussion of multiple modes of ventilation is beyond the scope of this section, for more extensive details on the topic please see the chapter on ventilation. In this section we do need to discuss the various modalities available for VAP (ventilation associated pneumonia) prevention, treatment of inhalation injury and ARDS.

## Ventilator associated pneumonia

The ABA guidelines for prevention, diagnosis, and treatment of ventilator-associated pneumonia (VAP) in burn patients were published in 2009 [69]. The guidelines are as follows:

► Mechanically ventilated burn patients are at high risk for developing VAP, with the presence of inhalation injury as a unique risk factor in this patient group.

► VAP prevention strategies should be used in mechanically ventilated burn patients.

► Clinical diagnosis of VAP can be challenging in mechanically ventilated burn patients where systemic inflammation and acute lung injury are prevalent. Therefore, a quantitative strategy, when available, is the preferable method to confirm the diagnosis of VAP.

► An 8-day course of targeted antibiotic therapy is generally sufficient to treat VAP; however, resistant *Staphylococcus aureus* and Gram-negative bacilli may require longer treatment duration.

► Any effort should be made to reduce length of intubation

## Inhalation injury

Inhalation injury is a significant confounder in burn injury increasing morbidity and mortality. There remains some controversy in the mode of ventilation used, however, we still need to establish diagnosis methodology and treatment modalities. The diagnosis ranges from history and physical findings, to bronchoscopic examination and serum marker measurements. Despite this variety there can be agreement that thermal injury associated with being in an enclosed space, loss of consciousness, and severe head and neck burns can have associated inhalation injury. The grading can be established by bronchoscopy but its relationship to possible mortality, length of ventilatory requirement, and need for tracheostomy remains unclear.

Asphyxiating gases such as carbon monoxide (CO), and cyanide (CN) are frequently associated with inhalation injury. The treatment for CO toxicity remains normobaric 100% $O_2$. The role of hyperbaric oxygen remains controversial, although both physiological data and some randomized-trial data suggest a potential benefit, in particular in terms of *reduction of c*ognitive sequelae: it has been included in the guidelines of the Undersea and Hyperbaric Medical Society [57, 104].

Cyanide toxicity associated with inhalation injury can be as result of burning of many household products, and it remains a diagnostic difficulty, as markers such as elevated blood lactate, elevated base deficit or metabolic acidosis used as evidence for cyanide poisoning in smoke or burn victims also represent under-resuscitation, coexisting traumatic injury, carbon monoxide poisoning or exposure to an oxygen-deficient atmosphere. Regardless, aggressive resuscitation and administration of 100% oxygen is indicated. The need for specific antidotes in cyanide poisoning is considered controversial in the U. S. [9, 19, 35], while it is widely accepted in Europe: intravenous hydroxocobalamine has become standard pre-hospital management in case of suspicion of cyanide poisoning [67] due to its improved safety profile for children and pregnant women [57, 90]. Aggressive supportive therapy aimed at the restoration of cardiovascular function augments the hepatic clearance of cyanide without specific antidotes and should be the first line of treatment. The role of cyanide poisoning in human smoke inhalation injury is undetermined, and lacks evidence.

Among other treatment modalities for inhalation injury $b_2$-agonist, nebulized heparin and NO but have not yet proven superiority. In an animal model treatment of inhalation injury with a $b_2$-agonist, albuterol, resulted in improved lung physiology by reducing pulmonary edema and lung vascular permeability to protein [73]. Although, these results are promising there's lack of evidence for its use in humans.

Inhalation injury results in airway obstructive casts, which are composed of mucus secretions, denuded airway epithelial cells, inflammatory cells, and fibrin [30]. The presence of fibrin solidifies the airway content forming the firm cast that is hard to remove by single cough or even by aggressive airway toilet. Therefore, prevention and/or dissolution of airway fibrin deposition is crucial in effective airway management. Nebulized heparin therapy has been demonstrated in animal and single-center studies to have potential efficacy in inhalation injury, particularly when combined with other anti-inflammatory agents and antithrombin [101].

Inhaled nitric oxide (NO) has been used as a therapeutic agent in pulmonary hypertension and to decrease intrapulmonary shunt [86]. Inhaled NO has been studied in animal models which have consistently shown reduction in pulmonary hypertension associated with inhalation injury, and variable reduction in shunting [91]. The studies in humans are small and limited, but invariably have shown improvement of PaO2/FiO2 ratio. There is no advantage in dosage above 20ppm. Given the current status of information available, the use of inhaled NO for inhalation injury should be restricted to patients that have failed conventional strategies with persistent refractory hypoxemia and PaO2/FiO2 ratios >80 [91].

## Renal failure and renal replacement therapy

Acute renal failure (ARF) is a major complication of burn injury. The incidence of ARF in burned patients has been reported to range from 1.2 to 20% and the incidence of ARF requiring renal replacement therapy (RRT) from 0.7 to 14.6% [70]. Although ARF is relatively rare, early diagnosis is important, as the mortality of burn patients with ARF has been reported from 50–100% [27, 44]. Applying the RIFLE classification to burn patients, Coca et al. found that the incidence of acute kidney injury was 27%, and it carried with it a mortality rate of 73% in the patients with the most severe acute kidney injury (requiring dialysis). Burn-related ARF can be divided into early and late ARF, depending on the time of onset with each having different etiologies [44]. Early ARF occurs during the first 5 days post-burn and its main causes are hypo-volemia, hypotonia and myoglobinuria. Prevention focuses on early aggressive fluid resuscitation and escharotomies or fasciotomies. Late ARF begins more than 5 days post-burn and is usually multi-factorial (generally caused by sepsis and/or nephrotoxic antibiotics) [44]. Regardless of the cause, there is mounting evidence that renal replacement therapy (RRT) should be instituted as early as possible in burn patients with renal dysfunction before the traditional criteria for RRT has been established [28]. Further to the discussion of RRT, is the choice in mode of delivery. CRRT (continuous renal replacement therapy) offers several potential advantages in the management of severe acute renal failure in burn patients. It is slow and continuous, consequently allowing for very efficient metabolic clearance and ultra-filtration of fluids, while minimizing hemodynamic compromise. Thus allowing for ongoing optimization of fluid and metabolic management [39]. There needs to be further studies to establish the triggers for instituting RRT in the burn patient with renal dysfunction followed by appropriate choice of modality (intermittent vs. continuous), dose and duration of therapy.

## Gastro-intestinal system

### GI complications/GI prophylaxis/enteral nutrition

The affect of thermal injury on the gastro-intestinal system was identified in 1970 with the description of Curling's ulcer [79]. Alterations in distribution of blood flow occur in the early post-burn period and are due to neurogenic and humoral release of catecholamines and prostanoids. During the initial hours, splanchnic blood flow is reduced, except for flow to the adrenals and to the liver. TXA$_2$ is likely to play a major role in gut dysfunction, promoting mesenteric vasoconstriction and decreasing gut blood flow. Poorly perfused organs shift towards anaerobic metabolism leading to acidosis. Aggressive fluid resuscitation restores perfusion to a great extent. But with over-enthusiastic fluid delivery, increasing intra-abdominal pressures and consequently abdominal compartment syndrome (ACS) becomes a matter of concern in both adult and pediatric burn patients [51, 71]. The Ivy index (250 ml/kg fluid resuscitation) is a cut-off value beyond which trouble is nearly certain. Abdominal pressures start rising, soon reaching the "gray zone" of 15–20 mmHg, and then the danger zone >20 mmHg, beyond which medical measures must be taken to reduce the IAP to avoid splanchnic organ ischemia. Figure 1 shows an example of progressive increase of intra-abdominal pressures associated with excessive fluid resuscitation in a young man with 95% TBSA burn resulting in a near arrest. Laparotomy is an extreme

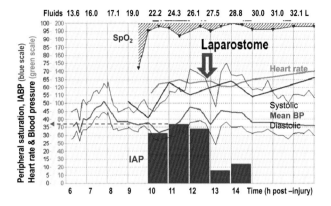

**Fig. 1.** Development of intra-abdominal hypertension (magenta bars) with pressure 37 mmHg 12 hours after injury in a young man burned 95% TBSA who had received 26.1 L of fluid resuscitation by that time (350 ml/kg in 12hrs). As a consequence several organ failures occur: cardiovascular (shock), respiratory (oxygenation) and renal (anuria) despite heavy vasopressor (norepinephrine) and inotropic (dobutamine) support

treatment tool, that indicates failure of medical management, or the combined presence of severe 3rd degree burns to the trunk and fluid resuscitation. IAP monitoring is essential for TBSA >30%.

Early enteral feeding should be initiated no later than 12 hours after injury. The benefits of this strategy are numerous: increasing blood flow to the splanchnic compartment before edema makes it impossible, maintaining pyloric function [84], maintaining intestinal motility, and reducing significantly infectious complications [63].

Indeed the gastrointestinal function, including the pyloric function, is depressed immediately after thermal injury. A true paralytic ileus will ensue for many days if the gastrointestinal tract is not used [84]. Opiates and sedatives, further depress the gastrointestinal function. Stress ulcer prophylaxis is mandatory (e.g. sucralfate, ranitidine or proton pump inhibitors), since the bleeding risk is elevated in burn injuries and may be life-threatening [79].

Due to the large doses of opioids and sedatives used during the early phase of treatment, constipation is frequent and may become critical with the development of ileus and intestinal obstruction by feces. Prevention should be initiated from admission using fiber containing enteral diets, lactulose (osmotic cathartic), and enemas when the other measures have failed.

Gut complications may be life threatening: in addition to the already mentioned ACS and constipation, the patients may develop Ogilvie syndrome, ischemic and non-ischemic bowel necrosis, and intestinal hemorrhage. A careful tight supervision of bowel function with daily examinations is therefore mandatory, particularly in perioperative periods with intra-operative hemorrhage leading to hypovolemia, which exposes the patient to gut hypo-perfusion and their threatened complications.

## Hepatic dysfunction

Severe burn injury causes numerous metabolic alterations, including hyper-glycemia, lipolysis, and protein catabolism [4]. These changes can induce multi-organ failure and sepsis leading to significant morbidity and mortality [21, 74]. Liver plays a significant role in mediating survival and recovery of burn patients, and preexisting liver disease is directly associated with adverse clinical outcomes following burn injury [53, 78, 102]. In the study by Price et al., they demonstrated that preexisting liver disease increased mortality risk from 6% to 27%, indicating that liver impairment worsens the prognosis in patients with thermal injury. Severe burn also directly induces hepatic dysfunction and damage, delaying recovery. More recently the work by Jeschke et al. [56] and Song et al. [93] has shed some light on the mechanism of the hepatic dysfunction following thermal injury, mainly by the up-regulation of the ER stress response, and increased cell death contributing to compromised hepatic function post-burn. Thus, one must not only be cognizant of the significant deleterious affects of hepatic dysfunction in the thermally injured patient as it has significant consequence in terms of multi-organ failure, morbidity and subsequent mortality of these patients; one can focus therapeutic modalities to alter this response and possibly improve outcome.

## Glucose control

There is no prospective adult trial addressing glucose management in major burns, but the retrospective studies suggest that toxic levels of hyperglycemia (>10 mmol/l) should be avoided and treated to prevent graft failure and infections (both increased with hyperglycemia) [41]. By contrast data are available in children: tight glucose control (90 to 120 mg/dl) has been shown to reduce infections and mortality [75]. Despite a demonstrated benefit of insulin administration on the maintenance of skeletal muscle mass, it is unknown if this effect translates to improved clinical outcomes in the thermally injured patient [8]. Optimal glycemic level remains uncertain: indeed feeding interruptions due to the procedures expose the patients to the risk of hypoglycemia. A good compromise is probably to opt for a glucose target 5–8 mmol/l (70–120 mg/dl) as in the majority of critically ill patients.

## Endocrine changes

### Stress response (Fig. 2)

In the post-burn state, pronounced hormonal and metabolic changes take place starting immediately after injury [7]. There is a tremendous increase in stress hormones after major burns, the increase being particularly marked during the first 2–3 weeks, but the alterations will persist for weeks and even months.

In response to the afferent stimuli from the burn wound, an intense sympatho-adrenal response is elicited. Catecholamine secretion contributes to arterial pressure maintenance, but also to a massive increase in cardiac after-load. The concentration of epinephrine and norepinephrine remains elevated for several days after injury and contributes to the integrated neuro-endocrine stress response.

Cortisol increases markedly, and the intensity of the response is modulated by optimization of pain control with good analgesia. However, the plasma value remains far above normal for at least 2 weeks. As with many other hormones, the circadian rhythm

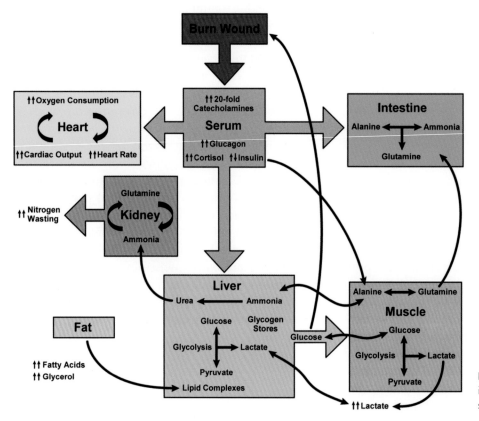

**Fig. 2.** Extensive organ involvement during the acute stress response

also changes. Aldosterone levels increase for several days. ACTH response frequently parallels the cortisol levels, and tends to be elevated for a few weeks. The increase in plasma rennin activity and aldosterone persist for several weeks.

Glucagon concentration is also increased after burn injury, contributing heavily to the hypermetabolic response, while insulin tends to remain within normal values, being paradoxically normal while plasma glucose concentration is elevated.

## Low T3 syndrome

The thyroid axis exhibits major abnormalities in the patients with major burns. The most constant finding is a "low T3 syndrome": TSH is generally normal, with low T3 levels, and T4 levels in the low-normal values, with elevated rT3 levels reflecting an altered de-iodination at the hepatic level. This activation step of thyroxin is under the control of a selenoenzyme, the 5-II de-iodinase: as the selenium status is strongly depressed in critically ill patients with an intense inflammatory response and even worse in those with negative selenium balances such as major burns and trauma patients, substitution of selenium is likely to improve the thyroid function. Indeed in critically ill trauma patients with a Low T3 syndrome, the alterations are improved by selenium supplementation with normalization of T3 levels [13]. The T3 and T4 concentrations are inversely related to the metabolic level.

## Gonadal depression

As a general rule, the gonadal axis is depressed in any patient with major burns. In men, post-burn changes in testosterone, 17β-estradiol are greater than in females, even during the first days. Plasma testosterone also decreases steeply in limited burn injury. The alterations last at least 4–5 weeks, but may persist for months in critically ill burned patients. The changes seem proportional to the severity of burns. A decreased pituitary stimulation causes lowered hormonal secretions from the testes. This change contributes to the low anabolic response and opens substitution perspectives. LH is more or less normal, LH-RH is decreased, FSH is low, and Prolactine is low to elevated.

In premenopausal females, amenorrhea is a nearly universal phenomenon, despite a near normal 17β-estradiol plasma concentration. Progesterone levels remains very low for many months after injury. Testosterone response is very different from that of males, with nearly normal concentrations in young females, and normal response to ACTH which elicits an increase in testosterone, while it decreases it men. Prolactine levels are also higher than seen in men.

In children, despite adequate nutritional support, severe thermal injury leads to decreased anabolic hormones over a prolonged period of time [52]. These changes contribute to stunting of growth observed after major burns. Female patients have significantly increased levels of anabolic hormones, which are associated with decreased pro-inflammatory mediators and hyper-metabolism, leading to a significantly shorter ICU length of stay compared with male patients

## Thermal regulation

Temperature regulation is altered with a "resetting" of the hypothalamic temperature above normal values. The teleological advantage of maintaining an elevated core temperature following burn injury is not fully understood. Major burns destroy the insulating properties of the skin, while the patients strive for a temperature of 38.0 to 38.5 °C [106]. Catecholamine production contributes to the changes in association with several cytokines, including interleukin-1 and interleukin-6. Any attempt to lower the basal temperature by external means will result in augmented heat loss, thus increasing metabolic rate.

Ambient temperature should be maintained between 28 and 33 °C to limit heat loss and the subsequent hyper-metabolic response [92]. Metabolic rate is increased as a consequence of several factors such as the catecholamine burst, the thermal effects of pro-inflammatory cytokines and evaporative losses from the wounds, which consumes energy, causing further heat loss. The evaporation causes extensive fluid losses from the wounds, approximating $4\,000\,ml/m^2/\%TBSA$ burns. Every liter of evaporated fluid corresponds to a caloric expenditure of about 600 kcal.

Finally, burned patients have frequent infections with febrile states, which may require additional free water delivery. On the other hand, extensively burned patients frequently experience hypothermia (defined as core temperature below 35°C) on admission, requiring active re-warming. Further surgery under general anesthesia, which inhibits the heat-conserving and heat-generating mechanisms, frequently results in hypothermia. Time to recover from hypothermia has been shown to be predictive of outcome in adults, with time to revert to normothermia being longer in non-survivors. Considering that hypothermia favors infections and delays wound healing, the maintenance of peri-operative normothermia is of utmost importance [33]. Tools include warming the ambient room temperature, intravenous fluid warming systems, and warming blankets.

Several centers use fluidized beds for the management of burns to the back, particularly during the 5–7 days following grafting, as it prevents maceration and dries the skin. The temperature of the bed is generally set at 38±0.5°C. However, this is contraindicated in the febrile patient, as it complicates fluid therapy due to largely unpredictable free water losses, and respiratory management due to the supine position. The patient may require additional 1–4 liters of free water per day (as D5W IV or enteral free water) to prevent dehydration. These additional requirements are difficult to assess in absence of bed-integrated weight scales. This further exposes the gut to dehydration with subsequent constipation.

## Metabolic modulation

A continued catabolic state results in weight loss, decrease in lean body mass, immunologic compromise, and poor or delayed wound healing with prolonged recovery times. Various efforts have been made to promote anabolism in the thermally injured patient.

### Propranolol

The massive catecholamine production associated with thermal injury heavily contributes to the intense catabolic response in major burn patients. The effects are through the intense stimulation of both alpha and beta receptors with subsequent cardiovascular, thermogenic and metabolic affects. Studies have shown that nonselective β-blockers efficiently reduce metabolic rate and protein catabolism, particularly in children and young adults, and to reduce the risk of liver steatosis [43, 68]. The metabolic advantages are observed with a 15–20% reduction of heart rate. The benefits are not as important in adults and elderly patients [4]. The limitations are the usual contraindications to b-blockade: early unstable resuscitation phase, incipient sepsis and asthmatic conditions. Treatment should be initiated as soon as resuscitation is completed (after 3–10 days depending on severity of burns), as it reduces the hypermetabolic response [20]. In adults starting doses are 10 mg 3×/day until achieving a 20% reduction in heart rate.

### Oxandrolone

Pharmacologic modulation of anabolism to counteract loss of lean body mass is beneficial in children with major burns [54]. Oxandrolone appears to be a promising anabolic agent although few outcome data are as yet available. A recent multicenter trial of early oxandralone administration in 81 patients seems promising [107]. Its use requires adaptation in case of renal failure and monitoring of liver function. The limited androgenic effects make its use possible in women.

### Recombinant human growth hormone

Recombinant human growth hormone (rhGH) therapy has been extensively investigated in GH-deficient children, where rhGH therapy improves nitrogen balance, increases body cell mass, and promotes bone formation [61]. These effects make rhGH a candidate for anabolism stimulation. Supplementation studies in burned pediatric patients have shown a decrease in donor-site healing times and length of hospital stay per %TBSA burns, and attenuation of hyper-metabolism and of inflammation particularly when used in combination with propranolol [55]. While safe in children, the use of rhGH in critically ill adult patients is not warranted, as it doubles mortality, mainly due to multiple organ dysfunction and septic shock [98].

## Insulin

Insulin is an anabolic hormone, promoting protein synthesis. High-dose intravenous glucose along with insulin has been shown to reduce the donor-site healing time of adolescent patients by 2 days [76]. However, recent data show that high loads of glucose promote de novo lipogenesis in the critically ill [100], questioning the rationale of providing large glucose along with insulin. In combination with data published several years ago, which reported increased liver fat deposits on postmortem evaluation in patients receiving large glucose loads [22], the de novo lipogenesis data indicate that using high glucose loads along with insulin should be restricted until further studies prove its safe use.

By actual knowledge total glucose administration (nutritional and delivered with drugs) should probably not exceed 6 g/kg BW/day, i. e. its maximal oxidation capacity.

## Electrolyte disorders

Burns is a condition where nearly any electrolyte abnormality can be observed. The causes for these disturbances are many and include fluid resuscitation with crystalloids, exudative and evaporative losses, impaired renal regulation, and responses to counter regulatory hormones.

## Sodium

During the first 24 hours, patients receive major amounts of sodium with their fluid resuscitation. Sodium accumulates in the interstitial space with edema. Despite this, hypernatremia occurring during the first 24 hours reflects under-resuscitation, and should be treated with additional fluid. Thereafter, mobilization of this fluid during the first weeks frequently results in hypernatremia and its resolution requires free water. Hypernatremia may also result from persistent evaporative losses from the wounds, particularly in case of treatment on a fluidized bed (contraindicated with severe hypernatremia) or in case of fever. Hypernatremia may also herald a septic episode.

## Chloride

During the early resuscitation and the surgical debridements of the burn wound, the patients tend to receive significant amounts of NaCl resulting in hyperchloremic acidosis [12]. The excess chloride is difficult to handle for the kidney, but the condition is generally resolves without further intervention.

## Calcium, phosphate and magnesium

Burns have high requirements for phosphate and magnesium in absence of renal failure. Those requirements start early, and are largely explained by 2 mechanisms: large exudative losses [11], and increased urinary excretion associated with acute protein catabolism and stress response.

Stimulation of sodium excretion is usually required and can usually be achieved by the simultaneous administration of free water (D5W IV or enteral water) along with furosemide with or without thiazide diuretics.

## Calcium

Total plasma calcium concentration consists of three fractions [23]: 15 % is bound to multiple anions (sulfate, phosphate, lactate, citrate), about 40 % is bound to albumin in a ratio of 0.2 mmol/L of calcium per 10 g/L of albumin, the remaining 45 % circulating as physiologically active ionized calcium. Calcium metabolism is tightly regulated. As albumin levels vary widely in burns and only ionized calcium is biologically active, only ionized calcium is a true indicator of status, as total plasma calcium determination is not a reliable indicator of calcium status: the use of conversion formula is unreliable:

$$[Ca]_{calculated} = Total\ [Ca]_{measured} + (0.2 \times (45 - [albumin]))$$

Hypocalcemia may occur during the early resuscitation phase, or in the context of massive peri-operative blood transfusion and requires intravenous supplementation using any form of available intravenous calcium formulation.

Hypercalcemia remains a poorly recognized cause of acute renal failure in patients with major burns that occurs as early as 3 weeks after injury [62]. The triad of hypercalcemia, arterial hypertension and acute renal failure is well known in other critical illnesses [40, 77], while the association of hypercalcemia and renal failure in patients with major burns is much less reported in the literature. In a recent retrospective study, hypercalcemia was shown to occur in 19% of the burned patients with hospital lengths of stay of more than 28 days, and was noted to be associated with an increased mortality [88].

In our own setting, 30% of patients developed hypercalcemia: median time to the first hypercalcemia value was 21 days [88]. Hypercalcemia may also occur in patients with smaller burns requiring a stay of more than 20 days in the ICU. Ionized calcium determination enabled earlier detection, while using total calcium determination 'with albumin correction' was only slightly sensitive, as shown by normal corrected values in 15 cases with ionized hypercalcemia.

Treatment of hypercalcemia includes hydration, volume expansion and early mobilization. As most causes of severe hypercalcemia depend on increased osteoclast activation, drugs that decrease bone turnover are effective [50]. The treatment of choice in cases that do not resolve with the simple measures relies on the bisphosphonates, pamidronate disodium and zoledronic acid, which are available in intravenous forms [37]. In burned children, acute intravenous pamidronate administration has been shown to help to preserve bone mass [60], achieving a sustained therapeutic effect on bone [81]. An alternative treatment of the latter in burns includes anabolic agents such as oxandrolone [61]. The bisphosphonates have been advocated in the prevention of heterotrophic ossification, a complication that occurs in 1.2% of burn patients.

## Bone demineralization and osteoporosis

Due to the substantial alterations of calcium and phosphorus metabolism and bone formation is reduced both in adults and children when burns exceed 40% TBSA. Bone mineral density is significantly lower in burned children compared with the same age normal children. Girls have improved bone mineral content and percent fat compared with boys [52]. The consequences are increased risk of fractures, decreased growth velocity and stunting [11]. The bone is affected by various means: alteration of mineral metabolism, elevated cytokine and corticosteroid levels, decreased growth hormone (GH), nutritional deficiencies, and intra-operative immobilization. Cytokines contribute to the alterations, particularly interleukin-1(and interleukin-6, both of which are greatly increased in burns and stimulate osteoblast-mediated bone resorption. The increased cortisol production in thermal injury, leads to decreased bone formation, and the low GH levels fail to promote bone formation [59], further exacerbating the situation. Various studies suggest that immobilization plays a significant role in the pathogenesis of burn-associated bone disease [58]. Alterations of magnesium and calcium homeostasis constitute another cause. Hypocalcemia and hypomagnesemia are constant findings, and ionized calcium levels remain low for weeks [97]. The alterations are partly explained by large exudative magnesium and phosphorus losses [11] A close monitoring of ionized calcium, magnesium, and inorganic phosphate levels is mandatory, since burn patients usually require substantial supplementation by intravenous or enteral routes.

## Micronutrients and antioxidants

Critically ill burned patients are characterized by a strong oxidative stress, an intense inflammatory response, and a hyper-metabolic state that can last months. Trace element (TE) deficiencies have repeatedly been described. The complications observed in major burns such as infections and delayed wound healing, can be partly attributed to TE deficiencies [16]. Plasma TE concentrations are low as a result of TE losses in biological fluids, low intakes, dilution by fluid resuscitation, and redistribution from plasma to tissues mediated by the inflammatory response. The large exudative losses cause negative TE balances. Intravenous supplementation trials show that early substitution improves recovery (IV doses: Cu 3.5 mg/d, Se 400–500 mcg/d, Zn 40 mg/d), reduces infectious complications (particularly nosocomial pneumonia) [14], normalize thyroid function, improve wound healing and shorten hospital length of stay [16]. The mechanisms underlying these improvements are a combination of antioxidant effects (particularly of selenium through restoration of glutathione peroxidase activity), but also immune (Cu, Se, Zn) and anabolic effects (Zn particularly).

High vitamin C requirements after major burns were identified already in the 40s, and have been confirmed since. Very interesting studies by Dubick et al. [34] and Tanaka et al. [99] have demonstrated that high doses of vitamin C administered during the first 24 hours after a major injury reduced the capillary leak, probably through antioxidant mechanisms, resulting in significant reductions in fluid resuscitation requirements. This has not yet become standard of clinical practice, but might do so in the coming years.

## Thrombosis prophylaxis

Hematological alterations observed after burns are complex and can last for several months and can be summarized as follows:

▶ uring the early phase after burns, fibrin split products increase.
▶ Dilution and consumption explain the early low PT values.
▶ The coagulation cascade is activated.
▶ Fibrin, factors V and VIII increase as part of acute phase response.
▶ Antithrombin deficiency is frequent [64, 72].
▶ Thrombocytosis develops when wounds are closing.

The risk of deep venous thrombosis and of pulmonary embolism is at least as high as in any other surgical condition [38]. In our CHUV experience, 13% of patients develop some form of thrombotic complication. Specific risk factors include central venous lines, prolonged bed-rest and an intense inflammatory state. Prophylaxis should be started from admission. Interruptions for surgery should be reduced to minimum and discussed with the surgical team.

## Conclusion

The critical care of the thermally injured patient, is complex and challenging for all involved. The result are however rather rewarding. The field has evolved tremendously over the last few decades and will continue to improve in-order to provide these challenging patients with the best care possible. Many questions remain in the etiology and thus treatment of these patients. Many of these can only be answered by the ongoing research in the field. This brief chapter highlights some of the important aspects of the care, and serves simply as a guide to the care of these patients.

## References

[1]  Agay D, Sandre C, Ducros V et al (2005) Optimization of selenium status by a single intra-peritoneal injection of Se in Se deficient rat: possible application to burned patient treatment. Free Rad Biol Med 39(6): 762–768
[2]  Alderson P, Bunn F, Lefebvre C et al (2004) Human albumin solution for resuscitation and volume expansion in critically ill patients. Cochrane Database Syst Rev 2004(4):CD001 208
[3]  Alvarado R, Chung KK, Cancio LC et al (2009) Burn resuscitation. Burns 35(1): 4–14
[4]  Arbabi S, Ahrns KS, Wahl WL et al (2004) Beta-blocker use is associated with improved outcomes in adult burn patients. J Trauma 56(2): 265–269; discussion 269–271
[5]  Arlati S, Storti E, Pradella V et al (2007) Decreased fluid volume to reduce organ damage: a new approach to burn shock resuscitation? A preliminary study. Resuscitation 72(3): 371–378
[6]  Arturson G, Jakobsson OP (1985) Oedema measurements in a standard burn model. Burns 12: 1–7
[7]  Arturson G, Bode G, Brizio-Molteni L et al (1990) Endocrinology of thermal trauma. Lea & Febiger, London
[8]  Ballian N, Rabiee A, Andersen DK et al (2010) Glucose metabolism in burn patients: The role of insulin and other endocrine hormones. Burns;e-pub:Jan 12
[9]  Barillo DJ, Goode R, Esch V (1994) Cyanide poisoning in victims of fire: analysis of 364 cases and review of the literature. J Burn Care Rehabil 15: 46–57
[10]  Belmonte Torras JA, Marin de la Cruz D, Sune Garcia JM et al (2006) [Burns produced by lighters]. An Pediatr (Barc) 64(5): 468–473
[11]  Berger MM, Rothen C, Cavadini C et al (1997) Exudative mineral losses after serious burns: A clue to the alterations of magnesium and phosphate metabolism. Am J Clin Nutr 65: 1473–1481

[12] Berger MM, Pictet A, Revelly JP et al (2000) Impact of a bicarbonated saline solution on early resuscitation after major burns. Intensive Care Med 26(9): 1382–1385

[13] Berger MM, Reymond MJ, Shenkin A et al (2001) Influence of selenium supplements on the post-traumatic alterations of the thyroid axis – a prospective placebo controlled trial. Intensive Care Med 27: 91–100

[14] Berger MM (2006) Acute copper and zinc deficiency due to exudative losses – substitution versus nutritional requirements. Burns 32: 393

[15] Berger MM, Eggimann P, Heyland DK et al (2006) Reduction of nosocomial pneumonia after major burns by trace element supplementation: aggregation of two randomised trials. Crit Care 10:R153:e-pub 2 Nov

[16] Berger MM, Shenkin A (2007) Trace element requirements in critically ill burned patients. J Trace Elem Med Biol 21 [Suppl 1]: $24–48

[17] Berger MM, Baines M, Raffoul W et al (2007) Trace element supplements after major burns modulate antioxidant status and clinical course by way of increased tissue trace element concentration. Am J Clin Nutr 85: 1293–1300

[18] Berger MM, Davadant M, Marin C et al (2010) Impact of a pain protocol including hypnosis in major burns. Burns 36(5): 639–646

[19] Borron SW, Baud FJ, Megarbane B, Chantal B (2007) Hydroxocobalamin for severe acute cyanide poisoning by ingestion or inhalation. Am J Emerg Med 25: 551–8

[20] Breitenstein E, Chioléro RL, Jéquier E et al (1990) Effects of beta-blockade on energy metabolism following burns. Burns 16: 259–264

[21] Brusselaers N, Monstrey SJ, Vandijck DM, Blot SI (2007) Prediction of morbidity and mortality on admission to a burn unit. Plast Reconstr Surg 120: 360–1; author reply 361

[22] Burke JF, Wolfe RR, Mullany CJ et al (1979) Glucose requirements following burn injury. Ann Surg 190: 274–285

[23] Bushinsky DA, Monk RD (1998) Electrolyte quintet: Calcium. Lancet 352(9124): 306–311

[24] Carlson DL, Horton JW (2006) Cardiac molecular signaling after burn trauma. J Burn Care Res 27(5): 669–675

[25] Carter EA, Tompkins RG, Babich JW et al (1996) Decreased cerebral glucose utilization in rats during the ebb phase of thermal injury. J Trauma 40(6): 930–935

[26] Cheatham ML, Malbrain ML, Kirkpatrick A et al (2007) Results from the International Conference of Experts on Intra-abdominal Hypertension and Abdominal Compartment Syndrome. II. Recommendations. Intensive Care Med 33(6): 951–962

[27] Chrysopoulos MT, Jeschke MG, Dziewulski P et al (1999) Acute renal dysfunction in severely burned adults. J Trauma 46: 141–144

[28] Chung KK, Juncos LA, Wolf SE et al (2008) Continuous Renal Replacement Therapy Improves Survival in Severely Burned Military Casualties With Acute Kidney Injury. J Trauma 64:S179 –S187

[29] Coca SG, Bauling P, Schifftner T et al (2007) Contribution of acute kidney injury toward morbidity and mortality in burns: a contemporary analysis. Am J Kidney Dis 49: 517–523

[30] Cox RA, Burke AS, Soejima K et al (2003) Airway obstruction in sheep with burn and smoke inhalation injuries. Am J Respir Cell Mol Biol 29: 295–302

[31] de Jonghe B, Lacherade JC, Sharshar T, Outin H (2009) Intensive care unit-acquired weakness: Risk factors and Prevention. Crit Care Med 37(10)[Suppl]: S309-S315

[32] Ding HQ, Zhou BJ, Liu L et al (2002) Oxidative stress and metallothionein expression in the liver of rats with severe thermal injury. Burns 28: 215–221

[33] Donner B, Tryba M, Kurz-Muller K et al (1996) [Anesthesia and intensive care management of severely burned children of Jehovah's Witnesses]. Anaesthesist 45(2): 171–517

[34] Dubick MA, Williams C, Elgjo GI et al (2005) High-dose vitamin C infusion reduces fluid requirements in the resuscitation of burn-injured sheep. Shock 24(2): 139–144

[35] Erdman AR (2007) Is hydroxocobalamin safe and effective for smoke inhalation? Searching for guidance in the haze. Ann Emerg Med 49: 814–816

[36] Etherington L, Saffle J, Cochran A (2009) Use of transesophageal echocardiography in burns:a retrospective review. J Burn Care Res 31(1): 36–39

[37] Evans RA, Lawrence PJ, Thanakrishnan G et al (1986) Immobilization hypercalcaemia due to low bone formation and responding to intravenous sodium sulphate. Postgrad Med J 62(727): 395–398

[38] Fecher AM, O'Mara MS, Goldfarb IW et al (2004) Analysis of deep vein thrombosis in burn patients. Burns 30(6): 591–593

[39] Forni JG, Hilton PJ (1997) Continuous hemofiltration in the treatment of acute renal failure. N Engl J Med 336: 1303–1309

[40] Forster J, Querusio L, Burchard KW et al (1985) Hypercalcemia in critically ill surgical patients. Ann Surg 202: 512–518

[41] Gore DC, Chinkes D, Heggers J et al (2001) Association of hyperglycemia with increased mortality after severe burn injury. J Trauma 51(3): 540–544

[42] Herndon DN, Hart DW, Wolf SE, Chinkes DL, Wolfe RR (2001) Reversal of catabolism by beta-blockade after severe burns. N Engl J Med 345: 1223–1229

[43] Herndon DN, Wolf SE, Chinkes DL et al (2001) Reversal of catabolism by beta-blockade after severe burns. N Engl J Med 345: 1223–1229

[44] Holm C, Horbrand F, von Donnersmarck GH et al (1999) Acute renal failure in severely burned patients. Burns 25: 171–178

[45] Holm C, Melcer B, Hörbrand F et al (2000) Intrathoracic blood volume as an endpoint in resuscitation of the severely burned: an observational study of 24 patients. J Trauma 48: 728–734

[46] Holm C, Mayr M, Tegeler J et al (2004) A clinical randomized study on the effects of invasive monitoring on burn shock resuscitation. Burns 30(8): 798–807

[47] Horton JW, Garcia NM, White DJ et al (1995) Postburn cardiac contractile function and biochemical markers of postburn cardiac surgery. J Am Coll Surg 181: 289–298

[48] Horton JW, White DJ, Maass DL et al (2001) Antioxidant vitamin therapy alters burn trauma-mediated cardiac NF-kappaB activation and cardiomyocyte cytokine secretion. J Trauma 50(3): 397–406

[49] Huang PP, Stucky FS, Dimick AR et al (1995) Hypertonic sodium resuscitation is associated with renal failure and death. Ann Surg 221: 543–557

[50] Inzucchi SE (2004) Management of hypercalcemia: diagnostic workup, therapeutic options for hyperparathyroidism and their common causes. Postgrad Med J 115(5): 27–36

[51] Ivy ME, Atweh NA, Palmer J et al (2000) Intra-abdominal hypertension and abdominal compartment syndrome in burn patients. J Trauma 49: 387–391

[52] Jeschke MG, Barrow RE, Mlcak RP et al (2005) Endogenous anabolic hormones and hypermetabolism: effect of trauma and gender differences. Ann Surg 241(5): 759–767

[53] Jeschke MG, Micak RP, Finnerty CC, Herndon DN (2007) Changes in liver function and size after a severe thermal injury. Shock 28: 172–177

[54] Jeschke MG, Finnerty CC, Suman OE et al (2007) The effect of oxandrolone on the endocrinologic, inflammatory, and hypermetabolic responses during the acute phase postburn. Ann Surg 246(3): 351–360; discussion 360–352

[55] Jeschke MG, Finnerty CC, Kulp GA et al (2008) Combination of recombinant human growth hormone and propranolol decreases hypermetabolism and inflammation in severely burned children. Pediatr Crit Care Med 9(2): 209–216

[56] Jeschke MG, Gauglitz GG, Song J, MD et al (2009) Calcium and ER Stress Mediate Hepatic Apoptosis after Burn Injury. J Cell Mol Med 13(8B):1857–1865

[57] Kealey GP (2009) Effects/Treatment of Toxic Gases. J Burn Care Res 30(1): 146–155

[58] Klein GL, Kikuchi Y, Sherrard DJ et al (1996) Burn-associated bone disease in sheep: roles of immobilization and endogenous corticosteroids. J Burn Care Rehabil 17: 518–521

[59] Klein GL, Wolf SE, Langman CB et al (1998) Effect of therapy with recombinant human growth hormone on insulin-like growth factor system components and serum levels of biochemical markers of bone formation in children after severe burn injury. J Clin Endocrinol Metab 83: 21–24

[60] Klein GL, Wimalawansa SJ, Kulkarni G et al (2005) The efficacy of acute administration of pamidronate on the conservation of bone mass following severe burn injury in children: a double-blind, randomized, controlled study. Osteoporos Int 16(6): 631–635

[61] Klein GL (2006) Burn-induced bone loss: importance, mechanisms, and management. J Burns Wounds 5:e5

[62] Kohut B, Rossat J, Raffoul W et al (2009) Hypercalcaemia and acute renal failure after major burns: An under-diagnosed condition. Burns 34(3): 360–366

[63] Lam NN, Tien NG, Khoa CM (2008) Early enteral feeding for burned patients: an effective method which should be encouraged in developing countries. Burns 34(2): 192–196

[64] Lavrentieva A, Kontakiotis T, Bitzani M et al (2008) Early coagulation disorders after severe burn injury: impact on mortality. Intensive Care Med 34(4): 700–706

[65] Lund T, Onarheim H, Reed RK (1992) Pathogenesis of edema formation in burn injuries. World J Surg 16: 2–9

[66] Marano MA, Fong Y, Moldawer LL et al (1990) Serum cachectin: tumor necrosis factor in critically ill patients with burns correlates with infection and mortality. Surg Gynecol Obstet 170: 32–38

[67] Mégarbane B, Delahaye A, Goldgran-Toledano D, Baud FJ (2003) Antidotal treatment of cyanide poisoning. J Chin Med Assoc 66: 193–203

[68] Morio B, Irtun O, Herndon DN et al (2002) Propranolol decreases splanchnic triacylglycerol storage in burn patients receiving a high-carbohydrate diet. Ann Surg 236(2): 218–225

[69] Mosier MJ, Pham TN (2009) American Burn Association Practice guidelines for prevention, diagnosis, and treatment of ventilator-associated pneumonia (VAP) in burn patients. J Burn Care Res 30(6): 910–928.

[70] Mustonen KM, Vuola J (2008) Acute Renal Failure in Intensive Care Burn Patients (ARF in Burn Patients). J Burn Care Res 29: 227–237.

[71] Namias N (2007) Advances in burn care. Curr Opin Crit Care 13(4): 405–410

[72] Niedermayr M, Schramm W, Kamolz L et al (2007) Antithrombin deficiency and its relationship to severe burns. Burns 33(2): 173–178

[73] Palmieri T, Enkhbaatar P, Bayliss R et al (2006) Continuous nebulized albuterol attenuates acute lung injury in an ovine model of combined burn and smoke inhalation. Crit Care Med 34: 1719–1724

[74] Pereira C, Murphy K, Herndon D (2004) Outcome measures in burn care: is mortality dead? Burns 30: 761–771

[75] Pham TN, Warren AJ, Phan HH et al (2005) Impact of tight glycemic control in severely burned children. J Trauma 59(5): 1148–1154

[76] Pierre EJ, Barrow RE, Hawkins HK et al (1998) Effects of insulin on wound healing. J Trauma 44: 342–345

[77] Popp M, Friedberg D, McMillan B (1980) Clinical characteristics of hypertension in burned children. Ann Surg 191: 473–478

[78] Price LA, Thombs B, Chen CL, Milner SM (2007) Liver disease in burn injury: evidence from a national sample of 31,338 adult patients. J Burns Wounds 7: e1

[79] Pruitt BA Jr, Foley F D, Moncrief J A (1970) Curling's ulcer: a clinical-pathology study of 323 cases. Ann Surg 172: 523–539

[80] Pruitt BA Jr (2000) Protection from excessive resuscitation: "pushing the pendulum back". J Trauma 49: 567–568

[81] Przkora R, Herndon DN, Sherrard DJ et al (2007) Pamidronate preserves bone mass for at least 2 years following acute administration for pediatric burn injury. Bone 41(2): 297–302

[82] Rainville P, Bao QV, Chretien P (2005) Pain-related emotions modulate experimental pain perception and autonomic responses. Pain 118(3): 306–318

[83] Rainville P (2008) Hypnosis and the analgesic effect of suggestions. Pain 134(1–2): 1–2

[84] Raff T, Hartmann B, Germann G (1997) Early intragastric feeding of seriously burned and long-term ventilated patients: a review of 55 patients. Burns 23: 19–25

[85] Richardson P, Mustard L (2009) The management of pain in the burns unit. Burns 35(7): 921–936

[86] Rossaint R, Falke KJ, Lopez F, Slama K, Pison U, Zapol WM (1993) Inhaled nitric oxide for the adult respiratory distress syndrome. N Engl J Med 328: 399–405

[87] Saffle JR (2007) The phenomenon of "fluid creep" in acute burn resuscitation. J Burn Care Res 28 (May/june):382–395

[88] Sam R, Vaseemuddin M, Siddique A et al (2007) Hypercalcemia in patients in the burn intensive care unit. J Burn Care Res 28: 742–746

[89] Shankar R, Melstrom KA Jr, Gamelli RL (2007) Inflammation and sepsis: past, present, and the future. J Burn Care Res 28(4): 566–571

[90] Shepherd G, Velez LI (2008) Role of hydroxocobalamin in acute cyanide poisoning. Ann Pharmacother 42: 661–669

[91] Sheridan RL (2009) Inhaled nitric oxide in inhalation injury. J Burn Care Res 30(1): 162–163

[92] Shiozaki T, Kishikawa M, Hiraide A et al (1993) Recovery from postoperative hypothermia predicts survival in extensively burned patients. Am J Surg 165: 326–330

[93] Song J, Finnerty CC, Herndon DN, Boehning D, Jeschke MG (2009) Severe burn–induced endoplasmic reticulum stress and hepatic damage in mice. Mol Med 15(9–10): 316–320

[94] Sparkes BG (1997) Immunological responses to thermal injury. Burns 23: 106–113

[95] Stucki P, Perez MH, Cotting J, Shenkin A, Berger MM (2010) Substitution of exudative trace elements losses in burned children. Critical Care 14: 439

[96] Sullivan SR, Friedrich JB, Engrav LH, Round KA, Heimbach DM, Heckbert SR, Carrougher GJ, Lezotte DC, Wiechman SA, Honari S, Klein MB, Gibran NS (2004) "Opioid creep" is real and may be the cause of "fluid creep". Burns 30(6): 583–90

[97] Szyfelbein SK, Drop LJ, Martyn JAJ (1981) Persistent ionized hypocalcemia in patients during resuscitation and recovery phases of body burns. Crit Care Med 9: 454–458

[98] Takala J, Ruokonen E, Webster NR et al (1999) Increased mortality associated with growth hormone treatment in critically ill adults. N Engl J Med 341: 785–792

[99] Tanaka H, Matsuda T, Miyagantani Y et al (2000) Reduction of resuscitation fluid volumes in severely burned patients using ascorbic acid administration. Arch Surg 135: 326–331

[100] Tappy L, Schwarz JM, Schneiter P et al (1998) Effects of isoenergetic glucose-based or lipid-based parenteral nutrition on glucose metabolism, de novo lipogenesis, and respiratory gas exchanges in critically ill patients. Crit Care Med 26: 860–867

[101] Tasaki O, Mozingo DW, Dubick MA, Goodwin CW, Yantis LD, Pruitt BA Jr (2002) Effects of heparin and lisofylline on pulmonary function after smoke inhalation injury in an ovine model. Crit Care Med 30: 637–43

[102] Thomas S, Wolf SE, Chinkes DL, Herndon DN (2004) Recovery from the hepatic acute phase response in the severely burned and the effects of long-term growth hormone treatment. Burns 30: 675–9

[103] Warden GD (1996) Fluid resuscitation and early management. In: Herndon D (ed) Total burns care. Saunders, London, pp 53–60

[104] Weaver LK (2009) Clinical practice. Carbon monoxide poisoning. N Engl J Med 360: 1217–1225

[105] Wibbenmeyer L, Sevier A, Liao J, Williams I, Light T, Latenser B, Lewis R 2nd, Kealey P, Rosenquist R (2010) The impact of opioid administration on resuscitation volumes in thermally injured patients. J Burn Care Res 31(1): 48–56

[106] Wolf SE, Debroy M, Herndon DN (1997) The cornerstones and directions of pediatric burn care. Pediatric Surgery International 12: 312–320

[107] Wolf SE, Edelman LS, Kemalyan N et al (2006) Effects of oxandrolone on outcome measures in the severely burned: a multicenter prospective randomized double-blind trial. J Burn Care Rehab 27(2): 131–139; discussion 140–141

[108] Zhang Q, Carter EA, Ma B et al (2008) Burn-related metabolic and signaling changes in rat brain. J Burn Care Res 29(2): 346–352

Correspondence: Mette M. Berger, Adult ICU and Burn Unit, CHUV, BH D8.612, 1011 Lausanne, Switzerland, E-mail: Mette.Berger@chuv.ch

# Treatment of infection in burns

Gerd G. Gauglitz[1], Shahriar Shahrokhi[2], Marc G. Jeschke[2]

[1] Department of Dermatology and Allergy, Ludwig Maximilian University, Munich, Germany
[2] Ross Tilley Burn Centre, Sunnybrook Health Sciences Centre, Department of Surgery, Division of Plastic Surgery, University of Toronto, ON, Canada

## Introduction

Infections remain a leading cause of death in burn patients. For patients with burn size greater than 40% TBSA, 75% of all deaths are due to infection [1]. Many features unique to burn patients make diagnosis and management of infection especially difficult. Burn injury represents the most extreme endpoint along the spectrum of traumatic injury and as such is associated with profound alterations in host defense mechanisms and immune function. These derangements predispose thermally injured patients to local and systemic invasion by microbial pathogens.

The burn wound represents a susceptible site for opportunistic colonization by organisms of endogenous and exogenous origin. A broad variety of patient factors such as age, immunosuppressed status, extent of injury, and depth of burn in combination with microbial factors such as type and number of organisms, enzyme and toxin production and motility determine the likelihood of invasive burn wound infection. Burn wound infections can be classified on the basis of the causative organism, the depth of invasion, and the tissue response. Diagnostic procedures and therapy must be based on an understanding of the pathophysiology of the burn wound and the pathogenesis of the various forms of burn wound infection.

The purpose of this chapter is to depict the diagnosis and management of burn wound infections, helping to provide the burn surgeon with a clinical guide to assist in clinical judgment.

## Clinical management strategies

Many of the clinical signs and symptoms used to diagnose infection in other settings are unreliable in the burn intensive care unit since they are often present even in the absence of true underlying infection. Advances in critical care such as earlier resuscitation and support of the hypermetabolic response have decreased burn mortality, but infections are still pervasive in severely burned patients and account for significant morbidity and mortality.

With regards to burn wound infection, the cornerstone of management continues to be aggressive early debridement of devitalized and infected tissue. Unfortunately, burn patients are rapidly colonized by nosocomial pathogens and foci of invasive infection must be identified and treated quickly with appropriate antimicrobial therapy. Additionally, other potential foci for invasive infection include the tracheobronchial tree, the lungs, the gastrointestinal tract, central venous catheters and the urinary tract. Once an infection is disseminated hematogenously and becomes established in a burn patient, it is very difficult to eradicate, even with large does of broad-spectrum antimicrobial therapy. Traditional thinking would argue for beginning broad-spectrum coverage at the first signs of infection and then narrowing the coverage as results of cultures come back. While this is clearly true for many critical ill patients, burn represents a unique situation, which may merit more aggressive management. New emerging strains of multiresitant organisms represent an ominous threat in the burn unit and monotherapy with conventional antimicrobials may be inadequate for some infections.

Time-related changes in the predominant flora of the burn wound from gram-positive to gram-negative recapitulate the history of burn wound infection. Treatment with two or more agents is becoming necessary in the management of these gram-negative invasive infections. Selection and dissemination of intrinsic and acquired resistance mechanisms increase the probability of burn wound colonization by resistant species such as *Pseudomonas aeruginosa*. Even so, effective topical antimicrobial therapy and early burn wound excision have significantly reduced the overall occurrence of invasive burn wound infections, individual patients, usually those with extensive burns in whom wound closure is difficult to achieve, may still develop a variety of bacterial and nonbacterial burn wound infections. Consequently, the entirety of the burn wound must be examined on a daily basis by the attending surgeon. Any change in wound appearance, with or without associated clinical changes, should be evaluated by biopsy. Quantitative cultures of the biopsy sample may identify predominant organisms but are not useful for making the diagnosis of invasive burn wound infection. Histologic examination of the biopsy specimen, which permits staging the invasive process, is the only reliable means of differentiating wound colonization from invasive infection. Identification of the histologic changes characteristic of bacterial, fungal, and viral infections facilitates the selection of appropriate therapy. A diagnosis of invasive burn wound infection necessitates change of both local and systemic therapy and, in the case of bacterial and fungal infections, prompt surgical removal of the infected tissue. Even after the wounds of extensively burned patients have healed or been grafted, burn wound impetigo, commonly caused by *Staphylococcus aureus*, may occur in the form of multifocal, small superficial abscesses that require surgical debridement. Current techniques of burn wound care have significantly reduced the incidence of invasive burn wound infection, altered the organisms causing the infections that do occur, increased the interval between injury and the onset of infection, reduced the mortality associated with infection, decreased the overall incidence of infection in burn patients, and increased burn patient survival.

## Pathophysiology of the burn wound

Thermal injury is associated with a state of generalized immunosuppression which is characterized by an impairment of host defense mechanisms and defects in humoral and cell-mediated immunity. There are several specific alterations in host defense which are intrinsic to the burn injury itself and which predispose these patients to microbial invasion. The most important intrinsic factor is breach of the mechanical barrier provided by the skin. The primary injury in burns results in irreversible tissue necrosis at the center of the burn due to exposure to heat, chemicals, or electricity. The extent of this injury is dependent on the temperature (or concentration) and the duration of exposure as well as the vascular supply and thickness of the injured skin [2].

A burn wound is characterized by three zones: a central zone of necrosis surrounded by a zone of ischemia and a third peripheral zone of hyperemia characterized by a reversible increase in blood flow [3].

While there is normal resident skin flora, invasive infection is rare through an intact epithelial barrier. The skin has bacteriostatic properties that normally limit the degree of colonization. The local microenvironment is not supportive for growth of microbial pathogens. This changes drastically with a severe burn trauma. The burn wound provides a warm and moist microenvironment in which bacterial proliferation is fostered. Microbial growth is rapid as once non-pathogenic organisms are now allowed to flourish. It is imperative to realize that the most important intrinsic factor is breach of the mechanical skin barrier, since this has implications for the overall approach to infection control. It is the fundamental and primary defect. Antimicrobial therapy and wound care can be viewed as temporizing measures to stave off infection until the primary defect is repaired.

In addition to these alterations in host defense, there are specific defects in humoral and cell-mediated immunity that occur following severe burn trauma, including impaired function of natural killer cells. The generalized immunosuppression is further characterized by specific alterations in B and T cell function.

## Diagnosis and management of specific infections

### Burn wound infection

The diagnosis and treatment of burn wound infection is based on early identification of an infected wound site. Clinically, burn wound infection is most often recognized based on gross appearance or conversion of a partial thickness to a full thickness wound. Most common local sign of invasive burn wound infection is the appearance of focal, multi-focal, or generalized dark brown, black, or violaceous discoloration of the wound [4]. The most reliable local sign is conversion of an area of partial thickness injury to full-thickness necrosis or the necrosis of previously viable tissue in an excised wound bed. Other signs of invasive burn wound infection include hemorrhagic discoloration of sub-eschar tissue, the presence of green pigment (pyocyanin) in subcutaneous fat, edema or violaceous discoloration of unburned skin (or both) at the margin of the burn, and the presence of initially erythematous and later black necrotic nodular lesions (ecthyma gangrenosa) in unburned skin. Local signs characteristic of burn wound infections caused by fungi include unexpectedly rapid separation of the eschar, presumably due to fat liquefaction, and rapid centrifugal spread of subcutaneous edema with central ischemic necrosis [5]. Vesicular lesions in healing or healed second degree burns and the presence of crusted serrated margins of partial-thickness burns of the face, particularly those involving the naso-labial area are characteristic of burn wound infections caused by herpes simplex virus type 1 (HSV-1)[6]. Once there is clinical suspicion of invasive burn wound sepsis, it is imperative to obtain quantitative wound cultures. Surface cultures are useful for identifying the organisms present on the burn wound and the predominant members of the burn wound flora, but even quantitative cultures are incapable of differentiating burn wound colonization from burn wound infection. Generally, a low quantitative bacterial count is a good indication that a burn wound infection is not present and wound cultures growing organisms at a quantitative count of greater than $1 \times 10^5$ organisms/gram of tissue are considered indicative of a wound at significant risk for invasive sepsis [7]. Thus, due to the limitations of cultures, the histologic examination of a burn wound biopsy is the most reliable and expeditious means of confirming a diagnosis of invasive burn wound infection. The most common pathogens include MSSA and MRSA species and *Pseudomonas aeruginosa*.

In the case of viral burn wound infections, the diagnosis may also be confirmed by histologic examination of scrapings from the cutaneous lesions. The specific histologic sign of burn wound infection is the presence of microorganisms in unburned tissue. Other histologic findings indicative of burn wound infection are the presence of hemorrhage in unburned tissue, small-vessel thrombosis and ischemic necrosis of unburned tissue, marked inflammatory changes in unburned tissue, dense bacterial growth in the sub-eschar space (a site of microbial proliferation prior to invasion), and intracellular viral inclusions (type A Cowdry bodies) typical for HSV-1 infections.

Generally, maintaining wounds at low contamination levels diminishes the frequency and duration of septic episodes caused by wound flora. This is accomplished by cleansing wound two to three times per day by immersing the wound in cleansing solutions. Some burn facilities still immerse patients in a tub to remove the debris and exudates that has accumulated between dressing changes, however most burn facilities no longer advocate this cleaning technique because of the potential seeding of surface bacteria to the open burn wound of other patients by an inadequately cleaned tube. It is imperative to note that wound cleansing can be painful, cause cooling and might be associated with hematogenous seeding leading to bacteremia. Therefore adequate monitoring is critical with this procedure. The entirety of the burn wound, those areas with intact eschar and those that have been excised, and even those that have been grafted, must be examined on at least a daily basis. Although donor site infections are rare, they occur most often in patients with massive burns, necessitating that donor sites on such patients be examined each day as well. The wound examination is best performed at the time of the daily burn wound cleansing or dressing change to identify infection in its earliest stages when pharmacologic intervention can control the infection and reduce the associated mortality. Even though topical antimicrobial agents play an important role in decreasing the incidence of burn wound infection, astute clinicians must be aware that antimicrobial therapy is not a substitute for aggressive debridement of grossly infected and devitalized tissue.

When invasive burn wound infection has been diagnosed, general supportive measures are employed to optimize cardiac and pulmonary function and to support other organ systems. Specific systemic antibiotic therapy is instituted based on the current results of the burn center's microbiology surveillance program and modified thereafter on the basis of the sensitivity tests of the individual patient's infecting organisms. Wound care must also be altered. If the causative organism is a bacterium, an antimicrobial dressing should be selected. This can range silver containing products such as Acticoat to solutions such as mafenide acetate. Mafenide acetate, which is water-soluble and readily diffuses into the eschar and underlying tissue, can reduce the microbial density of the burn wound and prevent further proliferation of organisms in the eschar and sub-eschar space. Sub-eschar clysis of a broadspectrum penicillin (one-half of the daily dose suspended in 150–1 000 ml saline) can be considered, using a No. 20 spinal needle to minimize the number of infusion sites [20].

## Cellulitis

Burn wound cellulitis of bacterial origin can be caused by a variety of organisms, but group A β-hemolytic streptococci are the most common offenders [8]. This infection is characterized by erythema, edema and hyperesthesia of unburned skin at the margins of the burn or donor site wound. If untreated, the lesions expand with variable rapidity with or without a lymphangitic component. There may be increased serous exudate from the wound bed, and if a β-hemolytic streptococcal infection involves a skin graft, the graft may be destroyed literally overnight. Progressively expanding cellulitis should be treated with topical application of antimicrobial dressing and systemic penicillin if it is caused by a group A β-streptococcus, or a broad-spectrum β-lactam antibiotic if specific cultures and sensitivity results are not available plus Vancomycin for MRSA coverage [8]. Antimicrobial dressings should be applied to the surface of the donor site until the infection is brought under control, consideration should be given to dressings with MRSA activity. If the donor site is not healed at that time, any open areas can be grafted if the defects are full thickness or covered with a biologic dressing if they are only partial thickness.

## Impetigo

Another form of burn wound infection that may occur following burn wound closure or grafting has been termed burn wound impetigo and is characterized by multifocal small superficial abscesses. This infection may lead to extensive destruction of previously adherent skin grafts or ulceration of spontaneously healed partial-thickness burns and healed split-thickness skin graft donor sites. It usually elicits little systemic response, although fever and leukocytosis may occur. The diagnosis, made on the basis of epithelial loss, is confirmed by cultures that commonly show growth of *Staphylococcus aureus*. Treatment consists in un-roofing all abscesses, meticulous cleansing of the infected areas with a surgical detergent disinfectant, and application of a topical antibacterial ointment, such as mupirocin. A disproportionate systemic response may indicate that the causative *Staphylococcus* is a producer of toxic shock syndrome toxin 1 (TSST-1), which can be confirmed by toxin assay and should be treated by intravenous administration of vancomycin [26].

## Catheter related infections

Infectious complications associated with intravenous and intra-arterial catheters represent a major problem irrespective of the constant attention to aseptic technique for insertion and appropriate maintenance [9]. The burned patient appears to be especially susceptible to this complication with catheter infection rates reported ranging from 8–57% [10, 11]. Central line sepsis is associated with prolonged indwelling central venous catheters. Meticulous sterile technique is essential during line placement to avoid introduction of potential pathogens. The use of antimicrobial coated catheters and rotation of the catheter site, tubing and apparatus every 72 hours have been reported to have a decrease in catheter infection rates, however these studies are flawed and more valid conclusions would be obtained with a prospective randomized study [12, 13]. All areas should be carefully prepped and draped with Betadine or Chlorhexidine solution and the physician gowned and gloved appropriately prior to insertion [14]. Central line sepsis may be primary in which the central line is the original focus of infection. It also may be secondary, in which case, the catheter tip is seeded and serves as a nidus for continued shedding of microorganisms into the blood stream. Signs of erythema or inflammation around the insertion site should alert the clinician to the potential for a line infection. However, it is important to realize that there may be a significant infection of the catheter tip even when skin surrounding the insertion site appears normal. Central lines can be associated with the development of both gram negative and gram-positive sepsis. The key concept to recognize is that central lines represent a foreign body and as such are prone to microbial seeding. There is significant controversy with regard to the frequency of line changes necessary to avoid catheter-related infection. Frequent line changes may actually increase the risk of central line sepsis. Once a catheter-related infection is suspected, the central venous line should be promptly removed and the tip cultured. Systemic antimicrobial therapy can be initiated for a short time, but generally once the source of infection has been removed the patient should improve quickly. Careful records of previously cannulated sites can allow for sequential venotomy, examination for ultra luminal pus and histologic examination for intimal colonization. Upon confirmation of the diagnosis, immediate operative excision is essential to prevent progressive sepsis. Entire excision of a vein to the port of entry into the central circulation may be required because of the tendency of phlebitis to migrate to vein valves, leaving an apparently normal vein in between the infected foci. The subcutaneous tissue and skin should be packed open where a grossly purulent vein is removed and allowed to granulate and close by secondary intention.

## Urinary tract infection

Urinary tract infections are usually associated with prolonged and often unnecessary catheterization, as it is rarely indicated to leave a catheter in place for more than a few days. Routine monitoring of urine from indwelling catheters should be done by needle aspirates on a regular basis two to three times a week. Urinary tract infections can generally be divided into upper and lower urinary tract infections. True pyelonephritis is very rare in thermally injured patients; however, lower urinary tract infection can occur as a result of a chronic indwelling Foley catheter. The diagnosis should be suspected when there are greater than $1 \times 10^5$ organisms cultured from urine specimen. Also urinalysis may reveal white cells and cellular debris associated with active infection. The most common organisms are gram-negative pathogens such as Escherichia coli. The appropriate treatment consists of either exchange or removal of the foley catheter and 7–10 day course of an antimicrobial with good gram-negative coverage. Fluroquinolones such as ciprofloxacin are often very effective for uncomplicated cases. Candiduria is often insignificant but may reflect active infection or septicemia, especially when mycelia can be demonstrated. When present, an active infection with Candida species usually responds well to low doses of fluconazole. If there is suspicion of an ascending infection, more aggressive treatment with prolonged systemic antimicrobials is warranted.

## Tracheobronchitis

Smoke inhalation injury is a chemical trancheobronchitis that results from the inhalation of the incomplete products of combustion and is often found in association with severe burn injury. Inhalation injury impairs the mucociliary transport mechanism and predisposes patients to colonization of the tracheobronchial tree by microorganisms. Additionally, direct cellular injury to the respiratory epitheli-

225

um results in the formation of extensive fibrinous casts composed of inflammatory exudates and sloughed cells. Increased bronchial blood flow leads to increased airway edema. As necrotic debris accumulates and airway edema is increased, patients become susceptible to post-obstructive atelectasis and pneumonia. There is no specific treatment for tracheobronchitis other than aggressive pulmonary toilet and supportive measures. It is important to realize, however, that an upper respiratory infection can quickly turn into a lower respiratory infection with significant mortality. Pneumonia has been shown to independently increase burn mortality by 40%, and the combination of inhalation injury and pneumonia leads to a 60% increase in deaths. Inhalation injury was also found to be associated with a twofold higher risk of developing nosocomial pneumonia than with burns alone. Children and the elderly are especially prone to pneumonia due to a limited physiologic reserve.

## Pneumonia

The diagnosis of pneumonia in severely burned patients is exceedingly problematic. During the acute phase of injury these patients demonstrate a hypermetabolic response characterized by increased basal metabolic rate and resetting of their hypothalamic temperature set point. The increased levels of catecholamines result in a hyperdynamic circulation. For these reasons, many of the usual signs and symptoms of pneumonia are unreliable in the severely burn patients. Fever, leucocytosis, tachycardia and tachypnea may all be present even in the absence of an infection. Sputum examination is rarely helpful since specimens are often contaminated with oropharyngeal flora. If sputum expectoration is chosen, examination should include a variety of criteria such as color, amount, consistency and odor of the specimen. Muco-purulent sputum is most commonly found with bacterial pneumonia or bronchitis. Scant or watery sputum is often related to viral and other atypical pneumonias. "Rusty" sputum indicates alveolar involvement and has been most commonly associated with pneumococcal pneumonia. Dark red, mucoid sputum suggests Friedlander's pneumonia caused by encapsulated K. I. Pneumonia. Foul-smelling sputum is associated with mixed anaerobic infections most commonly seen with as-

piration [14]. More invasive sampling techniques such as brochoalveolar lavage have been advocated; however, these have also been shown to be less than ideal for establishing a diagnosis of pneumonia. Radiographic findings can be helpful if they reveal lobar consolidation. Unfortunately, concomitant inhalation injury and changes in pulmonary vascular permeability more often result in diffuse nonspecific radiographic changes consistent with noncardiogenic pulmonary edema. Pneumonias can result from descending infection and have clearly been shown to increase the incidence and the mortality of nosocomial pneumonia in the burn population. Generally, patients with a significant inhalation injury and pneumonia develop atelectasis, ventilation-perfusion mismatch, arterial hypoxia and respiratory failure. Prolonged mechanical ventilation leads to inevitable barotraumas and further worsening of pulmonary status in these patients. Ventilator-associated pneumonia (VAP) specifically refers to pneumonia that develops more than 48 hours after intubation (late-onset VAP) in mechanically ventilated patients who had no clinical evidence suggesting the presence or likely development of pneumonia at the time of intubation. VAP that occurs within 48 hours of intubation is frequently the result of aspiration and usually yields a better prognosis than late-onset VAP, which is more often caused by antibiotic-resistant bacteria. While broncho-alveolar lavage has been to correlate better with the presence of trancheobronchitis than with radiographic evidence of true pneumonia, it is the best available tool. For this reason, a positive lavage in the appropriate clinical context mandates aggressive intervention. These nosocomial pneumonias are generally gram-negative infections and systemic antimicrobial therapy with multiple agents is generally required until the infection resolves clinically. Amikacain and piperacillin with tazobactam or ceftazidime are generally recommended for serious infections, but antibiotics should be selected on the basis of susceptibility patterns in each hospital. Once cultures are returned, antimicrobial coverage may be narrowed appropriately.

## Sepsis in the burn patient

Sepsis is one of the leading causes of morbidity and mortality in critically ill patients [15]. Severely burned patients are markedly susceptible to a variety of infectious complications [16]. Sepsis may result from seeding of the bloodstream from the burn wound, the respiratory tract, the gastrointestinal tract, and the urinary tract and central venous catheters. The burn wound and the lungs account for the vast majority of cases. The immunocompromised state of the burned patient is associated with multiple defects of the humoral and cellular components of both the nonspecific host defense system and the specific immune defense system and is markedly contributing to the increased susceptibility to infection. It is important to differentiate bacteremia from septicemia. Bacteremia refers to the presence of bacteria in the blood stream and may occur transiently after burn wound manipulation or excision. This transient bacteremia generally resolves and is not associated with any significant morbidity. Septicemia, however, implies a widespread response at the tissue level to bacteria or their products and toxins. Traditionally sepsis is categorized as gram-positive or gram-negative. Gram-negative sepsis is by far the most predominant in severely burned patients.

There are excellent criteria for the diagnosis of infection and sepsis in most patients, but the standard diagnoses for infection and sepsis really do not apply to burn patients [17]. Burn patients lose their primary barrier to microorganism invasion so they are constantly and chronically exposed to the environment. In response to this exposure, inflammatory mediators that change the baseline metabolic profile of the burn patient are continuously released. The baseline temperature is reset to about 38.5°C, and tachycardia and tachypnea persist for months in patients with extensive burns. Continuous exposure leads to significant changes in the white blood cell (WBC) count, making leukocytosis a poor indicator of sepsis.

The burn sepsis definition must therefore distinguish changes in patient status as the result of infection due to a microbial entity from the alterations secondary to the burn injury itself or associated events (such as inhalation injury). Several of these global changes are based on the fact that patients with extensive burns develop a hypermetabolic state that surpasses that of any other patient group.

Current definitions for sepsis and infection have many criteria (fever, tachycardia, tachypnea, leuko- cytosis) that are routinely found in patients with extensive burns, making these current definitions less applicable to the burn population. The diagnosis of sepsis is a clinical diagnosis. Laboratory studies are supportive. A patient who is adequately resuscitated and becomes hemodynamically unstable should alert the clinician to the possibility of either active bleeding or the development of septic shock. The five cardinal signs of sepsis are hyperventilation, thrombocytopenia, hyperglycemia, obtundation and hypothermia. Leucocytosis and fever are also important, but must be interpreted with caution in this setting. Based on the American Burn Association Consensus Conference to Define Sepsis and Infection in Burns, sepsis is defined by the criteria depicted in Tables 1 and 2 [17, 18].

A septic source can be documented as:

▶ 1) Burn wound biopsy with $> 10^5$ organisms/gm tissue and/or histologic evidence of viable tissue invasion

▶ 2) Positive blood culture

▶ 3) Urinary tract infection with $> 10^5$ organisms/ml urine of

▶ 4) Pulmonary infection

Local evidence of invasive wound infection includes black or brown patches of wound discoloration, rapid eschar separation, conversion of wounds to full thickness, spreading peri-wound erythema, punctate hemorrhagic subeschar lesions, and violaceous

**Table 1.** Definition of sepsis

| Burn | Modified ACCP/SCCM |
|---|---|
| ▶ At least 3 of the following:<br>• T > 38.5 or < 36.5 °C<br>• Progressive tachycardia<br>• Progressive tachypnea<br>• WBC > 12,000 or < 4,000<br>• Refractory hypotension<br>• Thrombocytopenia<br>• Hyperglycemia<br>• Enteral Feeding Intolerance<br>▶ AND<br>• Pathologic tissue source identified | ▶ At least 2 of the following:<br>• T > 38.5 or < 36.5°C<br>• HR>20% above NL for age<br>• RR > 20% above NL for age or PaCO2 < 32 torr<br>• WBC > 12,000 or < 4,000<br>▶ AND<br>• Bacteremia or fungemia<br>• Pathologic tissue source identified |

Hart et al. (2000) Determinants of skeletal muscle catabolism after severe burn. Ann Surg 233(4): 455–465

**Table 2.** Suggested ABA consensus

▶ At least 3 of the following parameters:
- > 38.5 or < 36.5 °C
- Progressive tachycardia > 90 bpm in adults or > 2 SD above age-specific norms in children
- Progressive tachypnea > 30 bpm in adults or > 2 SD above age-specific norms in children
- WBC > 12000 or < 4000 in adults or > 2 SD above age-specific norms in children
- Refractory hypotension: SBP < 90 mmHg, MAP < 70, or a SBP decrease > 40 mmHg in adult or < 2SD below normal for age in children
- Thrombocytopenia: platelet count < 100,000/μl in adults, < 2 SD below norms in children
- Hyperglycemia: plasma glucose > 110 mg/dl or 7.7 mM/l in the absence of diabetes
- Enteral feeding intolerance (residual > 150 ml/hr in children or 2 times feeding rate in adults; diarrhea > 2500 ml/day for adults or > 400 ml/day in children) 10

▶ AND
- Pathologic tissue source identified: > 105 bacteria on quantitative wound tissue biopsy or microbial invasion on biopsy.

Bacteremia or fungemia, or documented infection as defined by CDC

or black lesions in unburned tissue (ecthyma gangrenosum). When a patient exhibits signs and symptoms of sepsis, immediate institution of antibiotics is obligatory while awaiting confirmatory cultures. If a patient is already on antibiotics then the coverage should be broadened to include MRSA and Pseudomonas (i. e. Pip/Tazo plus Vancomycin in our institution). A delay of treatment for 3–4 days in a patient with a major burn results in an inordinately high morbidity. Specific antibiotic treatment should be administered if routine surveillance has identified the predominant organism. In addition to institution of antibiotic treatment, there should be a rapid aggressive attempt at source control.

Tight glycemic control is showing promise in decreasing infection rates in the intensive care unit. In a recent study in pediatric burn patients this finding has been upheld, is now being recommended and is an area of ongoing active research [19].

# The microbiology of burn wound infection

## Sources of organisms

Sources of organisms are found in the patient's own endogenous (normal) flora, from exogenous sources in the environment, and from healthcare personnel [20, 21]. Exogenous organisms from the hospital environment are generally more resistant to antimicrobial agents than endogenous organisms. Organisms associated with infection in burn patients include gram-positive, gram-negative, and viral and yeast/fungal organisms. The distribution of organisms changes over time in the individual patient and such changes can be ameliorated with appropriate management of the burn wound and patient.

The typical burn wound is initially colonized predominantly with gram-positive organisms, which are fairly quickly replaced by antibiotic-susceptible gram-negative organisms, usually within a week after the burn trauma. This wound flora may be replaced by yeasts, fungi and antibiotic-resistant bacteria, due to treatment with broad-spectrum antibiotics.

## Gram-positive organisms

Gram-positive organisms of particular concern include methicillin-resistant Staphylococcus aureus (MRSA), enterococci, group A b-hemolytic Streptococcus and coagulase negative Staphylococcus.

## Staphylococci

Staphylococcus aureus is the most frequently isolated pathogen from infected burn wounds and a leading cause for morbidity and mortality post burn [20, 21] Strains of S. aureus as well as other Staphylococcus species produce a wide variety of metabolites. Some are pathognomonic and also toxigenic, while those with minimal toxicity or no toxic effects at all, are of some diagnostic significance. An array of biproducts such as proteinases, collagenases and hyaluronidase digest the extra-cellular matrix, which serves as the structural integrity essential in wound healing [20]. Most of the human pathogens produce a- and ß-lysins. Some exotoxins, which are produced by the pathogenic strains of staphylococci, include a pyrogenic toxin, a dermo-necrotizing toxin, a lethal toxin, and leukocidin. These organisms can also produce an exotoxin, TSST-1 and enterotoxins A, B and C, which are risk factors for toxic shock syndrome in susceptible patients [20]. Toxic shock syndrome (TSS) was first described in 1978. The disease is characterized by sudden onset of fever, vomiting, diarrhea, shock, and a diffuse macular erythematous rash, followed by desquamation of the skin on the hand and feet as well as hyperemia of various mucous membranes. However, the role of TSS has not been completely elucidated in the burn patient. It has been our experience that while burn patients may be infected with a TSS potential S. aureus, no other serious or untoward complications have been observed. In fact treatment of their burn wounds was not any different than those patients infected with a nontoxic TSS S. aureus.

Another member of the Staphylococci genus, Staphylococcus epidermidis, is a resident of human skin and mucous membranes therefore also frequently associated with burn wound infection. S. epidermidis resembles S. aureus microscopically, and is tolerant to high NaCl concentrations as is S. aureus. Unlike S. aureus it is mannitol-, coagulase- and thermonuclease-negative. It is as pathogenic as S. aureus, and is the main pathogen for injuries such as subacute bacterial endocarditis or infected surgical prosthesis.

## Streptococci

Streptococci are catalase-negative and produce a variety of hemolytic activity in the presence of blood. Types of hemolysis produced on SBA are frequently used as an initial method to identify streptococci. ß-hemolytic streptococci, such as streptococcus pyogenes, ß-hemolytic streptococci group A and S. agalactiae ß-hemolytic streptococci group B are very virulent even in low concentrations and may lead to wound infection, failure of a primary closure, and loss of a skin graft. Enterococcus faecalis and Enterococcus faecium were first discovered in 1984 [22]. Since then 12 species have been classified within the Enterococcus group [22]. Due to their resistance third-generation cephalosporins enterococci present

today one of the most common pathogens responsible for burn wound infection. Enterococci are divided into three main groups based on specific biochemical reactions. Group I does not hydrolyze arginine but forms acid in a manitol, sorbitol and sorbose broth. The most common pathogen within this group is Enterococcus avium. E. faecalis and E. faecium, agents of Group II, hydrolyzes arginine and forms acid in mannitol and sorbitol broth only. Group III, including Enterococcus durans, is negative for all tests described above [22].

### Gram-negative organisms

The family of gram-negative organisms contains a distinctive group of etiologic pathogens commonly associated with burn wound infections. *Pseudomonas aeruginosa* was discovered 1960 and is the second most common pathogen within this group frequently associated with burn wound infections [21]. Because of its ability to survive in aqueous environments, these organisms have been become problematic in the hospital environment. Infections caused by this agent range from superficial skin infections to fulminant sepsis. *Pseudomonas aeruginosa* is the leading cause of nosocomial respiratory tract infection. Patients receiving ventilator assistance in the ICU have a 20-fold higher likelihood of developing nosocomial pneumonia caused by *Pseudomonas aeruginosa*. Wound infections due to *Pseudomonas aeruginosa* are particularly troublesome in burn patients. Even though the incidence of such infections has declined within this particular patient population, the high rate of sepsis following these wound infections is still strongly associated with the incidence of mortality in severely burned patients [22].

*Acinetobacter sp.* is part of the resident flora of the respiratory, skin, as well as the gastrointestinal and genitourinary tracts. These pathogens are frequently isolated from a diversity of clinical sources, including upper and lower respiratory tracts, urinary tract, surgical and burn wounds, and in bacteremia secondary to IV catheterization. Also occasional cases of septicemia or pneumonia have occurred in attenuated patients. Many of these patients who develop infections with this microorganism have had various manipulations including the use of respiratory therapy equipment, tracheal intubation, bladder or central venous line catheterization.

The most common and largest group of microorganisms, populating the burn wound environment along with the Staphylococcus sp. are *Enterobacteriaceae*. 12 sub-species have been identified within this family so far, including *Klebsiella, Serratia marcescens, Providencia species* and *Erwinia species* [8, 11, 23].

*Eschericia coli*, probably the most well known enteric pathogen, has been responsible for a wide diversity of infectious processes, such as appendicitis, cystitis, peritonitis, septicemia, and cholecystitis as well as surgical and burn wound sepsis and epidemic diarrhea. *Eschericia coli* can be differentiated from other members of *Enterobacteriacae* by its response to the classical IMVIC (indole, methyl red, Voges-Proskauer and citrate) reaction.

The *Klebsiella-Enterobacter* group (K-E) consists of gram-negative organisms that are either motile or non-motile. Fifty-one percent of moderately ill hospitalized patients were infected with either *K. pneumoniae, Enterobacter aerogenes* or *Enterobacter cloacae* isolated from their oropharyngeal space [1]. *K. pneumoniae* and are now considered a common pathogen causing nosocomial infections [22].

The remaining groups of enterics consist of three additional species: *Proteus, Providencia,* and *Morganella,* the latter frequently associated with wound infections or urinary tract infections. *Proteus mirabilis* and *Proteus vulgaris* are both found in massive concentrations in feces of patients receiving oral antibiotic therapy. Both pathogens are commonly leading to surgical and burn wound infections, intra-abdominal infections, as well as bacteremia and urinary tract infections.

## Anaerobes

The most repeatedly confronted organisms in this group, which may play a fearful role in surgical and burn wound infections are *Bacteroides spp.* and *Fusobacterium spp.* They are considered normal flora of the human body, beginning at the oropharyngeal cavity and ending at the gastrointestinal (GI) and urogenital tracts. Numerically they account for the major population in the oropharyngeal region in a 5:1 ratio over the aerobes and facultative anaerobes,

while in the urogenital and GI tract the ratio is more dynamic at a 1000:1 [22, 24]. Examining the current statistics of anaerobic infections related to locality, all but 2–5% of surgical wound infections in the oropharyngeal area are caused by the anaerobic flora [25, 26]. Those occurring in the GI and urogenital tract are only responsible for about 10–15% of the wound infections [27, 28]. Prior surgery, malignant neoplasms, arteriosclerosis, diabetes mellitus, prior antibiotic therapy, alcoholism, improper debridement, and steroid and immunosuppressive therapy are commonly major contributors associated in these types of wound infections [26, 27]. Specimens collected for anaerobic organisms should be placed in appropriate transport tubes void of atmospheric $O_2$ or remain in syringes with attached needles containing suspect aspirates sealed off with a rubber stopper. However, with the advent of the early excision and grafting, the incidence of anaerobic infections in the thermal injury has been significantly reduced; therefore anaerobic cultures are not economical. Culturing for these anaerobes would be futile, as they require vascular tissue for survival. Their presence would only be observed if such tissue were to remain.

Anaerobic infections in burned patients are usually associated with avascular muscle found in electrical injuries, frostbite, or cutaneous flame burns with concomitant crush-type injuries.

## Fungi

Until the advent of topical antimicrobial agents, fungal infections were not common in burned patients. However, the incidence of mycotic invasion has doubled since the implementation of topical antimicrobial agents to control bacterial colonization. The burn wound is the most commonly infected site, although local or disseminated fungal infections of the respiratory tract, urinary tract, GI tract, and vagina are increasingly common [29].

Fungi are generally isolated through the inoculation of both non-selective and selective culture media. The most commonly used non-selective media includes inhibitory mold agar and SABHI agar, which permit the enhanced growth of almost all fungi, including some of the more fastidious and slowly growing fungi. The most commonly utilized selective media include those containing antimicrobial agents such as penicillin (20 U/ml) plus streptomycin (40 U/ml) or gentamicin (5 µg/ml) plus chloramphenicol (16 µg/ml) to inhibit growth of bacteria. Media containing cyclohexamide (0.5 µg/ml) may also be utilized to inhibit growth of rapidly growing moulds that often overgrow slower growing dimorphic fungi; however, a medium without cyclohexamide should also be used, because this agent can inhibit the growth of some medically important fungi (e. g. *Cryptococcus neoformans* and *Aspergillus fumigatus*). Additionally, Sabouraud's dextrose or potato dextrose agar is used to allow for identification of fungi through their sporulation characteristics. Yeasts are identified on the basis of specific biochemical tests, whereas identification of moulds is based on growth rate, colony structure, microscopic appearance, dimorphism at different incubation temperatures, inhibition of growth by cyclohexamide, and a few biochemical tests [26].

*Candida sp.* are the most common nonbacterial colonizers of the burn wound, although true fungi such as *Aspergillus, Penicillium, Rhizopus, Mucor, Rhizomucor, Fusarium,* and *Curvularia* are not uncommon and have a much greater invasive potential than the yeasts [25].

Early diagnosis of fungal infection is difficult as clinical symptoms frequently mimic low-grade bacterial infections. Routine culture techniques may require 7 to 14 days for identifying fungal contaminants, with resultant delay in the initiation of treatment as these pathogens are frequently not recovered in culture [25]. In contrast to bacterial sepsis, venous blood cultures may not reflect the causative organism. Arterial blood cultures and retinal examination for characteristic candida lesions can be useful.

Unlike candida infections, true fungal infections occur early in the hospital course of patients with specific predisposing characteristics [30]. Most frequently, burned patients infected with fungi are exposed to spores in the environment by either rolling on the ground or jumping into surface water at the time of injury. Other environmental foci have been cited as the source of nosocomial fungal infection, including bandaging supplies left open to air, heating, and air conditioning ducts and floor drains [25]. Once colonized, broad non-branching hyphae ex-

tend into subcutaneous tissue, stimulating an inflammatory response. This phenomenon is diagnostic of fungal wound infection. Vascular invasion is common and often accompanied by thrombosis and avascular necrosis, clinically observed as rapidly advancing dark discolorations of the wound margins or well-described lesions. Systemic dissemination of the infection occurs with invasion of the vasculature.

## Infection control

The microorganisms initially populating the burned wound represent a mixture of endogenous resident flora and airborne contaminants seeded by contact with the environment and attending personnel. Burn patients are immunosuppressed and should be protected from exposure to environmental contaminants. The most effective means of decreasing exposure of burned patients to exogenous bacteria is strict observation of appropriate hand washing among the health care providers. Face masks waterproof gowns and gloves should be worn whenever direct contact with body fluids and wound exudates are unavoidable, thus protecting both the patient and the health care provider from inadvertent contamination. All dressing materials should be maintained as patient specific. IV pumps and poles, blood pressure devices, monitoring equipment, bedside tables and beds should be cleaned on at least a daily basis with antibacterial solutions. Many items such as blood pressure cuffs, stethoscopes, bedpans, if used on areas without dry, occlusive dressings, may need high-level disinfection as a semi-critical item or may need to be restricted to an individual patient.

Plants and flowers should not be allowed in units with burn patients because they harbor gram-negative organisms, such as Pseudomonas species, other enteric gram-negative organisms, and fungi. Many of these organisms are intrinsically resistant to multiple antibiotics, which may serve as reservoirs to colonize the burn wound [31]. Pediatric burn patients should also have policies restricting the presence of non-washable toys such as stuffed animals and cloth objects. These can harbor large numbers of bacteria and are difficult to disinfect. Toys should be nonporous and washable, designated for individual patient use, and thoroughly disinfected after use and before being given to another child to use. Paper items, such as storybooks and coloring books, should always be designated for single patient use and should be disposed of if they become grossly contaminated or when the child is discharged.

Terminal cleaning, following the discharge of the patient, should include the walls, ceiling, baseboards and floors. Mattresses should be covered with vinyl or other impermeable surface that allows culturing and cleaning without soiling, and be frequently inspected for cracks in their surfaces. At our institution we use air filters with 99.99% efficiency on 0.3 micron sized particles. They are changed regularly, cultured if clinically indicated by infection control monitoring.

All major burned patients should be housed within individual, self-contained positive pressure isolation rooms. However, common areas exist even within these units, predominantly the bathing or showering facilities. These areas should be conscientiously cleansed between patients with an effective bactericidal agent specifically directed at the bacteria, which are common to an individual unit.

## Pharmacological considerations in the treatment of burn infections

The timely and effective use of antimicrobials has revolutionized burn care by decreasing invasive wound infections. The untreated burn wound rapidly becomes colonized with bacteria and fungi because of the loss of normal skin barrier mechanisms. As the organisms proliferate to high wound counts ($>10^5$ organisms per gram of tissue), they may penetrate into viable tissue. Organisms then invade blood vessels, causing a systemic infection that often leads to the death of the patient. This scenario has become uncommon in most burn units because of the effective use of antibiotics and wound care techniques. The antimicrobials that are used can be divided into those given topically and those given systemically.

### Topical antimicrobial treatment

Available topical antibiotics can be divided into two classes: salves and soaks. Salves are generally applied directly to the wound with cotton dressings placed over them, and soaks are generally poured into cotton dressings on the wound. Each of these classes of antimicrobials has advantages and disadvantages. Salves may be applied once or twice a day but may lose their effectiveness between dressing changes. Frequent dressing changes can result in shearing with loss of grafts or underlying healing cells. Soaks remain effective because antibiotic solution can be added without removing the dressing; however, the underlying skin can become macerated.

Topical antibiotic salves include 11% mafenide acetate (Sulfamylon), 1% silver sulfadiazine (Silvadene), polymyxin B, neomycin, bacitracin, mupirocin, and the antifungal agent nystatin. No single agent is completely effective, and each has advantages and disadvantages. Silver sulfadiazine is the most commonly used. It has a broad spectrum of activity because its silver and sulfa moieties cover gram-positive, most gram-negative, and some fungal forms. Some *Pseudomonas* species possess plasmid-mediated resistance. Silver sulfadiazine is relatively painless on application, has a high patient acceptance, and is easy to use. Occasionally, patients complain of a burning sensation after it is applied, and, in a few patients, a transient leukopenia develops 3 to 5 days following its continued use. This leukopenia is generally harmless and resolves with or without treatment cessation.

Mafenide acetate is another topical agent with a broad spectrum of activity owing to its sulfa moiety. It is particularly useful against resistant *Pseudomonas* and *Enterococcus* species. It also can penetrate eschar, which silver sulfadiazine cannot. Disadvantages include painful application on skin, such as in second-degree wounds. It also can cause an allergic skin rash, and it has carbonic anhydrase inhibitory characteristics that can result in a metabolic acidosis when applied over large surfaces. For these reasons, mafenide sulfate is typically reserved for small full-thickness injuries.

Petroleum-based antimicrobial ointments with polymyxin B, neomycin, and bacitracin are clear on application, painless, and allow for easy wound observation. These agents are commonly used for treatment of facial burns, graft sites, healing donor sites, and small partial-thickness burns. Mupirocin is a relatively new petroleum-based ointment that has improved activity against gram-positive bacteria, particularly methicillin-resistant *S. aureus* and selected gram-negative bacteria. Nystatin either in a salve or powder form can be applied to wounds to control fungal growth. Nystatin-containing ointments can be combined with other topical agents to decrease colonization of both bacteria and fungus. The exception is the combination of nystatin and mafenide acetate; each inactivates the other.

Available agents for application as a soak include 0.5% silver nitrate solution, 0 025% sodium hypochlorite (Dakin's), 0.25% acetic acid, and mafenide acetate as a 5% solution. Silver nitrate has the advantage of being painless on application and having complete antimicrobial effectiveness. The disadvantages include its staining of surfaces to a dull gray or black when the solution dries. This can become problematic in deciphering wound depth during burn excisions and in keeping the patient and his or her surroundings clean of the black staining. The solution is hypotonic as well, and continuous use can cause electrolyte leaching, with rare methemoglobinemia as another complication. A new commercial dressing containing biologically potent silver ions (Acticoat) that are activated in the presence of moisture is available. This dressing holds the promise to retain the effectiveness of silver nitrate without the problems of silver nitrate soaks.

Dakin's solution (0.25% sodium hypochlorite) has effectiveness against most microbes; however, it also has cytotoxic effects on the healing cells of patients' wounds. Low concentrations of sodium hypochlorite (0 025%) have less cytotoxic effects while maintaining most of the antimicrobial effects. Hypochlorite ion is inactivated by contact with protein, so the solution must be continually changed. The same is true for acetic acid solutions, which may be more effective against *Pseudomonas*. Mafenide acetate soaks have the same characteristics of the mafenide acetate salve, except in liquid form.

## Systemic antimicrobial treatment (Table 3)

The major role of an antibiotic is to help the body eliminate an agent of infection in a burn patient. Systemic antimicrobial treatment must be thoughtfully considered in the care of the burn patient to prevent the emergence of resistant organisms. The burn wound will always be colonized with organisms until wound closure is achieved and administration of systemic antimicrobials will not eliminate this colonization but rather promote emergence of resistant organisms. The treatment of an infection is often begun based on empiric knowledge of the most common types of microbial infections seen in the burn population and the antimicrobial agents that are most efficacious in their treatment. If antimicrobial therapy is indicated to treat a specific infection, it should always be based on wound cultures that specifically identify the infecting organism, the colony counts and the sensitivity of that organism to specific antibiotics. Pathology studies of wound biopsies give us information on how invasive the infecting organism is in the body. A pharmaco-therapeutic regimen of antibiotics should follow known parameters about specific burn wound infections in order to potentiate each antibiotic agent's mechanism of action and pharmacokinetics while decreasing its side effects and systemic toxicities. Also, if antibacterial treatment is necessary, awareness should be heightened for the possibility of superinfection with resistant organisms, yeasts, or fungi. Systemic antimicrobials are indicated to treat documented infections, such as pneumonia, bacteremia, wound infection, and urinary tract infection. Empiric antimicrobial therapy to treat fever should be strongly discouraged because burn patients often have fever secondary to the systemic inflammatory response to burn injury. Prophylactic antimicrobial therapy is recommended only for coverage of the immediate perioperative period surrounding excision or grafting of the burn wound when if is used to cover the documented increase in risk of transient bacteremia. Treatment should be started immediately prior to the procedure and generally discontinued within 24h, assuming restoration of normal cardiovascular hemodynamics.

## Gram-positive bacterial infections

The three most common gram-positive organisms responsible for burn wound infections are *streptococci, staphylococci, and enterococci*.

233

**Table 3.** RTBC empiric therapy till speciation and sensitivity determines the antibiotic of choice

| | |
|---|---|
| **Surgical prophylaxis:** | Cefazolin<br>(Gentamicin 2 mg/kg or Vancomycin 1 g if PNC allergy) |
| **Clostridium difficile:** | Severe: Vanco 125 mg po qid × 10days<br>Milder: Flagyl 500 mg po tid × 10 days (change to above if not responding)<br>Recurrent episodes:<br>can add *Saccharomyces boulardii* 500 mg po bid |
| **Pyelonephritis** | Ampicillin + gent |
| **Sepsis** | Pip/Tazo (meropenem only if known resistance to other agents) |
| **Pneumonia:**<br>**If CAP** | <br>Ceftriaxone 1 g + azithromycin 500 mg IV daily × 5–7 days |
| **If nosocomial, empiric:** | Ceftriaxone<br>FQ: Levofloxacin preferred (Cipro has poor lung penetration) |
| **If aspiration suspected:** | Ceftriaxone ± Clindamycin<br>(ceftriaxone ok alone for basic oral anaerobes of minor aspiration) |
| **If VAP**<br>(i. e. pneumonia >48h after admission) | Pip/Tazo 3 375g IV q6h (4.5g IV q6h if *Pseudomonas aeruginosa*) |
| **Skin infections** | Cloxacillin or Ancef<br>Vancomycin or Clindamycin if PCN allergy<br>Vancomycin if MRSA |
| **Diabetic infections:** | Clindamycin + Cipro (or Septra) |
| **Necrotizing Fasciitis** | Penicillins + Clindamycin (added for first 3–5 days for aerobic/anaerobic) |
| **UTI** | Keflex or Nitrofurantoin or Bactrim (in that order)<br>(amoxicillin only if *E. coli* or *S. saprophyticus* confirmed as susceptible) |

## Streptococcal infections

β-hemolytic *streptococci* of group A or B (*Str. Pyogenes or Str. Agalactiae*) are most commonly seen in the first 72 hours post-burn. Cellulitis may develop due to streptococcal infections and usually respond to treatment with natural penicillins or first generation cephalosporins. The natural penicillins that consist of penicillin G and penicillin V and the first generation cephalosporins are bactericidal in action. Like many other β-lactam antibiotics, the antibacterial action results from inhibition of mucopeptide synthesis in the bacterial cell wall. Resistance to these antibiotics is caused by the production of β-lactamases and/or intrinsic resistance. B-lactamase enzymes inactivate these antibiotics by hydrolyzing their β-lactam ring. Intrinsic resistance can result from the presence of a permeability barrier in the outer membrane of an infecting organism or alteration in the properties of target enzymes (penicillin-binding proteins). In case of resistance or tolerance to natural penicillins or first generation cephalosporins, culture and sensitivity data should be utilized to appropriately treat the streptococcal infection.

## Staphylococcal infections

*Staphylococcus aureus* and *Staphylococcus epidermidis* are natural pathogens found on human skin and therefore the leading cause of infections in burn populations. With their ability to generate penicillinases these microbes break the penicillin β-lactam ring and make natural pencillins ineffective against these bacteria.

These types of infections are treated with penicillinase-resistant penicillins if they are termed "methicillin sensitive". These antibiotics included the parenteral antibiotics, nafcillin, methicillin, and oxacillin and the oral antibiotics, cloxacillin, dicloxacillin, nafcilllin and oxacillin. The penicillinase-resistant penicillins have a mechanism of action that is similar to other penicillins. They interfere with bacterial cell wall synthesis during active multiplication by binding to one or more of the penicillin-binding proteins. They inhibit the final transpeptidation step of peptidoglycan synthesis causing cell wall death and resultant bactericidal activity against susceptible bacteria. However, the Staphylococcal bacteria resistance pattern has become such that these penicillinase-resistant penicillin are no longer very effective against these organisms. Staphylococcal infections that are resistant to penicillinase-resistant penicillins are termed MRSA (methicillin resistant *Staphylococcus aureus*) or MRSE (methicillin-resistant *Staphylococcus epidermidis*).

Vancomycin alone or in combination with other antibiotics has been considered the treatment of choice for infections caused by methicillin-resistant staphylococci. Currently, 100% of all Staphylococcal isolates are susceptible to vancomycin at our hospital. Vancomycin is bactericidal and appears to bind to the bacterial cell wall, causing blockage of glycopeptide polymerization. This effect, which occurs at a site different from that affected by the penicillins, produces immediate inhibition of cell wall synthesis and secondary damage to the cytoplasmic membrane [32]. Vancomycin, however, is a time-dependent antimicrobial that requires that the serum level of this drug must remain at all times above the minimum inhibitory concentration (MIC) in order to provide adequate bactericidal activity.

The hypermetabolic burn patient exhibits an increased glomerular filtration rate and increased excretion of the renally cleared drug, vancomycin. Because of the wide interpatient variability of vancomycin elimination in a burn patient, the dosage must be individualized in order to provide an optimal time-dependent serum concentration. The peak and trough levels are derived from the MIC for a particular bacterial organism. The therapeutic peak level is approximately equivalent to 5–8 times the MIC and the trough concentration is equivalent to 1–2 times the MIC. The so-called therapeutic range most often quoted for vancomycin monitoring is peak levels of 30–40mcg/ml and trough levels of 5–10mcg/ml. Because vancomycin is a concentration independent, or time-dependent, antibiotic and because there are practical issues associated with determining a precise peak serum concentration with this multi-compartment antibiotic, most clini-

cians have abandoned the routine practice of determining peak serum concentrations.

The overall AUC/MIC value may be the pharmacodynamic parameter that best correlates with a successful outcome associated with the use of vancomycin, Prolonged exposure to serum levels close to the MIC are associated with the emergence of resistance; therefore it is important to maintain adequate serum concentrations in patients with fast or rapidly changing creatinine clearance such as burn patients. There are also certain body compartments in which penetration is poor, such as the lung and the CNS. It would, also, seem prudent to keep concentrations from being suboptimal in patients with pneumonia or meningitis, as well as in patients receiving dialysis for renal failure. The American Thoracic Society recently published guidelines for hospital-acquired, ventilator associated, and health care-associated pneumonia. These guidelines recommend vancomycin in concentrations of 15–20mcg/ml for the treatment of methicillin-resistant *Staphylococcus aureus* pneumonia [33]. These higher concentrations may be needed for sequestered infections or in situations where vancomycin penetration has been documented to be poor. Some clinicians recommend that these higher concentrations of vancomycin may be necessary in the treatment of staphylococcal infections as well.

In the burn patient, vancomycin is often used not only in combination with other ototoxic and nephrotoxic agents such as aminoglycosides, the loop diuretic, furosemide and the antifungal drug, amphotericin. Nephrotoxicity is manifested by transient elevations in the serum blood urea nitrogen (BUN) or serum creatinine and decreases in the glomerular filtration rate and creatinine clearance. Hyaline and granular casts and albumin may also be found in the urine.

Vancomycin should only be administered by slow intravenous infusions as this drug can cause an anaphylactoid reaction known as "Red Man's Syndrome". This reaction is characterized by a sudden decrease in blood pressure, which can be severe and may be accompanied by flushing and/or a maculopapular or erythematous rash on the face, neck, chest, and upper extremities; the latter manifestation may also occur in the absence of hypotension. Since this is not a true "allergic reaction", the patient may be pre-treated with acetaminophen and diphenhydramine before an extended infusion of vancomycin at least 90–120 minutes ahead.

For oral treatment of MRSA and MRSE Linezolid is the antibiotic of choice. Linezolid is a synthetic antibacterial agent of a new class of antibiotics, the oxazolidinones that has joined the armamentarium against MRSA and MRSE. Linezolid inhibits bacterial protein synthesis by binding to a site on the bacterial 23S ribosomal RNA of the 50S subunit and prevents the formation of a functional 70S initiation complex, which is an essential component of the bacterial translation process [32]. The results of time-kill studies have shown linezolid to be bacteriostatic against enterococci and staphylococci. For streptococci, linezolid was found to be bactericidal for the majority of the strains. In vitro studies, however, show that point mutations in the 23S ribosomal RNA are associated with linezolid resistance and have been reported with some strains of *Enterococcus faecium and Staphylococcus aureus* [32]. *S. aureus* and *S. epidermidis* both showed 96% susceptibility and *S. haemolyticus* showed 99% susceptibility to linezolid.

Side effects of linezolid include myelosupression (e. g. anemia leucopenia, pancytopenia and thrombocytopenia), which is generally reversible upon discontinuation of the drug, and *Clostridium difficile*-associated colitis. Linezolid is also a weak, nonselective, reversible inhibitor of monoamine oxidase (MAO) and may cause increased serotonin serum levels and serotonin syndrome in patients on various serotonin re-uptake inhibitors such as fluoxetine and sertraline.

Staphylococcal infections may also be treated with quinupristin/dalfopristin (Synercid®). Quinupristin/dalfopristin is bactericidal and inhibits bacterial protein synthesis by binding to different sites on the 50S ribosomal subunit thereby inhibiting protein synthesis in the bacterial cell [32]. We found *S. aureus* showed 97% susceptibility, *S. epidermidis* showed 99% susceptibility and *S. haemolyticus* showed 100% susceptibility to this drug.

Major adverse cardiovascular effects are seen when quinupristin/dalfopristin is given concomitantly with cytochrome P-450 isoenzyme 3A4 substrates such as cyclosporine, midazolam, and nifedipine that may cause QT prolongation [32]. The concomitant administration results in increased serum concentrations of those substrates and potentially prolonged/increased therapeutic or adverse effects. *Clostridium difficile*-associated diarrhea and colitis has also been reported with this drug ranging in severity from mild to life threatening. Adverse venous effects (e. g. thrombophlebitis) may occur; therefore, flushing infusion lines with 5% dextrose injection following completion of peripheral infusions is recommended. Do not flush with sodium chloride injection or heparin because of possible incompatibilities. Arthralgia and myalgia, severe in some cases, of unknown etiology have been reported. Some patients improved with a reduction in dosing frequency to every 12 hours [32].

## Enterococcal bacterial infections

The enterococcal microbial isolates most frequently isolated from burn wounds at our Hospital are *E. faecalis* and *E. faecium*. Most enterococcal bacteria are susceptible to vancomycin. At our institution all E. faecalis and E. faecium isolates showed 100% susceptibility to vancomycin. Vancomycin-resistant enterococci usually vancomycin-resistant *E. faecium,* or VRE, will require treatment with a combination of agents such as ampicillin and aminoglycosides. If this combination is not effective, the VRE may be treated with the quinupristin/dalfopristin (Synercid®) combination or linezolid. The reports in literature show that the use of quinupristin/dalfopristin resulted in resistance in one study and a superinfection in another study during the treatment of VRE infection [32]. In our institution *E. faecalis* showed 94% susceptibility and *E. faecium* showed 96% susceptibility to linezolid. Linezolid, however, is a bacteriostatic agent and resistance has been reported with some strains of *E. faecium.*

## Gram-negative bacterial infections

The most common gram-negative organisms in our hospital include *Pseudmonas aeruginosa, Echerichia coli, Klebsiella pneumoniae, Enterobacter cloacae and A. baumannii/haemolyticus.* The efficacy of the antibiotic arsenal varies based on the individual susceptibility of the microbial isolate. Synergy between different classes of antibiotics is often tested to determine efficacy for a multiply drug-resistant organism (MDRO's). The aminoglycosides and in particular, gentamicin, were historically the antibiotics of choice in the treatment of gram-negative infections. The synergistic activity with penicillinase-resistant penicillins and vancomycin in the treatment of staphylococcal infections further standardized its premier status before the advent of newer extended-spectrum penicillins, the fourth generation cephalosporins, the monobactams, the carbapenems and the quinolones. However, some gram-negative bacteria encountered in the burn unit are now resistant to all the aforementioned antibiotic classes and must now be treated with an old drug class, the polymixins.

Polymyxins are amphipathic molecules that interact with the lipopolysaccharide in the bacterial outer membrane; insertion of the antibiotic into the membrane disrupts it and releases lipopolysaccharide into the surrounding milieu. They also have potent antiendotoxic properties and antibacterial activity against P. aeruginosa and many of the Enterobacteriaceae [34].

Colistin, or polymyxin E, is a multicomponent polypeptide antibiotic comprised mainly of colistins A and B. It became available for clinical use in the 1960s. There are two forms of colistin available: Colistin sulfate for oral and topical use and colistimethate sodium for parenteral use [35]. Based on the studies of Storm et al., the polymyxins are bacteriostatic at low concentrations and bactericidal at high concentrations [36].

In early studies, Evans et al. and Nord and Hoeprich reported that at concentrations of 0.01 mcM/mL, polymyxin B sulfate was bactericidal for 88% of the P. aeruginosa strains [35, 37]. Full bactericidal activity against P. aeruginosa is not seen until the colistin concentration reaches 0.1 mcM/mL [35].

In susceptibility testing performed at the Galveston Shriners Hospital from 2005 to 2008, A. baumannii=haemlyticus, E. cloacae, E. coli, and K. pneumoniae all showed 100% susceptibility to colistin and polymyxin B, whereas P. aeruginosa showed 96% and 99% susceptibility to colistin and polymyxin B, respectively.

Nephrotoxicity and neurotoxicity are the most common adverse effects of colistin. Close monitoring of the dose-dependent nephrotoxicity and central nervous system toxicity associated with its systemic use therefore is necessary [38].

To investigate whether the use of colistin can moderate multi-resistant infections, and to elucidate whether it is associated with a greater number of adverse effects or a higher mortality rate in burn patients, Branski et al. reviewed 398 severely burned patients (burns >40% total body surface area [TBSA]) admitted to the Galveston Shriners Hospital between 2000 and 2006 who did not contract multi-drug-resistant gram-negative organisms during their hospital course and received the standard antibiotic regimen – vancomycin and piperacillin/tazobactam – served as controls (piperacillin/tazobactam; n=280) [38].

The treatment group consisted of patients who, during their acute hospital stay, developed infections with multi-drug-resistant gram-negative pathogens and were treated with vancomycin and colistin for at least three days (colistin; n=118). Colistin was given at a mean dose of 4.4±0.9 mg/kg divided into three (or, in rare cases, two) doses over 24h. Patients who required colistin therapy had a significantly larger average total and full-thickness burn than patients treated with piperacillin/tazobactam and vancomycin, and the mortality rate was significantly higher in the colistin group (p>0.05). However, there was no significant difference between the colistin and piperacillin/ tazobactam groups in the incidence of neurotoxicity, hepatic toxicity, or nephrotoxicity. The authors concluded that Colistin is a safe and efficacious antimicrobial therapy without a marked incidence of toxic side effects. The higher mortality rate in the colistin group at the Galveston Shriners Hospital indicates that multi-resistant organisms are aggressive and a major contributor to burn-related death. The significantly larger burns in the colistin group certainly are the main reason for this finding. This study indicates that treatment of the pediatric burn population with colistin can be safe, as it did not increase the overall incidence of adverse effects. However, colistin should be used only under close monitoring of renal function [38].

## Treatment of yeast and fungal infections

The five classes of systemic antifungal medications include the polyenes, the azoles, nucleosides, echinocandin, and allylamine. Thus there are 4 potential target sites in the fungal cell for the antifungal drugs to act. The allylamine antifungal, terbinafine, which is used primarily for management of dermatophytosis and onchomycosis, and ketoconazole which has been replaced by newer, less toxic triazole drugs will not be discussed.

## The Polyenes (Amphotericin B)

Amphotericin B, an amphoteric polyene macrolide, is an antifungal antibiotic. Conventional IV amphotericin N is used for the treatment of potentially life-threatening fungal infections including *aspergillosis*, North American *blastomycosis*, systemic *candidiasis, coccidioidomycosis, cryptococcosis, histoplasmosis, paracoccidioidomycosis, sporotrichosis*, and *zygomycosis* [32].

Amphotericin B usually is fungistatic in action at concentrations obtained clinically, but may be fungicidal in high concentrations or against very susceptible organisms. Amphotericin B exerts its antifungal activity principally by binding to sterols (e. g. ergosterol) in the fungal cell membrane. As a result of this binding, the cell membrane is no longer able to function as a selective barrier and leakage of intracellular contents occurs. Cell death occurs in part as a result of permeability changes, but other mechanisms also may contribute to the in vivo antifungal effects of amphotericin B against some fungi [32]. Amphotericin B is not active in vitro against organisms that do not contain sterols in their cell membranes (e. g. bacteria).

Binding to sterols in mammalian cells (such as certain kidney cells and erythrocytes) may account for some of the toxicities reported with conventional amphotericin B therapy. Nephrotoxicity is the major dose-limiting side effect reported with conventional IV amphotericin B and occurs to some degree in the majority of patients receiving the drug. Adverse renal effects include decreased renal function and renal function abnormalities such as azotemia, hypokalemia, hyposthenuria, renal tubular acidosis, and nephrocalcinosis [32]. Increased BUN and serum creatinine concentrations and decreased creatinine clearance, glomerular filtration rate, and renal plasma flow occur in most patients receiving conventional IV amphotericin.

Acute infusion reactions consisting of fever, shaking, chills, hypotension, anorexia, nausea, vomiting, headache, dyspnea, and tachypnea may occur 1–3 hours after initiating of IV infusions of conventional IV amphotericin B or other formulations such as amphotericin B cholesteryl sulfate, amphotericin B lipid complex, and amphotericin B liposomal. Acetaminophen, meperidine, antihistamines (e. g. diphenhydramine), or corticosteroids have been used for the treatment or prevention of these acute infusion reactions.

## Azole antifungals

The azole antifungals consist of the triazole antifungal oral and intravenous drugs, fluconazole, itraconazole and voriconazole and the imidazole oral drug, ketoconazole. These antifungal agents act by interfering with cytochrome P450 activity, decreasing ergosterol synthesis (the principal sterol in the fungal cell membrane), and inhibiting cell membrane formation [26].

The triazole antifungal drugs can be distinguished by differences in their spectrum of activity. Fluconazole is generally active in vitro against *Candida albicans*, many of the non-*albicans Candida* species, and *C. neoformans*. However it is not generally active against *Candida krusei* or *Aspergillus* species [26]. Itraconazole also has excellent anti-*Candida* activity, is more effective in vitro than fluconazole against the endemic fungi, *H. capsulatum, S. schenckii*, and *B dermatitidis* and has fungistatic activity against *Aspergillus* [26]. Voriconazole has up to 60-fold lower minimum inhibitory concentrations for *Candida* species (including resistant strains) than fluconazole, is fungicidal for *Aspergillus* and has some activity against *Fusarium* species and *Scedosporium apiospermum* [26]. None of the triazoles are active against the Zygomycetes.

In general, azole drugs are better tolerated than the amphotericin B formulations. Side effects of fluconazole, which are uncommon, include rash and elevations in liver function test results. In patients who receive prolonged courses of high-dose therapy, reversible alopecia and dry lips can occur. Potential side effects of itraconazole include peripheral edema, exacerbation of congestive heart failure (caused by a negative inotropic effect), hypokalemia, or rash [26]. Reported toxicities of voriconazole include elevations in liver function test results, rash, photosensitivity, and transient ocular toxicity, a unique phenomenon that has been studied extensively. The following visual disturbances have been described: blurred vision, photophobia, altered color vision, and perception of increased brightness of light. Up to one third of patients treated with voriconazole have describes such visual disturbances, which typically occur early in the course of therapy, begin 15–30 minutes after a dose, and resolve within 30 minutes [26]. No histopathologic changes have been seen in the retinas of treated patients, and there have been no permanent sequelae of voriconzole induced visual disturbances [26].

Because these azole drugs are metabolized by the hepatic cytochrome P450 system, a variety of interactions can occur between these agents and other medications, The azoles inhibit the metabolism of the sulfonyureasm warfarin, digoxin, phenytoin, cyclosporine, sirolimus, tacrolimus, omeprazole, and cisapride, resulting in increased serum concentrations of these medications and the potential for drug toxicity. Conversely, serum concentrations of the triazoles are decreased by rifampin, isoniazid, phenytoin, and fosphenytoin, as well as carbamazepine [39].

## Echinocandin antifungals

Caspofungin, an echinocandin antifungal, inhibits formation of ß 1, 3 glucan of the fungal cell wall. Caspofungin is effective in vitro against *Candida* species, including azole resistant isolates, and *Aspergillus* species.

Caspofungin therapy is usually well tolerated. Rash or GI toxicity occurs rarely. There are relatively few drug-drug interactions with caspofungin, which is neither an inducer nor an inibitor of the cytochrome P450 system. Caspofungin does reduce the area under the curve and peak serum concentrations of tacrolimus by 20% to 25%, so tacrolimus serum concentrations should be monitored in patients taking caspofungin [26]. Cyclosporin increases the area under the curve of caspofungin by 35% [26]. It is suggested that caspofungin and cyclosporine not be co-administered.

## Nucleoside analog antifungal (Flucytosine)

Flucytosine, the only available nucleoside analog, acts as an antifungal by disrupting pyrimidine metabolism in the fungal cell nucleus. Flucytosine is fungicidal in vitro against *Candida* species and *C. neoformans* but not against other commonly encountered fungi. Unfortunately, resistance emerges rapidly during flucytosine montherapy, so use of this drug s limited to combination therapy [26].

Flucytosine can cause bone marrow suppression and GI toxicity, although these side effects are seen less frequently with the current recommended dosage (100 mg/kg/day in 4 divided doses) than with the higher dosage that was used for many years (150 mg/kg/day in 4 divided doses). Flucytosine does not have any significant drug interactions.

## Conclusion

Current techniques of burn patient management and burn wound care have reduced not only the incidence of invasive burn wound infections but also the occurrence of all infections in burn patients. Even so, infection in sites other than the burn wound, principally the lungs, remains the most common cause of death in burn patients [40]. The use of effective topical antimicrobial therapy, early burn wound excision, the availability of effective biologic dressings, the wound monitoring and surveillance program described above, and the overall improvements in the care of critically ill patients over the past four decades have each made a contribution to the reduction in morbidity and the improved survival of burn patients, including those who develop infections.

## References

[1]  Murray CK (2007) Infections in burns. J Trauma 62 [6 Suppl]: S73

[2]  Singer AJ, Brebbia J, Soroff HH (2007) Management of local burn wounds in the ED. Am J Emerg Med 25(6): 666–671

[3]  Jackson DM (1953) [The diagnosis of the depth of burning.]. Br J Surg 40(164): 588–596

[4]  Pruitt BA, Jr, Lindberg RB, McManus WF, Mason AD, Jr (1983) Current approach to prevention and treatment of Pseudomonas aeruginosa infections in burned patients. Rev Infect Dis 5 [Suppl 5]: S889–897

[5] Pruitt BA, Jr (1984) The diagnosis and treatment of infection in the burn patient. Burns Incl Therm Inj 11(2): 79–91

[6] Foley FD, Greenawald KA, Nash G, Pruitt BA, Jr (1970) Herpesvirus infection in burned patients. N Engl J Med 282(12): 652–656

[7] McManus AT, Kim SH, McManus WF, Mason AD, Jr, Pruitt BA, Jr (1987) Comparison of quantitative microbiology and histopathology in divided burn-wound biopsy specimens. Arch Surg 122(1): 74–76

[8] Pruitt BA, Jr, McManus AT, Kim SH, Goodwin CW (1998) Burn wound infections: current status. World J Surg 22(2): 135–145

[9] Hamory BH (1989) Nosocomial sepsis related to intravascular access. Crit Care Nurs Q 11(4): 58–65

[10] Samsoondar W, Freeman JB, Coultish I, Oxley C (1985) Colonization of intravascular catheters in the intensive care unit. Am J Surg 149(6): 730–732

[11] Maki DG, Jarrett F, Sarafin HW (1977) A semiquantitative culture method for identification of catheter-related infection in the burn patient. J Surg Res 22(5): 513–520

[12] Franceschi D, Gerding RL, Phillips G, Fratianne RB (1989) Risk factors associated with intravascular catheter infections in burned patients: a prospective, randomized study. J Trauma 29(6): 811–816

[13] Smallman L, Burdon DW, Alexander-Williams J (1980) The effect of skin preparation and care on the incidence of superficial thrombophlebitis. Br J Surg 67(12): 861–862

[14] Ramzy PI, Herndon DN, Wolf SE, Irtun O, Barret JP, Ramirez RJ et al (1998) Comparison of wound culture and bronchial lavage in the severely burned child: implications for antimicrobial therapy. Arch Surg 133(12): 1275–1280

[15] Calandra T, Cohen J (2005) The international sepsis forum consensus conference on definitions of infection in the intensive care unit. Crit Care Med 33(7): 1538–1548

[16] Pruitt BA, Jr (1990) Infection and the burn patient. Br J Surg 77(10): 1081–1082

[17] Greenhalgh DG, Saffle JR, Holmes JH 4th, Gamelli RL, Palmieri TL, Horton JW et al (2007) American Burn Association Consensus Conference to Define Sepsis and Infection in Burns. J Burn Care Res 28(6): 776–780

[18] Hart DW, Wolf SE, Chinkes DL, Gore DC, Mlcak RP, Beauford RB et al (2000) Determinants of skeletal muscle catabolism after severe burn. Ann Surg 232(4): 455–465

[19] Pham TN, Warren AJ, Phan HH, Molitor F, Greenhalgh DG, Palmieri TL (2005) Impact of tight glycemic control in severely burned children. J Trauma 59(5): 1148–1154

[20] Edwards-Jones V, Greenwood JE (2003) What's new in burn microbiology? James Laing Memorial Prize Essay 2000. Burns 29(1): 15–24

[21] Mayhall CG (2003) The epidemiology of burn wound infections: then and now. Clin Infect Dis 37(4): 543–550

[22] Murray PR, BAron EJ, Jorgensen JH et al (2003) Manual of clinical microbiology. 8th ed. ASM, Washington, DC

[23] Robson MC (1979) Bacterial control in the burn wound. Clin Plast Surg 6(4): 515–522

[24] Baron S (1996) Medical microbiology, 4th edn. University of Texas Medical Branch, Galveston, Texas

[25] Becker WK, Cioffi WG, Jr, McManus AT, Kim SH, McManus WF, Mason AD et al (1991) Fungal burn wound infection. A 10-year experience. Arch Surg 126(1): 44–48

[26] Woods GLaG, Y (1993) Diagnostic pathology of infectious diseases, 1st edn. Lea & Febiger, Malvern, Pennsylvania

[27] Mandell GL, Bennett, JE, Dolin R (2004) Principles and practice of infectious diseases, 6th edn. Churchill Livingstone, New York

[28] Koneman EW, Allen SD, Janda WM, Schrekenberger C, Winn WC (1997) Color atlas and textbook of diagnostic microbiology, 5th edn. Lippincott-Raven Publishers, Philadelphia, Pennsylvania

[29] Sheridan RL (2005) Sepsis in pediatric burn patients. Pediatr Crit Care Med 6[3 Suppl]: S112–129

[30] Spebar MJ, Pruitt BA, Jr (1981) Candidiasis in the burned patient. J Trauma 21(3): 237–239

[31] Kates SG, McGinley KJ, Larson EL, Leyden JJ (1991) Indigenous multiresistant bacteria from flowers in hospital and nonhospital environments. Am J Infect Control 19(3): 156–161

[32] McEvoy GK (2003) American Hospital Formulary Service. In: Bethesda MD (ed) American Society of Health-System Pharmacists: American Society of Health-System Pharmacists

[33] Rybak MJ (2006) The pharmacokinetic and pharmacodynamic properties of vancomycin. Clin Infect Dis 42 [Suppl 1]: S35–39

[34] Gallagher JJ W-BN, Villarreal C et al (2007) Treatment of infection in burns. In: Herndon DN (ed) Total burn care, 3rd edn. WB Saunders, Philadelphia, pp 136–176

[35] Evans ME, Feola DJ, Rapp RP (1999) Polymyxin B sulfate and colistin: old antibiotics for emerging multiresistant gram-negative bacteria. Ann Pharmacother 33(9): 960–9967

[36] Storm DR, Rosenthal KS, Swanson PE (1977) Polymyxin and related peptide antibiotics. Annu Rev Biochem 46: 723–763

[37] Nord NM, Hoeprich PD (1964) Polymyxin B and Colistin. A critical comparison. N Engl J Med 270: 1030–1035

[38] Branski LK, Al-Mousawi A, Rivero H, Jeschke MG, Sanford AP, Herndon DN (2009) Emerging infections in burns. Surg Infect (Larchmt) 10(5): 389–397

[39] Lacy CF, Armstrong LL, Goldman MP, Lance LL (2003) Drug information handbook. 11 edn. Lexi-Comp Inc., Hudson, OH

[40] Pruitt BA, Jr, McManus AT (1992) The changing epidemiology of infection in burn patients. World J Surg 16(1): 57–67

Correspondence: Gerd G. Gauglitz, M.D., MMS, Department of Dermatology and Allergy, Ludwig-Maximilians-University Munich, Frauenlobstraße 9–11, 80337 Munich, Germany, E-mail: Gerd.Gauglitz@med.uni-muenchen.de

# Acute treatment of severely burned pediatric patients

Gerd G. Gauglitz[1,3], Marc G. Jeschke[2]

[1]Shriners Hospitals for Children, University of Texas Medical Branch Galveston, TX, USA
[2]Ross Tilley Burn Centre, Sunnybrook Health Sciences Centre, Department of Surgery, Division of Plastic Surgery, University of Toronto, ON, Canada
[3]Department of Dermatology and Allergy, Ludwig Maximilians University, Munich, Germany

## Introduction

Over 440 000 children receive medical attention for burn injuries each year in the US [1]. Children younger than 14 years of age account for nearly half of all emergency department–treated thermal burns [2]. With approximately 1100 children dying of burn-related injuries in the United States every year [2] severe burns represent the third most common cause of death in the pediatric patient population [3] and account for a significant number of hospital admissions in the United States [2, 4]. The devastating consequences of burns have been recognized by the medical community and significant amounts of resources and research have been dedicated, successfully improving these dismal statistics: Recent reports revealed a dramatic decline in burn-related deaths and hospital admissions in the USA over the last 20 years; mainly due to effective prevention strategies, decreasing the number and severity of burns [5–7]. Advances in therapy strategies, based on improved understanding of resuscitation, more appropriate infection control and improved treatment of inhalation injury, enhanced wound coverage and better support of hypermetabolic response to injury, have further improved the clinical outcome of this unique patient population over the past years. While other chapters within this book mostly summarize the general treatment of burn victims, this article is focusing on current and emerging therapeutic strategies for the acute treatment of severely burned pediatric patients.

## Initial management of the burned child

In general, initial management of the burned child should be the same as for any other burn or trauma patient, with special attention directed to the airway, breathing, circulation and cervical spine immobilization according to the guidelines of the American College of Surgeons Committee on Trauma and the Advanced Trauma Live Support Center [8]. The algorithms for trauma evaluation should be diligently applied to the burn patient and the primary survey begins with the ABCs (airway, breathing, circulation) and the establishment of an adequate airway as described elsewhere in this book [9]. Note worth to mention is to provide adequate pain control and relieve the patient from pain and stress. Pain medications should be carefully administered not to overdose and induce adverse side effects. In addition, the amount of pain medication should be reasonable and be based on the burn size and subjective pain of the patient [10]. Dosing of pain medication needs to be according to pediatric guidelines.

## Fluid resuscitation

Severe burn causes significant hemodynamic changes, which must be managed carefully to optimize intravascular volume, maintain end-organ tissue perfusion and maximize oxygen delivery to tissues [11]. Massive fluid shifts after severe burn injury result in the sequestration of fluid in both burned and non-burned tissue [12]. Release of pro-inflammatory mediators early post-burn, such as histamine, bradykinin and leukotriene leads to increased microvascular permeability, generalized edema and burn shock, a leading cause for mortality in severely burned patients [13–15]. Early and accurate fluid resuscitation of patients with major burns is thus critical for survival [16]. Calculations of fluid requirements are based on the amount of body surface involved in second or third degree burns (not first degree burns). The "Rule of Nines" (Fig. 1a) is commonly utilized to estimate the body surface area burned, but this does have limitations in the pediatric patient population where the head is proportionally larger than the body when compared to the adult. A more accurate assessment can be made of the burn injury, especially in children, by using the Lund and Browder chart, which takes into account changes brought about by growth (Fig. 1b). Many different fluid resuscitation formulas have been suggested, each of which can be used effectively to resuscitate a severe burn. The various formulas differ in the amount of crystalloid and colloid to be given, as well as in the tonicity of the fluid [11]. The American burn association has recently published practice guidelines on burn shock resuscitation in order to review the principles of resuscitation after burn injury, including type and rate of fluid administration, and the use of adjunct measures. It presents an excellent approach for the initial treatment of burn patients [17]. However, it is important to mention that there is no formula that will accurately predict the volume requirements of the individual patient: all resuscitation formulas are designed to serve as a guide only. The modified Brooke and Parkland (Baxter) formulas are the most commonly used early resuscitation formulas throughout the world [18]. They use 2–4 ml/kg/%BSA burn of Lactated Ringers solution respectively. The calculated needs are for the total fluids to be given over 24h [15]. In children, maintenance require-

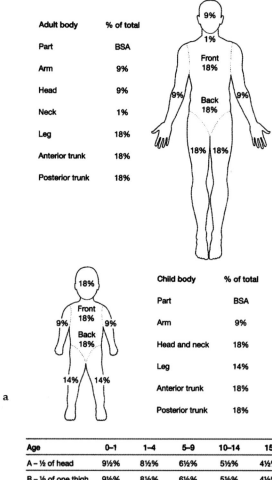

a

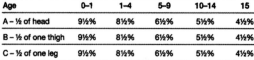

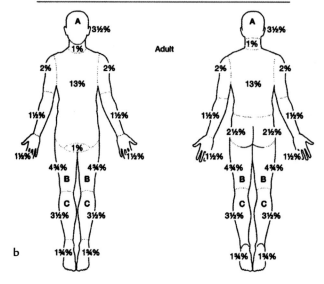

b

**Fig. 1.** a Estimation of burn size utilizing the rule-of-nines. b Estimation of burn size utilizing the Lund and Browder method

242

ments must be added to the resuscitation formula. For this reason, we recommend the Shriners Burns Hospital SBH-Galveston Formula, which calls for initial resuscitation with 5 000 ml/m² BSA burn/d + 2 000 ml/m² BSA/d of Lactated Ringers solution [19]. For both formulas, the first half is administered within the first 8 hours after the burn, and one-quarter in each of the next 16 hours. Intra-vascular volume status must be still reevaluated on a frequent basis during the acute phase. Fluid balance during burn shock resuscitation is typically measured by hourly urine output via an indwelling urethral catheter. It has been recommended to maintain urine output of approximately 0.5 cc/kg/h in adults [20] and between 0.5 and 1.0 ml/kg/h in patients weighing less than 30 kg [21], however, there have been no clinical studies identifying the optimal hourly urine output to maintain vital organ perfusion during burn shock resuscitation. Diuretics are generally not indicated during the acute resuscitation period. It is imperative to avoid over-aggressive resuscitation, particularly in small children under 4 years of age, which may potentially lead to increased extravascular hydrostatic pressure and pulmonary edema [22]. This is especially important in patients who have a concomitant inhalation injury, because they will also have increased pulmonary vascular permeability. Patients with high voltage electrical burns and crash injuries with myoglobin and/or hemoglobin in the urine have an increased risk of renal tubular obstruction. Therefore in these patients sodium bicarbonate should be added to IV fluids to alkalinize the urine, and urine output should be maintained at 1 and 2 cc/kg/h as long as these pigments are in the urine [23]. The addition of an osmotic diuretic such as mannitol may be needed to assist in clearing the urine of these pigments. Because large volumes of fluid and electrolytes are administered both initially and throughout the course of resuscitation, it is important to obtain baseline laboratory measurements of complete blood count, electrolytes, glucose, albumin, and acid-base balance [24]. Crystalloid, in particular lactated Ringer's solution, is the most popular resuscitation fluid currently utilized [19]. Proponents of the use of crystalloid solutions alone for resuscitation report that other solutions, specifically colloids, are not better and are certainly more expensive than crystalloids for maintaining intravascular vol-

ume following burn trauma [25]. Perel and Roberts identified 63 trials comparing colloid and crystalloid fluid resuscitation across a wide variety of clinical conditions and found no improvement in survival when resuscitated with colloids [26]. The use of albumin in burns and critically ill patients has recently been challenged by the Cochrane Central Register of Controlled Trials, which demonstrated no evidence that albumin reduces mortality in this particular patient population when compared with cheaper alternatives such as saline [27]. Vincent et al. showed in a cohort, multicenter, observational study that albumin administration was associated with decreased survival in a population of acutely ill patients when compared to those who did not receive any albumin at any time throughout their ICU stay. It is noteworthy that in this study albumin receiving patients were more severely ill than patients who did not receive any albumin [28]. Even though, most burn surgeons agree that burn patients with very low serum albumin during burn shock may benefit from albumin supplementation to maintain oncotic pressure [29].

## Sepsis

Sepsis is one of the leading causes of morbidity and mortality in critically ill patients [30]. Severely burned patients are markedly susceptible to a variety of infectious complications [31]. There are excellent criteria (fever, tachycardia, tachypnea, leukocytosis) for the diagnosis of infection and sepsis in most patients, however, the standard diagnoses for infection and sepsis do not really apply to burn patients, since these patients, according to the definitions of the ABA Consensus Conference to Define Sepsis and Infection in Burns, already suffer from a systemic inflammatory response syndrome (SIRS) due to their extensive burn wounds [32]. Consequently, experts in the field of burn care and/or research establish definitions and guidelines for the diagnosis and treatments of wound infection and sepsis in burns [Greenhalgh, 2007 #88]. However, it is important to realize that these definitions are sensitive but not specific screening tools to be used primarily for research purposes, and any direct application to the clinical setting must take into account the dynamic and continuous nature of the sepsis disease process and the static and categorical nature of the definitions. In addition, clinical parameters used to define SIRS and organ dysfunction are greatly affected by the normal physiologic changes that occur as children develop [33]. A description of pediatric-specific definitions for SIRS, sepsis, severe sepsis, and septic shock based on age-specific risks for invasive infections, age-specific antibiotic treatment recommendations, and developmental cardiorespiratory physiologic changes has been recently published by Goldstein et al. [34] and are summarized in Tables 1 and 2.

## Inhalation injury

Even though mortality from major burns has significantly decreased during the past 20 years, inhalation injury still constitutes one of the most critical concomitant injuries following thermal insult. Approximately 80% of fire-related deaths result not from burns but from inhalation of the toxic products of combustion and inhalation injury has remained associated with an overall mortality rate of 25% to 50% when patients require ventilator support for more than one week following injury [35, 36]. Early diagnosis of bronchopulmonary injury is thus critical fior survival and is conducted primarily clinically, based on a history of closed-space exposure, facial burns and carbonaceous debris in mouth, pharynx or sputum [37]. Evidenced based experience on diagnosis of inhalation injury, however, is rare. Chest X-rays are routinely normal until complications, such as infections have developed. The standard diagnostic method should be therefore bronchoscopy of the upper airway of every burn patient. Gamelli et al. established a grading system of inhalation injury (0, 1, 2, 3, and 4) derived from findings at initial bronchoscopy and based on Abbreviatcd Injury Score (AIS) criteria [38]. Bronchoscopic criteria that are consistent with inhalation injury included airway edema, inflammation, mucosal necrosis, presence of soot and charring in the airway, tissue sloughing or carbonaceous material in the airway. The treatment of inhalation injury should start immediately with the administration of 100% oxygen via face mask or nasal cannula. Maintenance of the airway is critical. As

**Table 1.** Definitions of systemic inflammatory response syndrome (SIRS), infection, sepsis, severe sepsis, and septic shock [32, 34]

| SIRS[1] |
|---|
| The presence of at least two of the following four criteria, **one of which must be abnormal temperature or leukocyte count:**<br>▶ Core[2] temperature of > 38.5 °C or > 36 °C.<br>▶ Tachycardia, defined as a mean heart rate > 2 SD above normal for age in the absence of external stimulus, chronic drugs, or painful stimuli; or otherwise unexplained persistent elevation over a 0.5- to 4-hr time period **OR for children > 1 yr old: bradycardia, defined as a mean heart rate > 10th percentile for age in the absence of external vagal stimulus, β-blocker drugs, or congenital heart disease; or otherwise unexplained persistent depression over a 0.5-hr time period.**<br>▶ Mean respiratory rate > 2 SD above normal for age or mechanical ventilation for an acute process not related to underlying neuromuscular disease or the receipt of general anesthesia.<br>▶ Leukocyte count elevated or depressed for age (not secondary to chemotherapy-induced leukopenia) or > 10% immature neutrophils. |

| Infection |
|---|
| A suspected or proven (by positive culture, tissue stain, or polymerase chain reaction test) infection caused by any pathogen OR a clinical syndrome associated with a high probability of infection. Evidence of infection includes positive findings on clinical exam, imaging, or laboratory tests (e. g. white blood cells in a normally sterile body fluid, perforated viscus, chest radiograph consistent with pneumonia, petechial or purpuric rash, or purpura fulminans) |

| Sepsis |
|---|
| SIRS in the presence of or as a result of suspected or proven infection. |

| Severe sepsis |
|---|
| **Sepsis plus one of the following: cardiovascular organ dysfunction OR acute respiratory distress syndrome OR two or more other organ dysfunctions. Organ dysfunctions are defined in Table 4.** |

| Septic shock |
|---|
| Sepsis **and cardiovascular organ dysfunction as defined in Table 4.** |

Modifications from the adult definitions are highlighted in boldface.
[1]See Table 2 for age-specific ranges for physiologic and laboratory variables
[2]Core temperature must be measured by rectal, bladder, oral, or central catheter probe

**Table 2.** Age-specific vital signs and laboratory variables (lower values for heart rate, leukocyte count, and systolic blood pressure are for the 5th and upper values for heart rate, respiration rate, or leukocyte count for the 95th percentile, [34])

| Age group | Heart Rate, Beats/Min | | Respiratory Rate, Breaths/Min | Leukocyte Count, Leukocytes × $10^3$/ mm$^3$ | Systolic Blood Tachycardia Bradycardia Pressure, mm Hg |
|---|---|---|---|---|---|
| | Tachycardia | Bradycardia | | | |
| Newborn: 0 days to 1 wk | >180 | >100 | >50 | >34 | > 65 |
| Neonate: 1 wk to 1 mo | >180 | >100 | >40 | >19.5 or>5 | > 75 |
| Infant: 1 mo to 1 yr | >180 | > 90 | >34 | >17.5 or>5 | >100 |
| Toddler and preschool: 2–5 yrs | >140 | N/A | >22 | >15.5 or>6 | > 94 |
| School age child: 6–12 yrs | >130 | N/A | >18 | >13.5 or>4.5 | >105 |
| Adolescent and young adult: 13 to >18 yrs | >110 | N/A | >14 | >11 or>4.5 | >117 |

NA, not applicable

mentioned above, if early evidence of upper airway edema is present, early intubation is required because the upper airway edema normally increases over 9 to 12 h. Prophylactic intubation without good indication however should not be performed.

Advances in ventilator technology and treatment of inhalation injury have resulted in some improvement in mortality. A multi-center, randomized trial in patients with acute lung injury and acute respiratory distress syndrome showed that mechanical ventilation with a lower tidal volume than traditionally utilized, resulted in decreased mortality and increased the number of days without ventilator use [39]. Pruitt's group showed that since the advent of high-frequency ventilation, mortality has decreased to 29% from 41% reported in an earlier study [40]. Management of inhalation injury consists of ventilatory support, aggressive pulmonary toilet, bronchoscopic removal of casts, and nebulization therapy [11]. Nebulization therapy can consist of heparin, α-mimetics, or polymyxin B and is applied between 2–6 times a day. Pressure-control ventilation with permissive hypercapnia is a useful strategy in the management of these patients and P $CO_2$ levels of as much as 60 mm Hg can be well tolerated if arrived at gradually. Prophylactic antibiotics are not indicated, but imperative with documented lung infections. Clinical diagnosis of pneumonia includes two of the following [32]: Chest x-ray revealing a new and persistent infiltrate, consolidation, or cavitation; sepsis (as defined in Table 3) and/or a recent change in sputum or purulence in the sputum, as well as quantitative culture. Clinical diagnosis can be modified after utilizing microbiologic data three categories according to the "American Burn Association Consensus Conference to Define Sepsis and Infection in Burns" [32]. Empiric choices for the treatment of pneumonia prior to culture results, should include coverage of methicillin-resistant *Staphylococcus aureus* and gram-negative organisms such as Pseudomonas and Klebsiella [41].

## Burn wound excision

Methods for handling burn wounds have changed in recent decades and are similar in adults and children. Early excision and closure of the burn wound has been probably the single greatest advancement in the treating patients with severe thermal injuries during the last twenty years; leading to substantially reduced resting energy requirements, subsequent improvement of mortality rates and substantially lower costs in this particular patient population [11, 42–45]. Early wound closure has been furthermore found to be associated with decreased severity of hypertrophic scarring, joint contractures and stiffness, and promotes quicker rehabilitation [11, 42].

Techniques of burn-wound excision have envolved substantially over the past decade. In general most areas are excised with a hand skin graft knife or powered dermatome. Sharp excision with a knife or electrocautery is reserved for areas of functional cosmetic importance such as hand and face. In partial

**Table 3.** Formulas for estimating caloric requirements in pediatric burn patients

| Formula | Sex/Age (years) | Equation (Daily Requirement in kcal) |
|---|---|---|
| WHO (155) | **Males** | |
| | 0–3 | $(60.9 \times W) - 54$ |
| | 3–10 | $(22.7 \times W) + 495$ |
| | 10–18 | $(17.5 \times W) + 651$ |
| | **Females** | |
| | 0–3 | $(61.0 \times W) - 51$ |
| | 3–10 | $(22.5 \times W) + 499$ |
| | 10–18 | $(12.2 \times W) + 746$ |
| RDA (156) | 0–6 months | $108 \times W$ |
| | 6 months–1 year | $98 \times W$ |
| | 1–3 | $102 \times W$ |
| | 4–10 | $90 \times W$ |
| | 11–14 | $55 \times W$ |
| Curreri junior (157) | >1 | $RDA + (15 \times \%BSAB)$ |
| | 1–3 | $RDA + (25 \times \%BSAB)$ |
| | 4–15 | $RDA + (40 \times \%BSAB)$ |
| Galveston infant (158) | 0–1 | $2\,100 \text{ kcal/m2 BSA} + 1\,000 \text{ kcal/m}^2 \text{ BSAB}$ |
| Galveston revised (75) | 1–11 | $1\,800 \text{ kcal/m2 BSA} + 1\,300 \text{ kcal/m}^2 \text{ BSAB}$ |
| Galveston adolescent (159) | 12+ | $1\,500 \text{ kcal/m2 BSA} + 1\,500 \text{ kcal/m}^2 \text{ BSAB}$ |

WHO = World Health Organization
RDA = Recommended Dietary Allowance (US)
BSA = Body Surface area

%BSAB = Percentage of Total Body Surface area Burned
BSAB = Body surface area Burned

thickness wounds an attempt is being made to preserve viable dermis, where as in full thickness injury all necrotic and infected tissue must be removed leaving a viable wound bed of either fascia, fat or muscle [46]. The following techniques are mainly utilized:

Tangential excision. This technique first described Janzekovic in the 1970s requires repeated shaving of deep dermal partial thickness burns using a Braithwaite, Watson or Goulian or dermatome set at depth 5–10/1,000 inch until a viable dermal bed is reached, which is manifested clinically by punctuate bleeding from the dermal wound bed [46].

Full thickness excision. A hand knife such as the Watson or powered dermatome is set at at 15–30/1,000 inch and serial passes are made excising the full thickness wound. Excision is aided by traction on the excised eschar as it passes through the knife or dermatome. Adequate excision is signaled by a viable bleeding wound bed, which is usually fat [46].

Fascial excisison. This technique is reserved for burn extending down to through the fat into muscle, where the patient presents late with large infected wounds and inpatients with life-threatening invasive fungal infections. It involves surgical excision of the full thickness of the integument including the subcutaneous fat down to the fascia using Goulian knives and number 11 blades. Unfortunately, fascial excision is mutilating and leaves a permanent contour defect, which is near impossible to reconstruct. Lymphatic channels are excised in this technique and peripheral lymphyedema may develop [46].

Most patients can be managed with layered excisions that optimize later appearance and function. Published estimates of the amount of bleeding associated with these operations range within 3.5 to 5% of the blood volume for every 1% of the body surface excised [47, 48]. The control of blood loss is one of the main determinants for outcome [49]. Therefore several techniques should be applied to control blood loss. Local application of fibrin or thrombin spray, topical application of epinephrine 1:10 000–1:20 000, epinephrine soaked lab-pads (1:40 000), and immediate electrocautery of the blood vessel can control blood loss [50]. The use of a sterilized tourniquet can also limit blood loss [51]. Lastly, pre-excisional tumescence with epinephrine saline can be used on trunk, back, extremities, but not fingers.

## Burn wound coverage

Various biological and synthetic substrates have been employed to replace the injured skin post-burn. Autografts from uninjured skin remains the mainstay of treatment for many patients. Since early wound closure using autograft may be difficult when full-thickness burns exceed 40% total body surface area (TBSA), allografts (cadaver skin) frequently serve as skin substitute in severely burned patients. While this approach is still commonly used in burn centers throughout the world, it bears considerable risks, including antigenicity, cross-infection as well as limited availability [52]. Xenografts have been used for hundreds of years as temporary replacement for skin loss. Even though these grafts provide a biologically active dermal matrix, the immunologic disparities prevent engraftment and predetermine rejection over time [53]. However, both xenografts and allografts are only a mean of temporary burn wound cover. True closure can only be achieved with living autografts or isografts. But the widespread use of cultured autografts is frequently hampered by poor long term clinical results, exorbitant costs and fragility and difficult handling of these grafts [53–55]. Alternatively, dermal analogs have been made available for clinical use in recent years. Integra© was approved by the United States Food and Drug administration for use in life-threatening burns and has been successfully utilized in immediate and delayed closure of full-thickness burns, leading to reduction in length of hospital stay, favorable cosmetics, and improved functional outcome in a prospective and controlled clinical study [56–59]. Our group recently conducted a randomized clinical trial utilizing Integra™ in the management of severe full-thickness burns of ≥50% TBSA in a pediatric patient population comparing it to standard autograft-allograft technique, and found Integra© to be associated with attenuated hepatic dysfunction, improved resting energy expenditure and improved aesthetic outcome post-burn [60]. Alloderm™, an acellular human dermal allograft, has been advocated for the management of acute burns. Small clinical series and case reports suggest that Alloderm™ may be useful in the treatment of acute burns [61–64]. Tissue engineering technology is advancing rapidly. Fetal constructs have recently been successfully trialed by Hohlfeld et al. [65] and the bilaminar skin substitute of Boyce [66] is now routine in clinical use and promise spectacular results [50]. Advances in stem cell culture technology are expected to deliver full cosmetic restoration for burn patients [67].

## Metabolic response and nutritional support

The response to burn injury, known as hypermetabolism, occurs most dramatically following severe burn its modulation constitute an ongoing challenge for successful burn treatment [68]. Increases in oxygen consumption, metabolic rate, urinary nitrogen excretion, lipolysis and weight loss are directly proportional to the size of the burn [69]. Metabolic rates of burned children can dramatically exceed those of other critical care or trauma patients and cause marked wasting of lean body mass within days after injury [10]. Failure to circumvent the subsequent large energy and protein requirements may result in impaired wound healing, organ dysfunction, susceptibility to infection and death [70]. Thus, adequate nutrition is imperative for the treatment of severely burned patients. Due to the significant increase in energy expenditure post-burn, high-calorie nutritional support was thought to decrease muscle metabolism [71]. However, a randomized, double blinded, prospective study performed by our group found that aggressive high-calorie feeding with a combination of enteral and parenteral nutrition was associated with increased mortality [72]. Most authors therefore recommend adequate calorie intake via early enteral feeding and avoidance of overfeeding to attenuate the catabolic response after injury [10, 11]. Different formulations have been developed to address the specific energy requirements of burned adult and pediatric patients [73–75]. In children, formulas based on body surface area are more appropriate because of the greater body surface area per kilogram. The formulas change with age based on the body surface area alterations that occur with growth (Table 3).

247

Since essential fatty acid deficiency is a well-documented complication in hospital patients receiving long-term nutritional supplements, most intensive care units (ICUs) provide a significant amount of caloric requirements as fat [76]. This has been shown to reduce the requirements for carbohydrates and can improve glucose tolerance significantly, which is often altered in the patient post-burn [70]. However, several studies showed that increased fat administration may lead to increased complications, including hyperlipidemia, hypoxemia, fatty liver infiltration, higher incidence of infection and higher postoperative mortality rates in the burned patient population [77–79]. We found in a large cohort of severely burned children that patients receiving a low fat/high carbohydrate diet (Vivonex® T. E. N.) displayed a significantly lower incidence of hepatic fatty metamorphosis upon autopsy when compared to milk fed patients. These patients furthermore displayed a significantly lower incidence of sepsis when compared to children receiving a high fat diet, demonstrated prolonged survival and had significantly shorter stays in the ICU as well as markedly decreased length of stay in the ICU per % TBSA. Based on these findings, we would recommend that nutritional regimes for treatment of post-burn patients include diets with a significantly reduced proportion of fat as the source of total caloric intake.

In addition, various vitamins, minerals and other micronutrients are required for nutrition following burns. Diminished gastrointestinal absorption, increased urinary losses, altered distribution and altered carrier protein concentrations following severe burn may lead to a deficiency in many micronutrients if not supplemented. These deficiencies in trace elements and vitamins (Cu, Fe, Se, Zn, vitamins C and E) have been repeatedly described in major burns since 1960 [80–82], leading to infectious complications, delayed wound healing and stunting in children [83]. However, evidence-based practice guidelines are currently unavailable for the assessment and provision of micronutrients in burn patients. Enhancing trace element status and antioxidant defences by selenium, zinc, and copper supplementation has been shown to decrease the incidence of nosocomial pneumonia in critically ill, severely burned children in two consecutive, ran-

domised, double-blinded, supplementation trials [84]. Caution should be used to avoid toxicities that can result in gastrointestinal tolerance as well as antagonistic reactions. A complete listing of micronutrients, their functions and supplementation protocols is beyond the scope of this chapter; excellent reviews are available [85–87].

## Modulation of the hormonal and endocrine response

Severe burn injury leads to significant metabolic alterations, characterized by a hyperdynamic circulatory response associated with increased body temperature, glycolysis, proteolysis, lipolysis and futile substrate cycling [88–90]. These responses are present in all trauma, surgical, or critically ill patients, but the severity, length and magnitude is unique for burn patients [10]. Modification of adverse components of the hypermetabolic response, particularly protein catabolism, seems desirable. Recombinant growth hormone, insulin-like growth factor, anabolic steroids, beta-adrenergic blockade and beta-adrenergic supplementation are under active investigation.

### Recombinant human growth hormone

Daily intramuscular administration of recombinant human growth hormone (rhGH) at doses of 0.2 mg/kg as a daily injection during acute burn care has favorably influenced the hepatic acute phase response [91, 92], increased serum concentrations of its secondary mediator IGF-I [93], improved muscle protein kinetics, maintained muscular growth [94, 95], decreased donor site healing time by 1.5 days [96], improved resting energy expenditure and decreased cardiac output [97]. These beneficial effects of rhGH are mediated by insulin-like growth factor (IGF)-I and patients receiving treatment, demonstrated 100 % increases in serum IGF-I and IGF-binding protein (IGFBP)-3 relative to healthy individuals [98, 99]. However, in a prospective, multicenter, double-blind, randomized, placebo-controlled trial involving 247 patients and 285 critically ill non-burned patients Takala et al. found that high doses of rhGH (0.10 +/− 0.02 mg/kg BW) were associated with increased morbidity and mortality [99]. Others demonstrated growth hormone treatment to be associated with hyperglycemia and insulin resistance [100, 101]. However, neither short nor long-term administration of rhGH was associated with an increase in mortality in severely burned children [97, 102].

## Insulin-like growth factor

Because IGF-I mediates the effects of GH, the infusion of equimolar doses of recombinant human IGF-1 and IGFBP-3 to burned patients has been demonstrated to effectively improve protein metabolism in catabolic pediatric subjects and adults with significantly less hypoglycemia than rhGH itself [103, 104]. It attenuates muscle catabolism and improves gut mucosal integrity in children with serious burns [104]. Immune function is effectively improved by attenuation of the type 1 and type 2 hepatic acute phase responses, increased serum concentrations of constitutive proteins, and vulnerary modulation of the hypercatabolic use of body protein [104–107]. However, studies by van den Berghe et al. [108] indicate the use of IGF-1 alone is not effective in critically ill patients without burns.

## Oxandrolone

Treatment with anabolic agents such as oxandralone, a testosterone analog which possesses only 5% of its virilizing androgenic effects, improves muscle protein catabolism via enhanced protein synthesis efficiency [109], reduce weight loss and increases donor site wound healing [110]. In a prospective randominized study Wolf et al. demonstrated that administration of 10 mg of oxandralone every 12 hours decreased hospital stay [111]. In a large prospective, double-blinded, randomized single-center study, oxandrolone given at a dose of 0.1 mg/kg every 12 hours shortened length of acute hospital stay, maintained LBM and improved body composition and hepatic protein synthesis [112]. The effects were independent of age [113]. Long-term treatment with this oral anabolic during rehabilitation in the outpatient setting is more favorably regarded by pediatric subjects then parenteral anabolic agents. Oxandrolone successfully abates the effects of burn asso-

ciated hypermetabolism on body tissues and significantly increases body mass over time, lean body mass at 6, 9, and 12 months after burn, and bone mineral content by 12 months after injury vs unburned controls [114]. Patients treated with oxandrolone show few complications relative to those treated with rHGH. However, it must be noted that although anabolic agents can increase lean body mass, exercise is essential to developing strength [115].

## Propranolol

Beta-adrenergic blockade with propranolol represents probably the most efficacious anti-catabolic therapy in the treatment of burns. Long-term use of propranolol during acute care in burn patients, at a dose titrated to reduce heart rate by 15 to 20%, was noted to diminish cardiac work [116]. It also reduced fatty infiltration of the liver, which typically occurs in these patients as the result of enhanced peripheral lipolysis and altered substrate handling. Reduction of hepatic fat results from decreased peripheral lipolysis and reduced palmitate delivery and uptake by the liver [79, 117], producing smaller livers that adversely affect diaphragmatic function less frequently. Stable isotope and serial body composition studies showed that administration of propranolol reduces skeletal muscle wasting and increases lean body mass post-burn [118, 119]. The underlying mechanism of action of propranolol is still unclear, however, its effect appears to occur due to an increased protein synthesis in the face of a persistent protein breakdown and reduced peripheral lipolysis [120]. Recent data suggests that administration of propanolol given at 4 mg/kg BW/q24 also markedly decreased the amount of insulin necessary to decrease elevated glucose level post-burn (unpublished data). Propranolol may thus constitute a promising approach to overcome post-burn insulin resistance.

## Glucose control

One prominent component of the hypermetabolic response post-burn is insulin resistance [121]. Stress-induced insulin resistance and its associated hyper-

249

glycemia results from both, an increase in hepatic gluconeogenesis and an impaired insulin-mediated glucose transport into skeletal muscle cardiac muscle, and adipose tissue [122, 123], leading to elevated blood glucose levels in association with normal or elevated serum insulin concentrations [124, 125]. Both are of serious clinical concern, as hyperglycemia is frequently linked to impaired wound healing, increased number of infectious complications and increased incidence of mortality in those patients [126–128]. Thus, recent studies have focused on elucidating potential treatment options in order to overcome insulin resistance induced hyperglycemia in the acute period following surgery or medical illness.

## Insulin

Insulin represents probably one of the most extensively studied therapeutic agents and novel therapeutic applications are constantly being found. Besides its ability to decrease blood glucose via mediating peripheral glucose uptake into skeletal muscle and adipose tissue and suppressing hepatic gluconeogenesis, insulin is known to increase DNA replication and protein synthesis via control of amino acid uptake, increase fatty acid synthesis and decreased proteinolysis [129]. The latter makes insulin particular attractive for the treatment of hyperglycemia in severely burned patients since insulin given during acute hospitalization has been shown to improve muscle protein synthesis, accelerate donor site healing time, and attenuate lean body mass loss and the acute phase response [130–137]. In addition to its anabolic actions, insulin was shown to exert totally unexpected anti-inflammatory effects potentially neutralizing the pro-inflammatory actions of glucose [134, 135]. These results suggest a dual benefit of insulin administration: reduction of pro-inflammatory effects of glucose by restoration of euglycemia and a proposed additional insulin-mediated anti-inflammatory effect [138]. Van den Berghe et al. confirmed the beneficial effects of insulin in large recent milestone study. Insulin administered to maintain glucose at levels below 110 mg/dl decreased mortality, incidence of infections, sepsis and sepsis-associated multi-organ failure in surgically critically ill patients [139]. They also found intensive insulin therapy to

significantly reducing newly acquired kidney injury, accelerating weaning from mechanical ventilation and accelerating discharge from the ICU and the hospital [140]. The authors further showed that insulin given during the acute phase not only improved acute hospital outcomes but also improved long-term rehabilitation and social reintegration of critically ill patients over a period of 1 year, indicating the advantage of insulin therapy [141, 142]. However, since strict blood glucose control in order to maintain normoglycemia was required to obtain the most clinical benefit, a dialogue has emerged between those who believe that tight glucose control is beneficial for patient outcome and others who fear that high doses of insulin may lead to increased risks for hypoglycemic events and its associated consequences in these patients [139]. In fact, a recent multi-center trial in Europe (Efficacy of Volume Substitution and Insulin Therapy in Severe Sepsis [VISEP]) investigated the effects of insulin administration on morbidity and mortality in patients with severe infections and sepsis [143]. The authors found that insulin administration did not affect mortality but the rate of severe hypoglycemia was 4-fold higher in patients receiving intensive insulin therapy when compared to the conventional therapy group [143]. Another large multi-center study examined the use of a continuous hyperinsulinemic, euglycemic clamp throughout ICU stay and found a dramatic increase in serious hypoglycemic episodes [144]. The ideal target glucose range therefore has not been found and several groups are currently undertaking clinical trials in order to define ideal glucose levels for the treatment of ICU and burned patients: A study by Finney et al. suggests glucose levels of 140 mg/dl and below [145], while the Surviving Sepsis Campaign recommend to maintain glucose levels below 150 mg/dl [146]. However, maintaining a continuous hyperinsulinemic, euglycemic clamp in burn patients is particularly difficult since these patients are being continuously fed large caloric loads via enteral feeding tubes in an attempt to maintain euglycemia. Since burn patients require weekly operations and daily dressing changes, enteral nutrition needs occasionally to be stopped, which may lead to disruption of gastrointestinal motility and increased risk of hypoglycemia [10].

## Metformin

Metformin (Glucophage), a biguanide, has recently been suggested as an alternative means to correct hyperglycemia in severely injured patients [147]. By inhibiting gluconeogenesis and augmenting peripheral insulin sensitivity, metformin directly counters the two main metabolic processes which underlie injury-induced hyperglycemia [148–150]. In addition, metformin has been rarely associated with hypoglycemic events, thus possibly eliminating this concern associated with the use of exogenous insulin [151]. In a small randomized study reported by Gore et al. metformin reduced plasma glucose concentration, decreased endogenous glucose production and accelerated glucose clearance in severely burned [147]. A follow-up study looking at the effects of metformin on muscle protein synthesis, confirmed these observations and demonstrated an increased fractional synthetic rate of muscle protein and improvement in net muscle protein balance in metformin treated patients [150]. Metformin may thus, analogous to insulin, have efficacy in critically injured patients as both, an antihyperglycemic and muscle protein anabolic agent. Despite the advantages and potential therapeutic uses, treatment with metformin, or other biguanides, has been associated with lactic acidosis [151, 152]. To avoid metformin-associated lactic acidosis, the use of this medication is contraindicated in certain diseases or illnesses in which there is a potential for impaired lactate elimination (hepatic or renal failure) or tissue hypoxia – and should be used with caution in subacute burn patients.

## Novel therapeutic options

Other ongoing trials in order to decrease post-burn hyperglycemia include the use of Glucagon-Like-Peptide (GLP)-1 and PPAR-γ agonists (e. g. pioglitazone, thioglitazones) or the combination of various anti-diabetic drugs. PPAR-γ agonists, such as fenofibrate, have been shown to improve insulin sensitivity in patients with diabetes. Cree et al. found in a recent double-blind, prospective, placebo-controlled randomized trial that fenofibrate treatment significantly decreased plasma glucose significantly decreased plasma glucose concentrations by improv-

ing insulin sensitivity and mitochondrial glucose oxidation [153]. Fenofibrate also led to significantly increased tyrosine phosphorylation of the insulin receptor (IR) and IRS-1 in muscle tissue after hyperinsulinemic-euglycemic clamp when compared to placebo treated patients, indicating improved insulin receptor signaling [153].

## Long-term responses

Despite adequate and rapid treatment immediately post-bun burn injury is associated with long-term consequences. Recent studies show that inflammation, hypermetabolism, catecholamines, and cortisol are increased for up to 3 years post-burn (unpublished data). This data indicate the local and systemic effects of a burn are not limited to the 95 % healed stage. A burn continues to plague and impair patients over a prolonged time. The Glue grant group investigated in a recent study the persistence of genomic changes after burn and found that the genome of white blood cells is altered for up 12 months post-burn indicating the profound changes with a burn injury (manuscript submitted for publication). We therefore initiated several studies to determine whether the long-term effects can be alleviated [10, 71, 88, 109, 154]. We found that administration of anabolic agents such as oxandrolone, growth hormone, or propranolol can improve long-term outcomes. Furthermore, in an unpublished study we found that exercise can tremendously improve strength and rehabilitation of severely burned patients. In summary, a burn is not limited to the acute phase. It is a process that continues over a long time and requires a patient specific treatment plan in order to improve patient outcome.

## Conclusion

Children younger than 14 years of age account for approximately 50 % of all emergency department-treated thermal burns. With nearly 1100 children dying of burn-related injuries in the United States every year severe burns still represent the third most common cause of death in the pediatric patient population. However, novel concepts and techniques have been proposed and significantly improved over the past 30 years resulting in a considerable decline in burn-related deaths and hospital admissions in the USA over the last years. The adequate and rapid institution of fluid resuscitation maintains tissue perfusion and prevents organ system failure. Sepsis is successfully controlled by early excision of burn wounds and topical antimicrobial agents. Patients suffering from sustained an inhalation injury require additional fluid resuscitation, humidified oxygen, and, occasionally, ventilatory support. Enteral tube feeding is commenced early in order to control stress ulceration, maintain intestinal mucosal integrity, and provide fuel for the resulting hypermetabolic state. Beta-adrenergic blockade is recommended by many burn units as the most effective anti-catabolic treatment. Tight glucose control has been shown to prevent several critical illness-associated complications, including blood stream infections, anemia and acute renal failure. Through the use of aggressive resuscitation, nutritional support, infection control, surgical therapy, and early rehabilitation, as well as multidisciplinary collaboration, better psychological and physical results can be achieved for burn children.

## References

[1] Palmieri TL, Greenhalgh DG (2002) Topical treatment of pediatric patients with burns: a practical guide. Am J Clin Dermatol 3(8): 529–534

[2] Nelson KJ, Beierle EA (2005) Exhaust system burn injuries in children () J Pediatr Surg 40(4):E43–46

[3] Foglia RP, Moushey R, Meadows L et al (2004) Evolving treatment in a decade of pediatric burn care. J Pediatr Surg 39(6): 957–960; discussion 957–960

[4] Miller SF, Bessey PQ, Schurr MJ et al (2006) National Burn Repository 2005: a ten-year review. J Burn Care Res 27(4): 411–436

[5] Brigham PA, McLoughlin E (1996) Burn incidence and medical care use in the United States: estimates, trends, and data sources. J Burn Care Rehabil 17(2): 95–107

[6] Wolf S (2007) Critical Care in the Severely burned: organ support and management of complications. In: Herndon DN (ed) Total burn care, 3 edn. Saunders Elsevier, London

[7] Thombs BD, Bresnick MG (2008) Mortality risk and length of stay associated with self-inflicted burn injury: evidence from a national sample of 30,382 adult patients. Crit Care Med 36(1): 118–125

[8] Trauma ACoSCo (1993) Resources of Optimal Care of the Injured Patient.. In: American College of surgeons. Chicago

[9] Nadkarni V, Hazinski MF, Zideman D et al (1997) Paediatric life support. An advisory statement by the Paediatric Life Support Working Group of the International Liaison Committee on Resuscitation. Resuscitation 34(2): 115–127

[10] Herndon DN, Tompkins RG (2004) Support of the metabolic response to burn injury. Lancet 363(9424): 1895–1902

[11] Ramzy PI, Barret JP, Herndon DN (1999) Thermal injury. Crit Care Clin 15(2): 333–352, ix

[12] Fodor L, Fodor A, Ramon Y et al (2006) Controversies in fluid resuscitation for burn management: literature review and our experience. Injury 37(5): 374–379

[13] Carvajal HF (1994) Fluid resuscitation of pediatric burn victims: a critical appraisal. Pediatr Nephrol 8(3): 357–366

[14] Youn YK, LaLonde C, Demling R (1992) The role of mediators in the response to thermal injury. World J Surg 16(1): 30–36

[15] Warden GD (1992) Burn shock resuscitation. World J Surg 16(1): 16–23

[16] Wolf SE, Rose JK, Desai MH et al (1997) Mortality determinants in massive pediatric burns. An analysis of 103 children with > or = 80% TBSA burns (> or = 70% full-thickness). Ann Surg 225(5): 554–565; discussion 565–559

[17] Pham TN, Cancio LC, Gibran NS (2008) American Burn Association practice guidelines burn shock resuscitation. J Burn Care Res 29(1): 257–266

[18] Holm C (2000) Resuscitation in shock associated with burns. Tradition or evidence-based medicine? Resuscitation 44(3): 157–164

[19] Warden GD (2007) Fluid resuscitation and early management. In: Herndon DN (ed) Total burn care. 3rd edn. Saunders Elsevier, London, pp 107–116

[20] Baxter CR, Shires T (1968) Physiological response to crystalloid resuscitation of severe burns. Ann N Y Acad Sci 150(3): 874–894

[21] Schwartz SI (1979) Supportive therapy in burn care. Consensus summary on fluid resuscitation. J Trauma 19(11 Suppl): 876–877

[22] Gore DC, Hawkins HK, Chinkes DL et al (2007) Assessment of adverse events in the demise of pediatric burn patients. J Trauma 63(4): 814–818

[23] Mlcak R (1999) Pre-Hospital care and emergency management of burn victims. In: Wolf SE, Herndon DN (eds) Burn care. Landes Bioscience, Austin, TX, pp 5–13

[24] Fabri PJ (1986) Monitoring of the burn patient. Clin Plast Surg 13(1): 21–27

[25] Pruitt BA Jr, Mason AD Jr., Moncrief JA (1971) Hemodynamic changes in the early postburn patient: the influence of fluid administration and of a vasodilator (hydralazine). J Trauma 11(1): 36–46

[26] Perel P, Roberts I (2007) Colloids versus crystalloids for fluid resuscitation in critically ill patients. Cochrane Database Syst Rev(4): CD000 567

[27] Alderson P, Bunn F, Lefebvre C et al (2004) Human albumin solution for resuscitation and volume expansion in critically ill patients. Cochrane Database Syst Rev(4): CD001 208

[28] Vincent JL, Sakr Y, Reinhart K et al (2005) Is albumin administration in the acutely ill associated with increased mortality? Results of the SOAP study. Crit Care 9(6):R745–754

[29] Warden GD (2007) Fluid resuscitation and early management. In: Herndon DN (ed) Total burn care, 3 edn. Saunders, New York City, pp 107–118

[30] Calandra T, Cohen J (2005) The international sepsis forum consensus conference on definitions of infection in the intensive care unit. Crit Care Med 33(7): 1538–1548

[31] Pruitt BA, Jr (1990) Infection and the burn patient. Br J Surg 77(10): 1081–1082

[32] Greenhalgh DG, Saffle Jr, Holmes JHt et al (2007) American Burn Association consensus conference to define sepsis and infection in burns. J Burn Care Res 28(6): 776–790

[33] Brilli RJ, Goldstein B (2005) Pediatric sepsis definitions: past, present, and future. Pediatr Crit Care Med 6 (3 Suppl): S6–8

[34] Goldstein B, Giroir B, Randolph A (2005) International pediatric sepsis consensus conference: definitions for sepsis and organ dysfunction in pediatrics. Pediatr Crit Care Med 6(1): 2–8

[35] Jeschke MG, Mlcak RP, Finnerty CC et al (2007) Burn size determines the inflammatory and hypermetabolic response. Crit Care 11(4):R90

[36] Thompson PB, Herndon DN, Traber DL et al (1986) Effect on mortality of inhalation injury. J Trauma 26(2): 163–165

[37] Sheridan RL (2002) Burns. Crit Care Med 30(11 Suppl): S500–514

[38] Endorf FW, Gamelli RL (2007) Inhalation injury, pulmonary perturbations, and fluid resuscitation. J Burn Care Res 28(1): 80–83

[39] Ventilation with lower tidal volumes as compared with traditional tidal volumes for acute lung injury and the acute respiratory distress syndrome (2000) The acute respiratory distress syndrome network. N Engl J Med 342(18): 1301–1308

[40] Rue LW 3rd, Cioffi WG, Mason AD et al (1993) Improved survival of burned patients with inhalation injury. Arch Surg 128(7): 772–778; discussion 778–780

[41] Nugent NH, Herndon DN (2007) Diagnosis and treatment of inhalation injury. In: Herndon DN (ed) Total burn care. Saunders & Elsevier, London, pp 262–272

[42] Atiyeh BS, Dham R, Kadry M et al (2002) Benefit-cost analysis of moist exposed burn ointment. Burns 28(7): 659–663

[43] Lofts JA (1991) Cost analysis of a major burn. N Z Med J 104(924): 488–490

[44] Munster AM, Smith-Meek M, Sharkey P (1994) The effect of early surgical intervention on mortality and cost-effectiveness in burn care, 1978–91. Burns 20(1): 61–64

[45] Chan BP, Kochevar IE, Redmond RW (2002) Enhancement of porcine skin graft adherence using a light-activated process. J Surg Res 108(1): 77–84

[46] Dziewulski P, Barret JP (1999) Assessment, operative planning and surgery for burn wound closure. In: Wolf SE, Herndon DN (eds) Burn care. Landes Bioscience, Austin, Tx, pp 19–52

[47] Budny PG, Regan PJ, Roberts AH (1993) The estimation of blood loss during burns surgery. Burns 19(2): 134–137

[48] Housinger TA, Lang D, Warden GD (1993) A prospective study of blood loss with excisional therapy in pediatric burn patients. J Trauma 34(2): 262–263

[49] Jeschke MG, Chinkes DL, Finnerty CC et al (2007) Blood transfusions are associated with increased risk for development of sepsis in severely burned pediatric patients. Crit Care Med 35(2): 579–583

[50] Muller M, Gahankari D, Herndon DN (2007) Operative wound management. In: Herndon DN (ed) Total burn care, 3 edn. Saunders, New York City, pp 177–195

[51] Sheridan RL, Szyfelbein SK (1999) Staged high-dose epinephrine clysis is safe and effective in extensive tangential burn excisions in children. Burns 25(8): 745–748

[52] Blome-Eberwein S, Jester A, Kuentscher M et al (2002) Clinical practice of glycerol preserved allograft skin coverage. Burns 28 [Suppl 1]: S10–12

[53] Garfein ES, Orgill DP, Pribaz JJ (2003) Clinical applications of tissue engineered constructs. Clin Plast Surg 30(4): 485–498

[54] Bannasch H, Fohn M, Unterberg T et al (2003) Skin tissue engineering. Clin Plast Surg 30(4): 573–579

[55] Pellegrini G, Ranno R, Stracuzzi G et al (1999) The control of epidermal stem cells (holoclones) in the treatment of massive full-thickness burns with autologous keratinocytes cultured on fibrin. Transplantation 68(6): 868–879

[56] Tompkins RG, Burke JF (1990) Progress in burn treatment and the use of artificial skin. World J Surg 14(6): 819–824

[57] Burke JF, Yannas IV, Quinby WC Jr et al (1981) Successful use of a physiologically acceptable artificial skin in the treatment of extensive burn injury. Ann Surg 194(4): 413–428

[58] Yannas IV, Burke JF, Orgill DP et al (1982) Wound tissue can utilize a polymeric template to synthesize a functional extension of skin. Science 215(4529): 174–176

[59] Yannas IV, Burke JF, Warpehoski M et al (1981) Prompt, long-term functional replacement of skin. Trans Am Soc Artif Intern Organs 27: 19–23

[60] Branski LK, Herndon DN, Pereira C et al (2007) Longitudinal assessment of Integra in primary burn management: a randomized pediatric clinical trial. Crit Care Med 35(11): 2615–2623

[61] Tsai CC, Lin SD, Lai CS et al (1999) The use of composite acellular allodermis-ultrathin autograft on joint

area in major burn patients-one year follow-up. Kaohsiung J Med Sci 15(11): 651–658

[62] Lattari V, Jones LM, Varcelotti JR et al (1997) The use of a permanent dermal allograft in full-thickness burns of the hand and foot: a report of three cases. J Burn Care Rehabil 18(2): 147–155

[63] Wainwright D, Madden M, Luterman A et al (1996) Clinical evaluation of an acellular allograft dermal matrix in full-thickness burns. J Burn Care Rehabil 17(2): 124–136

[64] Sheridan R, Choucair R, Donelan M et al (1998) Acellular allodermis in burns surgery: 1-year results of a pilot trial. J Burn Care Rehabil 19(6): 528–530

[65] Hohlfeld J, de Buys Rocssingh A, Hirt-Burri N et al (2005) Tissue engineered fetal skin constructs for paediatric burns. Lancet 366(9488): 840–842

[66] Supp DM, Boyce ST (2005) Engineered skin substitutes: practices and potentials. Clin Dermatol 23(4): 403–412

[67] Branski LK, Gauglitz GG, Herndon DN et al (2009) A review of gene and stem cell therapy in cutaneous wound healing. Burns 35(2): 171–180

[68] Wolfe RR, Herndon DN, Jahoor F et al (1987) Effect of severe burn injury on substrate cycling by glucose and fatty acids. N Engl J Med 317(7): 403–408

[69] Herndon DN, Curreri PW (1978) Metabolic response to thermal injury and its nutritional support. Cutis 22(4): 501–506, 514

[70] Saffle JR, Graves C (2007). Nutritional support of the burned patient. In: Herndon DN (ed) Total burn care, 3rd edn. Saunders Elsevier, London, pp 398–419

[71] Hart DW, Wolf SE, Chinkes DL et al (2003) Effects of early excision and aggressive enteral feeding on hypermetabolism, catabolism, and sepsis after severe burn. J Trauma 54(4): 755–761; discussion 761–754

[72] Herndon DN, Barrow RE, Stein M et al (1989) Increased mortality with intravenous supplemental feeding in severely burned patients. J Burn Care Rehabil 10(4): 309–313

[73] Curreri PW, Richmond D, Marvin J et al (1974) Dietary requirements of patients with major burns. J Am Diet Assoc 65(4): 415–417

[74] Allard JP, Pichard C, Hoshino E et al (1990) Validation of a new formula for calculating the energy requirements of burn patients. JPEN J Parenter Enteral Nutr 14(2): 115–118

[75] Hildreth MA, Herndon DN, Desai MH et al (1990) Current treatment reduces calories required to maintain weight in pediatric patients with burns. J Burn Care Rehabil 11(5): 405–409

[76] Demling RH, Seigne P (2000) Metabolic management of patients with severe burns. World J Surg 24(6): 673–680

[77] Garrel DR, Razi M, Lariviere F et al (1995) Improved clinical status and length of care with low-fat nutrition support in burn patients. JPEN J Parenter Enteral Nutr 19(6): 482–491

[78] Mochizuki H, Trocki O, Dominioni L et al (1984) Optimal lipid content for enteral diets following thermal injury. JPEN J Parenter Enteral Nutr 8(6): 638–646

[79] Barret JP, Jeschke MG, Herndon DN (2001) Fatty infiltration of the liver in severely burned pediatric patients: autopsy findings and clinical implications. J Trauma 51(4): 736–739

[80] Cuthbertson DP, Fell GS, Smith CM et al (1972) Metabolism after injury. I. Effects of severity, nutrition, and environmental temperatue on protein potassium, zinc, and creatine. Br J Surg 59(12): 926–931

[81] Shakespeare PG (1982) Studies on the serum levels of iron, copper and zinc and the urinary excretion of zinc after burn injury. Burns Incl Therm Inj 8(5): 358–364

[82] Berger MM, Cavadini C, Bart A et al (1992) Cutaneous copper and zinc losses in burns. Burns 18(5): 373–380

[83] Berger MM, Raffoul W, Shenkin A (2008) 'Practical guidelines for nutritional management of burn injury and recovery'-A guideline based on expert opinion but not including RCTs. Burns 34(1): 141–143

[84] Berger MM, Eggimann P, Heyland DK et al (2006) Reduction of nosocomial pneumonia after major burns by trace element supplementation: aggregation of two randomised trials. Crit Care 10(6):R153

[85] Prelack K, Dylewski M, Sheridan RL (2007) Practical guidelines for nutritional management of burn injury and recovery. Burns 33(1): 14–24

[86] Gamliel Z, DeBiasse MA, Demling RH (1996) Essential microminerals and their response to burn injury. J Burn Care Rehabil 17(3): 264–272

[87] Gottschlich MM, Mayes T, Khoury J et al (2004) Hypovitaminosis D in acutely injured pediatric burn patients. J Am Diet Assoc 104(6): 931–941, quiz 1031

[88] Hart DW, Wolf SE, Mlcak R et al (2000) Persistence of muscle catabolism after severe burn. Surgery 128(2): 312–319

[89] Reiss E, Pearson E, Artz CP (1956) The metabolic response to burns. J Clin Invest 35(1): 62–77

[90] Yu YM, Tompkins RG, Ryan CM et al (1999) The metabolic basis of the increase of the increase in energy expenditure in severely burned patients. JPEN J Parenter Enteral Nutr 23(3): 160–168

[91] Jeschke MG, Herndon DN, Wolf SE et al (1999) Recombinant human growth hormone alters acute phase reactant proteins, cytokine expression, and liver morphology in burned rats. J Surg Res 83(2): 122–129

[92] Wu X, Herndon DN, Wolf SE (2003) Growth hormone down-regulation of Interleukin-1beta and Interleukin-6 induced acute phase protein gene expression is associated with increased gene expression of suppressor of cytokine signal-3. Shock 19(4): 314–320

[93] Jeschke MG, Chrysopoulo MT, Herndon DN et al (1999) Increased expression of insulin-like growth factor-I in serum and liver after recombinant human growth hormone administration in thermally injured rats. J Surg Res 85(1): 171–177

[94] Aili Low JF, Barrow RE, Mittendorfer B et al (2001) The effect of short-term growth hormone treatment on growth and energy expenditure in burned children. Burns 27(5): 447–452

[95] Hart DW, Herndon DN, Klein G et al (2001) Attenuation of posttraumatic muscle catabolism and osteopenia by long-term growth hormone therapy. Ann Surg 233(6): 827–834

[96] Herndon DN, Barrow RE, Kunkel KR et al (1990) Effects of recombinant human growth hormone on donor-site healing in severely burned children. Ann Surg 212(4): 424–429; discussion 430–421

[97] Branski LK, Herndon DN, Barrow RE et al (2009) Randomized Controlled Trial to Determine the Efficacy of Long-Term Growth Hormone Treatment in Severely Burned Children. Ann Surg 250(4): 514–523

[98] Klein GL, Wolf SE, Langman CB et al (1998) Effects of therapy with recombinant human growth hormone on insulin-like growth factor system components and serum levels of biochemical markers of bone formation in children after severe burn injury. J Clin Endocrinol Metab 83(1): 21–24

[99] Takala J, Ruokonen E, Webster NR et al (1999) Increased mortality associated with growth hormone treatment in critically ill adults. N Engl J Med 341(11): 785–792

[100] Demling RH (1999) Comparison of the anabolic effects and complications of human growth hormone and the testosterone analog, oxandrolone, after severe burn injury. Burns 25(3): 215–221

[101] Gore DC, Honeycutt D, Jahoor F et al (1991) Effect of exogenous growth hormone on glucose utilization in burn patients. J Surg Res 51(6): 518–523

[102] Ramirez RJ, Wolf SE, Barrow RE et al (1998) Growth hormone treatment in pediatric burns: a safe therapeutic approach. Ann Surg 228(4): 439–448

[103] Moller S, Jensen M, Svensson P et al (1991) Insulin-like growth factor 1 (IGF-1) in burn patients. Burns 17(4): 279–281

[104] Herndon DN, Ramzy PI, DebRoy MA et al (1999) Muscle protein catabolism after severe burn: effects of IGF-1/IGFBP-3 treatment. Ann Surg 229(5): 713–720; discussion 720–712

[105] Spies M, Wolf SE, Barrow RE et al (2002) Modulation of types I and II acute phase reactants with insulin-like growth factor-1/binding protein-3 complex in severely burned children. Crit Care Med 30(1): 83–88

[106] Jeschke MG, Herndon DN, Barrow RE (2000) Insulin-like growth factor I in combination with insulin-like growth factor binding protein 3 affects the hepatic acute phase response and hepatic morphology in thermally injured rats. Ann Surg 231(3): 408–416

[107] Cioffi WG, Gore DC, Rue LW 3rd et al (1994) Insulin-like growth factor-1 lowers protein oxidation in patients with thermal injury. Ann Surg 220(3): 310–316; discussion 316–319

[108] Langouche L, Van den Berghe G (2006) Glucose metabolism and insulin therapy. Crit Care Clin 22(1): 119–129, vii

[109] Hart DW, Wolf SE, Ramzy PI et al (2001) Anabolic effects of oxandrolone after severe burn. Ann Surg 233(4): 556–564

[110] Demling RH, Orgill DP (2000) The anticatabolic and wound healing effects of the testosterone analog oxandrolone after severe burn injury. J Crit Care 15(1): 12–17

[111] Wolf SE, Edelman LS, Kemalyan N et al (2006) Effects of oxandrolone on outcome measures in the severely burned: a multicenter prospective randomized double-blind trial. J Burn Care Res 27(2): 131–139; discussion 140–131

[112] Jeschke MG, Finnerty CC, Suman OE et al (2007) The effect of oxandrolone on the endocrinologic, inflammatory, and hypermetabolic responses during the acute phase postburn. Ann Surg 246(3): 351–360; discussion 360–352

[113] Demling RH, DeSanti L (2001) The rate of restoration of body weight after burn injury, using the anabolic agent oxandrolone, is not age dependent. Burns 27(1): 46–51

[114] Murphy KD, Thomas S, Mlcak RP et al (2004) Effects of long-term oxandrolone administration in severely burned children. Surgery 136(2): 219–224

[115] Suman OE, Thomas SJ, Wilkins JP et al (2003) Effect of exogenous growth hormone and exercise on lean mass and muscle function in children with burns. J Appl Physiol 94(6): 2273–2281

[116] Baron PW, Barrow RE, Pierre EJ et al (1997) Prolonged use of propranolol safely decreases cardiac work in burned children. J Burn Care Rehabil 18(3): 223–227

[117] Aarsland A, Chinkes D, Wolfe RR et al (1996) Beta-blockade lowers peripheral lipolysis in burn patients receiving growth hormone. Rate of hepatic very low density lipoprotein triglyceride secretion remains unchanged. Ann Surg 223(6): 777–787; discussion 787–779

[118] Gore DC, Honeycutt D, Jahoor F et al (1991) Propranolol diminishes extremity blood flow in burned patients. Ann Surg 213(6): 568–574

[119] Herndon DN, Hart DW, Wolf SE et al (2001) Reversal of catabolism by beta-blockade after severe burns. N Engl J Med 345(17): 1223–1229

[120] Pereira CT, Jeschke MG, Herndon DN (2007) Beta-blockade in burns. Novartis Found Symp 280: 238–251

[121] Tredget EE, Yu YM (1992) The metabolic effects of thermal injury. World J Surg 16(1): 68–79

[122] Jahoor F, Herndon DN, Wolfe RR (1986) Role of insulin and glucagon in the response of glucose and alanine kinetics in burn-injured patients. J Clin Invest 78(3): 807–814

[123] Gearhart MM, Parbhoo SK (2006) Hyperglycemia in the critically ill patient. AACN Clin Issues 17(1): 50–55

[124] Xin-Long C, Zhao-Fan X, Dao-Feng B et al (2007) Insulin resistance following thermal injury: an animal study. Burns 33(4): 480–483

[125] Zauner A, Nimmerrichter P, Anderwald C et al (2007) Severity of insulin resistance in critically ill medical patients. Metabolism 56(1): 1–5

[126] Guvener M, Pasaoglu I, Demircin M et al (2002) Perioperative hyperglycemia is a strong correlate of postoperative infection in type II diabetic patients after coronary artery bypass grafting. Endocr J 49(5): 531–537

[127] McCowen KC, Malhotra A, Bistrian BR (2001) Stress-induced hyperglycemia. Crit Care Clin 17(1): 107–124

[128] Christiansen C, Toft P, Jorgensen HS et al (2004) Hyperglycaemia and mortality in critically ill patients. A prospective study. Intensive Care Med 30(8): 1685–1688

[129] Pidcoke HF, Wade CE, Wolf SE (2007) Insulin and the burned patient. Crit Care Med 35(9 Suppl):S524–530

[130] Ferrando AA, Chinkes DL, Wolf SE et al (1999) A submaximal dose of insulin promotes net skeletal muscle protein synthesis in patients with severe burns. Ann Surg 229(1): 11–18

[131] Pierre EJ, Barrow RE, Hawkins HK et al (1998) Effects of insulin on wound healing. J Trauma 44(2): 342–345

[132] Thomas SJ, Morimoto K, Herndon DN et al (2002) The effect of prolonged euglycemic hyperinsulinemia on lean body mass after severe burn. Surgery 132(2): 341–347

[133] Zhang XJ, Chinkes DL, Wolf SE et al (1999) Insulin but not growth hormone stimulates protein anabolism in skin would and muscle. Am J Physiol 276(4 Pt 1):E712-E720

[134] Jeschke MG, Klein D, Bolder U et al (2004) Insulin attenuates the systemic inflammatory response in endotoxemic rats. Endocrinology 145(9): 4084–4093

[135] Jeschke MG, Klein D, Herndon DN (2004) Insulin treatment improves the systemic inflammatory reaction to severe trauma. Ann Surg 239(4): 553–560

[136] Jeschke MG, Rensing H, Klein D et al (2005) Insulin prevents liver damage and preserves liver function in lipopolysaccharide-induced endotoxemic rats. J Hepatol 42(6): 870–879

[137] Klein D, Schubert T, Horch RE et al (2004) Insulin treatment improves hepatic morphology and function through modulation of hepatic signals after severe trauma. Ann Surg 240(2): 340–349

[138] Dandona P, Chaudhuri A, Mohanty P et al (2007) Anti-inflammatory effects of insulin. Curr Opin Clin Nutr Metab Care 10(4): 511–517

[139] van den Berghe G, Wouters P, Weekers F et al Intensive insulin therapy in the critically ill patients. N Engl J Med 2001;345(19): 1359–1367

[140] Van den Berghe G, Wilmer A, Hermans G et al (2006) Intensive insulin therapy in the medical ICU. N Engl J Med 354(5): 449–461

[141] Ellger B, Debaveye Y, Vanhorebeek I et al (2006) Survival benefits of intensive insulin therapy in critical illness: impact of maintaining normoglycemia versus glycemia-independent actions of insulin. Diabetes 55(4): 1096–1105

[142] Ingels C, Debaveye Y, Milants I et al (2006) Strict blood glucose control with insulin during intensive care after cardiac surgery: impact on 4-years survival, dependency on medical care, and quality-of-life. Eur Heart J 27(22): 2716–2724

[143] Brunkhorst FM, Engel C, Bloos F et al (2008) Intensive insulin therapy and pentastarch resuscitation in severe sepsis. N Engl J Med 358(2): 125–139

[144] Langouche L, Vanhorebeek I, Van den Berghe G (2007) Therapy insight: the effect of tight glycemic control in acute illness. Nat Clin Pract Endocrinol Metab 3(3): 270–278

[145] Finney SJ, Zekveld C, Elia A et al (2003) Glucose control and mortality in critically ill patients. JAMA 290(15): 2041–2047

[146] Dellinger RP, Levy MM, Carlet JM et al (2008) Surviving Sepsis Campaign: international guidelines for management of severe sepsis and septic shock: 2008. Crit Care Med 36(1): 296–327

[147] Gore DC, Wolf SE, Herndon DN et al (2003) Metformin blunts stress-induced hyperglycemia after thermal injury. J Trauma 54(3): 555–561

[148] DeFronzo RA, Goodman AM (1995) Efficacy of metformin in patients with non-insulin-dependent diabetes mellitus. The Multicenter Metformin Study Group. N Engl J Med 333(9): 541–549

[149] Stumvoll M, Nurjhan N, Perriello G et al (1995) Metabolic effects of metformin in non-insulin-dependent diabetes mellitus. N Engl J Med 333(9): 550–554

[150] Gore DC, Herndon DN, Wolfe RR (2005) Comparison of peripheral metabolic effects of insulin and metformin following severe burn injury. J Trauma 59(2): 316–323

[151] Bailey CJ, Turner RC (1996) Metformin. N Engl J Med 334(9): 574–579

[152] Luft D, Schmulling RM, Eggstein M (1978) Lactic acidosis in biguanide-treated diabetics: a review of 330 cases. Diabetologia 14(2): 75–87

[153] Cree MG, Zwetsloot JJ, Herndon DN et al (2007) Insulin sensitivity and mitochondrial function are improved in children with burn injury during a randomized controlled trial of fenofibrate. Ann Surg 245(2): 214–221

[154] Przkora R, Herndon DN, Suman OE et al (2006) Beneficial effects of extended growth hormone treatment after hospital discharge in pediatric burn patients. Ann Surg 243(6): 796–801; discussion 801–793

[155] Kleinman RE, Barness LA, Finberg L (2003) History of pediatric nutrition and fluid therapy. Pediatr Res 54(5): 762–772

[156] Dietary Reference Intakes, Food and Nutrition Board, Institute of Medicine (2002) In: National Academy Press

[157] Day T, Dean P, Adams M et al (1986) Nutritional requirements of the burned child: The Curreri Junior formula. Proceedings of the American Burn Association 18: 86

[158] Hildreth MA, Herndon DN, Desai MH et al (1993) Caloric requirements of patients with burns under one year of age. J Burn Care Rehabil 14(1): 108–112

[159] Hildreth M, Herndon D, Desai M et al (1989) Caloric needs of adolescent patients with burns. J Burn Care Rehabil 10: 523–526

Correspondence: Gerd G. Gauglitz, M.D., MMS, Department of Dermatology and Allergology, Ludwig Maximilians University, Frauenlobstraße 9–11, 80 337 Munich, Germany, E-mail: gerd.gauglitz@med.uni-muenchen.de

# Adult burn management

Peter Dziewulski[1], Jorge-Leon Villapalos[2], Joan Pere Barret[3]

[1] St Andrews Centre for Plastic Surgery and Burns, Chelmsford, Essex, UK
[2] Chelsea and Westminster Hospital Burns Service, London, UK
[3] Val D'Hebron Hospital, Barcelona, Spain

## Introduction

The management of the adult burn is a complex and multi- faceted endeavour. The burn injury and wound cause both local and systemic effects mediated by the host responses of inflammation, regeneration, and repair. Initial physiological derangement can give rise to shifts in fluids, electrolytes and proteins within body compartments necessitating formal fluid resuscitation in large burns. Following on from this initial physiological derangement subsequent metabolic, hematological, immunological and endocrine disturbances can occur making the care of these patients a difficult and challenging task. The sequelae and in general the severity of the injury is dependant on the aetiology, the size of the burn and the anatomical depth of tissue destruction. Management of the burn wound is key to attenuation of systemic sequelae and the aim of care is to achieve early durable and sound healing. This must be achieved whilst managing the multi system nature of the illness [1].

## Epidemiology and aetiology

Burn injury represents a major cause of morbidity and mortality with large societal and economic implications. There are variation in incidence and aetiology that relate to age and geography. The annual incidence of patients with severe burn injury in Europe has been reported as being between 0.2 and 2.9/10,000 inhabitants. There are no similar estimates from the developing world however it is widely recognised that the burden of burn injury in this setting is much more common. A higher incidence has been associated with lower socioeconomic status and in ethnic minorities.

The incidence of adult burn injury in Europe and North America has decreased over the past 30 years and has been related to increasing socioeconomic status and reduction of injury at work. Adults account for over half of all injuries admitted to hospital with the growth of the elderly population in the Western world being reflected in the increasing numbers of elderly patients being hospitalised. The majority of adult burn injuries (50–75%) occur in males and are often related to work, this ratio changes in children and the elderly with a more even sex distribution.

The commonest causes of burn injury in adults include flame (~45%), scald (~40%), contact injury (~10%) and chemical and electrical (~5%). These ratios change with scalds in children accounting for up to 80% and in the elderly. Flame burns are more common in men, whereas scalds are more frequent in women. Up to one third of adult injuries are work related. Self immolation injury accounts for a small but significant cohort of burn patients as they tend to be large body surface area injuries [2].

## Classification

A burn is defined as coagulative destruction of the surface layers of the body.

The skin is made up of the epidermis and dermis with the adenexal structures such as the hair follicles, sweat and sebaceous glands residing in the deeper parts of the dermis. These adenexal structures are important as they are the source of proliferating epithelial cells (keratinocytes), which resurface wound after the skin has been injured. Loss of the barrier function of the skin allows invasion of microorganisms and systemic sepsis.

Burn injury to the skin can be classified as partial or full thickness. If the epidermis and the superficial part of the dermis have been injured (superficial partial thickness injury), the majority of adenexal structures are preserved, epithelialisation is rapid (10–14 days) and the risk of hypertrophic scarring is low. If the burn extends down into the deeper parts of the dermis more adenexal structures are destroyed, epithelialisation is slower (3–6 weeks) and there is a high incidence of hypertrophic scarring. Full thickness burns involve destruction all constituents of the skin and usually will require surgical intervention to achieve wound healing.

Depth of burn injury classification quantifies the amount of tissue damage in anatomical terms. Depth is divided into partial and full thickness skin loss, with partial thickness burns being sub-divided into superficial and deep types.

Erythema (1st degree burn) involves the epidermis only, usually with no blistering although desquamation can occur later on.

Superficial partial thickness (2nd degree) burns involve the epidermis and part of the dermis sparing a significant proportion of hair follicles, sebaceous and sweat glands.

Deep partial thickness (2nd degree) burns destroy a larger proportion the dermis and associated of hair follicles, sebaceous and sweat glands.

Full thickness (3rd degree) burns destroy all of the epidermis, dermis and all adnexal structures

The depth of anatomical tissue destruction is an important determinant of wound healing.

Erythema (1st degree burns) usually resolves in a few days without any untoward effects. Superficial partial thickness wounds will heal spontaneously by re-epithelialisation from epidermal remnants within two weeks and leave few or no scars.

Deep partial thickness (2nd degree burns) wounds heal by a mixture of granulation, wound contraction and epithelialization from epidermal remnants and the wound edge. If left to heal spontaneously these wounds take 2–4 weeks or longer to heal and are associated with a high incidence of disfiguring hypertrophic scarring and scar contracture. These wounds often need skin grafting.

Full thickness wounds (3rd degree burns) require surgical intervention and split thickness skin grafting. This invariably leads to hypertrophic scarring particularly at the edges of the grafts (marginal hypertrophy).

If left to heal spontaneously these wounds granulate, contract and epithelialise from the wound margins. This process is prolonged, leaves the wound susceptible to invasive infection, and leads to significant functional and aesthetic deformity.

Burn wounds that require skin grafts have a higher incidence of scar hypertrophy if the grafting is performed after 14 days of injury and the wound has no viable dermal elements. Burn wounds that are not going to heal within two weeks should be debrided and covered with autologous split skin grafts to minimize hypertrophic scarring [3, 4].

## Pathophysiology

The necrotic tissue resulting from a burn is known as eschar. It separates slowly from underlying viable tissue and is a good substrate for microorganisms. If left untreated it becomes colonized, contaminated and eventually infected. Infection attracts white blood cells that can digest the interface and cause separation of the eschar from the underlying viable tissue. Topical antimicrobial agents reduce bacterial proliferation in the wound and will increase the time to eschar separation.

The initial local effect of a burn injury can be divided histologically into three differential zones of tissue damage and blood flow [5].

1. The zone of necrosis represents tissue necrosis centrally due to destruction of cells and tissues by the burn injury.

2. The zone of ischemia–represents an ongoing microvascular injury that surrounds the zone of necrosis. Following burn injury to the skin inflammatory mediators are released via the arachidonic acid pathway and inflammatory cells. These include histamine, prostaglandins (PGE$_2$), prostacyclins (PGI$_2$), leucotrienes, thromboxanes, kinins, serotonin, catecholamines, free O$_2$ radicals and platelet activating factor. Local action of these inflammatory mediators includes increase in microvascular permeability giving rise to oedema formation, microvascular stasis and thrombosis. These actions can lead to progressive injury and cell death leading to clinical deepening of the burn wound.

This process can be influenced by desiccation, infection and hypoperfusion of the burn wound. There is ongoing interest into the manipulation of this area of injury to preserve viable tissue and prevent progression of tissue necrosis.

3. The zone of inflammation (hyperaemia) surrounds zone of ischemia and is manifested by increased vascular permeability with extravasation of fluid from the intravascular to the interstitial space leading to oedema.

## Assessment of the burn wound

Key to management of the adult burn patient is the formulation of a treatment plan. The burn wound must be assessed clinically before a treatment plan can be formulated. The depth of the burn wound, the size of the burn and the anatomical site of injury are all vitally important factors that must be assessed and considered in the treatment plan.

### Depth of burn

This is determined mainly by clinical wound inspection. Determining the depth of the burn wound can be difficult. In general superficial partial thickness wounds are pink, moist, blistered, blanch on pressure and are very painful. Deep partial thickness burns will either be white or red with fixed staining. They do not blanch on pressure. Full thickness burns characteristically have a leathery appearance and are insensate. It is usually easy to diagnose a very superficial burn or a full thickness burn. Deep dermal burns can be a little more difficult to assess and are often indeterminate on first assessment. Techniques such as Laser Doppler scanning can give an estimate of dermal blood flow and depth of burn injury. Healing times and timing of surgical have been correlated to the incidence of hypertrophic scarring. Wounds that heal spontaneously within 14 days have a very low incidence of hypertrophic scarring [3]. Surgical intervention is associated with a higher incidence of hypertrophic scarring up to 3 weeks following injury [4].

### Size of the burn

This is usually represented as percent of total body surface area (%TBSA) injured using
a) Wallace's "Rule of Nines" useful for initial rapid estimation in the emergency setting
b) Lund and Browder Chart for a more precise estimation
c) Patient's palm ~ 1 % of their body surface.

## Initial management of the burn wound

A general systematic approach must be undertaken to manage fluid resuscitation, smoke inhalation and other injuries in the first instance. Maintenance of the airways, breathing and establishing venous access are paramount and are discussed in other chapters.

Following assessment of the depth, size and anatomical distribution of wound the following procedures should be considered:

### First aid

Cooling the burn wound soon after the injury (within 30 minutes) is beneficial in removing heat from the wound and limiting tissue damage. It can also reduce early oedema and protein extravasation. Care must be taken, as prolonged or excessive cooling can be detrimental and lead to hypothermia. Irrigating the wound in a drench shower for at least 20 minutes is essential in chemical injury to dilute the chemical [6].

### Burn blisters

There is ongoing debate about management with evidence of blister fluid having both beneficial and deleterious effects. In general blisters should be removed if large, over joints and if they produce functional impairment. Small intact blisters can be left in situ to act as a biological dressing. One of the key indications for blister removal is that the dermal wound beneath can be inspected and the depth diagnosed [7].

## Escharotomy

Escharotomy is required in circumferential full thickness burns of chest, limbs or digits.

In limbs/digits such burns impair circulation, produce distal ischemia and can lead to compartment syndromes, digital and limb loss. Circumferential full-thickness chest burns can restrict chest wall excursion and impair ventilation.

Such burns require mid-axial escharotomies performed either at bedside or in the operating room. A scalpel or electrocautery device can be used to incise through the full thickness burns down to bulging fat. The incisions should extend into adjacent non burned or less deeply burned tissue. Since the wounds are full thickness, minimal analgesia or anaesthesia should be required, but extension into less damaged tissue can be very painful. Current humane practice involves anaesthesia for this procedure. The decision to perform escharotomy is a clinical one. In a full thickness burn an escharotomy incision should improve outcome with minimal risk as the area will require excision and grafting later on during treatment.

## General care of the adult burn patient

Adult patients with major burn injuries must be managed in a dedicated facility used to looking after such complex problems. Patients requiring Intensive Care support should be managed in a Burn ICU. Recent analysis of the effects of burn centre volume and mortality revealed a complex relationship not only dependent on patient characteristics but also where the patient was treated [8].

Fluid resuscitation using Parkland formula is currently standard care and although fluid resuscitation is the cornerstone of acute burn management it is apparent that in most centres patients today are receiving more fluid per percent total body surface area (TBSA) giving rise to the concept of 'fluid creep'. It has been show that patients receiving larger volumes of resuscitation fluid are prone to increased complications and mortality [9].

Burn patients with respiratory failure may require ventilation using lung protective ventilation strategies designed to minimise shear and stress forces in the alveoli. Pressure limited low tidal volume ventilation is the currently favoured strategy although high frequency percussive ventilation based strategies are becoming increasingly popular especially for rescue ventilation. A recent trial comparing the two strategies showed similar clinical outcomes in burn patients with respiratory failure however a higher percentage of low tidal volume strategy patients required rescue ventilation [10].

Vascular access in adult burn patients can be a significant challenge. Obviously central venous catheters represent a risk in terms of catheter related blood stream infections. Central venous catheters in burn patients are usually change after about 7 days following insertion either to a new site or over a guide wire. A recent study showed no difference in the incidence of catheter-related bloodstream infections between lines placed by new site or by guide wire exchange. Subset analysis of adults in this study revealed rewires having less catheter related blood stream infections compared to new sites [11].

Other studies have shown the incidence of sepsis increasing with increasing number of central line days and increasing number of central line changes. No statistically significant difference in the incidence of sepsis between upper-and lower-body central line sites was demonstrated [12].

Other intensive care bundles routinely undertaken in general intensive care practise may also have benefits in care of critically ill burn patients. These included protocols for deep venous thrombosis prophylaxis, stress ulcer prophylaxis, daily weaning parameters, sedation holidays, elevation of the head-of-bed up at 30 degrees and tight glucose control. Implementing these care bundles into the burn critical care setting was associated with reduction in ventilator associated pneumonias, and blood stream infection rates and lower mortality [13].

The hypermetabolic response in critically ill burn patients is characterized by hyperdynamic circulatory, catabolic and immune system responses. Energy and protein requirements are massive during critical illness and inadequate replacement can lead to multiorgan failure, increased susceptibility to infection, and death. Attenuation of the hypermetabolic response using pharmacologic modalities is an essential part of care of the severely injured adult burn patients.

Current modalities include beta-adrenergic blockade with propranolol, growth hormone, insulin-like growth factor, oxandralone and intensive insulin therapy [14].

Early nutritional support is an essential component of burn care to prevent ileus, stress ulceration, the effects of hypermetabolism and should be initiated as soon as possible following admission. Multicentre analysis has demonstrated that patients fed within 24hrs of injury had no increase in complications and a lower rate of wound infections and shorter ICU length of stay [15]. There are a variety of techniques in assessing nutritional requirements ranging from formulae based on the age and weight and the percentage burn to the use of indirect calorimetry and the respiratory quotient. Nutrition is usefully provided using high energy, high protein enteral feeds via the nasogastric or nasojejunal route.

Pain control in the burn population is an essential part of care yet control of pain remains a difficult task that is often inadequately performed. The adverse sequelae of inadequate pain control in the burn population have long been recognised. Burn pain is dynamic and has a peripheral and central component. A therapeutic plan for pain control must be dynamic and flexible to address background, breakthrough, procedural and post-operative pain. Regular, ongoing and documented pain assessment is key in directing this process. The simple analgesic paracetamol (acetaminophen) has both anti-pyretic and opioid-sparing properties and justly deserves its place in the pharmacological treatment of every burn patient Opioid analgesics provide the backbone of analgesia to burn patients but must be used judiciously (Fig. 1). Other centrally acting drugs such as ketamine and gabapentin are increasingly being used as opioid sparing adjuncts. Non-pharmacological methods such as distraction therapy can also play a role. Pain specialists must be integral part of the modern burn multi-disciplinary team and pain control must be given a high clinical priority [16].

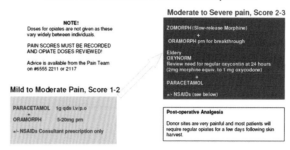

**Fig. 1.** Acute pain guidelines (courtesy of Dr P Richardson MB FRCA)

## Treatment planning

As with all areas in medicine treatment planning is key to successful outcome. Initially the size, site, and depth of the burn wound must be assessed whilst simultaneously undertaking initial urgent measures. A burn wound treatment plan must be formulated. This management plan will include conservative and surgical options depending on the individual patient and the type and site of the wound.

Treatment planning depends on the assessment of the factors described in Fig. 2.

In general, for superficial partial thickness wounds a more conservative approach is undertaken. A more aggressive surgical approach is best

---

**Treatment Planning – Patient Factors to Assess**

- Patient age

- Burn size

- Burn depth

- Anatomical distribution of injury

- Patient's general condition

- Co-morbid factors.

**Fig. 2.** Patient factors to assess for treatment planning

for deeper wounds, to improve outcome and reduce morbidity in smaller injury and to improve survival in bigger injuries. This based on the surgical principle that excision of dead tissues saves lives.

## Superficial partial thickness wound

The aim of management of this type of wounds is to promote rapid spontaneous re-epithelialisation with the minimum number of painful dressing changes and to prevent infection which can lead to deepening of the wound and subsequent increased risk of hypertrophic scarring.

The wounds can be treated either with biological or semi biological dressings, with topical antimicrobials, with standard dressings either impregnated or free from a topical agent or by exposure

### Biological/Semi biological dressings

Biological dressings can be defined as the use of human or animal tissue for temporary wound covering. A semi biological dressing refers to where a component of the dressing is derived from such tissue (i. e. collagen).

Biobrane® is a semibiological dressing made up of a fenestrated silicone layer bonded to a nylon mesh that has bee impregnated with Type I porcine collagen. It has been used in burn care for the past twenty years since its development. In randomised controlled studies its use has been shown to reduce pain, in patient stay and time to healing [17,18].

In patients presenting within 24h of their injury, following admission and stabilisation the patient's burns blisters are cleaned, debrided and all burned epithelium is removed under sedation or anaesthesia. Biobrane® is then applied to the wound in a circumferential fashion around the limb or trunk so that it is closely adherent to the wound. The Biobrane® is secured by either by stapling it to itself or the use of sterile Hypafix® tape. Care is taken not to staple the Biobrane® to the patient as this can cause granulomas and the staples are painful to remove. The Biobrane® is then wrapped with a standard dressing of rolled gauze covered by elastic bandages. The dressings are removed at 24–48 hrs to inspect the wound. Oral antibiotics with staphylococcal coverage are given for five

days. If the Biobrane® is adherent after the first day, no further dressings are required. As re-epithelialisation occurs in 10–14 days the Biobrane® spontaneously separates from the healed wound. If wound infection supervenes, the Biobrane® rapidly becomes non adherent and can trap any exudate produced by the wound. For this reason Biobrane® is not used in patients presenting more than 24–36h following their injury and in larger wounds (>40% TBSA). Biobrane® is also relatively expensive compared to common topical antimicrobials.

### Topical antimicrobials

Silver has been used as an antimicrobial agent for some time. Numerous silver containing dressings are currently used for the management of burn wounds.

Traditionally topical Silvadene/Flammazine (1% Silver Sulfadiazine) is the usual alternative for these wounds. After cleaning the wound and debridement of the blisters, Silvadene is applied topically to the wound which is then covered with rolled gauze and elasticated bandage. The Silvadene dressings are changed once or twice daily until re-epithelialisation occurs and the wound is healed. This method requires frequent dressing changes, which can be a painful.

Acticoat® is a nanocrystalline silver dressing that can provide sustained release of silver for up to 7 days [19]. A randomised controlled trial compared Acticoat® to Silver Sulfadiazine demonstrated Acticoat® to have better antimicrobial activity compared to silver sulfadiazine [20]. Other studies have suggested Acticoat® has fewer adverse effects and reduces healing times. It is easy to apply and requires low frequency of dressing changes makes it an ideal dressing in burn wounds [21]. It is the method of choice for patients presenting late after injury with a colonized wound.

### Biological dressings

Biological dressings such as allograft skin, xenograft skin (porcine), human amnion can all be used in a similar fashion to Biobrane® to physiologically close the wound while re-epithelialisation occurs. The problems associated with the use of these products include availability, collection, storage, transmission of infection and cost [22].

## Other dressings

Conventional dressings such as Vaseline gauze or silicone sheets (Mepitel®) can be used to cover the wound while re-epithelialization takes place. After application, these dressings need frequent changes, which can be painful. These types of dressing are useful for small burns (less than 5% TBSA). Synthetic dressings such as Duoderm®, Omniderm® Tegaderm® and hydrocolloids have all been used with success to dress such wounds. However a recent Cochrane review recently highlighted the paucity of high quality Randomised Controlled Trials on dressings for superficial and partial thickness burn injury. The authors summarised that available evidence was of limited usefulness in aiding clinicians to choosing suitable treatments [23].

## Exposure

After cleaning and debridement, wounds are left open in a warm dry environment o crust over. The coagulum formed separates as re-epithelialization proceed underneath. Advantages of this method are comfort and no need for dressing changes. Disadvantages of this method include prolonged inpatient treatment, specialized ward and nursing requirements and higher infection rates. This technique is now not commonly used apart from the treatment of specialized areas such as the face, genitalia and perineum.

## Large partial thickness wounds

In large superficial partial thickness injury (>40% TBSA) there is a higher risk of wound contamination, infection and subsequent organ dysfunction and morbidity.

The use of allograft applied within 24 hours of the injury is thought to improve outcome [24]. Under anaesthesia the wound is cleaned and all blisters and non adherent epidermis removed. Allograft split skin grafts meshed 2:1 are placed over the open dermal wound and secured with staples. It is important not to open up the mesh on the allograft as this can

lead to desiccation, infection and deepening of the underlying wound. A standard graft dressing is applied. A mid-dermal burn injury can be debrided with a dermatome at a depth of 10–15/1000 inch and allograft applied. This wound should then go on to heal spontaneously with the allograft spontaneously separation as the wound epithelialises. There should not be incorporation of the allograft into the wound unless the wound is deeper.

Xenograft skin can be used in a similar fashion to the allograft [25], but does not usually adhere as well, leaving the wound open to desiccation, infection with associated pain.

Biobrane® can be used in the same way as for smaller injuries. There is a higher rate of wound infection which can lead to loss of the Biobrane® and deepening of the burn wound.

Topical antimicrobials such as silver sulfadiazine or Acticoat® can be used for this type of wound in a similar manner to that described above. It is the treatment of choice for wounds that present late and are colonized, as by definition the wounds should heal spontaneously. The dressing changes can be painful and are an ordeal for the patient. There is a high incidence of wound sepsis, which can lead to deepening of the burn wound, which may then necessitate skin grafting.

## Deep partial thickness wound

Deep partial thickness burns are associated with significant morbidity in terms of time to healing, infective complications and subsequent scarring. Conservative management leading to spontaneous healing usually involves prolonged and painful dressing changes and the resultant scar is invariably hypertrophic leading to cosmetic and functional disfigurement and disability. An early surgical approach that tries to preserve dermis and achieve prompt wound healing is usually the optimal treatment method.

### Total wound excision

Burns that are deemed to be deep partial thickness in nature are best tangentially excised and the wound covered with autologous split skin grafts [26]. The grafts usually require meshing and the amount of wound that can be closed with autograft depends on the donor sites available and the mesh ratio used. Cosmetically and functionally sensitive areas such as the face and hands need thicker sheet autograft for wound closure.

If the burn size is large or if donor sites are scarce, then temporary wound closure with allograft, xenograft or other biological or semi-biological dressings may be required to close the rest of the wound while the donor sites heal. Standard graft dressings are applied. The grafted areas can be inspected five days later. Early inspection of the wound is recommended if there was late presentation or colonization of the excised burn wound. The authors prefer to undertake this type of total wound excision in one stage but the availability of enough surgeons is critical. Alternatively this can be done in two or three stages within the first five days following the burn. Patients with large burns need to return to the operating room for further grafting when their donor sites are healed. This is usually done on a weekly basis.

### Serial wound excision and conservative management

This method is employed for larger burns where donor sites are scarce. The surgical technique is similar to that given above but the amount of burn wound excised is the amount that can be covered by meshed split skin grafts from the available donor sites.

Unexcised areas are treated with topical antimicrobials until donor sites have healed and can be reharvested, usually 7–14 days later. The unhealed areas of burn wound are susceptible to invasive wound infection before they are excised and this treatment method has a higher morbidity and mortality compared to early excision. The use of the topical antimicrobial flamacerium (silver sulfadiazine and cerium nitrate) has been reported as decreasing episodes of invasive wound infection, morbidity and mortality with this method of treatment [27].

Alternatively wounds can be treated with Acticoat® with alternate day to weekly dressing changes or with daily or twice daily applications of silver sulfadiazine until wound healing is achieved. This may take up to 4–6 weeks and involve the patient in prolonged and painful periods of dressing

changes. There is a higher incidence of invasive wound infection using this method with associated deepening of the wound. Once healed there is a much higher incidence of hypertrophic scarring which can be functionally and cosmetically disabling. This method is usually reserved for patients who are thought to be unfit for surgical intervention and for smaller burns in functionally and cosmetically unimportant areas.

## Full thickness burns

Full thickness burns will not heal spontaneously unless very small and invariably require skin grafting. The necrotic tissue usually requires excision and the resultant wound requires closure to reduce the risks of invasive infection and systemic sepsis. Prompt excision and wound closure reduces morbidity and mortality inpatients with such injuries.

### Excision and autografting

By definition full thickness injuries will not heal spontaneously and require wound closure with split thickness autografts. On presentation it is usually best to excise these wounds in a tangential fashion and obtain wound closure with split thickness autograft. Meshed autograft is used if larger areas need closure, whereas sheet autograft is used for functionally and cosmetically sensitive areas such as the hands and face. Grafts are secured to the wounds by staples or absorbable sutures and are dressed in the standard fashion. Grafts and wounds are inspected on the second day if the initial wound was infected or heavily colonized or on the fifth day if not.

### Topical antimicrobials

In patients who are elderly or unfit for surgical intervention, conservative management with topical antimicrobials can be used. The antimicrobial agent–Acticoat® or silver sulphadiazine–is applied regularly until the burn eschar separates and a granulating wound is present. This usually takes approximately three to four weeks to occur and sometimes longer. This granulating wound can then be covered with autograft to achieve wound closure. In certain cases small wounds less than 5 cm diameter can be left to heal spontaneously by wound contraction and epithelialization from the wound margins. This method of treatment usually results in a higher incidence of invasive wound sepsis, a longer inpatient stay in the burn unit and a longer time to wound healing. It is not recommended except in the special circumstances given above.

## Large full thickness burns

In larger injuries (>10%TBSA) the treatment of choice is total excision of the burn wound and physiologic wound closure with split skin autograft, allograft and/or synthetic skin substitutes. This early aggressive surgical approach has been shown to improve mortality in selected adult patient groups with such injury [28–30] (Fig. 3).

It is a major surgical undertaking to do this in one sitting with the larger burns (greater 40% TBSA) and needs a coordinated approach from the surgical and anesthetic teams (Fig. 4). The timing of surgery post injury is critical as blood loss in the 24h post burn has been shown to be half that of surgery after this time [31]. In centers when numerous surgeons and anaesthetists are not available, total wound ex-

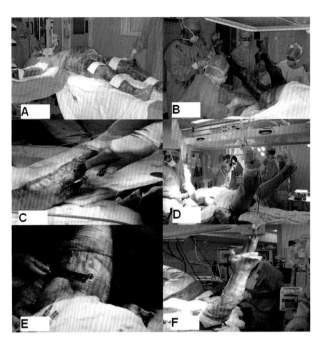

**Fig. 4.** Total Burn Wound Excision. A Patient completely exposed on operating table; B Total body prep with povidone iodine (Note thermal ceiling to maintain temperature); C Infiltration with Adrenaline solution (1/1x106); D Two surgical teams – limbs elevated. E Wound excision; F Temporary wound closure with Biobrane®

cision can be staged over two to three operations removing the wound within five days of the injury.

The type of wound excision depends on the state of the burn wound. Those patients presenting immediately following their injury usually have an uncolonized wound, which can be excised in a tangential fashion with a skin graft knife.

Those patients presenting late five or more days after injury will have a colonized or infected wound. Attempts to preserve subcutaneous fat in these cases usually fail and can lead to invasive systemic sepsis; therefore fascial excision is usually preferred.

After total wound excision the whole wound must be physiologically closed with auto- or allograft or a synthetic skin substitute like Integra®. In large and massive burns special techniques such as overlay grafting are used to cover large wound areas with widely meshed autograft [32] (Fig. 5). In these burns where wound closure cannot be achieved primarily with autograft, the patient returns to the operating room when the donor sites are ready for reharvesting at which time allograft is changed and further autograft

# Wound Treatment Programme

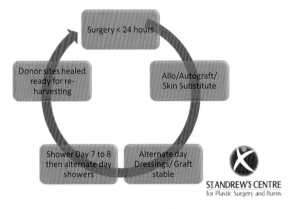

**Fig. 3.** Wound Treatment Programme for Major Burn Injury (courtesy Mr. M Lloyd MRCS). 1) Following admission total/near total wound excision is undertaken within 24hrs of injury. 2) Wound closure achieved with auto/allograft or skin substitute 3) Wound care until donor sites are healed 4) Process repeated

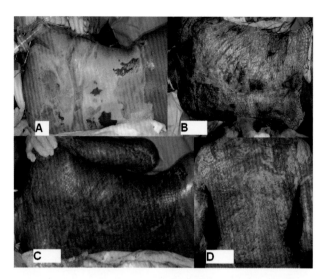

**Fig. 5.** Sandwich Grafting Technique. A Full thickness burn back; B Following excision and application 4:1 Autograft with 2:1 allograft overlay; C Allograft separated, autograft taken, interstices epithelialising; D Healed wound

is applied. This is usually done in stages on a weekly basis until the whole wound is closed with autograft.

## Serial excision

A more traditional conservative surgical approach has been described above for deep partial thickness burns and entails excision of as much of the wound that can be covered with available autograft. The un-excised areas of burn are treated with topical anti-microbials until the donor sites are ready to be re-harvested. This method of treatment has a higher morbidity and mortality in larger injuries and has generally been abandoned in the author's service but is still popular worldwide and is indeed the standard of care in many institutions.

Topical antimicrobials and autografting of a granulating wound used to be popular but in general has been abandoned for more aggressive surgical approaches described above.

It is only suitable for smaller burns in patients who are unfit for surgical debridement of the burn wound. It is not recommended for younger, fit patients with larger injuries.

## Mixed depth burn

Although the descriptions above have described specific depths of burn, in clinical practice most burns are mixed depth with areas of superficial partial, deep partial and full thickness injury in adjacent area. Treatment of such wound depends on the mixture of each component part of the injury, as one will usually predominate. In general superficial partial thickness areas should be left to epithelialize while the areas of deeper injury require excision and wound closure.

## Donor sites

Pre-operative planning is essential prior to burn surgery. In particular choice of donor sites to be used, anatomical areas to be debrided, and the technique used for debridement. It is essential to estimate the amount of autograft that will be required, which areas are priorities for autograft coverage and any required mesh ratios.

In smaller burns where donor sites and available graft is plentiful, the focus is to minimize donor site morbidity and to maximize functional and cosmetic outcome. Sheet grafts are preferred and care must be taken to preferentially harvest cosmetically hidden areas such as the upper thighs, buttocks and scalp. In young females skin should be harvested from either the buttock or the upper inner aspect of the thighs. In young males the upper outer aspect of the thigh can be used in addition. The scalp is an attractive donor site, as subsequent hair growth completely hides the scars.

In patients with major burn injury choice of donor sites is limited and skin grafts should be harvested from any available site as priority is given to cover large areas with available autograft in the smallest number of operations.

## Techniques of wound excision

It is accepted that removal of necrotic devitalized tissue saves lives and is key to wound healing and closure. The technique used to excise the burn wound depends on the depth and extent of injury. Preservation of viable dermis is important in partial thickness injury whereas in full thickness injury all necrotic and infected tissue must be removed. The aim of debridement is to leave a viable wound bed of fat, fascia or muscle that will accept a skin graft.

Tangential excision of the burn wound was described by Janzekovic in the1970s [26] and involves repeated shaving of partial thickness burns in a tangential fashion using a skin graft knife or dermatome until a viable dermal bed is reached. This is manifested clinically by punctate bleeding. The more numerous the bleeding vessels in the wound bed, the more superficial the wound. Hemostasis is obtained with hot soaks and electrocautery and the wound is ready for grafting.

A hand skin graft knife or powered dermatome can be used to make serial passes across the wound to excise the full thickness wound. Excision can be aided by traction on the excised eschar as it passes through the knife or dermatome. Adequate excision is signaled by a viable bleeding wound bed, which is usually fat. The fat underneath must be viable and can be distinguished by its colour (red fat being dead fat), punctate hemorrhages, and thrombosed vessels. These appearances are all indicative of inadequate excision and necessitate further wound excision. After hemostasis the wound is ready for grafting.

Full thickness excision can also be achieved using sharp excision with a knife or with electrocautery. The plane of excision runs between viable and nonviable tissue, and an attempt is made to preserve viable subdermal structures and fat. This more controlled type of wound excision is used where contour preservation is important such as the face or where subcutaneous structures such as the dorsal veins in the hand require preservation.

Water jet hydro surgery (Versajet®) has been described and popularize for burn wound excision mainly in partial thickness injury [33]. Most reports have been anecdotal case series with only one comparative study. Authors cite precision and dermal preservation as the main benefits associate with this technique but accept longer surgical time as a drawback. The only randomized trial assessing this technology reported equivalent adequacy of debridement and shorter surgical time for the Versajet® [34].

Fascial excision is reserved for deep burns extending down through the fat into muscle, late pres-

entation infected wounds and for failed initial surgery in patients with life-threatening invasive infections [35]. It involves surgical excision of the full thickness of the integument including the subcutaneous fat down to fascia. It is done with electrocautery and offers excellent control of blood loss and leaves a wound bed of fascia, which is an excellent bed for graft take. Unfortunately fascial excision is mutilating and leaves a permanent contour defect.

Avulsion can be used for some, deeper wounds particularly those treated conservatively. The necrotic eschar can be avulsed from the underlying viable tissue with minimal blood loss.

Occasionally primary amputation must be considered in management of the burn wound. It is usually reserved for high voltage electrical injuries or very deep thermal injuries with extensive muscle involvement and rhabdomyolysis which is life threatening. In general, limb salvage is attempted if possible with preservation of length to try and maximize function. Amputation in these cases is reserved for patients who have an ischemic limb or refractory invasive infection following repeated debridement. In other circumstances amputation is undertaken only if all other measures to preserve a useful functioning limb have failed.

## Blood loss

Blood loss during burn surgery can be massive and pre-operative planning and preparation is required. The amount of blood required can be estimated. It depends on timing of the surgery post injury and the area of wound that requires excision and autografting.

The approximate blood loss in ml per $cm^2$ burn excised in patients with burns >30 TBSA is estimated as [31]:

| Day post injury | Estimated blood loss (ml/cm²) |
|---|---|
| 0–1 | 0.4 |
| 1–2 | 0.6 |
| 2–16 | 0.75 |
| >16 | >0.5 |

Blood and blood products must be ordered and present in the operating theatre prior to the commencement of surgery. Incorporating this into the WHO patient safety checklist should minimize complications of blood loss [36].

Blood loss during surgery can also be minimized by the use of sterile limb tourniquets, infiltration of the eschar and donor sites with $1/10^6$ solution of adrenaline (1 mg in 1,000 ml N saline) and warm topical phenylephrine (2% solution) soaked dressings. It is possible to debride and excise significant wounds (>30%) without the need for blood transfusion.

## Antibiotics

The reported incidence of nosocomial infections varies at 63–240 per 100 patients and 53–93 per 1000 patient days. Infections precede multiple organ failure and are independently associated with adverse outcomes and increased mortality.

The wound plays a major role as the site of infection with rapid contamination and colonization with Gram positive bacteria, mainly staphylococci. The moist burn wound is a perfect site for proliferation of bacteria. Gram negative bacterial infections are thought to result from bacterial translocation from the gut. Burn patients are known to be immune-compromised and often require intensive care support making them prone to ventilator associated pneumonia and catheter related infections.. In general the consensus view in the current literature that prophylaxis with systemic antibiotics should not be given to patients with severe burns based on the lack of evidence, no obvious benefit and risk of adverse effects. However a recent meta-analysis of antibiotic prophylaxis indicated a reduction in the mortality risk in burn patients although the methodological quality of the data analysed was weak [37].

It is our practice to give antibiotic prophylaxis to patients undergoing surgical procedures. The antibiotic given and duration of therapy depend on the time since the injury, the surgical procedure being undertaken and microbiological surveillance and advice.

## Anatomical considerations

The sequence of areas to be autografted is variable depending on the surgeon's individual preference.

In general the authors try to cover the posterior trunk, anterior trunk, lower limbs, upper limbs, and head and neck in order. This sequence maximizes the area covered with autograft early in the course and allows for earlier ambulation. Areas not covered with autograft have allograft placed, which is removed when autograft is available at subsequent operations.

In general sheet grafts should be used whenever possible, however this not possible in burns over 30% TBSA. Care must be taken when mesh grafts are used as contracture can occur in the line of the interstices.

Mesh graft interstices on the trunk and breast should be placed horizontally. Care should be taken to preserve the breast or breast bud, especially in females, and to place enough skin with minimal mesh expansion into the infra mammary folds and the sternal area to try and reduce subsequent breast deformity. The umbilicus should be preserved if possible.

The buttocks are difficult to manage and skin graft take is poor. They are prone to faecal soiling and shearing and can be the site of repeated bouts of invasive wound sepsis. It is often worth autografting them in the first operation, but graft take can be disappointing. If the grafts fail it is then best to leave the area for a time when the patient can be nursed prone while the grafts take. This is usually done after all other areas are healed. It is not usually necessary to perform a colostomy to prevent fecal soiling as the faecal stream can be diverted with a rectal tube. The perineum and genitalia are usually managed conservatively with grafting of any unhealed areas later on in the course of surgical treatment.

Mesh graft interstices on the limbs should run longitudinally along the line of the limb except at the joints. At the knee, ankle, axilla, elbow and wrist joints graft expansion should be minimized if possible and the direction of the interstices should be the same as the axis of rotation of the joint i. e. perpendicular to the longitudinal axis of the limb.

The skin on the sole of the foot is glabrous skin and is very thick and specialized. It will commonly re-epithelialize despite what initially seems a full thickness injury. The sole of the foot is best treated conservatively until it is apparent that spontaneous re-epithelialization will not occur. In contrast the skin on the dorsal aspect of the foot is very thin and often requires grafting. It is important not to use widely meshed skin in this area as any significant hypertrophic scarring can cause difficulties with weight bearing ambulation and fitting of shoes.

The burnt hand requires attention to detail must to achieve optimal functional and cosmetic results. The volar aspect of the hand is covered with specialized glabrous skin, which usually heals and it is best to avoid grafting it if possible. The dorsal skin is thin and usually requires grafting in deep burns. In general, sheet graft is preferable to mesh graft and is best secured with absorbable sutures. Mesh interstices should run longitudinally along the hand and digits. The key to functional success is early mobilization of the hand. Initially after grafting the hand is dressed and splinted in the position of safety with the metacarpophalangeal joints flexed at 70–90°, the interphalangeal joints at 180°, the wrist in neutral or slightly extended and the thumb flexed and adducted at the metacarpophalangeal joint. The grafts are inspected at five days and, if stable, mobilization can be started. If sheet grafts are used they can be exposed with no dressing during mobilization during the day with splintage at night.

In patients with large burns, repeated application of allograft may be required until it is time to autograft the hands. It can be very difficult to maintain the position of safety of the hand during this phase and K-wires through the metacarpophalangeal and interphalangeal joints may be required to maintain the joints in optimal position.

The face and neck are areas that are both cosmetically and functionally important and are discussed in greater detail later on in the book. Deeper burns of the face will often benefit from early excision and autografting. Medium to thick sheet split skin autograft should be used for the face and applied in cosmetic units to place marginal scars in natural skin crease lines. If available, donor sites should be above the neck for optimum color and texture match. The scalp is an excellent donor site for grafts destined for the face. The use of skin substitutes like Integra® have been describes as giving superior cosmetic outcomes.

Early excision and closure of eyelid burns reduces the incidence of corneal injury secondary to exposure and should be a priority. When applying autograft to the eyelids thick split thickness graft should be used and overcorrection should be performed putting more skin in than seems to be needed as contraction can lead to corneal exposure.

## Skin replacement

Following wound excision it is vital to obtain wound closure. Wound closure can be permanent using autologous split skin graft or temporary using allograft or skin substitutes. Physiological closure of the burn wound reduces invasive infection, evaporative water loss, heat loss, pain and promotes wound healing. Temporary skin substitutes are used to achieve physiological wound closure following excision until donor sites have regenerated and are ready for harvesting. In general all these coverings buy time while the donor sites heal [38].

### Autograft

In general autologous split skin grafts are the gold standard for resurfacing burns. However they have limitations and attempts are being made to resolve some of these by the development of skin substitutes. Split skin grafts can be harvested either as split thickness or full thickness grafts. Full thickness grafts tend not to be used for acute burns, as the donor sites requires closure, do not regenerate and are limited and their use is usually reserved for postburn reconstruction.

Split skin grafts take more easily, and are the mainstay for wound closure. Split skin grafts can be harvested either with a hand knife or with a powered dermatome. Skin grafts can be used as sheet grafts or can be meshed using expansion ratios of 1:1, 2:1, 3:1, 4:1, 6:1 and 9:1. Other skin expansion techniques such as the Meek technique have also been described as being beneficial.

### Allograft

Allograft skin is a vital skin substitute and its use has been a key factor in improvement in the mortality associated with extensive burns [39]. Allograft skin is usually harvested from cadaveric donors after appropriate donor selection and screening for communicable disease, and consent from relatives has been

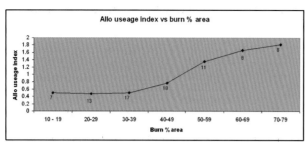

**Fig. 6.** Allograft Usage Index. Amount allograft used in cm² per % Burn TBSA

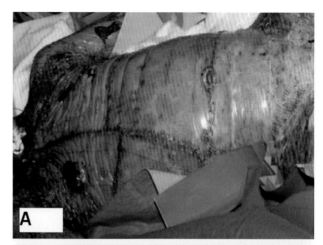

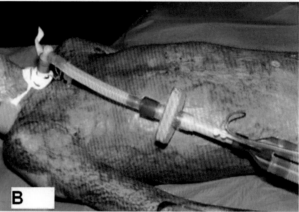

**Fig. 7.** Use of Integra® in Patient with 70% TBSA Burn. A Following application, Integra® Revascularised; B Following Autografting, Wound Healed

obtained. Strict exclusion criteria are applied to ensure safety for transplantation.

Allograft skin is usually harvested, collected, screened, processed, and distributed by a regional tissue bank. Allograft is analogous to blood, and it is important to use this vital resource responsibly. The amount can be estimated by determining the body surface area and burn size in cm². Recent analysis of total allograft use has produced an allograft index to aid planning [40] (Fig. 6).

Allograft skin can also be obtained from living donors, usually parents or relatives of burned children. It is usually harvested immediately prior to its use on the burn victim and is used fresh. In view of the reliable supplies of good quality allograft skin provided by tissue banks, this method is used infrequently.

Allograft skin can be used either as sheet or meshed graft. It is mainly used meshed 2:1, and care is taken not to expand the interstices to prevent desiccation, infection and necrosis of the underlying wound. Meshing the allograft allows any hematoma and seroma drainage. Sheet allograft tends to be used to cover cosmetic areas such as the face as even with unexpanded mesh granulation tissue can grow through the interstices and leave a permanent pattern.

## Integra®

Integra® is an acellular bilaminar structure that provides wound closure with permanent dermal replacement [41]. It is made of an upper silicone layer that acts as a temporary epidermis providing control of evaporative water loss acting as a barrier to microorganisms. The bottom layer is a cross linked matrix of bovine collagen and chondroitin-6-sulphate. This becomes incorporated into the wound and is termed a 'neodermis'. This skin substitute is used to replace dermis in full-thickness burns in an attempt to modulate post burn hypertrophic scarring.

After excision of the burn Integra® is applied to the wound in a similar fashion to autograft. Care is taken to avoid wrinkles or pleats in the Integra® and it is secured to the wound with either skin staples or sutures. Non-shear dressings are then applied and silver based dressings are applied to the covered areas on a regular basis to try and limit contamination, colonization and infection of the Integra® covered wounds. The Integra® should be inspected daily during this time. Any collections occurring under the matrix should be aspirated and sent for microbiological culture. If any purulent material appears under the Integra® or if it becomes non adherent, then it should be removed, the underlying wound cultured and the Integra® replaced with allograft skin.

The collagen/chondroitin-6-sulfate matrix is vascularised by host cells over the next three weeks or so and the artificial dermis is gradually replaced with a 'neodermis' which is pink and flat. No granulation tissue should be seen. When the 'neodermis' looks vascularised and has a healthy pink colour, the silastic covering can be removed and very thin epidermal autografts (2–4/1000 inch), containing epidermis only can be harvested and applied. This provides epidermal cover for the 'neodermis' and produces permanent wound closure (Fig. 7). The grafts are susceptible to loss at this stage and silver based dressings are applied over a non-shear dressing.

Integra® has been extensively studied and has produced encouraging results both in single centre studies and in a multi-centred randomized controlled trial [41]. Studies have reported less hypertrophic scarring with a much more pliable resultant scar and a reduced requirement for secondary reconstructive procedures [42], however, this concept has never been demonstrated fully even with over 20 years of use. Integra® is expensive, but when successful it has been shown to provide a durable, long-term result, with some suggestion of reduced hypertrophic scarring and pruritus [42].

Integra has also been used in post burn reconstruction, especially for in patients who have limited availability of donor sites [43].

## Matriderm®

Recently synchronous application of dermal substitutes and skin graft has been established as a standard procedure. Matriderm®, a bovine based collagen I, III, V and elastin hydrolysate based dermal substitute has been used with simultaneous application of split-thickness skin graft [44] (Fig. 8). This approach obviates the need for a second procedure for application of autograft. In a recent pilot study 20 wounds in 10 patients with severe burns were treated with either simultaneous transplantation of Matriderm® and split thickness autograft or split thickness autograft alone after appropriate excision of the burn

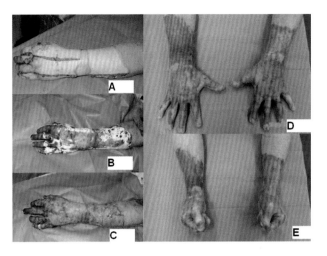

**Fig. 8.** Matriderm® for Deep Burn to Hand. A Deep burn to left hand; B Following excision and application of Matriderm®; C Following application autograft over Matriderm®; D Post Op picture at 3 months including right hand treated with autograft alone; E Good early functional result

wound. The study concluded that simultaneous application of a dermal matrix is safe and feasible, yielding significantly better results with respect to skin elasticity [45]. A similar Integra® one stage collagen based single stage dermal replacement product has also been produced but at the time of writing is not widely available.

## Other skin replacements

Alloderm® is a commercially available form of de-epidermalised de-cellularised sterile human dermis. It can be used as a dermal replacement for acute care and for post burn reconstruction [46]. In acute cases the burn wound is excised and prepared as usual. Alloderm® is applied to the wound and a thin (epidermal) split skin graft is applied over it. This bilayered graft is secured and managed as skin graft. The dermal portion must be initially revascularised from the wound bed before vascularisation of the epidermal graft. This makes the technique prone to epidermal loss due to desiccation and infection prior to vascularisation of the epidermal graft. The amount of wound covered is usually limited to the amount of autologous split skin available for harvest. This has limited its success in the management of acute burns especially those involving a large surface area. It has been used more successfully in post burn reconstruction.

Amnion is the inner layer of tissue that surrounds the foetus in utero, and contains amniotic fluid. Both the inner amnion and the outer chorion layers have been used for many years, but amnion is preferred because it is immunologically privileged and less antigenic. Amnion is commonly used by Ophthalmologists to cover damaged corneas as it is immunologically privileged tissue and does not stimulate rejection. Amnion can control evaporative fluid loss and is effective in reducing bacterial counts. It also contains many growth factors that stimulate epithelial proliferation and has antiangiogenic properties.

In view of these specific factors its main use in burn care has been in partial thickness wounds such as donor sites and partial thickness burns [47]. It has not been extensively used following wound excision. Like any allogeneic material the risk of disease transmission must be recognised and managed. The limited availability, small size and fragility limit its usefulness in burn care. The majority of reports on its use in burn care have come from the developing world.

Although a variety of xenograft (sheep skin, frog skin) has been described as being used as a skin substitute, the only commercially available product is obtained from domestic swine. It has been processed in a number of ways to reduce antigenicity and prolong adherence. Processing has included irradiation, lyophilisation, glutaraldehyde-crosslinking and impregnation with silver. Porcine xenograft is available as either de-epidermalised dermis or complete skin. Depending on processing it can be stored in a refrigerator or at room temperature. Porcine skin xenografts have many of the same advantages as allograft skin. They can reduce evaporative water loss, limit infection, and encourage autologous epidermal growth. Porcine xenografts adhere to the wound be but will not vascularise. They are useful as a temporary covering for partial thickness burns, donor sites, and medical desquamating skin conditions but are not useful for excised full thickness wounds. They have a prolonged shelf life, are easy available and are relatively inexpensive when compare to human cadaveric allograft [48].

## Cultured skin substitutes

Using tissue culture techniques, epidermal cells (keratinocytes) can be grown in a laboratory and then used to assist wound closure [49]. From a 1 cm$^2$ autologous biopsy, enough cells can be cultured in approximately 3–4 weeks to cover 1 m$^2$ body surface area. Sheets of these cultured epithelial autografts or CEAs, have been used by burn surgeons for over 20 years [50].

These cells can be cultured commercially for patients with large burn injuries, however, the cost is significant. This technique only produces the epidermal layer for wound closure and, although there have been many reports of successful use of CEA to close burn wounds, a number of problems limit their use. The lag time of 3 weeks from biopsy to production of adequate quantities allows wound colonization and granulation tissue to develop leading to low take rates compare to split skin grafts. Once applied, the grafts are very fragile and often-prolonged immobilization of the patient is required. Even after successful take, the grafted areas remain fragile and blister easily due to poor and delayed basement membrane formation. Attempts to overcome some of these problems have been to graft the CEA onto an allograft dermal bed as described by Cuono in 1986 [51]. Initially after wound excision, allograft is used for temporary wound closure while CEA are produced. When ready, the epidermal portion of the engrafted allograft is removed using a dermatome or dermabrasion leaving a viable dermal allograft bed behind onto which the CEA are applied. This technique has been reported as having better CEA take with improved basement membrane formation and less fragility and blistering [51].

More recently the use of sub-confluent, autologous keratinocyte suspensions sprayed onto excised wounds has been described. This promising technique has been used directly to treat partial thickness wounds and excised wounds after excision. It has also been used to augment epithelialisation by treating interstices of widely meshed skin grafts and also skin graft donor sites. Initial results have been promising and many burn surgeons have moved from using sheets of CEA to this subconfluent suspension technique [52]. However confirmation of the superiority of this technique has yet to be confirmed by a multi-centred trial.

In general the use of CEA should be reserved for patients with massive burns with extremely limited donor sites or major burns where donor sites are limited, difficult to harvest and cosmetically and functionally important (face, hands feet, genitalia). A review of patients surviving massive burn injury showed that patients treated with CEA had a longer hospital stay, required more operations, and had a higher treatment costs compared to a comparative group of patients treated with conventional techniques [52].

## Skin graft take

By definition a graft is completely removed from its donor site, loses its blood supply and requires revascularization when applied to the wound bed. Split skin grafts take on wound beds by adherence, plasmatic imbibition and revascularization. When a split skin graft is applied to a wound bed, rapid adherence is a good sign implying that the graft will take. Adherence is due to fibrin bonds, which are weak at first and can be disrupted by shear, hematoma or seroma. If serous fluid starts to leak through mesh interstices or fenestration's immediately after graft application and the graft is adherent, good take is ensured.

Over the first 48 h the graft survives by plasmatic imbibition, that is, absorption of fluid into the graft due to accumulation of osmotically active metabolites and denatured matrix proteins. This fluid may contribute to cell nutrition and may keep vascular channels within the graft open until it is revascularised. Thin grafts survive this process better than thicker ones. The graft is revascularized over a period of 3–4 days with vessel anastomoses between the wound bed vasculature and existing vessels within the graft (inosculation) and by direct fibrovascular ingrowth from the wound bed into the graft matrix forming new vascular channels.

In the initial stages graft revascularization can be prevented or disrupted by graft shear, hematoma or seroma formation. Graft shear can be minimized by non shear dressings, pressure dressings, exposure or graft quilting. Hematoma can be minimized by meticulous hemostasis following wound excision. Mesh grafting or fenestration will allow drainage of hematoma or seroma.

Adherence and subsequent take depend on the wound bed, thus freshly excised wounds take graft well with fascia better than fat. Fresh granulating wounds also take grafts well but chronic granulating wounds and contaminated wounds have poorer graft takes due to proteolytic enzymes in the wound that can be produced by both bacteria and cells within the wound itself. In chronic granulating wounds it is not uncommon to see 'ghosting' of skin where initial graft take is good but then the grafts slowly 'dissolve' over a period of days. They can be salvaged by wound care with topical antimicrobials.

Following take the graft goes through a number of stages to achieve maturation. Initially there is epithelial hyperplasia and thickening which leads to scaling and desquamation. The epithelial appendages such as sweat and sebaceous glands do not survive grafting but can regenerate in thicker grafts. The grafts are dry and require moisturizing until these functions return. Grafts tend to be re-innervated over a period of time with sensation developing within a month but continued improvement can occur for several years.

Pigmentation of grafts can be troublesome, particularly inpatients with dark skin. Grafts can be hypo- or hyperpigmented and it is difficult to predict which. In general, grafts harvested from the lower half of the body tend to be paler and can become yellow if placed above the clavicle.

The main problem with grafts is that of hypertrophic scarring and contraction. All grafts will be surrounded by a marginal hypertrophic scar. Interstices in mesh grafts will develop hypertrophic scarring and in widely meshed graft will give an unsightly appearance. The amount of wound contraction depends on the proportion of dermal thickness within the graft. Thus areas where there is no dermis, such as at the margin of grafts and in grafts interstices, hypertrophic scarring and wound contraction are inevitable. Wound contraction around mobile areas and anatomical landmarks can lead to contractures resulting in deformity and impairment of function.

## Rehabilitation and outcome

Burn rehabilitation starts on admission to the burn service. Having a significant burn is frightening, disorientating and painful. Positioning, splintage, and control of oedema are essential to maintain range of motion and function. Active mobilization and promoting functional activities are also vital and should commence on admission. Respiratory care and rehabilitation to maintain spontaneous ventilation, coughing and expectoration are important to minimize the need for mechanical ventilation and its associated complications.

Consistent repetitive and motivational education is a vital part of patient care. Patients are encouraged to share responsibility for their own management and to optimise their rehabilitative opportunities [53]. Well motivated patients can surpass expectations with regards to their functional recovery whereas poorly motivated patients can end up with poor functional outcomes despite best efforts [54]. Early exercise has been shown to be beneficial following paediatric burn injury, significantly enhancing lean mass and strength, without exacerbation of postburn hypermetabolism [55]. This work need to be repeated in an adult population to demonstrate benefit in this patient group.

Outcome following burn injury in adults has been traditionally defined in terms of mortality and length of stay. Crude mortality data are not helpful in assessing individual services performance and the Lethal Dose 50% is the recommended assessment tool. This can be obtained by probit analysis of mortality data and signifies the %TBSA burn at which 50% of the patients admitted to the service die. This data is available from North America where young adults (age 16 -65 yrs) have an LD50 of approximately 80% TBSA and middle aged adults have an LD50 of over 50% TBSA[56]. Unfortunately this data is not commonly available outside North America [57].

Length of stay is a good global surrogate measure for outcome and quality of care. If patients are admitted in a timely fashion, undergo adequate fluid resuscitation, have appropriate early surgical excision and grafting, receive satisfactory nutritional and critical care support, have good wound care and have timely physical and psychosocial rehabilitation, they will ready for discharge in a relatively short time frame. It is accepted that one day per percent burn as a goal for length of stay in their more significant injuries.

However delays may reflect complex rehabilitation, psychological or social issue that may be a barrier to discharge.

More sophisticated measurement of outcome in burns patients is complex and multi-faceted. As increased numbers of burned injured survive a more comprehensive assessment of outcome deserves high priority. Domains of assessment have been described that provide such a global view. These include (i) skin; (ii) neuromuscular function; (iii) sensory and pain; (iv) psychological function; (v) physical role function; (vi) community participation; and (vii) perceived quality of life [58]. There are many and varied measurement tools that have been used to assess these domains however further investigation is required to identify the best tools and new tools that can provide easily measurable and reproducible assessment of outcome.

## Future care

Despite significant advances in burn care leading to improved survival over the past 30 years, burn injury still represents a major challenge in clinical care. Improved fluid resuscitation, respiratory care, critical care and wound management have all contributed to decreases in morbidity and mortality. However limited donor sites, infectious complications, the systemic inflammatory response leading to organ dysfunction can lead to significant morbidity and prolonged in patient stay. It has been postulated that Stem Cell therapy has the potential to modify systemic response and enhance wound healing.

Embryonic and adult stem cells have the ability to differentiate into various tissue types and a prolonged self-renewal capacity. Bone marrow, peripheral blood, umbilical cord blood, adipose tissue, skin and hair follicles, have all been utilized to isolate stem cells. Beneficial effects include acceleration of healing of acute and chronic wounds [59].

Gene therapy, initially developed for treatment of congenital defects, holds potential for enhancing wound healing and repair by modifying genes encoding for growth factors or cytokines. The majority of gene delivery systems are based on viral transfection, naked DNA application, high pressure injection, or liposomal vectors. Recently, the combination of gene and stem cell therapy has emerged as a promising approach for treatment of chronic and acute wounds [60].

In the future combinations of such novel approaches should have beneficial effects on outcome in the management of adult burn patients.

## References

[1] Mosier MJ, Gibran NS (2009) Surgical excision of the burn wound. Clin Plast Surg 36(4): 617–625

[2] Brusselaers N, Monstrey S, Vogelaers D, Hoste E, Blot S (2010) Severe burn injury in europe: a systematic review of the incidence, etiology, morbidity, and mortality. Critical Care 14:R188

[3] Deitch EA, Wheelahan TM, Rose MP, Clothier J, Cotter (1983) Hypertrophic burn scars: analysis of variables. J Trauma 23(10): 895–898

[4] McDonald WS, Deitch EA (1987) Hypertrophic skin grafts in burned patients: a prospective analysis of variables. J Trauma 27(2): 147–150

[5] Jackson DM (1953) The diagnosis of the depth of burning. Br J Surg 40: 588

[6] Cuttle L, Pearn J, McMillan JR, Kimble RM (2009) A review of first aid treatments for burn injuries. Burns 35(6): 768–775

[7] Sargent RL (2006) Management of blisters in the partial-thickness burn: an integrative research review. J Burn Care Res 27(1): 66–81

[8] Light TD, Latenser BA, Kealey GP, Wibbenmeyer LA, Rosenthal GE, Sarrazin MV (2009) The effect of burn center and burn center volume on the mortality of burned adults–an analysis of the data in the National Burn Repository. J Burn Care Res 30(5): 776–782

[9] Klein MB, Hayden D, Elson C, Nathens AB, Gamelli RL, Gibran NS, Herndon DN, Arnoldo B, Silver G, Schoenfeld D, Tompkins RG (2007) The association between fluid administration and outcome following major burn: a multicenter study. Ann Surg 245(4): 622–628

[10] White CE, Bell DG, Schwacha MG, Wanek SM, Wade CE, Holcomb JB, Chung KK, Wolf SE, Renz EM, Allan PF, Aden JK, Merrill GA, Shelhamer MC, King BT (2010) High-frequency percussive ventilation and low tidal volume ventilation in burns: a randomized controlled trial. Crit Care Med 38(10): 1970–1977

[11] O'Mara MS, Reed NL, Palmieri TL, Greenhalgh DG (2007) Central venous catheter infections in burn patients with scheduled catheter exchange and replacement. J Surg Res 142(2): 341–350

[12] Still JM, Law E, Thiruvaiyaru D, Belcher K, Donker K (1998) Central line-related sepsis in acute burn patients. Am Surg 64(2): 165–170

[13] Wahl WL, Arbabi S, Zalewski C, Wang SC, Hemmila MR (2010) Intensive care unit core measures improve infectious complications in burn patients. J Burn Care Res 31(1): 190–195

[14] Williams FN, Herndon DN, Jeschke MG (2009) The hypermetabolic response to burn injury and interventions to modify this response. Clin Plast Surg 36(4): 583–596

[15] Mosier MJ, Pham TN, Klein MB, Gibran NS, Arnoldo BD, Gamelli RL, Tompkins RG, Herndon DN (2011) Early enteral nutrition in burns: compliance with guidelines and associated outcomes in a multicenter study. J Burn Care Res 32(1): 104–109

[16] Richardson P, Mustard L (2009) The management of pain in the burns unit. Burns 35(7): 921–936

[17] Barret JP, Dziewulski P, Ramzy PI, Wolf SE, Desai MH, Herndon D (2000) Biobrane versus 1% silver sulfadiazine in second-degree pediatric burns. Plast Reconstr Surg 105(1): 62–65

[18] Whitaker IS, Mallinson P, Drew PJ (2008) Biobrane: a versatile tool in the armamentarium of the reconstructive and burns surgeon. Plast Reconstr Surg 121(3): 152e–153e

[19] Khundkar R, Malic C, Burge T (2010) Use of Acticoat dressings in burns: what is the evidence Burns 36(6): 751–758

[20] Tredget EE, Shankowsky HA, Groeneveld A, Burrell R (1998) A matched-pair, randomized study evaluating the efficacy and safety of Acticoat silver-coated dressing for the treatment of burn wounds. J Burn Care Rehabil 19(6): 531–537

[21] Silver GM, Robertson SW, Halerz MM, Conrad P, Supple KG, Gamelli RL (2007) A silver-coated antimicrobial barrier dressing used postoperatively on meshed autografts: a dressing comparison study. J Burn Care Res 28(5): 715–719

[22] Jones I, Currie L, Martin R (2002) A guide to biological skin substitutes. Br J Plast Surg 55(3): 185–193

[23] Wasiak J, Cleland H, Campbell F (2008) Dressings for superficial and partial thickness burns. Cochrane Database Syst Rev (4):CD002106

[24] Naoum JJ, Roehl KR, Wolf SE, Herndon DN (2004) The use of homograft compared to topical antimicrobial therapy in the treatment of second-degree burns of more than 40% total body surface area Burns 30(6): 548–551

[25] Bukovcan P, Koller J (2010) Treatment of partial-thickness scalds by skin xenografts–a retrospective study of 109 cases in a three-year period. J Acta Chir Plast 52(1): 7–12

[26] Janzekovic Z (1970) A new concept in the early excision and immediate grafting of wounds. J Trauma 10: 1103–1108

[27] Garner JP, Heppell PS (2005) Cerium nitrate in the management of burns. Burns 31(5): 539–547

[28] Tompkins RG, Remensnyder JP, Burkr JF et al (1988) Significant reduction in mortality for children with burn injuries through the use of prompt eschar excision. Ann Surg 208 (5): 577–585

[29] Ong YS, Samuel M, Song C (2006) Meta-analysis of early excision of burns. Burns 32(2): 145–150

[30] Herndon DN, Barrow RE, Rutan RL, Rutan TC, Desai MH, Abston S (1989) A comparison of conservative versus early excision. Therapies in severely burned patients. Ann Surg 209(5): 547–552

[31] Desai MH, Herndon DN, Broemeling L, Barrow RE, Nichols RJ Jr, Rutan RL (1990) Early burn wound excision significantly reduces blood loss. Ann Surg 211(6): 753–759

[32] Alexander JW, MacMillan BG, Law E, Kittur DS (1981) Treatment of severe burns with widely meshed skin autograft and meshed skin allograft overlay. J Trauma 21(6): 433–438

[33] Klein MB, Hunter S, Heimbach DM, Engrav LH, Honari S, Gallery E, Kiriluk DM, Gibran NS (2005) The Versajet water dissector: a new tool for tangential excision. J Burn Care Rehabil 26(6): 483–487

[34] Gravante G, Delogu D, Esposito G, Montone A (2007) Versajet hydrosurgery versus classic escharectomy for burn débridment: a prospective randomized trial. J Burn Care Res 28(5): 720–724

[35] Mosier MJ, Gibran NS (2009) Surgical excision of the burn wound. Clin Plast Surg 36(4): 617–625

[36] Surgical Safety Checklist. The World Health Organization. http://www.who. int/patientsafety/safesurgery/en/

[37] Avni T, Levcovich A, Ad-El DD, Leibovici L, Paul M (2010) Prophylactic antibiotics for burns patients: systematic review and meta-analysis. BMJ 340:c241

[38] Pham C, Greenwood J, Cleland H et al (2007) Bioengineered skin substitutes for the management of burns: A systematic review. Burns 33: 946–957

[39] Leon-Villapalos J, Eldardiri M, Dziewulski P (2010) The use of human deceased donor skin allograft in burn care. Cell Tissue Bank 11(1): 99–104

[40] Horner CWM, Atkins J, Simpson L, Philp B, Shelley O, Dziewulski P (2010) Estimating the usage of allograft in the treatment of major burns. Burns (In Press) doi:10 1016

[41] Heimbach DM, Warden GD, Luterman A, Jordan MH, Ozobia N, Ryan CM, Voigt DW, Hickerson WL, Saffle JR, DeClement FA, Sheridan RL, Dimick AR (2003) Multicenter postapproval clinical trial of Integra dermal regeneration template for burn treatment. J Burn Care Rehabil 24(1): 42–48

[42] Sheridan RL, Heggerty M, Tompkins RG et al (1994) Artificial skin in massive burns–results at ten years. Eur J Plast Surg 17: 91–93

[43] Jeng JC, Fidler PE, Sokolich JC et al (2007) Seven years' experience with Integra as a reconstructive tool. J Burn Care Res 28(1): 120–126

[44] Haslik W, Kamolz LP, Nathschläger G, Andel H, Meissl G, Frey M (2007) First experiences with the collagen-elastin matrix Matriderm as a dermal substitute in severe burn injuries of the hand. Burns 33(3): 364–368

[45] Ryssel H, Gazyakan E, Germann G, Ohlbauer M (2008) The use of MatriDerm in early excision and simultaneous autologous skin grafting in burns–a pilot study. Burns 34(1): 93–97

[46] Callcutt RA, Schurr MJ, Sloan M et al (2006) Clinical experience with Alloderm A one- staged composite dermal/epidermal replacement utilizing processed cadaver dermis and thin autografts. Burns 32(5): 583–658

[47] Kesting MR, Wolff KD, Hohlweg-Majert B et al (2008) The role of allogenic amniotic membrane in burn treatment. J Burn Care Res 29(6): 907–916

[48] Saffle JR (2009) Closure of the excised burnwound: Temporary skin substitutes. Clin Plastic Surg 36: 627–641

[49] Green H, Kehinde O, Thomas J (1979) Growth of cultured human epidermal cells into multiple epithelia suitable for grafting. Proc Natl Acad Sci USA 76: 5665–5668

[50] Wood FM, Kolybaba ML, Allen P (2006) The use of cultured epithelial autograft in the treatment of major burn injuries: a critical review of the literature. Burns 32(4): 395–401

[51] Cuono C, Langdon R, McGuire J (1986) Use of cultured epidermal autografts and dermal allografts as skin replacement after burn injury. Lancet 1: 1123–1124

[52] Wood FM, Kolybaba ML, Allen P (2006) The use of cultured epithelial autograft in the treatment of major burn wounds: eleven years of clinical experience. Burns 32(5): 538–44. Epub 2006 Jun 14

[53] Edgar D, Brereton M (2004) Rehabilitation after burn injury. BMJ 329(7461): 343–345

[54] Wade RG, Dziewulski P, Philp BM (2010) The role of an ingestible telemetric thermometer in preventing exertional heat stroke, for a patient with healed massive burns running the 2007 London marathon. Burns 36(6):e119–125

[55] Al-Mousawi AM, Williams FN, Mlcak RP, Jeschke MG, Herndon DN, Suman OE (2010) Effects of exercise training on resting energy expenditure and lean mass during pediatric burn rehabilitation J Burn Care Res 31(3): 400–408

[56] Saffle JR, Davis B, Williams P (1995) Recent outcomes in the treatment of burn injury in the United States: a report from the American Burn Association Patient Registry. J Burn Care Rehabil 16(3 Pt 1): 219–232

[57] Rashid A, Khanna A, Gowar JP, Bull JP (2001) Revised estimates of mortality from burns in the last 20 years at the Birmingham Burns Centre. Burns 27(7): 723–730

[58] Falder S, Browne A, Edgar D, Staples E, Fong J, Rea S, Wood F (2009) Core outcomes for adult burn survivors: a clinical overview. Burns 35(5): 618–641

[59] Butler KL, Goverman J, Ma H, Fischman A, Yu YM, Bilodeau M, Rad AM, Bonab AA,Tompkins RG, Fagan SP (2010) Stem cells and burns: review and therapeutic implications. J Burn Care Res 31(6): 874–881

[60] Branski LK, Gauglitz GG, Herndon DN, Jeschke MG (2009) A review of gene and stem cell therapy in cutaneous wound healing. Burns 35(2): 171–180

Correspondence: P. Dziewulski FFICM FRCS FRCS(Plast), St Andrews Centre for Plastic Surgery and Burns, Chelmsford, Essex, CM1 7ET, UK, E-mail: peter.dziewulski@meht.nhs.uk

# Burns in older adults

Tam N. Pham

University of Washington Burn Center, Harborview Medical Center, Seattle, WA, USA

## Introduction

Burn injury in older adults is expected to have a greater impact on regional burn centers in the next several decades as the population in high-income countries is progressively aging. In the United States, adults aged ≥ 55 are projected to represent 30% of the population by 2030 [1]. The appropriate age cut-off defining the older adult is debated, with a spectrum of age ≥ 45 to age ≥ 80 used in previous burn literature reports [2, 3]. Although this cut-off should ideally be based on biology, aging is a continuous process influenced by the individual's health lifestyle and co-morbid conditions. In fact, the often quoted age ≥ 65 is primarily based on the age at which one can obtain full pension benefits, a reflection of societal constructs rather than biological truths. It is generally agreed, however, that aged patients are vulnerable to burn injury, and that injured older adults have far worse treatment outcomes compared to young adults [4]. Specifically, the American Burn Association reports that the lethal burn area associated with 50% mortality ($LA_{50}$) in a 50 year-old patient is 50% TBSA [5]. In the United Kingdom, the reported $LA_{50}$ for patients aged ≥ 65 is 21% TBSA [6]. Furthermore, those who survive their injuries are at greater risk for long-term disability and loss of independence [7, 8]. It is thus imperative for all burn providers to become familiar with the injury epidemiology, pathophysiologic differences and acute management challenges in older patients.

## Burn injury epidemiology

Flame exposure in household fires, brush burning, and smoking-related injuries account for approximately 65% of older patients requiring admission to US burn centers, followed by scalds (estimated at 15–30%), and contact injuries (5%) [2, 3, 9, 10]. Injury incidences and etiologies may vary with the region of interest. For instance, scalds may represent 31% of older adults admitted to a burn center in France, compared to 66% in Hong Kong [11, 12]. Interestingly, the higher incidence of burns in older adults in high-income countries has not yet been described in low- and middle-income countries, perhaps due to different population demographics and under-reporting [13]. Analysis of patients aged ≥ 55 in the US National Burn Repository (NBR) corroborates the epidemiologic and injury data reported by regional burn centers [14]. Most burns in adults ≥55 occur in the home (56%). The incidence of burns sustained in residential institutions is negligible in the youngest group (age 55–64), but rises to 5.5% in patients 75 and older. Mean burn severity is 9.6% TBSA with a 5.1% full-thickness component and does not significantly vary among age categories. Men comprise the majority of injuries (1.4:1 ratio),

**Table 1.** Common mortality prediction models

| Model/Author | Year | Origin | Formula/Method |
|---|---|---|---|
| "Baux rule" [120] | 1961 | Hôpital Saint-Antoine, Paris, France | Empirically derived: Sum of **age** + TBSA approximates mortality. Survival is very unlikely if score > 75 |
| "Modified Baux rule" [121] | 1979 | St Mary's Hospital, Wisconsin, USA | Probit analysis: Sum of **age** + TBSA predicts > 50% mortality if score exceeds 95 |
| Zawacki [122] | 1979 | University of Southern California, USA | Probit analysis: Probability of death = 0 036 (**age**) + 0 037 (TBSA) + 0 028 (full-thickness) + 0.40 (prior lung disease) + 0.52 (abnormal PaO2) + 0.56 (airway edema) |
| Abbrev. Burn severity Index (ABSI) [123] | 1982 | University of Virginia, USA | Logistic regression: $p(death) = 1/(1+e^{-s})$, where S is the composite score based on the following risk factors: sex (0–1), **age category** (1–5), inhalation injury (0–1), full-thickness burn (0–1), burn extent (1–10). |
| Ryan [124] | 1998 | Massachusetts General Hospital, USA | Logistic regression: -5.89 + 2.58 (number of risk factors) = logit for death.<br>Risk factors: **age > 60**, TBSA > 40, inhalation injury. |
| O'Keefe [125] | 2001 | Parkland Hospital, Texas, USA | Logistic regression: $p(death) = 1/(1+e^{-z})$, where Z= -6 3898 + 0 0462 (TBSA) + 0 0408 (full-thickness) + 22 (inhalation injury) + 0 0046 (if female) + 0 7066 (if aged 30–59) + 3 7128 (**if aged ≥ 60**) + 1 804 (if female and aged 30–59) + 0 4055 (if female and **aged ≥ 60**) |
| McGwin Jr. [126] | 2008 | University of Alabama, USA | Logistic regression, Logit for death = -7 3406 + (0 0556 × **age**) + (0 0654 ×TBSA) + (0. 1. 3340 × Inhalation Injury) + (0 2052 × Co-existent Trauma) + (0 5177 × Pneumonia) |
| "Revised Baux" [127] | 2010 | University of Vermont, USA | rBaux = **Age** + TBSA + 17(if inhalation injury present). rBaux to be fitted into nomogram to derive predicted mortality |

but the proportion of injured women increases with age. Women actually outnumber men in patients aged 75 and over. Older age remains an important risk factor for death after burn injury, as evidenced by commonly derived mortality prediction models (Table 1). Although several centers have reported improved outcomes in recent years, survival in older adults still lags far behind that in younger cohorts [10, 15, 16]. According to current US data, the adjusted odds ratios for death is 2.3 (95 % CI 2.1–2.7) for the 65–74 age group, and 5.4 (95 % CI 4.8–6.1) in the ≥ 75 group, compared to patients aged 55–64 [14].

There are multiple barriers to injury control in older adults. In the case of house fires, a low median income is associated with both a higher rate of fires and a higher rate of injuries once a fire has occurred. Certain types of homes (mobile homes, rental properties) and exposures (smoking, alcohol impairment) are strongly associated with burn injury. Individuals living in homes without a functioning smoke detector are more than eight times as likely to have an injury related to a house fire. Fires by arson, however, may be less likely to cause injury [17, 18]. The practice of burning brush, trash and other debris occurs predominantly in rural communities for logistical, cost, and convenience reasons. Residential burning disproportionately injures older men who use fuel as an accelerant, where safety education and implementation of alternative waste management practices may help reduce the incidence of injuries [19–21]. Hot water scalds continue to occur despite multiple educational programs and legislative interventions to reduce home water temperatures. Aging-related host factors predisposing to tap water scald injuries include not following recommendations, decreased mobility, impaired sensorium, and diabetic neuropathy, whereas environmental factors include lack of access to water temperature controls in some buildings, or living in buildings exempt from current law [22–26].

There are few available epidemiologic data on non-accidental burn injuries in aging adults, since these types of injuries are frequently under-reported [27]. Under-reporting of physical abuse and neglect occurs when the older adult is dependent on the abuser for care, feels shame or guilt from the event, or has impaired cognitive abilities. A British review of burns occurring in residential care facilities reported that inadequate staff supervision accounted for the majority of injuries, commonly from hot water scalds and contact with radiators [28]. In both types of injuries, residents with dementia and impaired mobility sustained burns because they were left unsupervised for variable periods of time. Appropriate recognition and management of non-accidental burns is challenging, as these injuries are associated with higher mortality rates when compared to accidental burns with similar characteristics [29, 30]. The recommended approach is to use a protocol for assessment, reporting and intervention in a multidisciplinary environment when elder abuse is suspected [31].

## Pathophysiologic changes and implications for burn therapy

### Aging

The aged skin is responsible for delayed wound healing in older adults. The dermis progressively thins with age, with a decrease in collagen content and extracellular matrix. The aging dermis has reduced microcirculation, macrophages and fibroblasts. In contrast, epidermal thickness is preserved with age, although there is flattening of the dermal-epidermal junction (rete ridges), making the epidermis more prone to shearing. Aging alters all phases of wound healing, from hemostasis and inflammation, to proliferation and resolution [32]. The rate of epidermal turnover is reduced by 50% after age 65, with fewer epidermal-lined skin appendages to permit re-epithelialization [33, 34]. Additionally, some environmental exposures can contribute to premature skin aging, such as tobacco smoking, sun exposure, and alcoholism-induced nutritional deficiencies [35]. Diabetes, chronic anticoagulation, and steroid immunosuppression are frequent comorbidities that predispose to premature skin aging and impaired wound healing. Clinically, burn providers often observe that even shallow-appearing partial thickness burn wounds in older adults can have significantly delayed re-epithelialization. In patients undergoing excision and grafting, delayed healing in donor sites and grafted wounds limits our ability to achieve early and complete wound closure.

Age-related changes in multiple organ systems contribute to the decreased physiologic reserve in older adults. Cardiac index decreases 1% per year whereas systemic vascular resistance rises 1% per year. Maximal heart rate and responses to adrenergic stimulation are also reduced with age [36]. Increased cardiovascular system stiffness (in the heart, arteries and arterioles) leads to an increased in pulse wave velocity and resetting of the baroreflex, thus causing the resting systolic pressure to rise. The aging cardiovascular system is more susceptible to the effects of hypovolemia, with a greater reduction in stroke volume and arterial systolic pressures. Respiratory performance decreases with age because of reduced chest wall compliance, decreased diaphragm strength, and alveolar airspace enlargement. Both forced vital capacity (FVC) and forced expiratory volume in 1 second ($FEV_1$) decrease over time [37]. Progressive renal deterioration is marked by a decrease in kidney size after age 50, with morphological changes often accelerated in the setting of diabetes and hypertension. Functionally, the age-dependent reduction in glomerular filtration rate (GFR) renders aging kidneys susceptible to second physiologic insults during critical illness [38]. Cognitive performance declines with age, although the underlying mechanisms are not fully characterized. Recent research indicates that brain tissue atrophy with aging may be concentrated in the loss of white matter fibers, resulting in altered relationships between cortical regions. This phenomenon has been termed "cortical disconnection", a deficit in integration between different networks [39, 40].

Aging also causes progressive loss of lean body mass, weakened muscle strength and reduced physical function [41]. Frailty itself is an important risk factor for injuries from falls, and poor hospitalization outcomes [42, 43]. Post-burn hyperdynamic and hypermetabolic responses are relatively blunted in older adults, although these patients still suffer from persistent catabolism, and loss of lean body mass[44, 45] Together, these factors constitute an enormous barrier to physical recovery in older patients. Early provision of nutritional support, maintenance of warm ambient temperatures, and control of infection are important strategies to mitigate the catabolic state. Pharmacologic agents to modulate hypermetabolism in older adults may achieve a similar benefit to those demonstrated in children with severe burns [46–49]. Oxandrolone, a testosterone analog with weak virilizing potential, is a promising agent for it induces anabolism in both older men and women after only two weeks of therapy [50]. The non-selective beta-blocker propranolol reduces tachycardia, energy expenditure, substrate cycling, and prevents fatty acid infiltration of the liver in severely burned children, but its application has not yet been reported in older adults with burns [45, 48]. This strategy is particularly appealing since aged patients do not tolerate tachycardia well. However, beta-adrenergic blockade must be balanced against the risks of inducing bradycardia and hypotension. The benefits of exercise regimens for older patients are numerous, including improved general health, faster hospitalization recovery in multiple conditions, and reduced repeat injuries [51–53]. The combination of anabolic agent supplementation and exercise should be a core component of a comprehensive rehabilitation plan, but thus far remains to be validated in older adults with burns.

Important changes in the aged host immune responses may partially account for post-injury complications and a higher susceptibility to infections. Aging alters antigen presentation, cytokine production, phagocyte activity and chemotaxis in multiple innate immune cells [54, 55]. Senescence also affects cell-mediated immunity with atrophy of the thymus, reduced naïve T-cells, and decreased T-cell memory [56]. At baseline, healthy older adults exhibit a chronic inflammatory state, characterized by higher circulating levels of pro-inflammatory mediators (TNF-α, IL-1, IL-6). This condition has been termed "inflamm-aging", and presumably arises from repeated exposure to antigens and other sources of cell stress [57]. After injury, early organ dysfunction develops more frequently in older adults with burns. It typically begins with acute lung and kidney injury, followed by deterioration in multiple organ systems [58]. Recent findings in a mouse burn injury model provide a potential mechanistic explanation for a higher incidence of pulmonary dysfunction in the aged host: burn-injured aged mice have protracted neutrophil infiltration and chemokine production in the lung compared younger mice [59]. Animal models of aging and sepsis demonstrate that the aged host immune response to infectious challenges is markedly altered. Aged mice respond poorly to either endotoxin challenge or cecal ligation and puncture (CLP) [60]. Turnbull et al. reported that aged mice have 70% mortality with CLP compared to 20% in young mice, and that antibiotic therapy initiated 12 hours after CLP does not significantly improve survival in older mice [61]. Although a burn + sepsis model in aged animals has not yet been reported, patient outcomes data give ample evidence that this combination is a strong risk factor for late-onset multiple organ dysfunction syndrome (MODS) and death [62, 63].

## Comorbidities

The relationship between injury and comorbidity is synergistic. Conditions such as smoking, physical disability, and altered sensorium are clear predisposing factors to burn injury [64, 65]. Additionally, the incidence of pre-injury comorbidities may be as high as 85% and frequently complicates the care of older burn patients [6]. Co-morbidities comprise a heterogeneous set of conditions, each with a different impact on burn management. Chronic obstructive lung disease and smoking strongly predict the development of pulmonary complications in older adults with burns [66]. Cardiac dysfunction may alter the timing of surgical procedures and can delay liberation from mechanical ventilation. The optimization of patients with systolic and diastolic heart dysfunction, or rhythm abnormalities may require additional diagnostic tests and invasive monitoring [67]. In contrast, well-managed comorbidities prior to injury may actually constitute a survival advantage: Arbabi et al. reported that older burn patients taking a beta-blocker prior to injury had better survival than those not treated with beta-blocker [68]. Whether this results from a biological effect of beta-blocker or simply better pre-injury care remains to be clarified. At the opposite end of the spectrum, patients on oxygen therapy who continue to smoke may be difficult to wean from mechanical ventilation following inhalation injury [69]. Burn injury may also uncover comorbidities not diagnosed prior to the event. At autopsy, approximately 75% of patients aged ≥65 have evidence of ischemic heart disease [15]. Demling noted a 61% incidence of pre-existing protein energy malnutrition in hospitalized burn patients >65 years old, associated with twice the hospital mortality rate compared to well-nourished patients [70]. Given their disparity, the impact of pre-existing conditions on burn outcomes is only beginning to be elucidated [71, 72]. Severe burn injuries are unlike elective surgery situations where preoperative optimization is possible, yet much work can be done to address co-morbidities in the intensive care unit, on the acute care ward, and at the time of hospital discharge. Preoperative optimization, however, is advisable with smaller size burns, for which the risks of the surgical procedure may outweigh the benefits of early wound closure. The contribution of geriatric specialists to the burn multidisciplinary care team model is another potential area for investigation, as it has already shown to benefit older patients with trauma and hip fractures [73, 74].

## Acute management challenges

### Fluid resuscitation

Recent publications on fluid administration highlight the phenomenon of excess fluid administration compared to prediction formulas, and describe the associated complications of elevated compartment pressures and acute lung injury [75–77]. Despite that, the incidence of acute kidney injury following resuscitation remains unacceptably high, and disproportionately affects aged patients [58, 78]. These data reinforce the adage that aged patients are less able to tolerate either over- or under-resuscitation because of limited cardiopulmonary reserve. However, what constitutes a proper resuscitation remains unclear as there is lack of agreement among providers on the type and composition of fluids for aged burn patients [44, 79]. A recent multicenter observational study found that age was inversely related to volume of fluid administered, meaning that providers likely limited fluid infusion in aged patients [76]. A commonly cited rationale is the concern for excess

edema formation in the lung. Accumulation of extravascular lung water (EVLW) as a result of high volume resuscitation is often posited, yet has not been proven to occur following burns [80, 81]. There are two potential explanations for this finding: first, that central hydrostatic pressures do not become elevated despite high volume administration during burn resuscitation, and second, that EVLW accumulation is more closely associated with direct lung injury from inhalation, or secondary lung injury from shock and sepsis, rather than changes in Starling forces during resuscitation [82, 83]. In the absence of convincing data to guide proper resuscitation in aged adults, it is prudent to initiate resuscitation for all adults according to weight and burn size according to standard formulas, and subsequently adjust according to individual patient response.

### Burn excision

Early excision has reduced mortality and decreased length of stay in pediatric and adult patients [84, 85]. Early excision in older adults, however remains controversial as multiple centers have indicated a lack of improvement in mortality, infection rates, and length of stay [11, 86–89]. Delayed wound healing and poor graft take are important limitations to wound closure in older patients. Despite harvesting thin grafts, it is often not possible to safely re-harvest from the same donor sites within several weeks. Interstices in expanded mesh grafts are slow to fill, and both grafted beds and donor sites are more prone to infection. In 1987, Herd et al. argued for a prospective randomized trial of early excision in older patients, given the lack of benefit at the authors' institution [88]. In contrast, others have reported that older adults generally tolerate surgical excision well, and several centers have noted improved survival with an early excision approach [3, 6, 90–92]. The definition of early excision has also varied in the literature, with a range of 72 hours to 7 days post-injury. In 2010, this issue remains one of the major unanswered questions in modern burn care, where the results of a well-conducted prospective evaluation could potentially alter care paradigms throughout the world. Our current practice at the University of Washington Burn Center is to perform surgical excision following completion of fluid resuscitation, and before 7 days in older patients with burns ≥ 20% TBSA. Our rationale for early excision is that older patients do not tolerate burn wound sepsis and that removal of the burn wound is essential for survival [33, 92].

## Pain and sedation

Appropriate pain management in aging adults has been historically hampered by two contradictory, yet widely held beliefs: first, that pain perception decreases with age, and second, that chronic pain in geriatric patients is so prevalent that it is assumed to be part of "normal aging". Pain research in older adults has proliferated over the past 20 years. It has helped characterize the complex and diverse causes of geriatric pain. Although older patients report decreased acute pain perception in certain circumstances, such as that associated with acute myocardial infarction, they are at increased risk of neuropathic pain with tissue injury, temporal summation and persistent hyperalgesia [93, 94]. Older patients are more likely to become disabled by pain than younger adults [95]. Pathways to adaptation to chronic pain perception may also differ middle age and older patient groups [96]. Thus pain does not simply increase or decrease with age. Rather different types of pain are affected differently by aging. The current framework conceptualizes geriatric pain as a disease associated with an underlying condition, rather than an unavoidable part of aging [97].

Pain assessment and treatment are both challenging in this population. Multiple studies have established that the standard visual analog scale (VAS) has limited value in older patients [98, 99]. Instead, pain experts currently recommend using numeric rating scales (NRS), verbal description scales (VDS), or the McGill Pain Questionnaire [97]. Observational scales become necessary when cognitive impairment or mechanical ventilation preclude self-reporting. Numerous observational measurements have been specifically developed for older patients over the past 20 years [100]. Whether these tools can be validated for older burn patients or a new scale should be developed remains a topic for investigation. Burn providers are also appropriately cautious when using pharmacologic agents to relieve pain in older adults [101]. Common side-effects of non-steroidal inflammatory agents are GI bleeding and renal

toxicity. The initial opioid analgesic dose for acute pain should be 25–50% of that in younger adults and carefully titrated upwards to achieve comfort [102]. Titration is paramount as undertreated pain is a risk factor for acute delirium and postoperative cognitive dysfunction (POCD) [103]. Barbiturates, benzodiazepines, and tricyclic antidepressants are other classes of agents that require caution in older patients because of decreased clearance and side effects. Pharmacists and geriatricians' expertise can contribute greatly to the multidisciplinary team in carefully titrating medications and minimizing of polypharmacy.

Acute delirium in the intensive care unit is an active area of research, with nearly 2,000 published manuscripts in the past 4 years. Criteria to diagnose acute delirium are 1) the acute onset of mental status change or fluctuating course, 2) inattention, and 3) disorganized thinking or altered level of consciousness [104]. Although providers easily recognize hyperactive delirium in agitated patients who pose a danger to themselves and their environment, hypoactive delirium is much more common and under-recognized. In this instance, the patient appears apathetic, withdrawn, and has decreased responsiveness. Acute delirium disproportionately affects older hospitalized patients because of pain, infection, inadequate sedation and intrinsic host factors such as mild dementia. Deeper sedation and higher severity of illness are other recognized risk factors for delirium. Data from surgical and mixed-ICU indicate that acute delirium is a risk factor for death and poor longterm outcomes [105, 106]. The benzodiazepine lorazepam has been implicated as an independent risk factor for delirium, whereas the newer sedation agent dexmedetomidine appears to decrease the incidence of delirium [107]. Until now, few pain and sedation studies have enrolled burn patients aged ≥ 65. However, we anticipate that future research will clarify the roles of traditional pharmacologic relief of pain, newer agents for sedation, and non-pharmacologic approaches to improve the care of older burn patients.

## End of life decisions

Not infrequently in the burn intensive care unit, providers withhold or withdraw life-sustaining therapies in aged patients when the extent of injury precludes the possibility of survival, or when the patient's deterioration indicates a lack of response to medical interventions [92, 108, 109]. Defining futility for the older burn patient should be based on the providers' own experiences, the available literature, and taking into account recent advances that may push the hope for survival [2, 10]. Mortality models are highly useful tools to estimate mortality among groups based on injury and patient characteristics (Table 1) yet do not discriminate well between individual survivors and non-survivors. Mortality models are derived from the recent past data; they are not rules to be strictly observed in order to repeat past achievements in survival. Thus, mortality models alone should not decide who should undergo aggressive treatment and who should not [110]. Focusing our research efforts not only on hospitalization but also long-term outcomes of older burn patients is critically important [111]. A better understanding of the functionality and quality of life of older adults with burns will also help guide medical professionals' decisions regarding aggressiveness of care, and counseling patients and family members about expected outcomes.

Unless they require mechanical ventilation, severely burn patients can remain alert and cooperative during acute resuscitation. Severely injured patients should be allowed to participate in a shared-decision making process when possible. Shared decision means that the physician discusses with the patient the nature and likely outcome of the patient's condition, the ramifications of treatment alternatives, and most importantly aims to achieve a consensus about treatment most consistent with the patient's values. Shared decision respects the principle of patient autonomy, and has gradually replaced the more traditional paternalistic approach in the US and other countries [112, 113]. Shared decision is essential as providers may otherwise be unduly influenced by their own values. Although some providers may forego treatment for themselves if given a low chance of survival, many prospective older patients would choose to undergo aggressive treatment nevertheless [114, 115]. In patients who are not able to participate, providers must rely on the substitute judgment of family members or a designated surrogate in the shared decision process. In decisionally-impaired patients who lack a surrogate, physicians must provide substitute judgment based on advance directives (if available), or their best estimate of the likelihood for survival and rehabilitation for each individual circumstance. Advance directives, however, are not always helpful as their wording may be too general or vague to address the specific circumstances of illness or injury [116, 117].

Both the process by which end of life decisions are made, and the quality of the communication between providers and family members can contribute to a positive experience [118, 119]. Convening a family conference can be an opportunity for families to receive information in an unhurried manner, present their views, and obtain reassurance that pain and suffering will be alleviated during intensive care [110]. If withdrawal of life support is chosen, the provider should explain the stepwise process of withdrawal to family members before it is initiated. Providers should also offer families available hospital services such as spiritual care and bereavement when available.

## Summary of key points and recommendations

► Older adults are disproportionately affected by burn injury, especially in high-income countries.
► Specific age-related physiologic changes and comorbidities contribute to worse hospitalization outcomes in older compared to younger burn patients.
► Acute fluid resuscitation in aged patients should proceed along the same guidelines as younger patients.
► Early excision is recommended in older adults with severe burns, although hospitalization outcomes remain far inferior to that of younger adults.
► Pain management in geriatric burn patients is challenging because it is often under-diagnosed and undertreated.
► Pharmacologic pain treatment should be initiated at smaller doses and carefully titrated for comfort.
► Older patients are at high-risk for acute delirium, a risk factor for worse hospitalization and long-term outcomes.

► Age alone should not be a criterion to forego acute resuscitation. Each case should be individually assessed for the potential for survival and rehabilitation.

► Good communication between providers, patients and surrogates improves the quality of intensive care. End of life decisions should be made following a shared-decision making model.

# References

[1] www.census.gov. Accessed 01/15/2010

[2] Pomahac B, Matros E, Semel M et al (2006) Predictors of survival and length of stay in burn patients older than 80 years of age: does age really matter? J Burn Care Res 27(3): 265–269

[3] Saffle JR, Larson CM, Sullivan J, Shelby J (1990) The continuing challenge of burn care in the elderly. Surgery 108(3): 534–543

[4] Keck M, Lumenta DB, Andel H, Kamolz LP, Frey M (2009) Burn treatment in the elderly. Burns 35(8): 1071–1079

[5] Miller SF, Bessey P, Lentz CW, Jeng JC, Schurr M, Browning S (2008) National burn repository 2007 report: a synopsis of the 2007 call for data. J Burn Care Res 29(6): 862–870; discussion 871

[6] Khadim MF, Rashid A, Fogarty B, Khan K (2009) Mortality estimates in the elderly burn patients: the Northern Ireland experience. Burns 35(1): 107–113

[7] Larson CM, Saffle JR, Sullivan J (1992) Lifestyle adjustments in elderly patients after burn injury. J Burn Care Rehabil 13(1): 48–52

[8] Manktelow A, Meyer AA, Herzog SR, Peterson HD (1989) Analysis of life expectancy and living status of elderly patients surviving a burn injury. J Trauma 29(2): 203–207

[9] Chipp E, Walton J, Gorman DF, Moiemen NS (2008) A 1 year study of burn injuries in a British Emergency Department. Burns 34(4): 516–520

[10] Macrino S, Slater H, Aballay A, Goldfarb IW, Caushaj PF (2008) A three-decade review of thermal injuries among the elderly at a regional burn centre. Burns 34(4): 509–511

[11] Ho WS, Ying SY, Chan HH (2001) A study of burn injuries in the elderly in a regional burn centre. Burns 27(4): 382–385

[12] Lumenta DB, Hautier A, Desouches C et al (2008) Mortality and morbidity among elderly people with burns–evaluation of data on admission. Burns 34(7): 965–974

[13] Forjuoh SN (2006) Burns in low- and middle-income countries: a review of available literature on descriptive epidemiology, risk factors, treatment, and prevention. Burns 32(5): 529–537

[14] Pham TN, Kramer CB, Wang J et al (2009) Epidemiology and outcomes of older adults with burn injury: an analysis of the National Burn Repository. J Burn Care Res 30(1): 30–36

[15] Pereira CT, Barrow RE, Sterns AM et al (2006) Age-dependent differences in survival after severe burns: a unicentric review of 1,674 patients and 179 autopsies over 15 years. J Am Coll Surg 202(3): 536–548

[16] Lionelli GT, Pickus EJ, Beckum OK, Decoursey RL, Korentager RA (2005) A three decade analysis of factors affecting burn mortality in the elderly. Burns 31(8): 958–963

[17] Istre GR, McCoy MA, Osborn L, Barnard JJ, Bolton A (2001) Deaths and injuries from house fires. N Engl J Med 344(25): 1911–1916

[18] Warda L, Tenenbein M, Moffatt ME (1999) House fire injury prevention update. Part I. A review of risk factors for fatal and non-fatal house fire injury. Inj Prev 5(2): 145–150

[19] Barillo DJ, Stetz CK, Zak AL, Shirani KZ, Goodwin CW (1998) Preventable burns associated with the misuse of gasoline. Burns 24(5): 439–443

[20] Wibbenmeyer LA, Amelon MA, Loret de Mola RM, Lewis R, 2nd, Kealey GP (2003) Trash and brush burning: an underappreciated mechanism of thermal injury in a rural community. J Burn Care Rehabil 24(2): 85–89

[21] Wibbenmeyer LA, Kealey GP, Young TL et al (2008) A prospective analysis of trash, brush, and grass burning behaviors. J Burn Care Res 29(3): 441–445

[22] Alden NE, Bessey PQ, Rabbitts A, Hyden PJ, Yurt RW (2007) Tap water scalds among seniors and the elderly: socio-economics and implications for prevention. Burns 33(5): 666–669

[23] Erdmann TC, Feldman KW, Rivara FP, Heimbach DM, Wall HA (1991) Tap water burn prevention: the effect of legislation. Pediatrics 88(3): 572–577

[24] Thomas KA, Hassanein RS, Christophersen ER (1984) Evaluation of group well-child care for improving burn prevention practices in the home. Pediatrics 74(5): 879–882

[25] Ehrlich AR, Bak RY, Wald-Cagan P, Greenberg DF (2008) Risk factors for fires and burns in homebound, urban elderly. J Burn Care Res 29(6): 985–987

[26] Leahy NE, Hyden PJ, Bessey PQ, Rabbitts A, Freudenberg N, Yurt RW (2007) The impact of a legislative intervention to reduce tap water scald burns in an urban community. J Burn Care Res 28(6): 805–810

[27] Greenbaum AR, Donne J, Wilson D, Dunn KW (2004) Intentional burn injury: an evidence-based, clinical and forensic review. Burns 30(7): 628–642

[28] Harper RD, Dickson WA (1995) Reducing the burn risk to elderly persons living in residential care. Burns 21(3): 205–208

[29] Thombs BD (2008) Patient and injury characteristics, mortality risk, and length of stay related to child abuse by burning: evidence from a national sample of 15,802 pediatric admissions. Ann Surg 247(3): 519–523

[30] Modjarrad K, McGwin G, Jr, Cross JM, Rue LW, 3rd (2007) The descriptive epidemiology of intentional burns in the United States: an analysis of the National Burn Repository. Burns 33(7): 828–832

[31] Aravanis SC, Adelman RD, Breckman R et al (1993) Diagnostic and treatment guidelines on elder abuse and neglect. Arch Fam Med 2(4): 371–388

[32] Gosain A, DiPietro LA (2004) Aging and wound healing. World J Surg 28(3): 321–326

[33] Demling R, Pereira, C, Herndon D (2007) Care of geriatric patients. In: Herndon DN (ed) Total burn care, 3rd edn. Saunders , pp 496–501

[34] Goodson WH, 3rd, Hunt TK (1979) Wound healing and aging. J Invest Dermatol 73(1): 88–91

[35] Morita A (2007) Tobacco smoke causes premature skin aging. J Dermatol Sci 48(3): 169–175

[36] Chang TT, Schecter WP (2007) Injury in the elderly and end-of-life decisions. Surg Clin North Am 87(1): 229–245, viii

[37] Rossi A, Fantin F, Di Francesco V et al (2008) Body composition and pulmonary function in the elderly: a 7-year longitudinal study. Int J Obes (Lond) 32(9): 1423–1430

[38] Colloca G, Santoro M, Gambassi G (2010) Age-related physiologic changes and perioperative management of elderly patients. Surg Oncol 19(3): 124–130

[39] Tang Y, Nyengaard JR, Pakkenberg B, Gundersen HJ (1997) Age-induced white matter changes in the human brain: a stereological investigation. Neurobiol Aging 18(6): 609–615

[40] Barrick TR, Charlton RA, Clark CA, Markus HS (2010) White matter structural decline in normal ageing; a prospective longitudinal study using tract based spatial statistics. Neuroimagen 51(2): 565–577

[41] Cawthon PM, Fox KM, Gandra SR et al (2009) Do muscle mass, muscle density, strength, and physical function similarly influence risk of hospitalization in older adults? J Am Geriatr Soc 57(8): 1411–1419

[42] Hirsch CH, Sommers L, Olsen A, Mullen L, Winograd CH (1990) The natural history of functional morbidity in hospitalized older patients. J Am Geriatr Soc 38(12): 1296–1303

[43] Tinetti ME, Baker DI, King M et al (2008) Effect of dissemination of evidence in reducing injuries from falls. N Engl J Med 359(3): 252–261

[44] Bowser-Wallace BH, Cone JB, Caldwell FT, Jr (1985) Hypertonic lactated saline resuscitation of severely burned patients over 60 years of age. J Trauma 25(1): 22–26

[45] Herndon DN, Tompkins RG (2004) Support of the metabolic response to burn injury. Lancet 363 (9424): 1895–1902

[46] Demling RH, DeSanti L (2001) The rate of restoration of body weight after burn injury, using the anabolic agent oxandrolone, is not age dependent. Burns 27(1): 46–51

[47] Demling RH, DeSanti L (2003) Oxandrolone induced lean mass gain during recovery from severe burns is maintained after discontinuation of the anabolic steroid. Burns 29(8): 793–797

[48] Herndon DN, Hart DW, Wolf SE, Chinkes DL, Wolfe RR (2001) Reversal of catabolism by beta-blockade after severe burns. N Engl J Med 345(17): 1223–1229

[49] Jeschke MG, Finnerty CC, Suman OE, Kulp G, Mlcak RP, Herndon DN (2007) The effect of oxandrolone on the endocrinologic, inflammatory, and hypermetabolic responses during the acute phase postburn. Ann Surg 246(3): 351–360; discussion 360–352

[50] Sheffield-Moore M, Paddon-Jones D, Casperson SL et al (2006) Androgen therapy induces muscle protein anabolism in older women. J Clin Endocrinol Metab 91(10): 3844–3849

[51] Cecins N, Geelhoed E, Jenkins SC (2008) Reduction in hospitalisation following pulmonary rehabilitation in patients with COPD. Aust Health Rev 32(3): 415–422

[52] Flynn KE, Pina IL, Whellan DJ et al (2009) Effects of exercise training on health status in patients with chronic heart failure: HF-ACTION randomized controlled trial. Jama 301(14): 1451–1459

[53] Vogler CM, Sherrington C, Ogle SJ, Lord SR (2009) Reducing risk of falling in older people discharged from hospital: a randomized controlled trial comparing seated exercises, weight-bearing exercises, and social visits. Arch Phys Med Rehabil 90(8): 1317–1324

[54] Agrawal A, Agrawal S, Tay J, Gupta S (2008) Biology of dendritic cells in aging. J Clin Immunol 28(1): 14–20

[55] Gomez CR, Nomellini V, Faunce DE, Kovacs EJ (2008) Innate immunity and aging. Exp Gerontol 43(8): 718–728

[56] Haynes BF, Markert ML, Sempowski GD, Patel DD, Hale LP (2000) The role of the thymus in immune reconstitution in aging, bone marrow transplantation, and HIV-1 infection. Annu Rev Immunol 18: 529–560

[57] Franceschi C, Bonafe M, Valensin S et al (2000) Inflamm-aging. An evolutionary perspective on immunosenescence. Ann N Y Acad Sci 908: 244–254

[58] Mosier MJ, Pham TN, Klein MB et al (2010) Early acute kidney injury predicts progressive renal dysfunction and higher mortality in severely burned adults. J Burn Care Res 31(1): 83–92

[59] Nomellini V, Faunce DE, Gomez CR, Kovacs EJ (2008) An age-associated increase in pulmonary inflammation after burn injury is abrogated by CXCR2 inhibition. J Leukoc Biol 83(6): 1493–1501

[60] Saito H, Sherwood ER, Varma TK, Evers BM (2003) Effects of aging on mortality, hypothermia, and cytokine induction in mice with endotoxemia or sepsis. Mech Ageing Dev 124(10–12): 1047–1058

[61] Turnbull IR, Wlzorek JJ, Osborne D, Hotchkiss RS, Coopersmith CM, Buchman TG (2003) Effects of age on mortality and antibiotic efficacy in cecal ligation and puncture. Shock 19(4): 310–313

[62] Fitzwater J, Purdue GF, Hunt JL, O'Keefe GE (2003) The risk factors and time course of sepsis and organ dysfunction after burn trauma. J Trauma 54(5): 959–966

[63] Saffle JR, Sullivan JJ, Tuohig GM, Larson CM (1993) Multiple organ failure in patients with thermal injury. Crit Care Med 21(11): 1673–1683

[64] Ansari Z, Brown K, Carson N (2008) Association of epilepsy and burns – a case control study. Aust Fam Physician 37(7): 584–589

[65] Lewandowski R, Pegg S, Fortier K, Skimmings A (1993) Burn injuries in the elderly. Burns 19(6): 513–515

[66] Pham TN, Kramer CB, Klein MB (2010) Risk factors for he development of pneumonia in older adults with burn injury. J Burn Care Res31(1): 105–110

[67] Scott EC, Ho HC, Yu M, Chapital AD, Koss W, Takanishi DM, Jr (2008) Pre-existing cardiac disease, troponin I elevation and mortality in patients with severe sepsis and septic shock. Anaesth Intensive Care 36(1): 51–59

[68] Arbabi S, Ahrns KS, Wahl WL et al (2004) Beta-blocker use is associated with improved outcomes in adult burn patients. J Trauma 56(2): 265–269; discussion 269–271

[69] Edelman DA, Maleyko-Jacobs S, White MT, Lucas CE, Ledgerwood AM (2008) Smoking and home oxygen therapy–a preventable public health hazard. J Burn Care Res 29(1): 119–122

[70] Demling RH (2005) The incidence and impact of pre-existing protein energy malnutrition on outcome in the elderly burn patient population. J Burn Care Rehabil 26(1): 94–100

[71] Barret JP, Gomez P, Solano I, Gonzalez-Dorrego M, Crisol FJ (1999) Epidemiology and mortality of adult burns in Catalonia. Burns 25(4): 325–329

[72] Thombs BD, Singh VA, Halonen J, Diallo A, Milner SM (2007) The effects of preexisting medical comorbidities on mortality and length of hospital stay in acute burn injury: evidence from a national sample of 31,338 adult patients. Ann Surg 245(4): 629–634

[73] Fallon WF, Jr., Rader E, Zyzanski S et al (2006) Geriatric outcomes are improved by a geriatric trauma consultation service. J Trauma 61(5): 1040–1046

[74] Marcantonio ER, Flacker JM, Wright RJ, Resnick NM (2001) Reducing delirium after hip fracture: a randomized trial. J Am Geriatr Soc 49(5): 516–522

[75] Chung KK, Wolf SE, Cancio LC et al (2009) Resuscitation of severely burned military casualties: fluid begets more fluid. J Trauma 67(2): 231–237; discussion 237

[76] Klein MB, Hayden D, Elson C et al (2007) The association between fluid administration and outcome following major burn: a multicenter study. Ann Surg 245(4): 622–628

[77] Pham TN, Cancio LC, Gibran NS (2008) American Burn Association practice guidelines burn shock resuscitation. J Burn Care Res 29(1): 257–266

[78] Steinvall I, Bak Z, Sjoberg F (2008) Acute kidney injury is common, parallels organ dysfunction or failure, and carries appreciable mortality in patients with major burns: a prospective exploratory cohort study. Crit Care 12(5):R124

[79] Slater H, Gaisford JC (1981) Burns in older patients. J Am Geriatr Soc 29(2): 74–76

[80] Holm C, Tegeler J, Mayr M, Pfeiffer U, Henckel von Donnersmarck G, Muhlbauer W (2002) Effect of crystalloid resuscitation and inhalation injury on extravascular lungwater:clinicalimplications.Chest121(6): 1956–1962

[81] Tranbaugh RF, Lewis FR, Christensen JM, Elings VB (1980) Lung water changes after thermal injury. The effects of crystalloid resuscitation and sepsis. Ann Surg 192(4): 479–490

[82] Holm C, Mayr M, Tegeler J et al (2004) A clinical randomized study on the effects of invasive monitoring on burn shock resuscitation. Burns 30(8): 798–807

[83] Tranbaugh RF, Elings VB, Christensen JM, Lewis FR (1983) Effect of inhalation injury on lung water accumulation. J Trauma 23(7): 597–604

[84] Engrav LH, Heimbach DM, Reus JL, Harnar TJ, Marvin JA (1983) Early excision and grafting vs. nonoperative treatment of burns of indeterminant depth: a randomized prospective study. J Trauma 23(11): 1001–1004

[85] Herndon DN, Barrow RE, Rutan RL, Rutan TC, Desai MH, Abston S (1989) A comparison of conservative versus early excision. Therapies in severely burned patients. Ann Surg 209(5): 547–552; discussion 552–543

[86] Housinger T, Saffle J, Ward S, Warden G (1984) Conservative approach to the elderly patient with burns. Am J Surg 148(6): 817–820

[87] Kirn DS, Luce EA (1998) Early excision and grafting versus conservative management of burns in the elderly. Plast Reconstr Surg 102(4): 1013–1017

[88] Herd BM, Herd AN, Tanner NS (1987) Burns to the elderly: a reappraisal. Br J Plast Surg 40(3): 278–282

[89] Cutillas M, Sesay M, Perro G, Bourdarias B, Castede JC, Sanchez R (1998) Epidemiology of elderly patients' burns in the South West of France. Burns 24(2): 134–138

[90] Burdge JJ, Katz B, Edwards R, Ruberg R (1988) Surgical treatment of burns in elderly patients. J Trauma 28(2): 214–217

[91] Deitch EA (1985) A policy of early excision and grafting in elderly burn patients shortens the hospital stay and improves survival. Burns Incl Therm Inj 12(2): 109–114

[92] Anous MM, Heimbach DM (1986) Causes of death and predictors in burned patients more than 60 years of age. J Trauma 26(2): 135–139

[93] Mehta RH, Rathore SS, Radford MJ, Wang Y, Wang Y, Krumholz HM (2001) Acute myocardial infarction in the elderly: differences by age. J Am Coll Cardiol 38(3): 736–741

[94] Schmader KE (2002) Epidemiology and impact on quality of life of postherpetic neuralgia and painful diabetic neuropathy. Clin J Pain 18(6): 350–354

[95] Edwards RR (2006) Age differences in the correlates of physical functioning in patients with chronic pain. J Aging Health 18(1): 56–69

[96] Cook AJ, Brawer PA, Vowles KE (2006) The fear-avoidance model of chronic pain: validation and age analysis using structural equation modeling. Pain 121(3): 195–206

[97] Gagliese L (2009) Pain and aging: the emergence of a new subfield of pain research. J Pain 10(4): 343–353

[98] Herr KA, Mobily PR (1993) Comparison of selected pain assessment tools for use with the elderly. Appl Nurs Res 6(1): 39–46

[99] Jensen MP, Karoly P, Braver S (1986) The measurement of clinical pain intensity: a comparison of six methods. Pain 27(1): 117–126

[100] Zwakhalen SM, Hamers JP, Abu-Saad HH, Berger MP (2006) Pain in elderly people with severe dementia: a systematic review of behavioural pain assessment tools. BMC Geriatr 6: 3

[101] Honari S, Patterson DR, Gibbons J et al (1997) Comparison of pain control medication in three age groups of elderly patients. J Burn Care Rehabil 18(6): 500–504

[102] Pasero C, Manworren RC, McCaffery M (2007) PAIN Control: IV opioid range orders for acute pain management. Am J Nurs 107(2): 52–59; quiz 59–60

[103] Lynch EP, Lazor MA, Gellis JE, Orav J, Goldman L, Marcantonio ER (1998) The impact of postoperative pain on the development of postoperative delirium. Anesth Analg 86(4): 781–785

[104] Pun BT, Ely EW (2007) The importance of diagnosing and managing ICU delirium. Chest 132(2): 624–636

[105] Lat I, McMillian W, Taylor S et al (2009) The impact of delirium on clinical outcomes in mechanically ventilated surgical and trauma patients. Crit Care Med 37(6): 1898–1905

[106] Pisani MA, Kong SY, Kasl SV, Murphy TE, Araujo KL, Van Ness PH (2009) Days of delirium are associated with 1-year mortality in an older intensive care unit population. Am J Respir Crit Care Med 180(11): 1092–1097

[107] Riker RR, Fraser GL (2009) Altering intensive care sedation paradigms to improve patient outcomes. Crit Care Clin 25(3): 527–538, viii–ix

[108] Wibbenmeyer LA, Amelon MJ, Morgan LJ et al (2001) Predicting survival in an elderly burn patient population. Burns 27(6): 583–590

[109] Slater AL, Fassnacht-Hanrahan K, Slater H, Goldfarb IW (1991) From hopeful to hopeless... when do we write "do not resuscitate"? Focus Crit Care 18(6): 476–479

[110] Luce JM (2010) End-of-life decision-making in the intensive care unit. Am J Respir Crit Care Med 182(1): 6–11

[111] Lundgren RS, Kramer CB, Rivara FP et al (2009) Influence of comorbidities and age on outcome following burn injury in older adults. J Burn Care Res 30(2): 307–314

[112] Thompson BT, Cox PN, Antonelli M et al (2004) Challenges in end-of-life care in the ICU: statement of the 5th International Consensus Conference in Critical Care: Brussels, Belgium, April 2003: executive summary. Crit Care Med 32(8): 1781–1784

[113] White DB, Braddock CH, 3rd, Bereknyei S, Curtis JR (2007) Toward shared decision making at the end of life

in intensive care units: opportunities for improvement. Arch Intern Med 167(5): 461–467

[114] Danis M, Patrick DL, Southerland LI, Green ML (1988) Patients' and families' preferences for medical intensive care. Jama 260(6): 797–802

[115] Lloyd CB, Nietert PJ, Silvestri GA (2004) Intensive care decision making in the seriously ill and elderly. Crit Care Med 32(3): 649–654

[116] Malloy TR, Wigton RS, Meeske J, Tape TG (1992) The influence of treatment descriptions on advance medical directive decisions. J Am Geriatr Soc 40(12): 1255–1260

[117] Teno J, Lynn J, Wenger N et al (1997) Advance directives for seriously ill hospitalized patients: effectiveness with the patient self-determination act and the SUPPORT intervention. SUPPORT Investigators. Study to Understand Prognoses and Preferences for Outcomes and Risks of Treatment. J Am Geriatr Soc 45(4): 500–507

[118] A controlled trial to improve care for seriously ill hospitalized patients. The study to understand prognoses and preferences for outcomes and risks of treatments (SUPPORT). The SUPPORT Principal Investigators. Jama 1995;274(20): 1591–1598

[119] Teno JM, Fisher E, Hamel MB et al (2000) Decision-making and outcomes of prolonged ICU stays in seriously ill patients. J Am Geriatr Soc 48[5 Suppl]: S70–74

[120] Baux S (1961) Contribution a l'etude du traitement local des brulures thermigues etendues. Paris, France

[121] Stern M, Waisbren BA (1979) Comparison of methods of predicting burn mortality. Scand J Plast Reconstr Surg 13(1): 201–204

[122] Zawacki BE, Azen SP, Imbus SH, Chang YT (1979) Multifactorial probit analysis of mortality in burned patients. Ann Surg 189(1): 1–5

[123] Tobiasen J, Hiebert JM, Edlich RF (1982) The abbreviated burn severity index. Ann Emerg Med 11(5): 260–262

[124] Ryan CM, Schoenfeld DA, Thorpe WP, Sheridan RL, Cassem EH, Tompkins RG (1998) Objective estimates of the probability of death from burn injuries. N Engl J Med 338(6): 362–366

[125] O'Keefe GE, Hunt JL, Purdue GF (2001) An evaluation of risk factors for mortality after burn trauma and the identification of gender-dependent differences in outcomes. J Am Coll Surg 192(2): 153–160

[126] McGwin G, Jr., George RL, Cross JM, Rue LW (2008) Improving the ability to predict mortality among burn patients. Burns 34(3): 320–327

[127] Osler T, Glance L, Hosmer DW (2010) Simplified estimates of the probability of death after burn injuries: Extending and updating the Baux Score. J Trauma 68(3): 690–697

Correspondence to: Tam N. Pham, M.D., University of Washington Burn Center, Harborview Medical Center, 325 Ninth Avenue, Box 359 796, Seattle, WA, 98 104, USA, E-mail: tpham94@uw.edu

# Acute management of facial burns

Peter Dziewulski, Jorge-Leon Villapalos

St Andrews Centre for Plastic Surgery and Burns, Chelmsford, Essex, UK

## Introduction

The face is a unique and vitally important structure in humans and plays an irreplaceable role in human life. The face contains the organs of smell, sight, hearing and taste. It is involved in important physiological functions such as vision, respiration, feeding, and hearing but is also vital in communication, transmitting expressions and emotions, feelings and signifying individual identity. It is a complex structure of skin, muscle, fat, vessels, nerves draped around the facial skeleton. A facial burn can vary from being relatively minor to a severely debilitating and disfiguring injury.

Facial burns disrupt the anatomical and functional structures creating swelling, pain, deformity and following wound healing scars that are potentially disfiguring. They can distort anatomical structures and function that can lead to lasting physical and psychological impairment [1].

The management of facial burns includes assessment, airway control, wound management, scar management, rehabilitation and reconstruction [2]. Wound management can be conservative, operative or both, depending on the depth and extent of the burn.

Few areas of burn care can be more challenging than the management of facial burns. The outcome of a facial burn can be critical to a patient's daily existence and integral to positive self-esteem. The acute and reconstructive management of facial burns require a thoughtful, methodical treatment plan with the ultimate goal of optimal aesthetic and functional outcomes [3].

## Anatomy and pathophysiology

The face is an extremely complex anatomical structure consisting of skin, fat, and muscle, draped over the facial skeleton. It hosts important sphincter structures and vital sensory organs of sight, hearing, smell, taste and touch. Skin acts as a protective barrier against mechanical trauma, bacteria, noxious substances, heat, and ultraviolet radiation. Other important functions include sensation, immunologic surveillance, and heat and fluid homeostasis.

Cutaneous wound healing depends on epithelial cell proliferation and migration following injury from epidermal appendages. These include sebaceous glands, sweat glands, apocrine glands, and hair follicles. The face and scalp contain a high concentration of sebaceous glands and in general epithelial appendages in the facial are located in the deep dermis and in the sub-dermal fat. The deep location of the epithelial appendages and their density in the face provide it with a remarkable ability to re-epithelialise and heal spontaneously

In addition the thickness of facial skin varies which can have consequences on the depth of injury. Skin thickness varies based on anatomic location and on the sex and age of the individual. Eyelid and post auricular skin is very thin (approximately 0.5 mm thick). Men have thicker skin compared to women in all anatomic locations. Skin thickness varies with age with children having relatively thin skin. There is progressive thickening until the fourth or fifth decade of life following which the skin begins to thin again.

Mechanisms of facial burn injury are varied and are related to patient age and determine depth and outcome. In general the majority of partial thickness facial burns in children are following scald injury. In adults, usually males, the commonest cause is a flash burn and these tend to be partial thickness in nature and will often affect other exposed areas such as the hand. Full thickness facial burns tend to be flame related injuries in both children and adults usually as a result of a conflagration and are often associated with a large TBSA burn affecting other areas [2].

The characteristic edema secondary to release of inflammatory mediators both locally and systemically in bigger injuries can give rise to upper airway obstruction when associated with a facial burn. Not only is there a risk of upper airway compromise, there is also a well known association of facial burns with smoke inhalation injury.

As described elsewhere in this book the depth of burn injury is defined by the anatomical depth of tissue injury and is the major determinant of wound healing potential. Burn injury has traditionally been classified into epidermal, superficial partial thickness, deep partial thickness and full thickness burns. Each of these has differing potential for healing and for subsequent scar formation. Epidermal and superficial partial thickness burns should heal rapidly within 10–14 days and should not leave significant scarring. Deep partial thickness burns take over 3 weeks to heal and are associated with a high risk of hypertrophic scarring. Full thickness injury will not usually heal without surgical intervention.

Authors have correlated healing times to hypertrophic scarring [4, 5] and also to timing of surgery. Evidence shows that wounds healing within 14 days spontaneously have a very low incidence of hypertrophic scarring (>2%) and that surgical intervention is associated with a higher incidence of hypertrophic scarring up to 3 weeks following injury [5, 6].

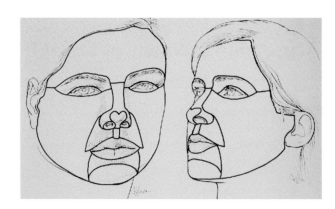

**Fig. 1.** Facial aesthetic units (Gonzalez-Ulloa 1987)

Most authors would now recommend timing of intervention between 10 to 21 days [5, 6]. However this data has been gathered and analyzed on burns occurring at all anatomical sites and as it is acknowledged that the face has improved healing potential further investigation is required into time to healing of facial burns in particular and subsequent scarring.

When considering facial burn injury it is vital to understand and remember the concept of aesthetic units and subunits first describe by Gonzalez Ulloa [7]. These units have consistent colour, texture, thickness and pliability, and can be divided into topographical subunits with a predictable contour which when used to plan placement of skin graft edges and subsequent scars can visually minimize the appearance of the scars (Fig. 1).

## Management

### General approach

The main goal in the management of facial burns is similar to that for all areas of the body.

The outcome of both facial and hand burns have a significant functional and psychosocial implication. Patients whose face and hands have been spared reintegrate more easily following burn injury. Deep burns of the face are devastating and requiring long-term psychosocial rehabilitation, physical therapy and multiple reconstructive procedures.

The aim of early wound healing, mobilization with preservation of form and function is as import-

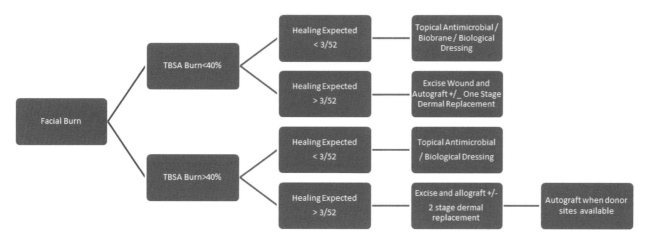

**Fig. 2.** Facial burn treatment algorithm

ant in the face as anywhere else. Specifically in the face the burn team should aim to maintain facial architecture and preserve normal facial subunits, with acceptable or good anatomical balance and symmetry and a dynamic facial expression.

In principle the treatment algorithm for facial burn injury is relatively straight forward (Fig. 2). Management depends on the depth and size of the wound and the age and comorbidities of the patient. Superficial partial thickness wounds are left to heal spontaneously and those that are obviously full thickness undergo surgical excision and resurfacing with autograft. Deep partial thickness injury is usually best dealt with by tangiential excision and grafting [8] although some authors would favour a more conservative approach followed by aggressive scar management recognizing the limitations of facial grafting being suboptimal in terms of colour, texture and cosmetic outcome [3].

However it is the group in between that represent the true challenge in terms of optimizing healing and minimizing scarring. Burns that are of intermediate or indeterminate depth that may or may not heal within 3 weeks pose a difficult clinical problem with regards to preservation of aesthetic units and the development of hypertrophic scar. Most burns are mixed depth and if treated conservatively will give rise to patchy areas of hypertrophic scars that cross aesthetic unit boundaries.

In general a consensus view suggests a delay in the excision of acute indeterminate facial burns until days 7 to 10 to allow better determination of the heal-

ing potential within a 3 week period. Adjunctive techniques such as the Laser Doppler that can help with burn depth estimation and potential for healing can be useful in this situation [9]. Once a decision is made to operate prevarication to 'see if it will heal' should be avoided as this usually leads to a prolonged period of wound dressing care with its attendant problems of pain infection and suboptimal scar formation.

Surgical excision of deep partial- and full-thickness burns must be carefully planned and undertaken following strict principles including maintenance and preservation of aesthetic units, sacrifice of less injured tissue to preserve aesthetic units, bloodless surgery techniques, the use of allograft and or skin substitutes to optimize autograft take and early intense scar management [10].

*Airway management*

Patients with facial burns will often have an associated upper airway injury and / or lower airway injury requiring intubation and ventilation either in the before or soon after admission to the burn service. These patients can often require long-term intubation and ventilation. The presence of an endotracheal/nasotracheal/tracheostomy tube or indeed any tube can cause associated problems when managing the facial injury. In particular pressure from the tube or tube ties can cause pressure necrosis especially in the alar or collumellar regions but also of the lip and of the cheeks.

293

It is our practice to use endo or naso tracheal tubes in patients with partial thickness burn injury that require short to medium term ventilation (> 14 days). Patients who have a pan facial full thickness burn, who require long term ventilation and have an associated major burn (> 60%) TBSA are usually managed with a tracheostomy [11]. This allows easy access to the face for wound and graft care, prevents shearing and allows the benefits of sedation reduction associated with tracheostomy. However this may increase the incidence of subsequent neck contracture when associated with a deep neck burn.

If an endo or naso tracheal intubation is preferred, the tube can be secured by standard tube tapes, however, these make wound care difficult and can rub against the cheek wound deepening it. Our preferred method in this circumstance is dental wiring or a trans-septal silk suture that secures the tube without the need for tapes. Other tubes can be secured in this way or alternatively to the endotracheal tube once it is secured.

## Facial burn wound management

### Initial wound care

Following admission patients with facial burns undergo cleaning with an antiseptic and debridement of debris and blisters. Superficial partial thickness wounds are cleaned twice daily and a topical antimicrobial is applied until epithelialization and healing occur. Deep burns are cleaned and dressed twice daily with Flammazine or Acticoat on alternate days until surgical excision is undertaken, usually within the first 5–7 days following admission. In indeterminate injury a topical antimicrobial such as twice daily Flammazine or alternate day Acticoat is applied until an assessment is made at or before day 10 to determine whether healing will occur by day 21. This cleaning and debridement may require a general anaesthetic in the operating theatre to adequately clean the wound, remove pseudo eschar and assess the underlying wound.

Conservative management is continued if the wound is believed to heal within 21 days, if not the patient is prepared for surgical debridement and wound closure. In male patients regular shaving of the beard area prevents excessive accumulation of hair and wound debris that if left can lead to folliculitis, infection and deepening of the wound.

### Topical agents

There are many topical agents that have been used in the management of facial burns. These include antiseptics, antimicrobial agents and dressings [12].

Antiseptics are topical agents designed to limit (bacteriostatic) or eliminate (bactericidal) the presence of microorganisms in the surgical wound. They are the mainstay of wound cleansing both following admission and afterwards during repeated wound bathing and cleaning. They include chlorhexidene and povidone iodine products that have similar anti gram-positive, gram-negative bactericidal and viricidal effects. The iodine-based antiseptics are also active against fungi, spores, protozoa, and yeasts. Iodine based preparations can be painful and irritating and in the past have been associated with toxicity [13].

Antimicrobial agents are topical agents that control and limit burn infection. The characteristics of the ideal prophylactic topical antimicrobial agent include a broad spectrum with long standing action, lack of toxicity and adequate local eschar penetration without systemic absorption. They should be inexpensive, and easy to apply and store. They need to provide a favorable wound healing environment and deliver a high concentration of active principle to a devitalized, devascularized and potentially necrotic wound [14]. The use of topical antimicrobials in facial burns is intended to limit bacterial colonization and invasive infection, which has a detrimental effect on the zone of stasis injury leading to deepening of the burn wound.

Silver preparations and silver sulfadiazine in particular are key products in burn surgery as they act on the potentially infected burn eschar limiting the extent of the non-viable tissue but can be irritant, stain the skin and can be absorbed systemically [15].

Silver sulfadiazine cream 1% (Flammazine1, Smith and Nephew; Silvadene1, King Pharmaceuticals) is a water-based cream containing the insoluble active principle silver sulfadiazine in micronized form. Fox introduced it in 1968 and at the time revolutionized burn wound management. It must be applied repeatedly at least every 12h with a layer thickness of about 3–5 mm and provides effective local antibacterial effect against gram-positive bacteria, gram-negative bacteria, viruses and fungal species such as candida albicans.

It can produce a transient consumptive leucopenia, methahemoglobinemia and is contraindicated in cases of sulfa allergy. Its use can produce a thick yellow pseudo-eschar that can make the differential diagnosis with full thickness burns difficult. It can delay wound healing due to keratinocyte and fibroblast inhibition rendering its use in facial burns questionable although the evidence in this group of patients is limited [16].

Comparison of the use of silver sulfadiazine against bio-engineered skin substitutes showed a significant decrease in wound care time, pain and re-epithelialization time in the skin substitute group [17]. A similar report comparing silver sulfadiazine and allografts found decreased re-epithelialization time and hypertrophic scar incidence in the allograft group [18].

Cerium nitrate can be combined with silver sulfadiazine (Flammacerium) and has excellent penetration, forms a hard eschar and reduces bacterial colonization with gram positive, gram negative and fungal species [19]. Its use has been popularized in Europe with varying results [20] and the results of a randomized controlled study comparing it to Flammazine in the management of facial burns are awaited (ClinicalTrials.gov IdentifierNCT00 297 752).

Acticoat (Smith and Nephew, Hull, UK) is a bilayered polyethylene nanocrystalline silver-based dressing attached to a soaking coat of polyester. It delivers silver at a regular rate to the wound once it becomes saturated with water, avoids the rapid neutralization of silver occurring in other silver-based preparations and limits the need for dressing changes. It needs to be kept hydrated with water. Acticoat is useful in the management of facial burns and is a successful alternative to traditional silver sulfadiazine [21]. It has been compared to silver sulfadiazine and was noted to reduce grafting requirements [22].

Neosporin, Polysporin and Bacitracin are commonly used antibiotic ointments in North America for the treatment of superficial burned areas. Their eschar penetration is limited. The Neosporin contains bacitracin (gram-positive activity) and neomycin and polymyxin B (gram-negative activity) [23].

Moist exposed burn ointment (MEBO) has been popularized in the Far East and Middle East recently. It contains herbs in a wax ointment but it is not clear what the active ingredient and comparative studies have shown varying results [24, 25].

Beta-Glucan preparations have been reported as reducing pain and promoting healing with Glucan-collagen being reported as being useful in partial thickness burns in children [26].

## Biological dressings

There are a number of biological and semi-biological dressings that can be used to physiologically close the burn wound to aid epithelialisation in partial thickness injury and to protect the deeper, excised wound from desiccation, infection and mechanical trauma [27].

Prior to application of any of these dressings the wounds need thorough cleaning, decontaminating and debridement of blisters, debris and devitalized tissue. This can only be adequately achieved in most cases under a general anaesthetic in a dedicated facility.

A popular semi-biological dressing Biobrane has been popularized in the management of superficial partial thickness wounds. It is a bilaminar dressing with an external silicone layer bonded to a nylon mesh impregnated with porcine collagen. It has been shown to have advantages over conventional open technique topical management in terms of ease of care, reduction in costs, decrease of pain and decrease in time to healing [28, 29] (Fig. 3).

Cadaver allograft can be used to physiologically close partial thickness wounds. to enhance epithelialsation and healing. A prospective study demonstrated cadaver allograft to be superior when compared to open treatment with silver sulphadiazine. in shallow and deep partial thickness burns [18].

Porcine skin xenografts can also be used for temporary physiological wound closure to promote epithelialisation and healing or as interim prior to autografting [27].

Human amnion can also be used a biological dressing to physiologically close the wound and pro-

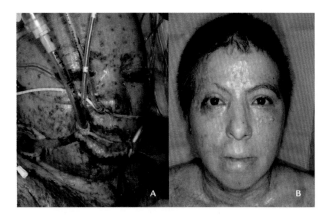

**Fig. 3.** Indeterminate depth facial burn treated conservatively with Biobrane.
A  Following biobrane application;
B  At 3 months

mote epithelialisation and healing. A recent randomized controlled study comparing amnion to standard topical antimicrobial care showed a reduction in healing time, reduction in the amount of re-applications of facial dressings in the amnion group, but no difference in scarring [30].

A recent literature review compared and analyzed bioengineered skin substitutes with biological dressings and topical management and found similar efficacy in the three options [31].

## Surgical burn wound excision of the face

Once the decision to operate is made surgical excision of the facial burn should proceed on the next available operating list if the patient's condition permits and there are no other areas with greater priority to excise.

A team used to undertaking such surgery must undertake the procedure. Preparation is of vital importantance. The operating theatre staff should be informed of the nature of the surgery and to ensure that homografts and skin substitutes are ordered and available. Blood must be cross matched preoperatively and be available in the operating theatre before commencing surgery as blood loss can be massive. Prior to commencing surgery the WHO patient safety checklist should be run through to minimize avoidable complications [32].

The operation is performed with the patient supine in the reverse Trendelemburg

position under general anesthesia. Prophylactic perioperative antibiotics are given.

The endotracheal tube should be suspended together with feeding tubes from an overhead hook to keep the tubes out of the operative field. Care must be taken to protect the eyes with silicone pads or temporary tarsorraphy stitches.

Depending on the size and the depth of the burn, facial burns can be excised and resurfaced either in one, two or multiple stages.

Isolated deep facial burns can be excised and autografted in one operation. A one-stage dermal skin substitute (Matriderm®/Integra®) may be considered in this type of injury to provide dermal replacement without prolonging inpatient stay. Immediate autografting is feasible if thorough debridement and meticulous hemostasis can be ensured [10].

In larger body surface area and deeper burns repeated debridement with cadaver allograft or skin substitute wound closure to ensure adequacy of debridement and hemostasis. This principle of repeated or second look surgery performed within 4–7 days allows for thorough and adequate debridement with re-excison of non viable tissue, perfect hemostasis and prevention of graft loss due to hematoma (Fig. 4).

Hemostasis is aided by subeschar infiltration of 1/1,000,000 solution of epinephrine and topical application of 2% phenylephrine soaked swabs. The authors believe this technique limits blood loss, and does not lead to over excision of the burn wound.

The aesthetic units that will not heal within 3 weeks of the injury are outlined with markers. These are surgically excised in a tangential fashion. In some aesthetic units small areas of normal skin or superficial wounds can be excised to conform to the unit.

If only a small area of an aesthetic unit is burned it can be debrided and grafted leaving the adjacent uninjured normal tissue. This may require reconstruction at a later stage.

In areas of mixed depth burn injury excision should aim to be at a uniform depth to remove any skin appendage remnants to prevent subsequent problems with buried hair follicles and associated pits, cysts and infection.

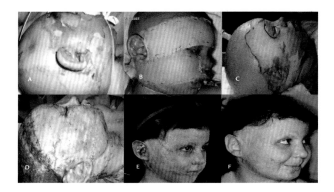

**Fig. 4.** Mixed deep partial thickness / Full thickness facial burn.
A   On admission;
B   Inital application of allograft;
C   5 days post injury it is apparent that healing will take
    > 3 weeks. Areas for excision marked;
D   Following debridement and split thickness skin grafting in
    cosmetic units. Scalp donor site;
E   Outcome at 3 months;
F   Outcome at 2 years

Adjuvant care includes post pyloric enteral nutrition using a naso-jejunal tube, which is continued until all grafts have taken and are stable, usually by day 7 postgrafting.

Continued postoperative intubation and ventilation in non-ventilated patients can be considered for 48 h to preserve integrity of the grafted areas [33].

## Wound closure

Depending on the size and depth of the injury as described above a single or staged approach is taken to wound closure. Following excision and appropriate hemostasis the wound is covered with either autograft or cadaver allograft. The grafts are tailored to match aesthetic units, with graft seams placed in the boundaries of units. Grafts are secured with staples or absorbable sutures.

Following wound excision cadaver allograft can be used as a good test of wound bed viability as they will vascularise. Xenografts and Biobrane can be used in a similar fashion for temporary wound closure but they do not revascularise and do not test wound viability.

Following excision and application of cadaveric allograft, further surgery is undertaken 4 to 7 days later for definitive wound closure. If the allograft is adherent and re-vascularized, then the wound is ready for autografting. If the allografts are non-adherent they are removed and the underlying wound re-excised and re-allografted. This process is repeated until the allograft is adherent. If donor sites are limited in a major burn injury, repeated application of allograft may be require until adequate suitable donor sites become available. An alternative approach is to use a two-stage dermal regeneration template (Integra®) to close the wound and wait for donor site availability for second stage grafting

Split-thickness autografts are preferably harvested from the scalp to optimize texture and colour match with facial skin. In larger burn, if the scalp is burnt and if the entire face must be grafted, other donor sites must be considered. In these circumstances larger donor sites obtained from the same area should be used to ensure similar texture and colour of the grafted skin. Powered dermatomes set at 10–12 /100ths inch provide the best quality skin and the use of a 4 inch dermatome in a child and a 6 inch dermatome in an adult will ensure grafts of adequate width to resurface aesthetic units.

Biosynthetic skin substitutes or dermal regeneration templates have been popularized in recent years in the management of full thickness facial burns and have become the standard of care for these injuries in some centres particularly for pan-facial burn injury [34]. One-stage dermal regeneration templates (Matriderm®/Integra®) can be considered for small or isolated full thickness facial burns. In larger burns associated with pan-facial injury a two-stage technique has benefits as it closes the burn wound until precious donor sites become available. The use of dermal templates may also have benefits in children by limiting skin graft donor site morbidity by taking thinner grafts, which are usually harvested at 6–8/100ths inch.

## Special areas and adjacent of the face

### Eyelids

Burns to the eyelids are very common in patients with facial burn injury. Eyelid injury can signify or lead to underlying ocular damage and subsequent

297

blindness. All patients with periorbital burns should undergo ocular exam on admission using fluorescein and Wood's lamp to to show up any epithelial conjunctival loss. Early involvement of patients with corneal injury is essential. The presence of uninjured skin in the crow's feet is a reliable clinical sign indicating absence of corneal injury [35]. Initial management includes aggressive lubrication and topical antimicrobials to prevent corneal exposure and desiccation. Early excision and skin grafting with either thick split thickness or full thickness skin grafts for full thickness eyelid burns reduces exposure keratitis, conjunctivitis, and corneal ulceration and is best undertaken within 7 days [36]. In patients with severe large total body surface areas burns with limited donor sites temporary tarsorrhaphy may be required.. Temporary tarsorrhaphy is recommended to prevent ectropion and corneal exposure although traditional tarsorrhaphy techniques traumatise the tarsal plate, cut out after a time and can even traumatize the cornea.

Unfortunately despite early excision and grafting scar contracture during the acute phase can lead to ectropion and corneal ulceration. These patients will often require release and further grafting during their acute stay.

Reversible semi-permanent tarsorrhaphy techniques have been described in patients who develop conjunctivitis which can be used both laterally and medially to protect the conjunctiva [37]. The adhesion of the lower to the upper eyelid may also be helpful in counteracting scar contracture.

## Nose and ears

The nose and ears are facial appendages that consist of a cartilaginous / bony framework with closely applied overlying skin. This means that in deeper burns the underlying skeleton is exposed and or involved which can lead to vital tissue loss and structural support leading to subsequent deformity. These areas are subsequently a significant reconstructive challenge.

Ear management in the acute phase requires preservation of the cartilaginous structures by the judicious use of topical antimicrobials and avoidance of desiccation [38]. This has reduced the incidence of suppurative chondritis and its devastating

consequences. Some authors advocate the use of early debridement and flap cover to preserve ear cartilage and undertake this in patients with major injuries [39], although in practice most surgeons treat these injuries expectantly with grafting as when donor sites become available.

Nasal burn injury presents simpler problem, as therapeutic options are limited. Excision and resurfacing is usually undertaken at the same time as the rest of the face but it is not uncommon for the nasal cartilaginous skeleton to be involved and exposed leading to total or subtotal loss of the nose.

## Lips

Injuries to the lips are treated according to the different structures involved. Mucosal injury is usually managed conservatively and will heal spontaneous. Pain and contact bleeding are an issue and oral nutrition may not be tolerated necessitating tube feeding. The cutaneous portions of the lips are treated in conjunction with the rest of the face and are debrided and grafted at the same time for the same indications. Special attention must be paid in wound care to the hair bearing lip and beard area in males. Regular shaving to control hair growth and the build up of necrotic debris and exudate is important in the prevention of chronic folliculitis and infection.

## Scalp

Although the scalp is a distinct anatomical entity it is useful to consider management of burn injuries to this area at the same time as the face as the two commonly coexist. In general management of scalp burns is relatively conservative with meticulous wound care, topical antimicrobials and an expectant policy. This is because the scalp is a highly specialized area of skin, it has a very high density of hair follicles many of which are sub dermal and healing potential is much greater even in those injuries that clinically appear to be full thickness. In injuries that have the potential to heal, meticulous wound care including regular shaving of the scalp must be undertaken to prevent hair growth, clogging up with necrotic tissue and debris which leads to infection and chronic folliculitis. Not only is this painful and distressing for the patient it can lead to unnecessary alopecia. The wound care and shaving often has to be undertaken under general anaesthesia particularly in the paediatric patient.

Tangential excision of the scalp is usually accompanied by significant bleeding and most surgeons would avoid this in wounds that have undetermined healing potential. Formal excision is preferred once it is obvious that the injury has no healing potential and/or does not heal. In either case it is not uncommon for the calvarium to be exposed especially in those cases of catastrophic injury. Exposed calvarium poses a difficult management problem especially in a patient with a major burn injury [40]. Traditionally conservative wound care with topical antimicrobials has been used until there is sequestration of the outer table of calvarium leaving a granulating wound bed which is then skin grafted. Drilling holes in or burring off the outer table of skull, which promotes the granulation process, can accelerate this process. This can then be covered either with autograft, allograft or In tegra®.

Alternatively free tissue transfer may be used for these difficult cases and can be particularly useful in catastrophic facial burn injury.

## The neck

The neck should also be considered as an important area adjacent to the face. Burns in this area are generally treated to a similar fashion to other areas of the body. Surgical excision of deep burns is undertaken early and it is priority area for early autologous skin grafting to achieve early wound healing, particularly in the pre tracheal area if prolonged ventilation is predicted and a tracheostomy is being considered.

## Catastrophic injury

Facial burn injury that is both extensive and very deep involving destruction of important facial landmarks can be classified as being catastrophic. This type of injury is usually present in an extensive body surface area burn and its associated organ dysfunction and critical illness. Management of this type of injury involves repeated wound debridement, repeated allograft applications, the use of skin substitutes, the use of early microsurgical reconstruction

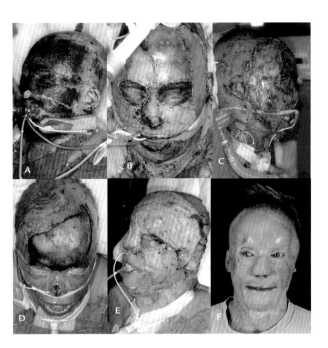

**Fig. 5.** Catastrophic complex facial burn in patient with 75% full thickness injury.
A On admission;
B Following excision at 5 days post burn and allograft application;
C Resurfacing with Integra;
D 2 months post injury, face healed but extensive area exposed calvarium;
E Coverage exposed calvarium and initial nasal reconstruction with LatissimusDorsi Free Flap and Integra
F Late appearance 3 years post burn following reconstruction with scalp tissue expansion, lip resurfacing with full thickness skin graft, Free Thoracodorsal Artery Perforator (TAP) Flap nasal reconstruction

for preservation of vital structures and tissue salvage. These injuries present an extremely complex challenge usually in the presence of an already complex injury, which requires significant effort in planning and execution to optimize appearance and function. This group of patients may suitable for reconstruction with composite allo-transplantation [41] (Fig. 5).

## Post healing rehabilitation and scar management

Rehabilitation of the burn patient begins on admission. This is as true for the patient with a facial burn as it is for any burn patient. The patient is assessed following admission by the whole multidisciplinary team including the surgical and therapy staff [42]. During the inpatient stay and treatment facial mobilisation, oral food and fluid intake (if possible) and the prevention of microstomia are important aspects of care. Following healing and prior to discharge the patient must be evaluated and a plan made as to ongoing therapy needs and scar management. The therapists must assess the face and document any areas of concern and potential for scar hypertrophy, deformity or developing contracture.

The most commonly used interventions include skin moisturizing, massage, pressure and topical applications of silicone. In particular patients are advised to avoid excessive sun exposure and to use sunscreen cream to prevent hyperpigmentation of the scars.

Silicone sheets have been used for many years to soften the scar, prevent contracture and increase mobility. The most likely mechanism of action is hydration of the scar by occlusion, thus improve the texture, thickness and colour of hypertrophic scars [43].

Massage is universally thought to be a key therapeutic intervention to encourage scar maturation, softening, pliability and fading. Few studies have been undertaken to evaluate the delivery, timing, intensity and duration of scar massage and have produced conflicting evidence as to efficacy [44]. Pressure therapy in the form of a mask or garment is usually indicated in deep partial thickness or full thickness burns following adequate wound healing or in more superficial injuries that begin to form scar hypertrophy. The evidence for the use of pressure is limited however most clinicians believe in the benefits of pressure in terms of the scar maturation process [45].

Facial pressure is difficult to achieve due to the complex convexities and concavities of the face. One option is to combine pressure garments and silicone inserts or sheeting. Another is to make custom made masks that can be lined with silicone. These masks have been traditionally made using a facial mold but more recently they have been made using computer aided design [46]. Both garments and masks can be total or partial depending on the distribution of the scar. Pressure therapy and scar management are usually continued until the scar matures fully or stops maturing and patients must be warned that this may take up to two years post injury.

Microstomia splints and nasal dilators can be inserted via the nasal and oral apertures of the pressure garment or mask. Compliance with therapeutic interventions and orthotic devices is often a problem, especially with oral splints. A variety of modalities must be used and tailored to the patient's needs and compliance.

## Outcome and reconstruction

The aim of both acute care and subsequent reconstruction in facial burn injury is the restoration of form and function and the amelioration of any discomfort.

In general burn injury gives rise to the following sequealae: hypertrophic scarring, scar contracture, skin colour and texture change and loss of body parts. Although these features apply to all patients, their combination results in unique injury patterns and disfigurement.

Donelan has defined characteristic sequaelae of facial burn injury to include: lower eyelid ectropion, short nose with alar flaring, short retruded upper lip, lower lip eversion and inferior displacement, flat facial features and loss of jaw line definition.

Donelan has classified facial burn categories into 2 general types: Type I – Normal facies with focal or diffuse scarring +/– contractures. Type II – Pan facial burn deformity with some / all stigmata of facial burn deformity [3].

Such characterisation and classification are useful in defining deformity and helpful in planning surgical interventions. Timing of intervention depends on the urgency of the problem and traditionally reconstructive surgery has been delayed until scar maturation is established although more recently early reconstruction has been advocated.

Planning reconstruction requires a realistic approach from both the patient and the surgeon to harmonise expectations with the probable outcomes following surgery. Facial burn reconstruction starts on admission and good primary care will often obviate the need for secondary reconstruction (Fig. 6).

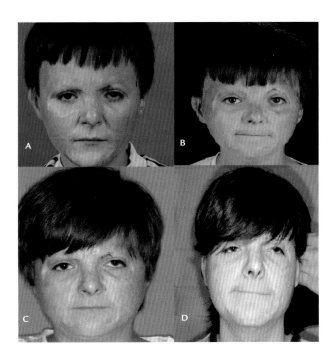

**Fig. 6.** Appearances of sheet grafting of face using aesthetic units over time.
A  2 years post injury;
B  4 years post injury;
C  6 years post injury;
D  8 years post injury

## Summary

Management of facial burns continues to be a difficult and challenging area in burn care. The strategy and options for treatment are debated, in particular about the timing of excisional surgery. For indeterminate depth burn injury a consensus view of topical antimicrobial treatment and observation undertaken until the burn declares itself in terms of healing within a three-week period. Once it is clear the wound will not heal within this time frame excisional surgery is indicated. Early excision and grafting are indicated for those injuries that are obviously full thickness to improve function and outcome.

## References

[1]  Ye EM (1998) Psychological morbidity in patients with facial and neck burns. Burns 24: 646–648

[2]  Klein MB, Moore ML, Costa B et al (2005) Primer on the management of face burns at the University of Washington. J Burn Care Rehabil 26: 2–6

[3]  Donelan MB (2006) Reconstruction of the head and neck. In: Herndon DN (ed) Total burn care. Saunders/Elsevier, London, pp 701–718

[4]  Deitch EA, Wheelahan TM, Rose MP, Clothier J, Cotter (1983) Hypertrophic burn scars: analysis of variables. J Trauma 23(10): 895–898

[5]  Cubison TC, Pape SA, Parkhouse N (2006) Evidence for the link between healing time and the development of hypertrophic scars (HTS) in paediatric burns due to scald injury. Burns 32(8): 992–999. Epub 2006 Aug 8

[6]  McDonald WS, Deitch EA (1987) Hypertrophic skin grafts in burned patients: a prospective analysis of variables. J Trauma 27(2): 147–150

[7]  Gonzalez Ulloa M (1987) Regional aesthetic units of the face. Plast Reconstr Surg 79: 489

[8]  Fraulin FO, Illmayer SJ, Tredget EE (1996) Assessment of cosmetic and functional results of conservative versus surgical management of facial burns. J Burn Care Rehabil 17: 19–29

[9]  Jaskille AD, Ramella-Roman JC, Shupp JW, Jordan MH, Jeng JC (2010) Critical review of burn depth assessment techniques: part II. Review of laser doppler technology. J Burn Care Res 31(1): 151–157

[10]  Friedstat JS, Klein MB (2009) Acute management of facial burns. Clin Plast Surg 36(4): 653–660

[11]  Aggarwal S, Smailes S, Dziewulski P (2009) Tracheostomy in burns patients revisited. Burns 35(7): 962–966

[12]  Leon-Villapalos J, Jeschke MG, Herndon DN (2008) Topical management of facial burns. Burns 34(7): 903–911

[13]  Khera SY et al (1999) A comparison of chlorhexidine and povidone-iodine skin preparation for surgical operations. Curr Surg 56: 341–343

[14]  Monafo WW, West MA (1990) Current treatment recommendations for total burn therapy. Drugs 40: 364–373

[15]  Atiyeh BS et al (2007) Effect of silver on burn wound infection control and healing: review of the literature. Burns 33: 139–148

[16]  Cooper ML et al (1991) The cytotoxic effects of commonly used topical antimicrobial agents on human fibroblasts and keratinocytes. J Trauma 31: 775–784

[17]  Demling RH, DeSanti L (1999) Management of partial thickness facial burns (comparison of topical antibiotics and bioengineered skin substitutes). Burns 25: 256–261

[18]  Horch RE et al (2005) Treatment of second degree facial burns with allografts-preliminary results. Burns 31: 597–602

[19] Garner JP, Heppell PSJ (2005) Cerium nitrate in the management of burns. Burns 31: 539–547

[20] Bowser BH et al (1981) A prospective analysis of silver sulfadiazine with and without cerium nitrate as a topical agent in the treatment of severely burned children. J Trauma 7: 558–563

[21] Dunn K, Edwards-Jones V (2004) The role of Acticoat™ with nanocrystalline silver in the management of burns. Burns 30 [Suppl 1]: S1–9

[22] Cuttle L, Naidu S, Mill J, Hoskins W, Das K, Kimble R (2007) A retrospective cohort study of Acticoat™ versus Silvazine™ in a paediatric population. Burns 33: 701–707

[23] Bessey PQ (2006) Wound care. In: Herndon DN (ed) Total burn care. Saunders, London, pp 127–135

[24] Ang ES et al (2000) The role of alternative therapy in the management of partial thickness burns of the face. Experience with the use of moist exposed burn ointment (MEBO) compared with silver sulphadiazine. Ann Acad Med Singapore 29: 7–10

[25] Zhang H et al (2005) Efficacy of moist exposed burn ointment on burns. J Burn Care Rehabil 26: 247–251

[26] Delatte SJ et al (2001) Effectiveness of beta-glucan collagen for treatment of partial thickness burns in children. J Pediatr Surg 36: 113–118

[27] Chester DL, Papini R (2004) Skin and skin substitutes in burn management. Trauma 6: 87–99

[28] Demling RH, De Santi L (2002) Closure of partial-thickness facial burns with a bioactive skin substitute in the major burn population decreases the cost of care and improves outcome. Wounds 14: 230–234

[29] Barret JP, Dziewulski P, Ramzy PI, Wolf SE, Desai MH, Herndon D (2000) Biobrane versus 1% silver sulfadiazine in second-degree pediatric burns. Plast Reconstr Surg 105(1): 62–65

[30] Branski LK et al (2008) Amnion in the treatment of pediatric partial-thickness facial burns. Burns 34: 393–399

[31] Pham C et al (2007) Bioengineered skin substitutes for the management of burns: a systematic review. Burns 33: 946–957

[32] Surgical Safety Checklist. The World Health Organization. http://www.who. int/patientsafety/safesurgery/en/

[33] Barret JP (2005) The face. In: Barret-Nerin JP, Herndon DN (eds) Principles and practice of burn surgery. Marcel Dekker, New York, pp 281–289

[34] Klein MB, Engrav LH, Holmes JH et al (2005) Management of facial burns with a collagen/glycosamino-glycan skin substitute–prospective experience with 12 consecutive patients with large, deep facial burns. Burns 31: 257–261

[35] Dancey A, Mein E, Khan M, Rayatt S, Papini R (2008) Is crow's feet sign a reliable indicator of corneal injury in facial burns? J Plast Reconstr Aesthet Surg 61(11): 1325–1327

[36] Barrow RE, Jeschke MG, Herndon DN (2000) Early release of third-degree eyelid burns prevents eye injury. Plast Reconstr Surg 105: 860–863

[37] Klein MB, Ahmadi AJ, Sires BS et al (2008) Reversible marginal tarsorrhaphy: a salvage procedure for periocular burns. Plast Reconstr Surg 121: 1627–1630

[38] Engrav LH, Richey KJ, Walkinshaw MD et al (1989) Chondritis of the burned ear: a preventable complication. Ann Plast Surg 23: 1–2

[39] Saito T, Yotsuyanagi T, Ezoe K, Ikeda K, Yamauchi M, Arai K, Urushidate S, Mikami M (2009) The acute surgical management of injury to the helix and antihelix in patients with large body surface area burns. J Plast Reconstr Aesthet Surg 62(8): 1020–1024

[40] Spies M, McCauley RL, Mudge BP, Herndon DN (2003) Management of acute calvarial burns in children. J Trauma 54(4): 765–769

[41] Pushpakumar SB, Barker JH, Soni CV, Joseph H, van Aalst VC, Banis JC, Frank J (2010) Clinical considerations in face transplantation. Burns 36(7): 951–958

[42] Edgar D, Brereton M (2004) Rehabilitation after burn injury. BMJ 329: 342–344

[43] Lyle WG (2001) Silicon gel sheeting. PRS 1079: 272–275

[44] Patiño O, Novick C, Merlo A, Benaim F J (1999) Massage in hypertrophic scars. Burn Care Rehabil 20(3): 268–271

[45] Engrav LH, Heimbach DM, Rivara FP, Moore ML, Wang J, Carrougher GJ, Costa B, Numhom S, Calderon J, Gibran NS (2010) 12-Year within-wound study of the effectiveness of custom pressure garment therapy. Burns 36(7): 975–983

[46] Rogers B et al (2003) Computerized manufacturing of transparent face masks for the treatment of facial scarring. J Burn Care Rehabil 24: 91–96

Correspondence: Jorge Leon Villapalos, St Andrews Centre for Plastic Surgery and Burns, Court Road, Broomfield, Chelmsford, Essex CM1 7ET, UK,
E-mail:Jorge.Leon-Villapa los@chelwest.nhs.uk

# Hand burns

Benjamin P. Amis[1], Matthew B. Klein[2]

[1] Resident, Department of Orthopaedic Surgery, University of Washington, Seattle, WA, USA
[2] David and Nancy Auth-Washington Research Foundation, Endowed Chair for Restorative Burn Surgery, Division of Plastic Surgery, University of Washington, Seattle, WA, USA

## Introduction

Loss of hand function is the leading cause of impairment following burn injury [18]. Over 80% of severe burns involve the hands [2]. In addition, superficial and partial-thickness burns are often incurred during routine occupational and recreational activities due to the hand's function as the primary point of physical contact during day-to-day activities. Even small hand burns could potentially impair function and quality-of-life.

Advances in acute burn care have made survival of previously fatal injuries possible and shifted the focus of burn care and research towards optimizing functional outcomes. Consequently, care for and restoration of hand function have received increased attention with a multidisciplinary team of burn surgeons, plastic surgeons, rehabilitation physicians, and physical and occupational therapists coordinating care at specialized burn centers to improve outcomes.

## Initial evaluation and history

Following trauma protocols, all patients presenting with burn injuries should undergo an initial evaluation focusing on systemic illness and life threatening injuries. Once this has been completed, the burn injury itself may be addressed. In evaluating hand burns, a careful history, including handedness, mechanism, and the circumstances surrounding the injury should be obtained. The date of the patient's last tetanus vaccination or booster should be documented and tetanus toxoid or immunoglobulin should be administered as necessary.

After a thorough history, the physical examination proceeds by classifying the extent and depth of burns. Other injuries, such as crush or laceration, occurring in conjunction with the burn should also be documented. The extent of the burn may be efficiently recorded using a hand diagram as well as distinctive markings to indicate the depth of the burn in each area and damaged or exposed underlying structures. The appearance of the hand should also be noted. Edema, especially on the dorsum of the hand and around the joints, may lead to a posture with decreased tension on the collateral ligaments (i. e. extension through the metacarpophalangeal joints and flexion through the interphalangeal joints). Corrective splinting and early motion may be required to minimize the risk of fixed contracture.

Particular attention should be paid to vascular perfusion, especially in the presence of circumferential burns. Decreased perfusion may be suspected if capillary refill is greater than 2–3 seconds or absent, radial or ulnar pulses are diminished, or the skin is cool to the touch. Areas of suspected vascular injury should be further evaluated with a Doppler ultrasound examination. Patients with circumferential forearm burns are at risk for vascular insufficiency or compartment syndrome when edema collects deep to an unyielding eschar resulting in decreased arterial flow and venous congestion. To prevent compartment syndrome, escharotomy or fasciotomy (as described below) should be performed to restore adequate perfusion.

## Initial wound management

During the initial evaluation of burn wounds, foreign material should be removed and thin or loose blisters should be debrided. An appropriate dressing is then applied. The choice of dressing is dependent on the depth of the burn with the goals of preventing infection, promoting re-epithelialization, avoiding water and heat loss, and keeping the wound moist. Additionally, the ideal dressing should be easy to apply and reduce pain.

Local wound care is the definitive treatment for superficial and superficial partial-thickness hand burns with the objective of optimizing re-epithelialization. We prefer an ointment with antimicrobial properties such as bacitracin and a non-adherent gauze dressing. For deeper burns that may form an eschar, we prefer silver sulfadiazine (Silvadene), which provides increased antibacterial protection and is soothing when applied. Silvadene forms a film or "pseudo-eschar" after application necessitating daily cleansing prior to repeat use. Sulfamylon (Mafenide) is preferred for infected burns due to sulfadiazine's poor eschar penetration. However, metabolic acidosis resulting from carbonic anhydrase inhibition is a potential side effect for which the treating physician must be vigilant. When epithelialization is imminent or occurring, the dressing may be switched to bacitracin and a non-adherent gauze. There is no evidence supporting the use prophylactic antibiotics.

## Escharotomy and fasciotomy

Deep extremity burns, particularly those that are circumferential, must be closely monitored for distal vascular insufficiency. Additionally, patients who sustain extensive burn injuries require large volumes of intravenous fluid and will develop significant soft tissue edema under the tight shell-like eschar. Decreased pulses or Doppler signals, cool extremities, or decreased capillary refill in this setting should be addressed immediately with escharotomy to increase distal perfusion [3]. Escharotomy may be performed under general anesthesia in the operating room or at the bedside in the intensive care unit with appropriate analgesia and sedation. Eschar is insensate and pain should be minimal during the procedure. A full release of the forearm may be achieved using either electrocautery or a scalpel to incise the eschar through two longitudinal incisions, radially and ulnarly, to the level of the 1st and 5th metacarpophalangeal joints. Furtherer decompression of the hand itself is achieved through longitudinal incisions between the metacarpals from the base of the hand to the head of the metacarpal taking care not to expose any tendons (Fig. 1). Digital escharotomy is avoided at our institution; however, one small case series suggests that it may decrease finger necrosis [24]. It is crucial that digital incisions be limited to the eschar itself as deeper incisions may expose underlying vital structures unnecessarily.

Compartment syndrome should be suspected in all patients but is less likely in patients with isolated thermal burns limited to superficial tissues. Electri-

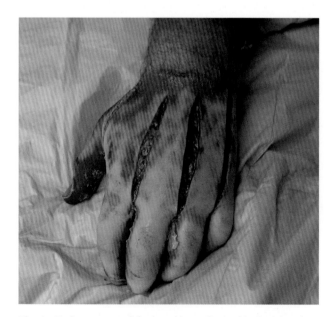

**Fig. 1.** Escharotomy of the hand is performed by incising the eschar in the intermetacarpal spaces. Care is taken not to unnecessarily expose underlying structures

cal burns and burns with an associated crush injury are more likely to result increased compartmental pressures and a resulting compartment syndrome. Deep muscle compartments are often more affected than superficial after electrical burns because bone has a very high resistance to the flow of electrical current. Neuropraxia following electrical shock can also complicate the initial assessment.

The diagnosis of compartment syndrome is generally clinical and heralded by the constellation of pain on passive stretch, paresthesias, pallor, paralysis, decreased pulses, and poikilothermia (the 6 P's). Systemic deterioration, including myoglobin induced metabolic acidosis, may be the only sign of compartment syndrome in an obtunded patient with myonecrosis. Although not specific to burns or electrical injuries, compartmental pressures of > 30 mmHg or within 10–20 mmHg or diastolic pressure are also diagnostic criteria of compartment syndrome. In the setting of suspected compartment syndrome, or failure of escharotomy to restore distal perfusion, dorsal and volar fascial incisions, including carpal tunnel release, should be made and the muscle compartments examined and debrided as necessary [3–5].

## Surgical management: Early excision and grafting

Early excision and grafting has been shown to reduce hypertrophic scarring and subsequent contractures leading to a reduced need for later reconstructions. Superficial and intermediate partial-thickness burns will often heal within 2 weeks and rarely require excision. However, deeper wounds that are expected to take longer to heal (i. e. longer than 21 days) should be carefully monitored for healing potential. Once clear that wounds will not heal in a timely fashion, plans for excision and grafting should be made. Given the relatively small surface area of the hand, timing of hand excision in a patient with extensive burns should be weighed against the need to remove large areas of eschar to prevent burn wound sepsis [10].

Excision and grafting is usually performed under general anesthesia with the use of a tourniquet to reduce blood loss. Excision is performed with the use of a Goulian knife to remove eschar to a depth of

healthy, bleeding tissue. For excision of web spaces and other areas in which the Goulian knife is difficult to maneuver, the Versajet (Smith and Nephew, London, UK) high-pressure water jet system is useful [15, 23] (Fig. 2). Excision on the dorsum of the hand should be performed carefully given the paucity of

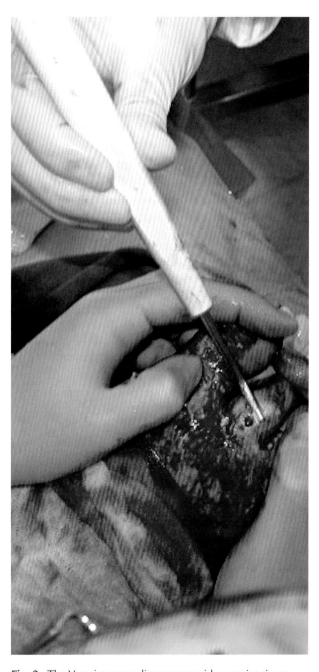

Fig. 2. The Versajet water dissector provides precise tissue excision and is particularly suited for use in areas of convexity or concavity

subcutaneous tissue and subsequent risk of exposing tendons. Small areas of exposed tendon may be covered with surrounding soft tissue to avoid the need for flap coverage. However, larger areas of exposed tendons and joints will not be amenable to grafting without the use of flap coverage [13]. Once excision is complete, the tourniquet should be deflated to assess tissue viability by observing bleeding. Epinephrine (concentration 1 : 10,000) soaked Telfa (Mansfield, MA) and laparotomy pads should be applied for ten minutes. The wound bed is then assessed for hemostasis and new Epinephrine soaked dressings replaced as needed to achieve a bloodless field. Electrocautery should be used sparingly and only on small focal areas of bleeding.

The majority of hand burns can be covered with split thickness skin grafts. In order to guide graft harvest, the wound bed should be templated and the template transposed to the planned donor site. The anterolateral thigh is the preferred donor location in adults and older children. The buttocks, taking care to remain beneath the diaper area, are harvested in younger children. A dermatome with the widest guard appropriate for the amount of skin needed helps to minimize the number of graft junctions. For the majority of the hand, 0.012 inch thick grafts are sufficient while 0.015–0.018 inch thick grafts are necessary for the palm [19]. Sheet grafts are preferred to meshed grafts to improve functional and cosmetic result. Full-thickness grafts harvested from the inguinal crease or the flank may be the most appropriate choice for small burns on both the dorsum of the hand and the palm [7, 25]. Grafts are affixed with absorbable sutures around the edges and fibrin glue applied to the wound bed. The edges of the graft are reinforced with Hypafix (Smith and Nephew, London, UK) and Mastisol (Ferndale Laboratories, Ferndale, MI). A dressing of non-adherent material, fine-mesh gauze, kerlex rolls, and a custom fabricated splint is applied. Of note, grafting should take place in the same position as splinting, attempting to maintain tension on the collateral ligaments and abduct the first webspace. The dressing is removed on post-operative day one and fluid collections are evacuated with a small incision in the graft. It is important to note that we do not make any pie-crusting incisions in the graft at the time of initial placement. The wound should be inspected daily until no fluid

collections are noted. The dressing is maintained until post-operative day five and then replaced with a lighter non-adherent dressing to allow for range of motion exercises [27]. The donor site, if properly harvested and dressed, should re-epithelialize spontaneously within two weeks. We prefer Mepilex AG (Molynycke Health Care, Norcross, GA), a silver-impregnated dressing, although a non-adherent gauze and bacitracin is also acceptable.

Two exceptions to early excision are palm burns, particularly in pediatric patients, and small burns. Palm burns are common in the pediatric population after contact with a stove or fireplace. These burns are usually deep partial-thickness or more superficial and heal well with conservative management. Avoiding excision will help to protect palmar sensation that is vital to overall hand function. It is critical that children with palm burns undergo aggressive range of motion therapy as these burns are prone to contracture particularly if a more conservative approach to excision is taken [9]. Parents must be instructed on how to adequately range the hand and the child should do so at least 10 times daily. Splints should only be used if early signs of contracture are noted. Small burns (either linear burns or less than the size of a small coin) should also be given a chance to heal without excision.

## Tissue flaps

Severe burns, especially on the dorsum of the hand where the skin is thin with little underlying subcutaneous tissue, are often not amenable to skin grafting due to exposed bone or tendon. When this situation arises, flap coverage is required. Additionally, digits sometimes require vascular soft tissue coverage to optimize function. Numerous soft tissue flaps have been described to provide durable coverage for areas for which skin grafting would not be appropriate. It is important to keep in mind associated injuries that should be treated at the time of grafting. For example, damage to extensor tendons or intra-articular burns may result in eventual joint contracture. In these cases, arthrodesis in the optimal position may facilitate a swifter functional recover.

**Local flaps.** The radial forearm fasciocutaneous or fascial flap, based on the radial artery, is an appropriate choice for local coverage when the donor site remains uninjured. An Allen's test, as well as Doppler examination of the superficial palmar arch, should be performed prior to raising the flap to ensure adequate perfusion of the hand. Skin grafting of the donor site in the case of a fasciocutaneous flap or recipient site in the case of a fascial flap will be necessary. The distally based posterior interosseous flap is a fasciocutaneous flap harvested from the dorsal aspect of the forearm and does not disrupt either of the major blood vessels perfusing the hand [1]. Although the flap's perfusing vessel is sometimes hypoplastic or absent, this flap is especially useful when there has been an injury to either the radial or ulnar artery.

**Distant flaps.** When local flaps are unavailable due to injury, distant flaps may be considered. The primary distant flaps used for hand coverage are the abdominal (random) or groin (pedicled) flaps [27]. In either case, a flap of Scarpa's fascia, subcutaneous tissue, and skin is templated, raised, and sutured onto the hand. The hand is left in-situ for 2–3 weeks after which the flap is divided (Fig. 3). Vascularization of the flap can be determined, when in doubt, using indocynanine-green fluorescence video angiography [21]. A variant of groin or abdominal flaps may be performed in which only Scarpa's fascia is transferred and skin grafted, leaving behind the groin or abdominal skin and subcutaneous tissue – the Crane procedure.

**Free tissue transfer.** Free tissue transfer may be necessitated when extensive burns prevent local or distant pedicled flaps. Numerous options exist including a contralateral radial forearm fascial flap, dorsalis pedis fascial flap, temporoparietal fascial flap, perforator flap (ex. thin anterolateral thigh perforator flap), and muscle flaps (ex. serratus anterior, rectus abdominus, or gracilis) [4, 13]. All have been used with success to provide durable, pliable coverage. Prior to considering a free tissue transfer, the viability of the recipient vessels must be evaluated to ensure that they have not also been damaged.

## Skin substitutes

Skin substitutes may be useful in cases of extensive burn injury where there is limited donor site to allow

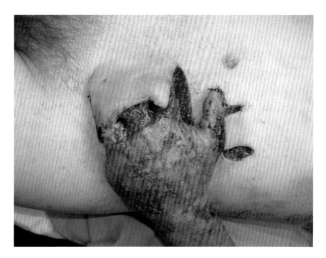

**Fig. 3.** A pedicled abdominal flap was used in this case to provide soft tissue coverage over exposed joints and tendons of the hand. In this case two separate flaps were used – one for the thumb and one for the digits

for the harvest of quality autografts for hand coverage. Skin substitutes are applied to the freshly excised wound bed and, as in the case of autograft, it is essential that the wound bed be viable and hemostatic prior to skin substitute placement. Depending on the skin substitute used, the autograft may be placed over the substitute in one operation or in a second procedure after the substitute has had adequate time to vascularize. Two popular skin substitutes are Integra (Integra Life Sciences, Plainsboro, NJ) which requires two procedures and Matriderm (Dr. Otto Suwelack Skin & Health Care AG, Billerbeck, Germany) which is a one-stage product. Each approach has relative benefits and drawbacks. A full discussion of skin graft substitutes is beyond the scope of this chapter; however, their use has been described in several small case series studies involving the hand [6, 11, 12, 16, 31].

## Amputation

Severe burns of the hand may result in injuries for which salvage is either impossible or impractical. The ultimate goal of treatment of hand burns is optimization of function. The loss of a digit may provide the patient with a more favorable outcome when compared to an insensate, painful, and stiff finger.

Delayed amputation is also sometimes required when all other treatments options have been exhausted or have failed. Length should be protected at all times. As is the case with all severe hand burns, realistic discussions about the goals of reconstruction should take place prior to embarking on a plan of treatment. In addition, an area of viable soft tissue on a digit which is to be amputated may be useful for coverage of other areas of the hand. For example, if the dorsal aspect of a digit is burned down through the tendon and joint, a filet flap from the volar aspect of the digit can be used to cover any exposed metacarpophalangeal joints or tendons.

## Hand therapy

Hand therapy is an integral component in the treatment of any hand injury. Surgical management of hand burns without proper post-operative hand therapy – including splinting, edema management, and range-of-motion exercises – preferably led by an experienced burn therapist, is likely to result in suboptimal results. Hand therapy should begin within 24-hours of injury. Edema management is initiated with elevation and proceeds to compressive wraps. Custom compressive gloves and sleeves should be fitted to the patient when there is no longer concern for a shear injury [17]. Any hand which begins to assume a clawed posture should be splinted in the intrinsic plus position with the wrist in 30 degrees of extension, the metacarpophalangeal joints in 70–90 degrees of flexion, and the interphalangeal joint in full extension to 15 degrees of flexion. The first webspace should also be held in an abducted position. This posture will maintain the collateral ligaments in tension and help to avoid fixed contractures. Palm burns, which are at significant risk of flexion contracture, should be splinted with all joints in full extension. Range of motion exercises should be withheld in the acute phase of graft or flap healing, but should be initiated as soon as possible thereafter, usually after five days in the case of split- or full-thickness skin grafting. If prolonged splinting is required, range of motion exercises out of the splint should occur several times a day. Night time only splinting should be considered and independent therapy should be encouraged. Passive range of motion should be performed on intubated patients daily. Patients should not be discharged from the hospital until they have demonstrated that they are self-sufficient with both hand therapy and wound care [20].

## Secondary reconstruction

Even optimal care of burned hands may result in excessive scarring and contracture. Hand contractures may be categorized as digital, palmar, dorsal, or syndactyly [14] (Fig. 4). Secondary reconstructions include scar release, rearranging or lengthening scar, and replacing deficient tissues with grafts or flaps. Treatment of contracted tissue should be initiated after the scar has fully matured, often a period of 12 months. The patient must also be mentally prepared to return to the operating room and participate in postoperative rehabilitation. In case of pediatric patients, parental compliance must also be assured. However, in some cases of severe contracture, early release and grafting should be considered.

The approach to secondary reconstruction begins with defining the problem or functional deficit. A discussion of realistic goals and expectations should follow. Physical therapy should be initiated to both improve contracture and demonstrate future compliance. Coverage options, both local and distant, should be inventoried. If two hands require sur-

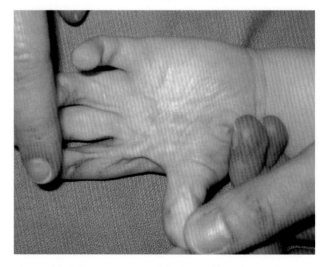

**Fig. 4.** Digital contractures of the burned hand extending from the palm to the digits

gery, only one should be addressed at a time. Surgeries with competing post-operative needs, such as prolonged immobilization and early motion, should also be performed separately. Standard plastic surgery techniques such as Z-plasty and Z-to-Y flap release are commonly performed to release hand contractures The Z-plasty is particularly well suited for web spaces and the Z-to-Y flap release is appropriate for small, linear contractures. Full-thickness skin grafts may be required after the release or excision of scar to accommodate for increased excursion. In cases of long-standing contracture, consideration of Kirschner wire fixation in extension for 3 weeks may help to prevent recurrence of contracture.

# References

[1]  Agir H, Sen C, Alagoz S et al (2007) Distally based posterior interosseous flap: primary role in soft-tissue reconstruction of the hand. Ann Plast Surg 59(3): 291–296

[2]  Anzarut A, Chen M, Shankowowsky H et al (2005) Quality-of-life and outcome predictors following massive burn injury. Plast Reconstr Surg 116(3): 791–797

[3]  Arnoldo B, Klein M, Gibran N (2006) Practice guidelines for management of electrical injuries. J Burn Care Res 27(4): 439–447

[4]  Baumeister S, Koller M, Dragu A et al (2005) Principles of microvascular reconstruction in burn and electrical burns injuries. Burns 31(1): 92–98

[5]  Burd A, Noronha F, Ahmed K et al (2006) Decompression not escharotomy in acute burns. Burns 32(3): 284–292

[6]  Callcut R, Schurr M, Sloan M et al (2006) Clinical experience with Alloderm: a one-staged composite dermal/epidermal replacement utilizing processed cadaver dermin and thin autografts. Burns 32(5): 583–588

[7]  Chandrasegaram M, Harvey J (2009) Full-thickness vs split-skin grafting in pediatric hand burns – a 10-year review of 174 cases. J Burn Care Res 30(5): 867–871

[8]  Edstrom L, Robson M, Macchiaverna J et al (1979) Prospective randomized treatments for burned hands: nonoperative vs. operative. Preliminary report. Scand J Plast Reconstr Surg 13(1): 131–135

[9]  Engrav L, Heimbach D, Reus J et al (1983) Early excision and grafting vs. nonoperative treatment of burns of indeterminate depth: a randomized prospective study. J Trauma 23(11): 1001–1004

[10]  Goodwin C, Maguire M, McManus W et al (1983) Prospective study of burn wound excision of the hands. J Trauma 23(6): 510–517

[11]  Haslik W, Kamolz L, Nathschlager G et al (2007) First experiences with collagen-elastin matrix Matriderm as a dermal substitute in severe burn injuries of the hand. Burns 33(3): 364–368

[12]  Heimbach D, Warden G, Luterman A et al (2003) Multicenter postapproval clinical trial of Integra dermal regeneration template for burn treatment. J Burn Care Rehabil 24(1): 42–48

[13]  Herter F, Ninkovic M (2007) Rotational flap selection and timing for coverage of complex upper extremity trauma. J Plast Reconstr Aesthet Surg 60(7): 760–768

[14]  Kamolz L, Kitzinger H, Karle B et al (2009) The treatment of hand burns. Burns 35(3): 327–337

[15]  Klein M, Hunter S, Hemiback D et al (2005) The Versajet water dissector: a new tool for tangential excision. J Burn Care Rehabil 26(6): 483–487

[16]  Lattari V, Jones L, Varcelotti J et al (1997) The use of permanent dermal allograft in full-thickness burns of the hand and foot: a report of three cases. J Burn Care Rehabil 18(2): 147–155

[17]  Lowell M, Pirc P, Ward R et al (2003) Effect of 3M Coban Self-Adherent Wraps on edema and function of the burned hand: a case study. J Burn Care Rehabil 24(4): 253–258

[18]  Luce E (2000) The acute and subacute management of the burned hand. Clin Plast Surg 27(1): 49–63

[19]  Mann R, Gibran N, Engrav L et al (2001) Prospective trial of thick vs standard split-thickness skin grafts in burns of the hand. Journal Burn Care Rehabil 22(6): 390–392

[20]  Moore M, Dewey W, Richard R (2009) Rehabilitation of the burned hand. Hand Clin 25(4): 529–541

[21]  Mothes H, Donicke T, Friedel R et al (2004) Indocyanine-green fluorescence video angiography used clinically to evaluate tissue perfusion in microsurgery. J Trauma 57(5): 1018–1024

[22]  Orgill D, Piccolo N (2009) Escharotomy and decompressive therapies in burns. J Burn Care Res 30: 759–768

[23]  Rennekampff H, Schaller H, Wisser D et al (2006) Debridement of burn wounds with a water jet surgical tool. Burns 32(1): 64–69

[24]  Salisbury R, Taylor J, Levine N (1976) Evaluation of digital escharotomy in burned hands. Plast Reconstr Surg 58(4): 440–443

[25]  Schwanholt C, Greenhalgh D, Warden G (1993) A comparison of full-thickness versus split-thickness autografts for the coverage of deep palm burns in the very young pediatric patient. J Burn Care Rehabil 14(1): 29–33

[26]  Scott J, Costa B, Gibran N et al (2008) Pediatric palm contact burns: a ten-year review. J Burn Care Res 29(4): 614–618

[27]  Smith M, Munster A, Spence R (1998) Burns of the hand and upper limb - a review. Burns 24(6): 493–505

[28]  Tambuscio A, Governa M, Caputo G et al (2006) Deep burn of the hands: Early surgical treatment avoids the need for late revision? Burns 32(8): 1000–1004

[29]  Tiwari A, Haq A, Myint F et al (2002) Acute compartment syndromes. Br J Surg 89(4): 397–412

[30] van Zuijlen P, Kreis R, Vloemans A et al (1999) The prognostic factors regarding long-term functional outcome of full-thickness hand burns. Burns 25(8): 709–714

[31] Wainwright D, Madden M, Luterman A et al (1996) Clinical evaluation of an acellular allograft dermal matrix in full-thickness burns. J Burn Care Rehabil 17(2): 124–136

Correspondence: Matthew B. Klein, M.D., M.S., FACS, David and Nancy Auth-Washington Research Foundation, Endowed Chair for Restorative Burn Surgery, Associate Director, University of Washington Burn Center, Program Director and Associate Professor, Division of Plastic Surgery, Harborview Medical Center, 325 9th Avenue, Box 359796, Seattle, WA 98104, USA, E-mail: mbklein@uw.edu

# Treatment of burns – established and novel technology

Ludwik K. Branski[1], Manuel Dibildox [2], Shahriar Shahrokhi[2], Marc G. Jeschke[2]

[1] Department of Plastic, Hand and Reconstructive Surgery Hannover Medical School, Hannover, Germany
[2] Ross Tilley Burn Centre, Sunnybrook Health Sciences Centre, Department of Surgery, Division of Plastic Surgery, University of Toronto, Toronto, ON, Canada

## Introduction

Burn trauma is one of the worst injuries suffered worldwide with an incidence of approximately 2 million cases annually [1]. Over the past decades, progress in the treatment of severe burn injuries has significantly decreased morbidity and mortality [2]. The improvements in survival have been most notable in the elderly patient population [3, 4]; however, survival has also improved in severely burned pediatric patients. Four major areas of advancement in burn care have been identified:

► Fluid resuscitation and early patient management
► Control of infection
► Modulation of the hyper-metabolic response
► Surgery and wound care.

Because of their extensive wounds, burn patients are chronically exposed to inflammatory mediators and microorganisms. With the advent of early burn wound excision and coverage [5], the risk of serious systemic infection originating from the burn wound has been reduced [6]. The current surgical approach to burn care is based on early excision of full-thickness burn tissue followed by early wound coverage, preferably with autologous skin graft. Early excision within the first 48hrs can significantly reduce blood loss and is safe and effective [7, 8]. In order to provide sufficient temporary wound coverage in large burns, allograft or xenograft can provide protection for many weeks until enough donor sites are available for grafting. In addition, widely meshed autografts have been utilized with allograft or xenograft overlay (sandwich technique) to provide adequate coverage. Repeated autografting can be performed within 7 to 10 days when donor sites have healed [9–11]. This approach, albeit still not implemented in many burn centers around the world, has been practiced for the last quarter century almost without change. During this time period, however, new approaches and devices, such as the use of fibrin sealant for autograft fixation [12, 13], the dermal substitute Integra® [14], cultured epidermal autografts (CEA) and cultured skin substitute (CSS) [15, 16], human amniotic [17], Biobrane® and similar biodressings [18], and stem cell and gene therapy have been successfully introduced or are currently being studied. This chapter introduces and discusses some of these exciting developments and gives an outlook on new ideas.

## Partial thickness burns

Partial thickness burns are divided into superficial and deep categories. The distinction between the two types of partial thickness burns is based on the depth of injury. Superficial partial thickness burns (from accidents such as immersion in an overheated bath tub water, flash flame burns, etc.) are erythematous and painful, blanch to touch, and often blister.

These wounds spontaneously re-epithelialize from retained epidermal structures in the rete ridges, hair follicles, and sweat glands within 7 to 14 days. After the wound has re-epithalialized, secondary scar maturation takes place that may result in hypo- or hyperpigmentation over the long term.

Deep dermal burns into the reticular dermis appear more pale and mottled, do not blanch to touch, but remain painful to pinprick. These burns can take up to four weeks for complete re-epithelialization from the hair follicles and sweat glands, often with severe scarring as a result of the loss of dermis. The epidermal layer in partial thickness burns usually sloughs off, leaving open raw skin with nerve endings exposed. Therefore, partial-thickness burns represent one of the most painful of the several categories of thermal injuries [19].

Historically, partial-thickness burns were treated conservatively by removing the damaged top layer of skin after the initial injury, followed by application of topical medications one to two times each day [20, 21]. These procedures, however, may cause severe pain and anxiety in patients, even with the use of pain medication.

## Synthetic and bio-synthetic membranes – biobrane, awbat, suprathel

To improve patient comfort, control infection, and increase the rate of re-epithelialization, alternatives for the treatment of partial-thickness burns have been developed. Semi-occlusive and synthetic membranes are the most important clinically applicable devices. These partly occlusive dressings allow re-epithelialization to occur beneath the dressing and eliminate the need for frequent dressing changes. There are several skin substitutes that are available commercially. Biobrane® is a biosynthetic wound dressing constructed of a silicone film with a nylon fabric partially embedded into the film. The fabric presents to the wound bed a complex 3-D structure of tri-filament thread to which collagen has been chemically bound. Blood and sera clot in the nylon matrix, thereby firmly adhering the dressing to the wound until epithelialization occurs. It controls vapor transfer, maintains a moist healing environment, and has been shown to be effective in the treatment of partial-thickness burns, particularly in pediatric patients, in numerous scientific publications since

**Table 1.** Common partial thickness burn wound dressings

| Dressing agent | Active substance | Presentation | Main use | Advantages | Disadvantages |
|---|---|---|---|---|---|
| Bacitracin | Bacitracin | Ointment | Superficial burns, skin grafts | Gram (+) coverage | No G(–) or fungal coverage |
| Polymyxin | Polymyxin B | Ointment | Superficial burns, skin grafts | Gram (–) coverage | No G(+) or fungal coverage |
| Mycostatin | Nystatin | Ointment | Superficial burns, skin grafts | Good fungal coverage | No bacterial coverage |
| Silvadene | Silver sulfadiazine | Ointment | Deep burns | Good bacterial and fungal coverage, painless | Poor eschar penetration, sulfa moiety, leucopenia, pseudoeschar formation |
| Sulfamylon | Mafenide acetate | Ointment and liquid solution | Deep burns | Good bacterial coverage, good eschar penetration | Painful, poor fungal coverage, metabolic acidosis |
| Dakin's | Sodium hypochlorite | Liquid solution | Superficial and deep burns | Good bacterial coverage, inexpensive and readily available | Very short half life |
| Silver | Silver nitrate, silver ion | Liquid solution, dressing sheets | Superficial burns | Good bacterial coverage, painless | Hyponatremia, dark staining of wounds and linens |

1982 [22–28]. A newer biosynthetic product, Awbat®, has been cleared by the FDA in 2009 and is now commercially available. Biobrane® and Awbat® are comparable constructs, as both feature a thin medical grade silicone membrane, good stretchabilty, and pores in the silicone membrane. Both have collagen peptides for the purpose of reacting with the fibrin in the wound to achieve good acute adherence. The main difference between the two membranes is the pore size and regularity – the approximate area of an Awbat pore is 88 sq. mm; the approximate area of a Biobrane pore is about 6.2 sq. mm, with Awbat about five times more porous than Biobrane. The greater porosity of Awbat is expected to result in improved transfer of exudate from the wound surface which may result in better acute adherence, and shorter healing time. As of now, however, there is only limited clinical experience with this new membrane [29, 30].

Suprathel® is produced from a synthetic copolymer mainly based on DL-lactide (>70%), the other components are trimethylenecarbonate and ε-caprolactone. The monomers are polymerized by a melting procedure. The final product is a porous membrane with an interconnected structure of pores between 2 and 50 um and an initial porosity of over 80%. It also boasts high plasticity and water permeability. It is applied to the wound bed with an overlay of paraffin or non-adherent gauze, and peels off within approximately two weeks as the re-epithelialization of the wound bed progresses [31]. Prospective randomized clinical studies in partial-thickness burns and on split-thickness donor sites showed mainly a reduction in pain, with wound healing times and long-term scar qualities comparable to other commercially available membranes [31–33].

## Biological membranes – amnion and others

Human amniotic membrane has been used for centuries as a biological wound dressing. In western medicine, amniotic membranes have been used since the beginning of the last century. The first reported use of amnion in burn wounds was by Sabella in 1913, shortly after Davis used amniotic membrane in skin transplantations in 1910 [34]. However, it soon became clear that amnion could not be used as a permanent skin transplant, but only as a temporary biological wound dressing. Many advantages of amnion as a temporary dressing have been reported, most notably alleviation of pain, the prevention of infection [35–38], acceleration of wound healing [34, 37, 39], and good handling properties [40]. The first use of amnion as a *temporary* skin substitute in burn wound care has been reported by Douglas in 1952 [41]. It has been subsequently used mainly in the treatment of partial thickness burns [36, 39, 42, 43].

In the last 20 years, literature addressing the use of amnion in chronic wounds and burns has increased significantly. In order to make amnion a standard dressing alternative, safe and reliable production methods had to be implemented. To meet these needs, in several countries amnion banks have been established alongside tissue banks [44–46].

Amnion has the advantage of being thin, adhesive but not sticking, easily moldable and removable. These qualities are of great importance especially in the pediatric population. In a study performed at the Shriners Hospital for Children – Galveston, amniotic burn dressings were compared to standard ointment and gauze controls [17]. The authors reported the same wound healing rate as with the standard dressing regimen and no increase in the rate of infections or impaired long-term cosmetic results after treatment with amniotic membrane. The conclusion was that amnion can be used safely for temporary wound coverage with the chief advantage of significantly less full dressing changes and therefore improved patient comfort.

Recently, there has been a push towards a standardization and commercial availability of amniotic membranes. Commercially available amniotic membranes can now be found in fresh frozen (Grafix©, Osiris Therapeutics, Inc.) and glycerol preserved form.

## Xenograft

Xenografts, also known as heterografts, are used to provide a temporary wound coverage and to ensure wound homeostasis. One of the first descriptions was by Lee in 1880 [47]. A Xenograft may be obtained from various animals, although pigs are the most common donors. Typically, porcine xenograft is distributed as a reconstituted product consisting of homogenized porcine dermis which is harvested with dermatomes, shaped into sheets and subsequently meshed, sterilized via radiation and stored frozen [48]. Xenograft can be used in the same manner as allograft, as an overlay for widely meshed autograft or as standalone coverage of partial thickness burns. Porcine xenograft can be used as a substitute for cadaveric skin allograft due to its structural and functional resemblance to human skin, efficacy in protecting the wound and reducing pain, bacterial overgrowth, and heat and fluid losses [49–52]. Zawacki et al. [53] showed that necrosis in the zone of stasis (the damaged but potentially viable area of thermally injured tissue surrounding irreversibly necrotic skin) could be avoided by optimal treatment of the wound with a biologic dressing such as xenograft, implying that application of xenograft on a debrided mid-dermal burn might prevent the need for excision and autografting. Porcine Xenografts have also been combined with silver to suppress wound colonization [54, 55]. They do not vascularize, and create a moist and semi-occlusive wound dressing that usually stays on the wound for over one week. It can be combined with local antimicrobial treatment, such as Sulfamylon or Silver Nitrate soaks. A common complication of porcine xenograft application is high fever, especially within 2 to 4 days after the application; this fever usually responds well to antipyretics, physical cooling, and wound soaks.

## Full thickness burns

Full thickness burns or deep dermal burns which do not heal within 14 to 21 days are best treated by full excision and coverage with autograft. This early excision and grafting has become the gold standard of burn care since the 1950's [5, 56, 57]. In severe burns, however, there is not enough uninjured skin left for a complete coverage of the excised burn with autograft. Dermal analogs, keratinocyte sheets and sprays, and complex full tissue transplantation methods have been developed as an alternative to the established techniques fo serial excision and grafting.

### Dermal analogs

The development of a burn wound coverage independent from autograft or homograft has been the goal of burn research around the world. The goal is to develop a "skin from the can", a fully functional composite graft that replaces dermis and epidermis and is available immediately for coverage of an excised burn. A first step in this direction was the development of dermal analogs. Integra™ (Integra LifeSciences Corporation, Plainsboro, NJ, USA) was created by a team lead by surgeon John Burke from the Massachusetts General Hospital and by scientist Ionnas Yannas from the Massachusetts Institute of Technology [58]. It is composed of bovine collagen and glucosaminoglycans that allow fibrovascular ingrowth. This dermal analog is placed over the wound bed after full thickness excision. The matrix is fully incorporated into the wound bed within 2 to 3 weeks and a split thickness autograft is placed over it. Except for a possible increased risk of infections, its use and long term results are favorable [14, 59]. Another dermal analog available for the treatment of full thickness burns is Alloderm® (LifeCell Corporation, The Woodlands, TX, USA). It consists of cadaveric dermis devoid of cells and epithelial elements. Its use is very similar to that of other dermal analogs and has shown favorable results [60, 61].

### Keratinocyte coverage

Cultured Epithelial Autograft (CEA) has become an important tool in the management of patients with massive burn injuries. In cases where full thickness burns involve more than 90% of the total body surface area, it may be the only choice for the patient, given that procurement of the uninvolved skin will not be sufficient to cover the body, even when extensive autograft expansion techniques are employed. The use of CEA involves obtaining two 2 × 6 cm specimens of unburned skin very early in the patient's course, preferably upon admission. The skin is then processed and cultured ex-vivo in the presence of murine fibroblasts that promote growth. The final product consists of sheets of keratinocytes 5 × 10 cm in size, 2 to 8 cells thick mounted on a petrolatum gauze.

While the CEA is made available, a process that usually takes up to three weeks, these critically ill patients need to be excised and temporarily covered with allograft or xenograft. Complications, such as wound infections and multiorgan failure, have to be treated aggressively to increase the chances of survival and eventual graft take.

The application of CEA can be difficult because of the fragility of the grafts, which has been described as having the consistency of wet tissue paper. CEA applied to areas of the back, buttocks, posterior lower extremities and other dependent areas are prone to shearing and graft loss. Once healed, the skin has a better cosmetic result when compared to healed wide-mesh autograft, but is associated with a longer hospital stay and more reconstructive procedures [62]. Recent studies have shown very variable results of CEA application. A single- center retrospective cohort study with over thirty severely burned patients showed an excellent survival and graft survival, although no control group was provided [15]. CEA used in conjunction with an allodermis base was reported to result in a graft take of over 72% [63].

## Keratinocyte suspension

Wood et al. concluded in their review of CEA use in extensive burns that its application ranges from useful to non-beneficial given its difficult handling and fragility, as well as lack of standardized application [64]. Because of these limitations, a technique consisting of a keratinocyte suspension delivered to the wound through an aerosol spray has been described [65].

In a porcine model by Reid et al. [66], wounds treated with a split thickness skin graft compared to wounds treated with this method plus the application of sprayed keratinocytes showed a significant decrease in contracture after healing took place. James et al. [67] later showed in a clinical trial that the addition of sprayed cultured autologous keratinocytes may help to clinically reduce the contraction of meshed autografts and reduce healing time. Also, the use of sprayed keratinocytes proved to be a versatile procedure that overcomes some of the limitations of the CEA sheets. In this study, split thickness skin was obtained from unburned areas, a keratinocyte cell suspension created, expanded during a 3 week period to a concentration of $10^7$ cells per ml and subsequently aerosolized to the wound at a density of $5 \times 10^5$ cells per cm$^2$.

One of the major drawbacks of this technique is the delay of application while the cell expansion

takes place. Zweifel et al. [68] reported a series of three patients where non-cultured autologous keratinocyte suspension was delivered to split and full-thickness burn wounds in an aerosol spray two days after admission. The results suggest a decrease in healing time and hypertrophic scarring. Recently, the group of Hartmann in Berlin reported good results with sprayed cultured epithelial autograft suspensions [69, 70].

## Facial transplantation

Severe facial burns can cause significant deformities that are technically challenging to treat. Traditional approaches with conventional treatment modalities are insufficient to address the esthetic and functional outcome. Following the lead set by the team in Amiens, France in 2005 [71], several other groups in Europe, China and USA have been able to meet this complex clinical challenge with the use of composite tissue allo-transplantation (CTA), which uses healthy facial tissue transplanted from donors for reconstruction thus allowing for the best possible functional and esthetic outcome. The techniques required to perform this procedure, have been developed over many years and are used routinely in reconstructive surgery. The immunosuppressive regimens necessary to prevent rejection have been previously developed for and used successfully in solid organ transplantation for many years [72, 73]. The psychosocial and ethical issues associated with this new treatment have some unique challenges, which need to be addressed by a dedicated team [74, 75].

The conventional treatment modalities offer little improvement in facial burn function and appearance, and often leave patients significantly debilitated. These patients often become socially and personally isolated, and many suffer from psychological disorders and phobias. These patients also tend to require multiple reconstructive procedures, in a setting, which there's minimal normal tissue (secondary to burn in other areas). Facial transplantation in such patients can offer the possibility of improved quality of life. Since the initial face transplant in 2005 there have been further 12 transplant procedures that will eventually reduce the knowledge gap, as the teams performing these new reconstructive procedures share the details responsible for their success and failure. Facial transplantation can improve the lives of those suffering with severe facial burn. It poses significant challenges, which, when overcome, may provide a promising treatment modality for the severe facial burn injury [76].

## Tissue engineering and stem cells

Despite the success of wound healing and skin grafting, transplanted skin lacks the flexibility and elasticity of normal skin. This has lead to the pursuit of a skin substitute that more closely resembles the dermal and epidermal structures of uninjured skin. A breakthrough in the use of dermal analogs and cultured epidermal autograft has been the development of combined dermal and epidermal skin replacements [22, 77]. For its preparation, fibroblasts and keratinocytes are obtained from the patient and cultured ex-vivo. These cells are then inoculated onto collagen-glycosaminoglycan substrates [78, 79]. Further culture and processing at an air-liquid interface provides liquid nutrient medium to the dermal substitute and air contact to the epidermal substitute, resulting in stratification and cornification of the keratinocyte layer [80, 81]. In the dermal layer, fibroblasts proliferate into the collagen substrate, degrade it, and generate new autologous dermal matrix. At the dermal-epidermal junction, collagen and basement membrane formation takes place in-vitro [78]. This increases the strength of the dermal-epidermal junction and decreases the development of epidermolysis and blistering frequently encountered with split thickness grafting or application of CEA.

New techniques have been employed to further improve these engineered skin replacements. The addition of melanocytes can decrease hypopigmentation and achieve better appearance and color matching [82]. Vascular endothelial growth factors and angiogenic cytokines have been introduced to induce a vascular growth in the transplanted skin, thus shortening healing time and preventing graft loss [82, 83].

A new approach in the management of burns and other conditions that involve skin loss is the use of stem cells. Several mechanisms have been described by which these cells play an important role in wound healing process, both locally and systemically.

In humans, stem cells can be found in the bone marrow, adipose tissue, umbilical cord blood and in the blastocystic mass of embryos [84]. Even though obtaining embryonic stem cells can involve the destruction of the human embryo and raise ethical questions, the ability to obtain these cells from other tissues without affecting the source has facilitated research in the field.

The promising characteristics of stem cells are plentiful. Given the clonicity and pluripotency, they can be used to regenerate dermis and expedite re-epithelialization [85]. Another important characteristic of stem cells is the lack of immunogenicity, which ultimately implies that the cells can be obtained from one source, processed, and then transplanted to a different host [86].

After an injury, bone marrow stem cells migrate to the site of injury and aid in the healing and regeneration process [87, 88]. While these cells are blood-borne and after they reach the affected tissue, they have the ability to control inflammation by decreasing pro-inflammatory cytokine release and upregulating anti-inflammatory cytokines, such as IL-10 [89].

Embryonic human stem cells can be differentiated into keratinocytes in vitro and then stratified into an epithelium that resembles human epidermis [90]. This graft can then be applied to open wounds on burn patients as a temporary skin substitute while autograft or other permanent coverage means becomes available. This application, however, is still in its early stages of experimental clinical application.

## Gene therapy and growth factors

Gene therapy, defined as the insertion of a gene into recipient cells, was initially considered only as a treatment option for patients with a congenital defect of a metabolic function or late-stage malignancy [91]. More recently, skin has become an important target of gene therapy research. This research is made possible due to the ease of fibroblast and keratinocyte harvest and cultivation, thus allowing for gene transfer testing *in vitro* and the use of skin cells as vehicles in gene transfer [92]. Skin is also easily accessible and the effects of therapy can be repeatedly monitored.

Gene transfer, using viral vectors, relies on the ability of viruses to carry and express their genes into host cells. Gene therapy vectors are developed by the

**Table 2.** Engineered skin substitutes

| Model | Description | Indications |
|---|---|---|
| *Acellular* | | |
| Biobrane (Bertek Pharmaceuticals, Morgantown, WV) | Very thin semipermeable silicone membrane bonded to nylon fabric | Temporary adherent wound covering for partial-thickness excised burns and donor sites |
| Integra (Integra Life Sciences, Plainsboro, NJ) | Bilayer structure; biodegradable dermal layer made of porous bovine collagen-chondroitin-6-sulfate matrix; temporary epidermal layer made of synthetic silicone polymer | Grafting of deep partial- or full-thickness burns; epidermal layer removed when donor sites available for autografting |
| Alloderm (LifeCell Corporation, Branchburg, NJ) | Structurally intact allogeneic acellular dermis; freeze-dried after cells were removed with detergent treatment; rehydrated before grafting | Dermal template for grafting to burns and other wounds; repair of soft tissue defects |
| Matriderm (Dr. Suwelack Skin & Health Care AG, Germany) | Non-cross linked bovine collagen and elastin matrix that allows cellular ingrowth and neovascularization | Template for dermal reconstruction in the treatment of full thickness burns |
| *Cellular-allogeneic* | | |
| Dermagraft (Advanced Biohealing, Westport, CT) | Cryopreserved allogeneic neonatal foreskin fibroblasts seeded on bioabsorbable polyglactin mesh scaffold;cells are metabolically active at grafting | Treatment of full-thickness chronic diabetic foot ulcers |
| Apligraf (Organogenesis/ Novartis, Canton, MA) | Bilayer; allogeneic neonatal foreskin fibroblasts and keratinocytes in bovine collagen gel | Treatment of chronic foot ulcers and venous leg ulcers; also used for burn wounds and EB |
| OrCel (Forticell Bioscience, Englewood Cliffs, NJ) | Bilayer; allogeneic neonatal foreskin fibroblasts and keratinocytes cultured in bovine collagen sponge | Treatment of split-thickness donor sites in patients with burn and surgical wounds in EB |
| *Cellular-autologous* | | |
| Epicel (Genzyme Biosurgery, Cambridge, MA) | Autologous keratinocytes cultured from patient skin biopsy, transplanted as epidermal sheet using petrolatum gauze support | Permanent wound closure in patients with burn with greater than 30% TBSA injury and in patients with congenital nevus |
| Epidex (Modex Therapeutiques, Lausanne, Switzerland) | Autologous keratinocytes isolated from outer root sheath of scalp hair follicles; supplied as epidermal sheet discs with a silicone membrane support | Treatment of chronic leg ulcers |
| TranCell* (CellTran Limited, Sheffield, UK)48 | Autologous keratinocytes cultured from patient skin biopsy, grown on acrylic acid polymer-coated surface; transplanted as epidermal sheets | Treatment of chronic diabetic foot ulcers |
| Cultured skin substitute* (University of Cincinnati/Shriners Hospitals, Cincinnati, OH)49–53 | Bilayer; autologous keratinocytes and fibroblasts cultured from patient skin biopsy, combined with degradable bovine collagen matrix | Permanent wound closure in patients with burn with greater than 50% TBSA injury; also used in patients with congenital nevus and chronic wound |

Adapted from [28]

**Table 3.** Review of stem cell nomenclature

| Cell | Source | Potency | Advantages | Disadvantages | Examples of utility |
|---|---|---|---|---|---|
| Embryonic stem cells | Inner cell mass of blastocyst | Pluripotent | Pluripotent Clonogenic | Teratogenic Ethical controversy | Knockout mouse |
| Umbilical cord blood stem cells | Umbilical cord blood | Pluripotent | Pluripotent Non-immunogenic Clonogenic | Limited supply with low yield | Bone marrow transplantation |
| Mesenchymal stem cells | Bone marrow stroma, blood | Multipotent | Autologous Accessible Clonogenic | Require time to culture Harvest invasive Limited supply | Parkinson's, myocardial remodeling, wound healing |
| Adipose-derived stem cells | Adipose tissue | Multipotent | Non-immunogenic Abundant supply Accessible Clonogenic | Processing required | Wound healing, tissue engineering |
| Resident progenitor cells | Numerous tissues/organs | Unipotent | Accessible Potential for transdifferentiation | Limited potency and clonogenicity | Re-epithelialization of wounds from hair follicular cells |

From Butler, Butler KL et al. (2010) Stem cells and burns: review and therapeutic implications. J Burn Care Res 31(6): 874–881

modification of different types of viruses. Retroviruses and lentiviruses are non-lytic replicators produced from the cellular membrane of an infected cell, which leaves the host cell relatively intact. The lytic replication method involves the release of virions with the collapse of the host cell after infection. Human adenoviruses, adeno-associated viruses and herpes simplex viruses are examples of lytic replicators. A large body of literature is now available which describes success and pitfalls in viral transfection of skin and wounds [93–107].

To summarize, viral vectors are the original and most established technology for gene delivery. A wide range of applications have been developed and many virus-mediated gene transfer models are successful. The production of viral vectors, however, is time and cost consuming, transfection efficacy is variable, and the risk of local or systemic infections, leading to fatal outcomes, remains a concern.

In 1995, Hengge et al. first described the direct injection of DNA coding for interleukin-8 genes [108]. By injecting naked genes into the skin, they found a significant recruitment of dermal neutrophils. However, the injection of naked DNA into the skin has been proven to have a low transfection efficacy and a high rate of initial degradation even before the injectate reaches the cytosol. Naked DNA

constructs are not likely to penetrate the cells due to their fragility in the extracellular environment, large size, and electrical charge [109].

Eriksson et al. (1998) modified the direct injection technique, termed "micro-seeding", which delivers naked DNA directly into target cells via solid needles mounted on a modified tattooing machine. Elevated levels of transferred DNA could be maintained for one to two weeks [110], but transfection was only observed in the superficial layers of skin with minimal penetration into deeper tissue. Another technique used to penetrate the cellular membrane employs the "gene gun". In this approach, 1–5 um gold or tungsten-coated particles carrying DNA plasmids are propelled into skin cells [107]. Gene transfer is mostly transient and reaches its highest expression between the first and the third day after injection [104–107]. *In vivo* transfection with epithelial growth factor (EGF) cDNA in porcine partial-thickness wounds has demonstrated an increase in the rate of wound healing and re-epithelization [111]. Recent studies in the rat model indicate that gene gun particle mediated transfection of different PDGF isomers significantly improved wound healing by increasing its tensile strength [107]. Differing results have been reported on the depth of transfection, with one study showing the gene gun technique primarily delivering particles no deeper than the epidermis with transfection rates of up to 10%. Gene expression in skin and muscle reached its peak 24 hours after application and remained detectable for at least 1 week with little tissue damage [112].

The technique of electroporation has been successfully used to accelerate the closure of diabetic and chronic wounds [113, 114]. Lee et al. describe the synergistic use of electroporation, where an electric field is applied to tissue, in combination with tissue growth factor-β1 (TGF-β1) cDNA in a diabetic mouse model [115]. In the group which received electroporation and gene transfer, the wound bed showed an increased rate of re-epithelialization, angiogenesis, and collagen synthesis. Apart from a transitional effect between the second and fourth day after wounding, the wound healing process itself was not significantly accelerated by the combined use of electric stimulation and gene transfer [115]. Marti et al. showed that electroporation and simultaneous administration of keratinocytes growth factor (KGF) plasmid DNA increased wound healing when compared to controls receiving no treatment (92% vs. 40% of the area healed) [116]. No significant improvement in comparison to administration of KGF plasmid DNA alone was observed. Taking into account these inconclusive results, the benefit of this concept remains in question.

Another reliable and efficient method is the cutaneous gene delivery with cationic liposomes. Cationic liposomes (CL) are synthetically prepared vesicles with positively charged surfaces that form loose complexes with negatively charged DNA to protect it from degradation in the wound environment. The net positive charge of the complex binds readily to negatively charged cell surfaces to facilitate uptake via endocytosis [117, 118]. Genes encapsulated in CL can be applied either topically or by direct injection [117, 119]. Alexander et al. used topical application of CL constructs containing the Lac Z-gene to induce transfection and expression in the epidermis, dermis, and hair follicles in shaved 4-week-old mice. Expression was observed as early as 6 hours after topical application, which persisted at high levels for 48 hours, and was detectable for seven days [120]. Several studies have been performed to determine CL gene transfer for growth factors [107, 121, 122]. Sun et al. administered fibroblast growth factor-1

(FGF-1) by topical application and subcutaneous injection to the injured skin of diabetic mice [122]. Transfection with FGF was found to increase tensile strength. In a preliminary study of IGF-I cDNA constructs applied to thermally injured rat skin, Jeschke et al.detected a transfection rate of 70–90% in myofibroblasts, endothelial cells and macrophages, including multinucleate giant cells [123]. In an *in vivo* approach, thermally injured rats treated with liposomal IGF-I cDNA significantly improved body weight and increased muscle protein when compared to burn controls. An accelerated rate of re-epithelialization of nearly 15% was observed when compared to naked IGF-I protein and IGF-I protein encapsulated in liposomes [118]. Furthermore, no evidence was found that the dermal injection of IGF-I cDNA-complexes led to transfection or increase in β-galactosidase or IGF-I expression in blood, liver, spleen or kidney, thus gene transfection and production of growth factors remains localized. Animals transfected with IGF-I cDNA increased their basal skin cell proliferation, suggesting that myofibroblasts, endothelial cells and macrophages, identified as transfected, produce biologically active IGF-I [123]. The same group performed the transfection of PDGF-cDNA in a large animal burn model via the liposomal vector. Gene transfer of liposomal PDGF-cDNA resulted in increased PDGF-mRNA and protein expression on days 2 and 4 post injection, accelerated wound re-epithelialization as well as graft adhesion on day 9. The authors concluded that liposomal cDNA gene transfer is possible in a porcine wound model, and by using PDGF-cDNA dermal and epidermal regeneration can be improved [124].

A potential problem of single growth factor gene therapy is that simply increasing the concentration may not promote all phases of wound healing. A single growth factor cannot counteract all the deficiencies of a burn wound, nor control the complexities of chronic wound healing. Lynch et al. demonstrated in a partial thickness wound healing model that the combination of PDGF and IGF-I was more effective than either growth factor alone [125], while Spruegel et al. found that a combination of PDGF and FGF-2 increased the DNA content of wounds in the rat better than any single growth factor [126]. Jeschke investigated the efficacy of KGF cDNA in combination with IGF-I cDNA compared to the same genes individually [127]. It was noted that this combination accelerated re-epithelization, increased proliferation, and decreased skin cell apoptosis compared to the single construct alone. The re-epithelialization in the burn model was over twice that of the untreated control with a significant improvement in cell survival. Applying genes at strategic time points of wound healing (sequential growth factor therapy) is therefore the next logical step in augmenting wound healing. Multiple groups worldwide are currently working towards this goal.

Other delivery routes including biomaterials [128], calcium phosphate transfection [129], diethyl-aminoethyl-dextran [130], and microbubble-enhanced ultrasound [131] have been investigated. Slow-release matrices [132] and gene-delivering gel matrices [133] are used for prolonged transgenic expression. The concept of a genetic switch is another exciting development, where transgenic expression in target cells can be switched 'on' or 'off', depending on the presence or absence of a stimulator such as tetracycline [134]. Bio-technological refinements, such as wound chamber technique [135], may also improve the efficacy of gene delivery to wounds. These new techniques need further studies to define their efficacy and clinical applicability. More studies are also needed to define growth factor levels in different phases of wound healing and to elucidate the precise timing of gene expression or down-regulation required to better augment wound healing and control of scar formation.

## Conclusion

In the past decades, the progress in treating severely burned patients has been a success story, leading to a significant decrease in ICU mortality and the long-term survival of severely burned patients. This development, however, has led to a set of new challenges for burn researchers – reduction of scarring, improvement of skin graft quality, and the creation of a pluristratified dermal and epidermal constructs for the coverage of an excised burn wound. Therefore, a continuous and critical re-evaluation of all aforementioned aspects of temporary and definitive burn wound coverage, the design of new molecular methodologies and animal models for the studies of un-

derlying pathophysiological mechanisms, the conduction of tightly controlled multi-center clinical studies with the use of new skin constructs, and, most importantly, an integration of all these efforts with the multidisciplinary stem cell research are paramount for the successful development of clinically applicable products.

## References

[1] Brigham PA, McLoughlin E (1996) Burn incidence and medical care use in the United States: estimates, trends, and data sources. J Burn Care Rehabil 17(2): 95–107

[2] Pereira C, Murphy K, Herndon D (2004) Outcome measures in burn care. Is mortality dead? Burns 30(8): 761–771

[3] National Burn Repository – 2005 Report2006, Chicago, IL: American Burn Association

[4] Barrow RE, Herndon DN (1988) Thermal burns, gender, and survival. Lancet 2(8619): 1076–1077

[5] Janzekovic Z (1970) A new concept in the early excision and immediate grafting of burns. J Trauma 10(12): 1103–1108

[6] Merrell SW et al (1989) The declining incidence of fatal sepsis following thermal injury. J Trauma 29(10): 1362–1366

[7] Herndon DN et al (1989) A comparison of conservative versus early excision. Therapies in severely burned patients. Ann Surg 209(5): 547–553

[8] Barret JP et al (1999) Total burn wound excision of massive pediatric burns in the first 24 hours post burn injury. Ann Burns Fire Disasters XIII(1): 25–27

[9] Barret JP et al (1999) Effect of topical and subcutaneous epinephrine in combination with topical thrombin in blood loss during immediate near-total burn wound excision in pediatric burned patients. Burns 25(6): 509–513

[10] Herndon DN et al (1990) Effects of recombinant human growth hormone on donor-site healing in severely burned children. Ann Surg 212(4): 424–9; discussion 430–1

[11] Herndon DN et al (1995) Characterization of growth hormone enhanced donor site healing in patients with large cutaneous burns. Ann Surg 221(6): 649–56; discussion 656–659

[12] Dyess D et al (1995) The use of fibrin sealant in burn treatment. In: Schlag G, HJ (eds) Fibrin sealing in surgical and non-surgical fields. Springer, Berlin, pp 120–127

[13] Mittermayr R et al (2006) Skin graft fixation by slow clotting fibrin sealant applied as a thin layer. Burns 32(3): 305–311

[14] Branski LK et al (2007) Longitudinal assessment of Integra in primary burn management: a randomized pediatric clinical trial. Crit Care Med 35(11): 2615–2623

[15] Carsin H et al (2000) Cultured epithelial autografts in extensive burn coverage of severely traumatized patients: a five year single-center experience with 30 patients. Burns 26(4): 379–387

[16] Herndon DN, Parks DH (1986) Comparison of serial debridement and autografting and early massive excision with cadaver skin overlay in the treatment of large burns in children. J Trauma 26(2): 149–152

[17] Branski LK et al (2007) Amnion in the treatment of pediatric partial-thickness facial burns. Burns 34(3): 393–399

[18] Barret JP et al (2000) Biobrane versus 1% silver sulfadiazine in second-degree pediatric burns. Plast Reconstr Surg 105(1): 62–65

[19] Gallagher JJ, Wolf SE, Herndon DN (2007) Burns. In: Townsend CM, Jr (ed) Sabiston Textbook of Surgery. Saunders Elsevier, Philadelphia

[20] Dhennin C (2002) [Methods of covering severe burns]. Soins 2002(669): 45–47

[21] Jones I, Currie L, Martin R (2002) A guide to biological skin substitutes. Br J Plast Surg 55(3): 185–193

[22] Bishop JF (1995) Pediatric considerations in the use of Biobrane in burn wound management. J Burn Care Rehabil 16(3 Pt 1): 331–3; discussion 333–334

[23] Cassidy C et al (2005) Biobrane versus duoderm for the treatment of intermediate thickness burns in children: a prospective, randomized trial. Burns 31(7): 890–893

[24] Demling RH (1995) Use of Biobrane in management of scalds. J Burn Care Rehabil 16(3 Pt 1): 329–330

[25] Lal S et al (2000) Biobrane improves wound healing in burned children without increased risk of infection. Shock 14(3): 314–8; discussion 318–319

[26] Lang EM et al (2005) Biobrane in the treatment of burn and scald injuries in children. Ann Plast Surg 55(5): 485–489

[27] Ou LF et al (1998) Use of Biobrane in pediatric scald burns–experience in 106 children. Burns 24(1): 49–53

[28] Whitaker IS, Prowse S, Potokar TS (2008) A critical evaluation of the use of Biobrane as a biologic skin substitute: a versatile tool for the plastic and reconstructive surgeon. Ann Plast Surg 60(3): 333–337

[29] Vandenberg VB (nn) AWBAT: early clinical experience. Eplasty 10: e23

[30] Woodroof EA et al: The Search for an Ideal Temporary Skin Substitute: AWBAT Plus, a Combination Product Wound Dressing Medical Device. Eplasty. 10

[31] Uhlig C et al (2007) Suprathel-an innovative, resorbable skin substitute for the treatment of burn victims. Burns 33(2): 221–229

[32] Schwarze H et al (2007) Suprathel, a new skin substitute, in the management of donor sites of split-thickness skin grafts: results of a clinical study. Burns 33(7): 850–854

[33] Schwarze H et al (2008)Suprathel, a new skin substitute, in the management of partial-thickness burn wounds: results of a clinical study. Ann Plast Surg 60(2): 181–185

[34] Maral T et al (1999) Effectiveness of human amnion preserved long-term in glycerol as a temporary biological dressing. Burns 25(7): 625–635

[35] Robson MC, Krizek TJ (1973) The effect of human amniotic membranes on the bacteria population of infected rat burns. Ann Surg 177(2): 144–149

[36] Robson MC et al (1973) Amniotic membranes as a temporary wound dressing. Surg Gynecol Obstet 136(6): 904–906

[37] Ninman C, Shoemaker P (1975) Human amniotic membranes for burns. Am J Nurs 75(9): 1468–1469

[38] Salisbury RE, Carnes R, McCarthy LR (1980) Comparison of the bacterial clearing effects of different biologic dressings on granulating wounds following thermal injury. Plast Reconstr Surg 66(4): 596–598

[39] Quinby WC, Jr et al (1982) Clinical trials of amniotic membranes in burn wound care. Plast Reconstr Surg 70(6): 711–717

[40] Gajiwala K, Gajiwala AL (2004) Evaluation of lyophilised, gamma-irradiated amnion as a biological dressing. Cell Tissue Bank 5(2): 73–80

[41] Douglas B (1952) Homografts of fetal membranes as a covering for large wounds; especially those from burns; an experimental and clinical study. J Tn State Med Assoc 45(6): 230–235

[42] Haberal M et al (1987) The use of silver nitrate-incorporated amniotic membrane as a temporary dressing. Burns Incl Therm Inj 13(2): 159–163

[43] Ramakrishnan KM, Jayaraman V (1997) Management of partial-thickness burn wounds by amniotic membrane: a cost-effective treatment in developing countries. Burns 23 [Suppl 1]: S33–36

[44] Ravishanker R, Bath AS, Roy R (2003) "Amnion Bank"–the use of long term glycerol preserved amniotic membranes in the management of superficial and superficial partial thickness burns. Burns 29(4): 369–374

[45] Tyszkiewicz JT et al (1999) Amnion allografts prepared in the Central Tissue Bank in Warsaw. Ann Transplant 4(3–4): 85–90

[46] Hennerbichler S et al (2007) The influence of various storage conditions on cell viability in amniotic membrane. Cell Tissue Bank 8: 1–8

[47] Lee EW(1880) Zoografting in a burn case. Boston Med Surg 103(260)

[48] Brennan, Mediskin© I, 2010, Brennan Medical LLC: St Paul, MO

[49] Bromberg BE, Song IC, Mohn MP (1965) The use of pig skin as a temporary biological dressing. Plast Reconstr Surg 36: 80–90

[50] Cohen IKDRFLWJ (1992) Wound healing: biochemical & clinical aspects. W. B. Saunders Co, Philadelphia, xxv, 630 p

[51] Fang Z (1991) Application of skin and skin substitutes to burns wounds. In: Leung P (ed) Burns treatment and research. World Scientific, Singapore, pp 97–106

[52] Forbes P (1969) Advances in the biology of skin hair growth Pergamon, Oxford, pp 419–432

[53] Zawacki BE (1974) Reversal of capillary stasis and prevention of necrosis in burns. Ann Surg 180(1): 98–102

[54] Ersek RA, Denton DR (1984) Silver-impregnated porcine xenografts for treatment of meshed autografts. Ann Plast Surg 13(6): 482–487

[55] Ersek RA, Navarro JA (1990) Maximizing wound healing with silver-impregnated porcine xenograft. Todays OR Nurse 12(12): 4–9

[56] Cope O et al (1947) Expeditious care of full-thickness burn wounds by surgical excision and grafting. Ann Surg 125(1): 1–22

[57] Jackson D et al (1960) Primary excision and grafting of large burns. Ann Surg 152: 167–89

[58] Burke JF et al (1981) Successful use of a physiologically acceptable artificial skin in the treatment of extensive burn injury. Ann Surg 194(4): 413–428

[59] Heimbach DM et al (2003) Multicenter postapproval clinical trial of Integra dermal regeneration template for burn treatment. J Burn Care Rehabil 24(1): 42–48

[60] Wainwright DJ (1995) Use of an acellular allograft dermal matrix (AlloDerm) in the management of full-thickness burns. Burns 21(4): 243–248

[61] Sheridan RL, Choucair RJ (1997) Acellular allogenic dermis does not hinder initial engraftment in burn wound resurfacing and reconstruction. J Burn Care Rehabil 18(6): 496–499

[62] Barret JP et al (2000) Cost-efficacy of cultured epidermal autografts in massive pediatric burns. Ann Surg 231(6): 869–876

[63] Sood R et al (2010) Cultured epithelial autografts for coverage of large burn wounds in eighty-eight patients: the Indiana University experience. J Burn Care Res 31(4): 559–568

[64] Wood F., Kolybaba ML, Allen P (2006) The use of cultured epithelial autograft in the treatment of major burn injuries: a critical review of the literature. Burns 32(4): 395–401

[65] Wood FM et al (2007) The use of a non-cultured autologous cell suspension and Integra dermal regeneration template to repair full-thickness skin wounds in a porcine model: a one-step process. Burns 33(6): 693–700

[66] Reid MJ et al (2007) Effect of artificial dermal substitute, cultured keratinocytes and split thickness skin graft on wound contraction. Wound Repair Regen 15(6): 889–896

[67] James SE et al (2010) Sprayed cultured autologous keratinocytes used alone or in combination with meshed autografts to accelerate wound closure in difficult-to-heal burns patients. Burns 36(3): e10–20

[68] Zweifel CJ et al (2008) Initial experiences using non-cultured autologous keratinocyte suspension for burn wound closure. J Plast Reconstr Aesthet Surg 61(11): e1–4

[69] Gerlach JC et al (2011) Method for autologous single skin cell isolation for regenerative cell spray transplantation with non-cultured cells. Int J Artif Organs 34(3): 271–279

[70] Hartmann B et al (2007) Sprayed cultured epithelial autografts for deep dermal burns of the face and neck. Ann Plast Surg 58(1): 70–73

[71] Devauchelle B et al (2006) First human face allograft: early report. Lancet 368(9531): 203–209

[72] Pomahac B et al (2011) Face transplantation. Curr Probl Surg 48(5): 293–357

[73] Pomahac B et al (2011) Restoration of facial form and function after severe disfigurement from burn injury by a composite facial allograft. Am J Transplant 11(2): 386–393

[74] Soni CV et al (2010) Psychosocial considerations in facial transplantation. Burns 36(7): 959–964

[75] O'Neill H, Godden D (2009) Ethical issues of facial transplantation. Br J Oral Maxillofac Surg 47(6): 443–445

[76] Pushpakumar SB et al (2010) Clinical considerations in face transplantation. Burns 36(7): 951–958

[77] Boyce ST, Glatter R, Kitzmiller WJ (1995) Treatment of chronic wounds with cultured cells and biopolymers: a pilot study. Wounds 1995(7): 24–29

[78] Boyce ST, Supp AP, Swope VB (2002) Vitamin C regulates keratinocyte viability, epidermal barrier, and basement membrane formation in vitro, and reduces wound contraction after grafting of cultured skin substitutes. J Investig Dermatol 118: 565–572

[79] Hansbrough JF et al (1989) Burn wound closure with cultured autologous keratinocytes and fibroblasts attached to a collagen-glycosaminoglycan substrate. JAMA 262(15): 2125–2130

[80] Boyce ST, Williams ML (1993) Lipid supplemented medium induces lamellar bodies and precursors of barrier lipids in cultured analogues of human skin. J Invest Dermatol 101(2): 180–184

[81] Prunieras M, Regnier M, Woodley DT (1983) Methods for cultivation of keratinocytes at the air-liquid interface. J Investig Dermatol 81: 28S–33S

[82] Swope VB et al (1997) Regulation of pigmentation in cultured skin substitutes by cytometric sorting of melanocytes and keratinocytes. J Invest Dermatol 109(3): 289–295

[83] Supp DM et al (2000) Enhanced vascularization of cultured skin substitutes genetically modified to overexpress vascular endothelial growth factor. J Invest Dermatol 114(1): 5–13

[84] Butler KL et al (2010) Stem cells and burns: review and therapeutic implications. J Burn Care Res 31(6): 874–881

[85] Wu Y et al (2007) Mesenchymal stem cells enhance wound healing through differentiation and angiogenesis. Stem Cells 25(10): 2648–2659

[86] Burd A et al (2007) Stem cell strategies in burns care. Burns 33(3): 282–291

[87] Korbling M, Estrov Z, Champlin R (2003) Adult stem cells and tissue repair. Bone Marrow Transplant 32 [Suppl 1]: S23–24

[88] Mansilla E et al (2006) Bloodstream cells phenotypically identical to human mesenchymal bone marrow

stem cells circulate in large amounts under the influence of acute large skin damage: new evidence for their use in regenerative medicine. Transplant Proc 38(3): 967–969

[89] Weil BR et al (2009) Stem cells in sepsis. Ann Surg 250(1): 19–27

[90] Guenou H et al (2009) Human embryonic stem-cell derivatives for full reconstruction of the pluristratified epidermis: a preclinical study. Lancet 374(9703): 1745–1753

[91] Hernandez A, Evers BM (1999) Functional genomics: clinical effect and the evolving role of the surgeon. Arch Surg 134(11): 1209–1215

[92] Khavari PA, Rollman O, Vahlquist A (2002) Cutaneous gene transfer for skin and systemic diseases. J Intern Med 252(1): 1–10

[93] Kozarsky KF, Wilson JM (1993) Gene therapy: adenovirus vectors. Curr Opin Genet Dev 3(3): 499–503

[94] Lu B et al (1997) Topical application of viral vectors for epidermal gene transfer. J Invest Dermatol 108(5): 803–808

[95] Silman NJ, Fooks AR (2000) Biophysical targeting of adenovirus vectors for gene therapy. Curr Opin Mol Ther 2(5): 524–531

[96] Bett AJ, Prevec L, Graham FL (1993) Packaging capacity and stability of human adenovirus type 5 vectors. J Virol 67(10): 5911–5921

[97] Liechty KW et al (1999) Adenoviral-mediated overexpression of platelet-derived growth factor-B corrects ischemic impaired wound healing. J Invest Dermatol 113(3): 375–383

[98] Badillo AT et al (2007) Lentiviral gene transfer of SDF-1alpha to wounds improves diabetic wound healing. J Surg Res 143(1): 35–42

[99] Deodato B et al (2002) Recombinant AAV vector encoding human VEGF165 enhances wound healing. Gene Ther 9(12): 777–785

[100] Galeano M et al (2003) Effect of recombinant adeno-associated virus vector-mediated vascular endothelial growth factor gene transfer on wound healing after burn injury. Crit Care Med 31(4): 1017–1025

[101] Chen S et al (2005) Efficient transduction of vascular endothelial cells with recombinant adeno-associated virus serotype 1 and 5 vectors. Hum Gene Ther 16(2): 235–247

[102] Carretero M et al (2004) A cutaneous gene therapy approach to treat infection through keratinocyte-targeted overexpression of antimicrobial peptides. FASEB J 18(15): 1931–1933

[103] Morgan JR et al (1987) Expression of an exogenous growth hormone gene by transplantable human epidermal cells. Science 237(4821): 1476–1479

[104] Eming SA et al (1995) Genetically modified human epidermis overexpressing PDGF-A directs the development of a cellular and vascular connective tissue stroma when transplanted to athymic mice–implications for the use of genetically modified keratinocytes to

modulate dermal regeneration. J Invest Dermatol 105(6): 756–763

[105] Eming SA et al (1998) Genetically modified human keratinocytes overexpressing PDGF-A enhance the performance of a composite skin graft. Hum Gene Ther 9(4): 529–539

[106] Eming SA et al (1996) Targeted expression of insulin-like growth factor to human keratinocytes: modification of the autocrine control of keratinocyte proliferation. J Invest Dermatol 107(1): 113–120

[107] Eming SA et al (1999) Particle-mediated gene transfer of PDGF isoforms promotes wound repair. J Invest Dermatol 112(3): 297–302

[108] Hengge UR et al (1995) Cytokine gene expression in epidermis with biological effects following injection of naked DNA. Nat Genet 10(2): 161–166

[109] Vogel JC (2000) Nonviral skin gene therapy. Hum Gene Ther 11(16): 2253–2259

[110] Eriksson E et al (1998) In vivo gene transfer to skin and wound by microseeding. J Surg Res 78(2): 85–91

[111] Nanney LB et al (2000) Boosting epidermal growth factor receptor expression by gene gun transfection stimulates epidermal growth in vivo. Wound Repair Regen 8(2): 117–127

[112] Dileo J et al (2003) Gene transfer to subdermal tissues via a new gene gun design. Hum Gene Ther 14(1): 79–87

[113] Baker LL et al (1997) Effects of electrical stimulation on wound healing in patients with diabetic ulcers. Diabetes Care 20(3): 405–412

[114] Gardner SE, Frantz RA, Schmidt FL (1999) Effect of electrical stimulation on chronic wound healing: a meta-analysis. Wound Repair Regen 7(6): 495–503

[115] Lee PY, Chesnoy S, Huang L (2004) Electroporatic delivery of TGF-beta1 gene works synergistically with electric therapy to enhance diabetic wound healing in db/db mice. J Invest Dermatol 123(4): 791–798

[116] Marti G et al (2004) Electroporative transfection with KGF-1 DNA improves wound healing in a diabetic mouse model. Gene Ther 11(24): 1780–1785

[117] Felgner PL, Ringold GM (1989) Cationic liposome-mediated transfection. Nature 337(6205): 387–388

[118] Jeschke MG et al (2000) Biodistribution and feasibility of non-viral IGF-I gene transfers in thermally injured skin. Lab Invest 80(2): 151–158

[119] Slama J, Davidson JM, Eriksson E (2001) Gene therapy of wounds. In: Falanga V (ed) Cutaneous wound healing. Taylor & Francis, London, pp 123–140

[120] Alexander MY, Akhurst RJ (1995) Liposome-mediated gene transfer and expression via the skin. Hum Mol Genet 4(12): 2279–2285

[121] Jeschke MG et al (1999) IGF-I gene transfer in thermally injured rats. Gene Ther 6(6): 1015–1020

[122] Sun L et al (1997) Transfection with aFGF cDNA improves wound healing. J Invest Dermatol 108(3): 313–318.

[123] Jeschke MG, Schubert T, Klein D (2004) Exogenous liposomal IGF-I cDNA gene transfer leads to endog-

enous cellular and physiological responses in an acute wound. Am J Physiol Regul Integr Comp Physiol 286(5): R958–966

[124] Branski LK et al (2010) Pre-clinical evaluation of liposomal gene transfer to improve dermal and epidermal regeneration. Gene Ther 17(6): 770–778

[125] Lynch SE et al (1987) Role of platelet-derived growth factor in wound healing: synergistic effects with other growth factors. Proc Natl Acad Sci USA 84(21): 7696–7700

[126] Sprugel KH et al (1987) Effects of growth factors in vivo. I. Cell ingrowth into porous subcutaneous chambers. Am J Pathol 129(3): 601–613

[127] Jeschke MG, Klein D (2004) Liposomal gene transfer of multiple genes is more effective than gene transfer of a single gene. Gene Ther 11(10): 847–855

[128] Shea LD et al (1999) DNA delivery from polymer matrices for tissue engineering. Nat Biotechnol 17(6): 551–554

[129] Fu H et al (2005) A calcium phosphate-based gene delivery system. J Biomed Mater Res A 74(1): 40–48

[130] Eriksson E (2000) Gene transfer in wound healing. Adv Skin Wound Care 13[2 Suppl]: 20–22

[131] Lawrie A et al (2000) Microbubble-enhanced ultrasound for vascular gene delivery. Gene Ther 7(23): 2023–2027

[132] Chandler LA et al (2000) Matrix-enabled gene transfer for cutaneous wound repair. Wound Repair Regen 8(6): 473–479

[133] Voigt M et al (1999) Cultured epidermal keratinocytes on a microspherical transport system are feasible to reconstitute the epidermis in full-thickness wounds. Tissue Eng 5(6): 563–572

[134] Gossen M, Bujard H (1992) Tight control of gene expression in mammalian cells by tetracycline-responsive promoters. Proc Natl Acad Sci USA 89(12): 5547–5551

[135] Breuing K et al (1992) Healing of partial thickness porcine skin wounds in a liquid environment. J Surg Res 52(1): 50–58

Correspondence: Ludwik K. Branski M.D., Department of Plastic, Hand, and Reconstructive Surgery, Hannover Medical School, Carl-Neuberg-Straße 1, 30625 Hannover, Germany, phone +49 511 532 8864, E-mail: branski@web.de

# Wound healing

David A. Brown[1], Nicole S. Gibran[1,2]

[1] University of Washington, Department of Surgery, USA
[2] University of Washington, Regional Burn Center, USA

## History of wound care

The science of wound healing occupies a central role in surgical history and continues to represent a common theme for all surgical subspecialties. As early as 1550 B. C., the Ebers Papyrus of ancient Egypt documents the use of a multitude of natural remedies in wound healing. The Egyptians observed that honey, now known to have hygroscopic and antibacterial properties, proved an effective wound dressing. Mild antiseptics such as frankincense, date-wine, turpentine, and acacia gum also found a place in the Egyptian pharmacopeia. The Egyptians are also credited with the first use of sutures for primary wound closure. In a strikingly early use of 20th century medicine, there is documentation of the application of sour or moldy bread to wounds, now understood to harbor antibiotic-producing fungus [1].

Galen of Pergamon, the celebrated surgeon and anatomist, undoubtedly derived a wealth of wound care experience from serving as a surgeon to the Roman gladiators. It was he who first emphasized the importance of maintaining a moist environment for wound healing, although not until recent times has it been understood that wound epithelialization is greatly enhanced in sufficiently hydrated wound beds [2].

The next major breakthroughs in wound care arrived almost two millennia later with the development of the germ theory of disease. Ignaz Phillip Semmelweis, a Hungarian obstetrician, noted that the incidence of puerperal infections was significantly lower when medical students on the ward washed their hands with soap and hypochlorite after attending cadaver dissection. Louis Pasteur stands among the first to apply the microbial theory of disease to healthcare applications. In addition to relating natural phenomena such as the souring of milk the fermentation of sugar to microorganisms, he developed a heat treatment (pasteurization) of milk that prevented the transmission of tuberculosis or typhoid. Robert Koch remains another giant of the era, having formulated a generalized set of criteria for microbial infections, now known as Koch's postulates [3].

Finally, the English surgeon Joseph Lister is widely credited as the father of antiseptic surgery. Lister's use of carbolic acid for surgical sterilization is said to derive from his observation that sewage treated with the chemical was less murky than without. He began treating surgical instruments and instituted hand-washing protocols with carbolic acid, which initially led to his suspension from practice, but eventually paved the way for institution of sterile technique in surgery [3].

## Types of wounds

The nature of the wound and the manner in which it may heal are fundamentally linked to the mechanism of insult. Injuries by physical agents may be broadly classified into four groups: mechanical trauma, thermal injury, chemical injury, electrical injury, and injury caused by ionizing radiation [4]. These may be considered primary wounds, in contrast to the subtypes of each group are listed in Table 1 with typical characteristics of the wound.

Mechanical injuries take on a variety of forms, such as abrasions, contusions, lacerations, incisions, and puncture wounds. Abrasions are caused by scraping or rubbing and result in removal of superficial skin layers. More severe forms of abrasions are

**Table 1.** Categories of wounds and various subtypes

| Category | Subtype | Wound characteristics |
|---|---|---|
| Mechanical | Abrasions | Removal of superficial skin layer(s) |
| | Contusions | Disruption of blood vessels and extravasations of blood into tissue |
| | Lacerations | Tissue disruption caused by blunt or sharp instrument, usually irregular |
| | Incisions | Tissue disruption caused by sharp instrument, usually linear |
| | Puncture wounds | Penetration of sharp instrument or projectile into tissue |
| Thermal | Superficial Partial thickness | Burns confined to epidermis Burns involving papillary (superficial) or reticular (deep) dermis |
| | Full thickness | Burns extending through dermis into subcutaneous tissue |
| Chemical | Alkali | Fat saponification, cellular dehydration, and deep tissue penetration |
| | Acid | Hard eschar, thermal injury, and electrolyte imbalances |
| | Hydrocarbons | Dissolution of cell membranes, typically superficial erythema & blistering |
| Electrical | Complex | Degrees of cutaneous & deep tissue injury associated with systemic complications |
| Radiation | Complex | Basal skin layer damage with short- and long-term sequelae |
| Chronic | Complex | Persistent inflammation and matrix degradation leading to non-healing |

avulsions, which involve detachment of skin and possibly underlying tissue, and degloving injuries, in which the blood supply to the detached tissue is compromised. Contusions, or bruises, are caused by blunt trauma and characteristically rupture blood vessels. Extravasation of blood into the affected tissue is evident by skin discoloration, which evolves over time based on the degradation of hemoglobin. Lacerations and incisions refer to tissue separation extending through the skin, with lacerations caused by accidental trauma and incisions caused by purposeful dissection. Puncture wounds are the result of sharp penetration through the skin by an instrument or a projectile. They may extend into deeper structures and/or produce a second wound at the exit site (through-and-through wounds).

Thermal injuries demonstrate a characteristic cutaneous injury pattern, which is divided into three zones based on blood perfusion and tissue viability: zone of coagulation, zone of stasis, and zone of hyperemia. The innermost zone of coagulation represents the irreversibly damaged, necrotic tissue without perfusion. Surrounding the necrotic tissue is an area of moderately burned tissue that may survive or progress to coagulative necrosis depending on the wound environment. This so-called zone of stasis is characterized by increased capillary permeability and vascular damage. The final zone of hyperemia is an area of intense vasodilatation and inflammation that contains viable tissue and is not usually at risk of progression to necrosis [5].

Electrical injuries produce a variety of cutaneous and extra-cutaneous damage that depend upon the strength (amperage), duration, and path of transmission through the body. If the contact time is brief, damage is relatively restricted to the cell membrane and non-thermal mechanisms will dominate the injury pattern. With longer contact time, thermal injury dominates and the entire cell is affected. Higher voltage burns are associated with a greater degree of systemic complications such as ventricular fibrillation, rhabdomyolysis, compartment syndrome, and renal failure [6].

Chemical injuries are grouped by the causative agent, with alkali burns generally known as the most severe. Alkali burns induce fat saponification, profound cellular dehydration, and formation of alkaline proteinates that cause deeper tissue damage.

Examples of alkalis include lime, cement, potassium hydroxide, and bleach. Acid injuries induce protein hydrolysis and do not penetrate tissue as readily as alkalis. However, acid reactions with skin are exothermic and may cause coincident thermal injury, and extensive acid injuries are associated with electrolyte imbalances. One acid worth noting is hydrofluoric acid due to its unique mechanism of injury and the ability to treat it with topical or systemic calcium. Finally, hydrocarbons such as organic solvents are capable of dissolving cell membranes and producing skin necrosis. Systemic absorption of hydrocarbons is associated with respiratory depression and hepatic toxicity [5].

Radiation injuries, which can be accidental or iatrogenic, are known to cause short- and long-term sequelae. The concept of acute radiation syndrome (ARS) was developed in recent years to describe the adverse effects of large doses of ionizing radiation on the skin. The basal skin layer is damaged, which results in inflammation, erythema, and desquamation. Blistering and ulceration may follow in days to weeks, and most wounds will heal normally, though larger doses may result in destruction of skin appendages, fibrosis, abnormal pigmentation, and ulceration or necrosis of exposed tissue. Acute ionizing radiation exposure is also associated with dysfunction of hematopoietic, gastrointestinal, and cerebrovascular, and systems [7].

## Mechanisms of wound healing

Wound healing is classically divided into four phases: hemostasis, inflammation, proliferation, and remodeling. Considerable overlap exists between each phase, and a combination of biochemical and cellular events contributes to the natural continuum of tissue repair.

### Hemostasis

The initial phase of wound healing is characterized by a coordinated effort between circulating platelets, soluble clotting factors, and vascular endothelium to stop hemorrhage by formation of a clot. The key sequences of events are divided into the (1) coagulation cascade and (2) platelet activation, although it is important to remember the fundamentally integrated nature of these processes.

Hemostasis is initiated by a chain reaction of soluble serum proteins to form an insoluble fibrin mesh. The coagulation cascade has been historically grouped into intrinsic and extrinsic pathways, which have since been renamed into the contact activation and tissue factor pathways, respectively. The initial reactions of the two enzyme cascades are unique with a final common pathway consisting of factors X, V, and thrombin. The primary pathway for blood coagulation is thought to be the tissue factor pathway, with the contact activation pathway playing a secondary role. The end result of the clotting cascade is the generation of fibrin, which serves to enhance platelet aggregation and structurally reinforce the ensuing platelet plug [4]. Topical fibrin sealants have been used clinically to promote hemostasis and even skin graft adhesion in burn wounds [8].

Disruption of normal endothelium exposes subendothelial collagen and thrombogenic extracellular matrix molecules, most notably von Willebrand factor (vWF). Platelets adhere to vWF via the glycoprotein (GP) Ib receptor, which strengthens the interaction between platelets and underlying extracellular matrix. Individuals with vWF deficiency are known to have von Willebrand disease, which stands as the most common hereditary coagulation deficiency. Likewise, mutations in the GPIb receptor result in Bernard-Soulier syndrome. Both of these conditions result in bleeding tendencies because of altered platelet adhesion to exposed subendothelium [4].

Platelet adhesion leads to platelet activation, invoking the release of stored granule contents. Environmental cues from the wound environment such as hypoxia and acidosis are known to enhance platelet degranulation [9]. Alpha-granules store a number of growth factors such as platelet factor-4 (PF4), platelet derived-growth factor, fibronectin, vWF, and fibrinogen [10]. Many of these substances serve to enhance platelet adhesion or activation. PF4 binds with high affinity to endothelial-derived heparin, which serves to inactive the molecule and promote coagulation. It is the PF4-heparin complex on platelet membranes to which antibodies bind in the syndrome of heparin-induced thrombocytopenia (HIT), which can lead to dangerously low levels of platelets with a paradoxical increase in thrombosis [4].

Dense granules harbor smaller molecules involved in platelet activation such as ADP, ATP, calcium, and serotonin. Release of these molecules into the platelet cytosol initiates a $G_q$-linked protein receptor cascade, which results in an increased cytosolic calcium concentration. The calcium activates protein kinase C, which, in turn, activates phospholipase A2 (PLA2), and eventually modifies the integrin membrane glycoprotein IIb-IIIa [4].

The platelet glycoprotein IIb-IIIa receptor deserves mention because of its relevance to cardiovascular medicine and disease. The natural ligand of GPIIb-IIIa is fibrinogen, which serves to link the coagulation cascade with platelet activation. Platelet activation leads to increasing its affinity to bind fibrinogen, which enhances platelet aggregation and clotting factor-mediated coagulation. The activated platelets change shape from spherical to stellate, and the fibrinogen cross-links with glycoprotein IIb-IIIa receptors in neighboring platelets to promote aggregation and eventual clot formation [4].

The GPIIb-IIIA receptor is the target of several antiplatelet agents including abciximab, eptifibatide, and tirofiban. Similarly, the drug clopidogrel is known to inhibit ADP binding to the GPIIb-IIIA receptor, which results in a reduced ability of platelets to aggregate and consequently form clots. Mutations in the GPIIb-IIIa receptor lead to Glanzmann's thrombasthenia, which leads to bleeding tendencies from impaired platelet aggregation [4].

## Inflammation

Vasoconstriction occurs at the wound site immediately after injury, which may be considered the beginning of the second event in wound healing: inflammation. Vasoconstriction is primarily mediated by catecholamines (epinephrine and norepinephrine), prostaglandin $F_{2\alpha}$, and thromboxane $A_2$. The contraction of blood vessels aids in platelet aggregation and hemostasis. Vasoconstriction is followed shortly by vasodilatation and increased vascular permeability, which allows access of inflammatory cells to the damaged tissue. Vasodilatation is mediated by prostaglandin $E_2$, prostacyclin, histamine, serotonin, and kinins [10]. Inflammatory cells undergo a three-stage process of rolling along the vascular endothelium, integrin-mediated adhesion to endothelial cells, and transmigration into the extracellular space [11].

Neutrophils are the first inflammatory cell to arrive at the wound and play a primary role in the phagocytosis of bacteria and tissue debris. A huge array of molecular signals serves as chemoattractant agents for neutrophils, including products of platelet degranulation, formyl methionyl peptides cleaved from bacterial proteins, and the degradation products of matrix proteins. Neutrophils are a major source of early cytokines in the systemic response to injury, including tumor necrosis factor (TNF)-α [5].

The second cell to arrive at the wound site is the monocyte, which undergo phenotypic changes into macrophages. Macrophages can be regarded as the "master cell" involved in wound healing because of their central role in phagocytosis, inflammatory cell recruitment, and systemic inflammation. Macrophages release a variety of growth factors such as transforming growth factor-β (TGF-β), platelet-derived growth factor (PDGF), and fibroblast growth factor (FGF), which induce fibroblast proliferation and extracellular matrix production [12]. Macrophages express specific receptors for IgG (Fc receptor), complement C3b (CR1 and CR3), and fibronectin (integrins) that facilitate recognition and phagocytosis of opsonized pathogens [13]. Importantly, macrophages also secrete cytokines such as IL-1 and TNF-α that modulate the systemic response to injury. Excessive production of TNF-α has been linked with multisystem organ failure as well as chronic non-healing ulcers [14]. Both IL-1 and TNF-α appear to play crucial roles in early wound healing, but may have an inhibitory effect on wound maturation if persistently elevated.

Emerging data also suggests a role for nerve-derived neuropeptides in wound repair. Stimulation of efferent nerves is known to induce local vasodilation and plasma extravasation in skin, which contributes to the local inflammatory response. The neuropeptide substance P, released from terminal endings of sensory nerves in response to noxious stimuli, is known to influence inflammatory cell chemotaxis [15, 16], angiogenesis [17, 18], and keratinocyte proliferation [19]. We have previously suggested that dysregulated neuroinflammation plays an important role in hypertrophic scarring, evident by increased levels of substance P and decreased levels of the regulating enzyme neutral endopeptidase [20], which is responsible the exuberant matrix production, hyperemia, and pruritus seen in this condition [21].

A robust but appropriate inflammatory response is essential to prepare the wound bed for subsequent migration of proliferative cells. However, an overzealous inflammatory response may inhibit the formation of granulation tissue and neovascularization. Experiments in mice constitutively expressing the chemotactic cytokine interferon-inducible protein 10 demonstrate that an intense inflammatory infiltrate inhibits angiogenesis and development of healthy granulation tissue [22]. Thus, as in all homeostatic systems, a careful balance of functionalized cellular and biochemical processes is essential to proper wound healing.

## Proliferation

The proliferative phase is characterized by the formation of granulation tissue, which is a pink, soft, highly vascularized platform for tissue formation. Granulation tissue is largely a product of two cell types: fibroblasts and vascular endothelial cells. Fibroblasts are evident at the wound site within 2–5 days and become the predominant cell type after the first week [4]. Migration of fibroblasts is driven by a number of chemokines secreted by macrophages including TNF-α, PDGF, FGF, and TGF-β. Fibroblasts begin to deposit collagen and other extracellular matrix molecules that strengthen the wound bed. Macrophages stimulate fibroblasts to produce FGF-7 (keratinocyte growth factor) and IL-6, which promote keratinocyte migration and proliferation. IL-6 is also potent stimulator of fibroblasts, which explains the decreased level found in aging fibroblasts and fetal wounds [23]. Although essential to normal wound healing, granulation tissue also harbors high bacterial counts and proteolytic activity, which may require that it is excised before skin grafting. Granulation tissue in a burn wound prevents epithelialization and likely leads to hypertrophic scar formation [24].

A number of other inflammatory cytokines may find clinical relevance in wound care. IL-8 is secreted by macrophages and fibroblasts early in wound healing and may have a stimulatory effect on keratinocytes and epithelialization. Topical application of IL-8 to human skin grafts in a chimeric mouse model enhanced keratinocyte proliferation and re-epithelialization [25]. Additionally, in both human and animal studies, wound strength and healing time has been improved with topical application of PDGF [26].

TGF-β is expressed by platelets and fibroblasts in the wound bed and plays an important role in collagen deposition and turnover. TGF-β is the most potent known stimulator of fibroblast proliferation and can accelerate wound healing in steroid-treated and irradiated animals [27]. Overexpression of TGF-β mRNA has been found in keloid and hypertrophic scars, whereas fetal wounds contain relatively little TGF-β [28]. This contrast between the heavily fibrotic scars of keloid and the scarless repair observed in utero may underscore the importance of TGF-β in the fibrotic response to tissue injury. A similar phenomenon has been observed in burn injuries, where higher levels of TGF-β correlate with excessive wound contraction [29]. Interestingly, exogenous application of TGF-β3 appears to reduce monocyte and macrophage recruitment to the wound site, resulting in less deposition of collagen and fibronectin in the early stages of wound healing and eventually less scarring [30]. A clinical formulation of TGF-β3 (Juvista) is currently undergoing evaluation in phase 2 trials for use in dermal scarring [31].

Coincident with fibroblast migration to the wound site is angiogenesis. Angiogenesis, or neovascularization, was historically considered a critical element of early wound healing to provide adequate transport of metabolites to and from the regenerating tissue; more recent data suggest that normal healing can occur when angiogenesis is inhibited and that most angiogenesis in the wound bed is not associated with increased blood flow to the wound [32].

Vascular endothelial cells in the wound bed arise from both preexisting blood vessels and endothelial progenitor cells (EPCs) in bone marrow. The most important regulators of angiogenesis are vascular endothelial growth factor (VEGF) and FGF-2. A dose-dependent effect of both VEGF and FGF-2 has been observed in angiogenesis [33]. VEGF is secreted as many different isoforms from a variety of stromal and mesenchymal cells, with the tyrosine kinase VEGF-receptor 2 emerging as the most preeminent in angiogenesis. VEGF/VEGFR2 signaling is involved in EPC migration from bone marrow, as well as promotion of endothelial cell proliferation and differentiation [34].

Hypoxia is a potent inducer of both angiogenesis and fibroblast proliferation. The major player in hypoxic gene expression has emerged as hypoxia-inducible factor 1 (HIF-1), a DNA-binding transcription factor that is known to alter gene transcription of a number of proteins involved in metabolism, angiogenesis, migration, and proliferation [35]. Cultured endothelial cells upregulate expression of several pro-angiogenic molecules when cultured in hypoxia, including endothelin-1, VEGF, and PDGF-β chain [36]. Fibroblast replication and longevity are increased in low oxygen tension culture [37], as is TGF-β secretion [36]. These observations highlight the contribution of hypoxia in the wound bed in proliferative cell signaling.

Recently, the role of T-lymphocytes in wound healing is under increased investigation. T-cells migrate into the wound bed during the late proliferative and early remodeling phase. Mice deficient in T- and B-cells have a reduced capacity to scar [38], though contradictory reports exist concerning the beneficial effects of CD4+ and CD8+ lymphocytes on wound healing [39, 40]. Additionally, a unique type of T-cell exists in the skin, known as dendritic epidermal T-cells, which are thought to modulate many aspects of wound healing such as inflammation, host defense, and maintenance of tissue integrity. Mice lacking or defective in dendritic epidermal T-cells show delayed wound closure and decreased keratinocyte proliferation at the wound site [41, 42].

## Epithelialization

Epithelialization is the third important concomitant event in wound repair and the most clinically significant evidence of wound closure. Keratinocytes migrate from wound edges and dermal appendages such as hair follicles, sweat glands, and sebaceous glands. Subsequent proliferation of these cells at the wound site provides a neo-epidermal covering. A discrete sequence of events has been identified in keratinocyte migration and proliferation, which involves disassembly of hemidesmosomes and desmosomes, retraction of intracellular tonofilaments and keratin filaments, and formation of focal contacts and cytoplasmic actin filaments [43]. The interplay between laminin, MMPs, integrins, and soluble growth factors has been extensively studied in this process [44].

Renewal of keratinocytes during normal homeostasis and wound repair is a defining feature of re-epithelialization. The upper region of hair follicles below the sebaceous gland (known as the bulge) contains multipotent progenitor cells that contribute to maintenance and renewal of epithelium [45, 46]. Additionally, epidermal cells are known to migrate from neighboring unwounded epidermis or from the infundibulum, the portion of the hair follicle between the epidermis and the sebaceous gland [47]. The role of epidermal appendages is especially evident in partial thickness burns, where advancement of the epidermal tongue is limited to approximately 1 cm from an epidermal appendage source. Full-thickness burns greater than 2 cm rarely heal other than by contraction.

The relative contributions of follicular stem cells and epidermal stem cells to re-epithelialization is debatable, although genetic analyses have confirmed that the epidermis has intrinsic capacity for self-renewal and does not depend on follicule-derived multipotent progenitor cells [48, 49]. Further evidence for this notion comes from reports of de novo hair follicle generation in the healing skin of adult mice [50]. This phenomenon, which has never been observed in human, is contingent upon Wnt-mediated signaling, which is also involved in pattern formation and the epithelial-mesenchymal transformation during embryogenesis [51]. Elucidation of the overlapping pathways in wound repair and development is a central principle of efforts toward scarless repair and skin regeneration.

## Remodeling

The remodeling phase depicts the replacement of granulation tissue with scar. A key feature of tissue remodeling that emerges during this stage of wound healing is the balance between ECM synthesis and degradation. While fibrogenic growth factors such as PDGF and FGF stimulate fibroblast matrix deposition, resident cells induce continuous degradation of extracellular matrix by matrix metalloproteases (MMPs). MMPs are a family of zinc-proteases that are capable of degrading a variety of ECM components such as collagen, fibronectin, proteoglycans, and laminin [52].

Collagen composition of the wound appears to follow a similar pattern as embryogenesis. Granulation tissue is comprised of a large amount of collagen III, which is gradually replaced by collagen I. Collagen I provides a higher degree of tensile strength to the developing scar, although the final tensile strength approaches only 70% of uninjured skin [53]. A morphological change in fibroblasts ensues during wound contraction, in which fibroblasts begin to express alpha-smooth muscle actin and adapt functions of smooth muscle cells. The resulting cell is termed a myofibroblast and serves to enhance wound contraction [5].

## Fetal wound healing

Fetal wound healing is typified by scarless healing and a paucity of inflammation. Epithelialization occurs more quickly with less neovascularization, and wounds heal faster than adult counterparts. Reticular collagen III is the predominant type of collagen in healed fetal wounds, in contrast to fibrilar collagen I in adult scars. Fetal skin wounds are also able to regenerate appendages such as hair follicles, sweat glands, and sebaceous glands. The transition from scarless to scarring repair appears to occur near the end of the second trimester, with the propensity for wound scarring increasing through neonatal to adult life [5].

Much of the research on fetal wound healing has focused on fibroblasts. Fetal fibroblasts exhibit different collagen expression profiles than adult fibroblasts (type III dominant), and produce comparatively more collagen in culture. Collagen expression falls to adult levels after 20 weeks gestation, concurrent with a sharp increase in MMP-1, MMP-3, and MMP-9 expression [54]. While fibroblasts appear to exhibit more vigorous activity in fetal wounds, minimal quantities of the potent fibroblast stimulant TGF-β have been noted. The hyaluronan-rich amniotic fluid environment may also provide a permissive milieu for fibroblast migration and proliferation [55]. Attempts to recapitulate the secrets of fetal wound healing in adults are ongoing, though the underlying mechanisms remain incompletely understood.

## Stem cells

In addition to resident epidermal stem cells in the skin, bone marrow-derived stem cells may contribute substantially to cutaneous wound healing. Bone marrow contains both hematopoietic (CD34+) and non-hematopoietic (mesenchymal) stem cells, which aid wound healing by direct contribution of cells as well as by paracrine signaling. A notable study, in which green fluorescent protein-labeled bone marrow stem cells were used to reconstitute the marrow of mice with cutaneous wounds, indicated that non-hematopoietic mesenchymal stem cells may contribute up to 15–20% of dermal fibroblasts in normal skin and healing cutaneous wounds [56]. Cells with a keratinocyte phenotype have also been traced to bone marrow origin [56, 57]. Evidence also exists that bone marrow-derived stem cells are involved in hair follicle regeneration [58]. Bone marrow stem cells expanded ex vivo have been shown to promote neovascularization [59], appendage regeneration [60], and accelerate wound closure [61].

Endothelial progenitor cells (EPCs) are derived from CD34+ hematopoietic stem cells in the bone marrow and contribute some proportion of endothelial cells to adult skin. Transplantation of EPCs enhances wound healing in mice [62], as does topical application of EPCs to ischemic ulcers in diabetic mice [63]. Interestingly, the mechanism is thought to involve paracrine signaling from EPCs instead of direct contribution of endothelial cells [62].

Fibrocytes are a newly-identified subpopulation of leukocytes that also arise in the bone marrow, which were originally identified by their rapid recruitment from peripheral blood to wound sites in mice [64]. Fibrocytes are significantly increased in the blood of burned patients in comparison to normal individuals, and appear to localize in the deeper papillary dermis[65]. The evidence to date points towards a prominent role for fibrocytes in the fibrosis associated with hypertrophic scarring [66]. These cells may also contribute to the myofibroblast population in wounds [67].

## Abnormal wound healing

### Impaired wound healing

A variety of local and systemic factors are implicated in abnormal wound healing, which impair tissue regeneration by interrupting each of the stages of wound healing. Physical impediments to wound closure may delay or prevent healing, such as the presence of foreign bodies or neoplasm; hematomas and seromas commonly cause failure of skin grafts. Excessive tension on a wound or surrounding edema may compress the vascular supply and lead to ischemia; recent data also implicate mechanical tension as a leading cause for hypertrophic scar formation [68]. Therapeutic radiation and repetitive trauma are also well-known detriments to wound healing. A summary of the classic factors that are known to impair wound healing is listed in Table 2.

Delivery of oxygen is especially important in the healing wound, and a variety of insults can disturb wound healing by evoking hypoxia. In addition to providing a substrate for ATP synthesis in aerobic cell metabolism, large quantities of oxygen are used by neutrophils for superoxide radical generation in oxidative killing. Furthermore, molecular oxygen itself is toxic to anaerobic microorganisms. Wound oxygenation is determined by blood perfusion, hemoglobin dissociation, local oxygen consumption, fraction of inspired oxygen, hemoglobin content, arterial oxygen tension, circulating blood volume, cardiac output, arterial inflow, and venous

drainage [70]. Disruption of vascular supply and depletion of oxygen can lead to wound hypoxia, which has been associated with systemic diseases such as connective tissue disorders and microvascular disease in diabetes mellitus. Tobacco smoking produces similar effects through nicotine-induced vasoconstriction and displacement of oxygen on hemoglobin with carbon monoxide [5].

Infection is another classic adversary of proper wound healing. Bacterial counts that exceed approximately $10^5$ organisms per gram of tissue will generally not heal by any means, including flap closure, skin graft placement, or primary intention [71]. The introduction of early excision and grafting for burn wounds has virtually eliminated burn wound sepsis, which was historically a leading cause of burn mortality. Endotoxin produced by gram-negative bacteria stimulates phagocytosis and collagenase expression, which contributes to matrix degradation and destruction of normal tissue. Bacteria are also known to accelerate protease production in macrophages (such as MMPs) while inhibiting protease inhibitor expression. This effect leads to increased matrix destruction and degradation of growth factors, which are characteristics of chronic non-healing wounds [72].

Nutritional status has a profound effect on wound healing as well. Serum albumin is thought to be one of the most accurate predictors of surgical morbidity and mortality, with levels below 2.1 g/dL associated with poorer outcomes [73]. Protein replacement has been shown to enhance wound healing [74], as has supplementation with the amino acids arginine, taurine, and glutamine [75, 76]. Whereas patients with large burns characteristically have albumin levels below 1.0 g/dL, there has been no conclusive demonstration that exogenous albumen will improve outcomes. Nevertheless, all efforts should be made to provide early enteral nutrition and to modulate the metabolic state. Some data suggest that the catabolic state can be modulated by propranolol in children [77], as well as by oxandrolone in children and adults [78,79].

Vitamin C (ascorbic acid) is an essential cofactor in proline and lysine hydroxylation during collagen synthesis, and supplementation of 100–1,000 grams per day may improve wound healing [76]. Vitamin A (retinoic acid) is required for wound epithelial-

**Table 2.** Local and systemic factors that impair wound healing. Adapted from [69]

| Local factors | Systemic factors |
|---|---|
| Tension | Connective tissue disorders |
| Foreign bodies | Hypothermia |
| Infection | Oxygen |
| Ischemia | Tobacco smoking |
| Hematoma and seroma | Malnutrition |
| Trauma | Jaundice |
| Edema | Age |
| Irradiation | Diabetes mellitus |
| | Uremia |
| | Steroids |
| | Chemotherapeutic agents |

ization, maintenance of normal epithelium, proteoglycan synthesis, and normal immune function. Oral retinoid therapy is well known to counteract the detrimental effects of corticosteroids on wound healing, possibly through promotion of TGF-β and IL-1 signaling [80]. Vitamin K deficiency will impede clot formation and hemostasis, while vitamin D is required for bone healing and calcium metabolism. Finally, vitamin E supplementation may serve an important role as an antioxidant in trauma patients. Early administration of vitamin E has been shown to reduce the incidence of organ failure and the length of ICU stay in critically ill surgical patients [81].

The dietary minerals associated with adverse wound healing are zinc and possibly iron. Zinc is an essential cofactor in RNA and DNA polymerases, and a deficiency can inhibit granulation tissue formation [82] and delay wound healing [83]. Supplementation with zinc was also reported to improve wound healing [75]. Iron is also a cofactor in DNA synthesis as well as proline and lysine hydroxylation. Although the role of iron in normal hematopoiesis is well established, chronically anemic patients do not appear to suffer from delayed wound healing [5, 84]. Selenium deficiency is known to cause hair and skin abnormalities in humans and rodents, though it has not been implicated in abnormal wound healing. Recent evidence has implicated selenoproteins in keratinocyte function and cutaneous development [85]. Based on the importance of hair follicles and keratinocytes in wound epithelialization, it may prudent to assume that adequate selenium is necessary for proper wound healing.

## Hypertrophic scars and keloids

Hypertrophic scar and keloids are the prime examples of proliferative scars, which are characterized by excessive collagen deposition. Whereas these two morphological aberrations can be difficult to differentiate, keloids are defined as scars that grow beyond the periphery of the original wounds and hypertrophic scars represent raised scars that remain confined to the boundaries of the original wound. Keloids rarely regress with time; hypertrophic scars frequently regress spontaneously. Keloids appear to have a strong genetic component, with more prevalence in dark-skinned patients of African, Asian, or Latin American descent. Hypetrophic scars, in contrast, are the result of prolonged inflammation and maybe frequently preventable [5]. Hypertrophic scars also tend to occur in pigmented individuals; they are more common in young people and rarely occur in the aged. Interestingly, they often develop in areas of the body where contraction occurs and rarely form on the scalp or the palms and soles.

In light of its potent effect on fibroblast proliferation and collagen deposition, it is perhaps not surprising that TGF-β plays a central role in proliferative scarring. Increased levels of the TGF-β1 isoform have been found in both keloids and hypertrophic scars [86]. Likewise, antibodies to TGF-β isoforms have been found to reduce fibrosis in hypertrophic scars [87]. Novel therapies for hypertrophic and keloid scars are in development that target ECM synthesis and fibroblast proliferation [88].

## Chronic non-healing wounds

Dysfunction of normal wound healing processes leads to chronic wounds. In particular, chronic wounds appear to have sustained inflammation with less matrix production. Chronic wounds exhibit higher levels of cytokines such as IL-1, IL-6, and TNF-α, with reduced levels of essential growth factors such as EGF and PDGF [14]. Higher levels of MMP-1, MMP-2, MMP-8, and MMP-9 have been demonstrated, with reduced levels of MMP inhibitors [89]. These non-healing wounds are prone to developing squamous cell carcinoma, originally reported in burn wounds by Marjolin. Marjolin ulcers tend to be very aggressive and should be highly suspected with non-healing burn wounds. Therapy includes complete local extirpation of the cancer with negative margins and lymphatic mapping [90]. Other conditions such as osteomyelitis, pressures sores, venous stasis ulcers, and hidradenitis have also been associated with wound malignancies [5]. Patients with impaired skin integrity due to burn injuries are at increased risk for decubitus ulcers, which constitute a closely monitored hospital-acquired complication.

A variety of burn dressings and skin substitutes are employed in the treatments of acute burns, which are listed in Tables 3 and 4 respectively.

## Conclusions

Wound healing remains an integral element of modern surgical science, contributing to both the function and form of wounds in all surgical patients but especially those with burn injuries. The biology of wound healing entails many integrated, parallel processes that lead to decontamination and closure of a wound. Restoration of tissue integrity relies on a careful balance between inflammation and proliferation, which is tipped in pathologic states of wound healing. Efforts are underway to unravel the mysteries of fetal wound repair and regeneration, which may lead to novel treatments for proliferative wounds or reduce scarring in normal adult wound healing.

**Table 3.** Examples of burn dressings, adapted from reference [91]. Products listed are registered trademarks: Jelonet®, Opsite®, Intrasite Gel®, Allevyn®, and Acticoat® (Smith & Nephew UK Limited, London, UK); Atrauman® (Hartmann, Homebush, Australia), Mepilex® (Molnlycke, Norcross, GA), Tegaderm® (3M, St. Paul, MN), Comfeel® and Biatain Adhesive® (Coloplast, Minneapolis, MN); DuoDERM®, Granuflex®, Aquacel®, Versiva®, Kaltostat®, and Aquacel Ag®, and Aquaform® (ConvaTec, Skillman, NJ); Actisorb® and Inadine® (Johnson & Johnson, New Brunswick, NJ)

| Dressing type | Examples | Clinical use |
|---|---|---|
| Low adherence dressings | Jelonet® (Smith & Nephew) Atrauman® (Hartmann) Mepilex® (Molnlycke) | Superficial and partial thickness burns with minimal exudate |
| Semi-permeable films | Opsite® (Smith & Nephew) Tegaderm® (3M) | Superficial and partial thickness burns with minimal exudate |
| Hydrocolloids | Comfeel® (Coloplast) DuoDERM® (ConvaTec) Granuflex® (ConvaTec) | Superficial and partial thickness burns in high range of motion areas |
| Hydrofibers | Aquacel® (ConvaTec) Versiva® ConvaTec) | Partial thickness burns with moderate exudate |
| Hydrogels | Aquaform® (ConvaTec) Intrasite Gel® (Smith & Nephew) | Small deep partial thickness burns with slough |
| Alginate | Kaltostat® (ConvaTec) | Skin graft donor sites |
| Foam/hydrocellular | Allevyn® (Smith & Nephew) Biatain Adhesive® (Coloplast) | Superficial and partial thickness burns with minimal exudate |
| Antimicrobials | Acticoat (Smith & Nephew) Actisorb® (Johnson & Johnson) Aquacel Ag® (ConvaTec) Inadine (Johnson & Johnson) Mepilex Ag (Molnyke) | Superficial and partial thickness burns with moderate exudate and/or evidence of infection |

**Table 4.** Examples of skin substitutes for burns wounds, adapted from reference [92]. Oasis® (Healthpoint LTD, San Antonio, TX), Transcyte® (Advanced BioHealing, Westport, CT), Biobrane® (Smith & Nephew UK Limited, London, UK), Apligraf® (Organogenesis, Canton, MA), OrCel® (Forticell Bioscience, Englewood Cliffs, NJ), Epicel® (Genzyme, Cambridge, MA), and Alloderm® (LifeCell, Branchburg, NJ), Integra® (Integra Life Sciences, Plainsboro, NJ) are registered trademarks

| Product | Composition | Clinical Uses |
|---|---|---|
| Human allograft | Cadaveric epidermis & dermis | Temporary coverage of large excised burns |
| Porcine xenograft | Porcine dermis | Temporary coverage of large excised burns |
| Human amnion | Placental amniotic membrane | Temporary coverage of large excised burns |
| Oasis® | Porcine intestine submucosa | Superficial burns, skin graft donor sites, chronic wounds |
| Biobrane® | Silicone and collagen-nylon bilayer | Partial thickness burns, temporary coverage of excised burns |
| Transcyte® | Allogenic dermis and silicone bilayer | Partial thickness burns, temporary coverage of excised burns |
| Apligraf® | Collagen matrix with human neonatal fibroblasts and keratinocytes | Permanent coverage of excised burns, chronic wounds |
| OrCel® | Collagen matrix with human neonatal fibroblasts and keratinocytes | Skin graft donor sites, chronic wounds |
| Epicel® | Cultured autologous keratinocytes | Deep partial thickness and full thickness burns |
| Alloderm® | Acellular human dermis | Soft tissue defects |
| Integra® | Silicone and collagen-glyco-saminoglycan bilayer | Deep partial thickness and full thickness burns |

# References

[1] Sipos P, Gyory H, Hagymasi K, Ondrejka P, Blazovics A (2004) Special wound healing methods used in ancient egypt and the mythological background. World J Surg 28: 211–216

[2] Forrest RD (1982) Early history of wound treatment. J Roy Soc Med 75: 198–205

[3] Lederberg J (2000) Infectious history. Science 288: 287–293

[4] Kumar V, Abbas AK, Fausto N (2005) Robbins and Cotran pathologic basis of disease. Elsevier Saunders, Philadelphia

[5] Townsend CM (2007) Sabiston textbook of surgery: Expert consult: Online & Print. Saunders

[6] Lee RC (1997) Injury by electrical forces: pathophysiology, manifestations, and therapy. Curr Probl Surg 34: 677

[7] Waselenko JK, MacVittie TJ, Blakely WF, Pesik N, Wiley AL, Dickerson WE, Tsu H, Confer DL, Coleman CN, Seed T (2004) Medical management of the acute radiation syndrome: recommendations of the Strategic National Stockpile Radiation Working Group. Ann Intern Med 140: 1037

[8] Foster K, Greenhalgh D, Gamelli RL, Mozingo D, Gibran N, Neumeister M, Abrams SZ, Hantak E, Grubbs L, Ploder B (2008) Efficacy and safety of a fibrin sealant for adherence of autologous skin grafts to burn wounds: results of a phase 3 clinical study. J Burn Care Res 29: 293

[9] Ramasastry SS (2005) Acute wounds. Clin Plast Surg 32: 195–208

[10] Singer AJ, Clark RAF (1999) Cutaneous wound healing. N Engl J Med 341: 738

[11] Ley K (1992) Leukocyte adhesion to vascular endothelium. J Reconstr Microsurg 8: 495–495

[12] Leibovich SJ, Ross R (1975) The role of the macrophage in wound repair. A study with hydrocortisone and anti-macrophage serum. Am J Pathol 78: 71–100

[13] Nwomeh BC, Olutoye OO, Diegelmann RF, Cohen IK (1997) Biology of wound healing. J Surg Pathol 2: 1–19

[14] Murphy MA, Joyce WP, Condron C, Bouchier-Hayes D (2002) A reduction in serum cytokine levels parallels healing of venous ulcers in patients undergoing compression therapy. Eur J Vasc Endovasc Surg 23: 349–352

[15] Helme RD, Eglezos A, Hosking CS (1987) Substance P induces chemotaxis of neutrophils in normal and capsaicin-treated rats. Immunol Cell Biol 65: 267–269

[16] Kavelaars A, Jeurissen F, Heijnen CJ (1994) Substance P receptors and signal transduction in leukocytes. Immunomethods 5: 41

[17] Ziche M, Morbidelli L, Masini E, Amerini S, Granger HJ, Maggi CA, Geppetti P, Ledda F (1994) Nitric oxide me-

diates angiogenesis in vivo and endothelial cell growth and migration in vitro promoted by substance P. J Clin Invest 94: 2036

[18] Ziche M, Morbidelli L, Pacini M, Geppetti P, Alessandri G, Maggi CA (1990) Substance P stimulates neovascularization in vivo and proliferation of cultured endothelial cells. Microvasc Res 40: 264–278

[19] Paus R, Heinzelmann T, Robicsek S, Czarnetzki BM, Maurer M (1995) Substance P stimulates murine epidermal keratinocyte proliferation and dermal mast cell degranulation in situ. Arch Dermatol Res 287: 500–502

[20] Scott JR, Muangman PR, Tamura RN, Zhu KQ, Liang Z, Anthony J, Engrav LH, Gibran NS (2005) Substance P levels and neutral endopeptidase activity in acute burn wounds and hypertrophic scar. Plast Reconstr Surg 115: 1095

[21] Scott JR, Muangman P, Gibran NS (2007) Making sense of hypertrophic scar: a role for nerves. Wound Repair Regen 15:S27-S31

[22] Luster AD, Cardiff RD, MacLean JA, Crowe K, Granstein RD (1998) Delayed wound healing and disorganized neovascularization in transgenic mice expressing the IP-10 chemokine. Proceedings of the Association of American Physicians 110: 183

[23] Liechty KW, Adzick NS, Crombleholme TM (2000) Diminished interleukin 6 (IL-6) production during scarless human fetal wound repair. Cytokine 12: 671–676

[24] Spyrou GE, Naylor IL (2002) The effect of basic fibroblast growth factor on scarring. Br J Plast Surg 55: 275–282

[25] Rennekampff HO, Hansbrough JF, Kiessig V, Doré C, Sticherling M, Schröder JM (2000) Bioactive interleukin-8 is expressed in wounds and enhances wound healing. J Surg Res 93: 41–54

[26] Smith PD, Kuhn MA, Franz MG, Wachtel TL, Wright TE, Robson MC (2000) Initiating the inflammatory phase of incisional healing prior to tissue injury. J Surg Res 92: 11–17

[27] Pierce GF, Mustoe TA, Lingelbach J, Masakowski VR, Gramates P, Deuel TF (1989) Transforming growth factor beta reverses the glucocorticoid-induced wound-healing deficit in rats: possible regulation in macrophages by platelet-derived growth factor. Proc Natl Acad Sci U S A 86: 2229

[28] Tredget EE, Wang R, Shen Q, Scott PG, Ghahary A (2000) Transforming growth factor-beta mRNA and protein in hypertrophic scar tissues and fibroblasts: antagonism by IFN-alpha and IFN-gamma in vitro and in vivo. J Interferon Cytokine Res 20: 143–152

[29] Gabriel VA (2009) Transforming growth factor-[beta] and angiotensin in fibrosis and burn injuries. J Burn Care Res 30: 471

[30] Shah M, Foreman DM, Ferguson MW (1995) Neutralisation of TGF-beta 1 and TGF-beta 2 or exogenous addition of TGF-beta 3 to cutaneous rat wounds reduces scarring. J Cell Sci 108: 985

[31] Occleston NL, Laverty HG, O'Kane S, Ferguson MWJ (2008) Prevention and reduction of scarring in the skin by Transforming Growth Factor beta 3 (TGF3): from laboratory discovery to clinical pharmaceutical. J Biomater Sci, Polym Ed 19: 1047–1063

[32] Tsou R, Fathke C, Wilson L, Wallace K, Gibran N, Isik F (2002) Retroviral delivery of dominant-negative vascular endothelial growth factor receptor type 2 to murine wounds inhibits wound angiogenesis. Wound Repair Regen 10: 222–229

[33] Nissen NN, Polverini PJ, Koch AE, Volin MV, Gamelli RL, DiPietro LA (1998) Vascular endothelial growth factor mediates angiogenic activity during the proliferative phase of wound healing. Am Journal Pathol 152: 1445

[34] Nagy JA, Dvorak AM, Dvorak HF (2007)VEGF-A and the induction of pathological angiogenesis. Annu Rev Pathol 2: 251–275

[35] Hopf HW, Gibson JJ, Angeles AP, Constant JS, Feng JJ, Rollins MD, Zamirul Hussain M, Hunt TK (2005) Hyperoxia and angiogenesis. Wound Repair Regen 13: 558–564

[36] Shweiki D, Itin A, Soffer D, Keshet E (1992) Vascular endothelial growth factor induced by hypoxia may mediate hypoxia-initiated angiogenesis. Nature 359: 843–845

[37] Packer L, Fuehr K (1977) Low oxygen concentration extends the lifespan of cultured human diploid cells. Nature 267: 423–425

[38] Gawronska B, Bogacki M, Rim JS, Monroe WT, Manuel JA (2006) Scarless skin repair in immunodeficient mice. Wound Repair Regen 14: 265–276

[39] Guo S, DiPietro LA (2010) Factors affecting wound healing. J Dent Res 89: 219

[40] Park JE, Barbul A (2004) Understanding the role of immune regulation in wound healing. Am J Surg 187:S11-S16

[41] Jameson J, Ugarte K, Chen N, Yachi P, Fuchs E, Boismenu R, Havran WL (2002) A role for skin gamma delta T cells in wound repair. Science 296: 747

[42] Mills RE, Taylor KR, Podshivalova K, McKay DB, Jameson JM (2008) Defects in skin {gamma}{delta} T cell function contribute to delayed wound repair in rapamycin-treated mice. J Immunol 181: 3974

[43] Santoro MM, Gaudino G (2005) Cellular and molecular facets of keratinocyte reepithelization during wound healing. Exp Cell Res 304: 274–286

[44] Martin P (1997) Wound healing–aiming for perfect skin regeneration. Science 276: 75–81

[45] Oshima H, Rochat A, Kedzia C, Kobayashi K, Barrandon Y (2001) Morphogenesis and renewal of hair follicles from adult multipotent stem cells. Cell 104: 233–245

[46] Taylor G, Lehrer MS, Jensen PJ, Sun TT, Lavker RM (2000) Involvement of follicular stem cells in forming not only the follicle but also the epidermis. Cell 102: 451–461

[47] Gurtner GC, Werner S, Barrandon Y, Longaker MT (2008) Wound repair and regeneration. Nature 453: 314–321

[48] Ito M, Liu Y, Yang Z, Nguyen J, Liang F, Morris RJ, Cotsarelis G (2005) Stem cells in the hair follicle bulge contribute to wound repair but not to homeostasis of the epidermis. Nat Med 11: 1351–1354

[49] Levy V, Lindon C, Harfe BD, Morgan BA (2005) Distinct stem cell populations regenerate the follicle and interfollicular epidermis. Dev Cell 9: 855–861

[50] Ito M, Yang Z, Andl T, Cui C, Kim N, Millar SE, Cotsarelis G (2007) Wnt-dependent de novo hair follicle regeneration in adult mouse skin after wounding. Nature 447: 316–320

[51] Wodarz A, Nusse R (2003) Mechanisms of Wnt signaling in development. Annu Rev Cell Dev Biol 14: 59

[52] Toy LW (2005) Matrix metalloproteinases: their function in tissue repair. Jo Wound Care 14: 20–22

[53] Lawrence WT (1998) Physiology of the acute wound. Clin Plast Surg 25: 321

[54] Peled ZM, Phelps ED, Updike DL, Chang J, Krummel TM, Howard EW, Longaker MT (2002) Matrix metalloproteinases and the ontogeny of scarless repair: the other side of the wound healing balance. Plast Reconst Surg 110: 801

[55] Dang C (2003) Fetal wound healing current perspectives. Clin Plast Surg 30(1): 13–23

[56] Fathke C, Wilson L, Hutter J, Kapoor V, Smith A, Hocking A, Isik F (2004) Contribution of bone marrow-derived cells to skin: collagen deposition and wound repair. Stem Cells 22: 812–822

[57] Brittan M, Braun KM, Reynolds LE, Conti FJ, Reynolds AR, Poulsom R, Alison MR, Wright NA, Hodivala-Dilke KM (2005) Bone marrow cells engraft within the epidermis and proliferate in vivo with no evidence of cell fusion. J Pathol 205: 1–13

[58] Deng W, Han Q, Liao L, Li C, Ge W, Zhao Z, You S, Deng H, Murad F, Zhao RCH (2005) Engrafted bone marrow-derived Flk-1+ mesenchymal stem cells regenerate skin tissue. Tissue engineering 11: 110–119

[59] Wu Y, Chen L, Scott PG, Tredget EE (2007) Mesenchymal stem cells enhance wound healing through differentiation and angiogenesis. Stem Cells 25: 2648–2659

[60] Chen L, Tredget EE, Wu PYG, Wu Y (2008) Paracrine factors of mesenchymal stem cells recruit macrophages and endothelial lineage cells and enhance wound healing. PLoS One 3: 1886

[61] Kwon DS, Gao X, Liu, YB, Dulchavsky DS, Danyluk AL, Bansal M, Chopp M, McIntosh K, Arbab AS, Dulchavsky SA (2008) Treatment with bone marrownderived stromal cells accelerates wound healing in diabetic rats. Int Wound J 5: 453–463

[62] Suh W, Kim KL, Kim JM, Shin IS, Lee YS, Lee JY, Jang HS, Lee JS, Byun J, Choi JH (2005) Transplantation of endothelial progenitor cells accelerates dermal wound healing with increased recruitment of monocytes/macrophages and neovascularization. Stem Cells 23: 1571–1578

[63] Barcelos LS, Duplaa C, Krankel N, Graiani G, Invernici G, Katare R, Siragusa M, Meloni M, Campesi I, Monica M (2009) Human CD133+ progenitor cells promote the healing of diabetic ischemic ulcers by paracrine stimulation of angiogenesis and activation of Wnt signaling. Circ Res 104(9): 1095–1102

[64] Bucala R, Spiegel LA, Chesney J, Hogan M, Cerami A (1994) Circulating fibrocytes define a new leukocyte subpopulation that mediates tissue repair. Mol Med 1: 71

[65] Yang L, Scott PG, Dodd C, Medina A, Jiao H, Shankowsky HA, Ghahary A, Tredget EE (2005) Identification of fibrocytes in postburn hypertrophic scar. Wound Repair Regen 13: 398–404

[66] Wang JF, Dodd C, Shankowsky HA, Scott PG, Tredget EE (2008) Deep dermal fibroblasts contribute to hypertrophic scarring. Lab Invest 88: 1278–1290

[67] Mori L, Bellini A, Stacey MA, Schmidt M, Mattoli S (2005) Fibrocytes contribute to the myofibroblast population in wounded skin and originate from the bone marrow. Expl Cell Res 304: 81–90

[68] Yagmur C, Akaishi S, Ogawa R, Guneren E (2010) Mechanical receptor-related mechanisms in Scar management: a review and hypothesis. Plast Reconst Surg 126: 426

[69] Souba WW, Fink MP, Jurkovich GJ, Kaiser LP, Pearce WH, Pemberton JH, Soper aNJ (2007) ACS surgery: principles & practice, 6th edn. WebMD Professional Publishing

[70] Ueno C, Hunt TK, Hopf HW (2006) Using physiology to improve surgical wound outcomes. Plast Reconst Surg 117: 59S

[71] Robson MC (1997) Wound infection: a failure of wound healing Caused by an imbalance of bacteria. Surg Clin North Am 77: 637–650

[72] Menke NB, Ward KR, Witten TM, Bonchev DG, Diegelmann RF (2007) Impaired wound healing. Clin Dermatol 25: 19–25

[73] Gibbs J, Cull W, Henderson W, Daley J, Hur K, Khuri SF (1999) Preoperative serum albumin level as a predictor of operative mortality and morbidity: results from the National VA Surgical Risk Study. Arch Surg 134: 36

[74] Jeschke MG, Herndon DN, Ebener C, Barrow RE, Jauch KW (2001) Nutritional intervention high in vitamins, protein, amino acids, and {omega} 3 fatty acids improves protein metabolism during the hypermetabolic state after thermal injury. Arch Surg 136: 1301

[75] Desneves KJ, Todorovic BE, Cassar A, Crowe TC (2005) Treatment with supplementary arginine, vitamin C and zinc in patients with pressure ulcers: a randomised controlled trial. Clin Nutr 24: 979–987

[76] Williams JZ, Abumrad NN, Barbul A (2002) Effect of a specialized amino acid mixture on human collagen synthesis. Ann Surg 236: 369–374

[77] Williams FN, Herndon DN, Kulp GA (2010)Propranolol decreases cardiac work in a dose-dependent manner in severely burned children. Surgery 149(2): 231–239

[78] Demling RH, Orgill DP (2000) The anticatabolic and wound healing effects of the testosterone analog oxandrolone after severe burn injury. J Crit Care 15: 12–17

[79] Pham TN, Klein MB, Gibran NS, Arnoldo BD, Gamelli RL, Silver GM, Jeschke MG, Finnerty CC, Tompkins RG, Herndon DN (2008) Impact of oxandrolone treatment on acute outcomes after severe burn injury. Injury 2: 4

[80] Wicke C, Halliday B, Allen D, Roche NS, Scheuenstuhl H, Spencer MM, Roberts AB, Hunt TK (2000) Effects of steroids and retinoids on wound healing. Arch Surg 135: 1265

[81] Nathens AB, Neff MJ, Jurkovich GJ (2003) Randomized, prospective trial of antioxidant supplementation in critically ill surgical patients. Nutr Clin Pract 18: 264

[82] Fernandez-Madrid F, Prasad AS, Oberleas D (1973) Effect of zinc deficiency on nucleic acids, collagen, and noncollagenous protein of the connective tissue. J Lab Clin Med 82: 951

[83] Andrews M, Gallagher-Allred C (1999) The role of zinc in wound healing. Adv Skin Wound Care 12: 137

[84] Macon WL, Pories WJ (1971) The effect of iron deficiency anemia on wound healing. Plast Reconst Surg 48: 399

[85] Sengupta A, Lichti UF, Carlson BA, Ryscavage AO, Gladyshev VN, Yuspa SH, Hatfield DL, Cobine P (2010) Selenoproteins are essential for proper keratinocyte function and skin development. PloS one 5: 199–209

[86] Colwell AS, Phan TT, Kong W, Longaker MT, Lorenz PH (2005) Hypertrophic scar fibroblasts have increased connective tissue growth factor expression after transforming growth factor-[beta] stimulation. Plast Reconst Surg 116: 1387

[87] Lu L, Saulis AS, Liu WR, Roy NK, Chao JD, Ledbetter S, Mustoe TA (2005) The temporal effects of anti-TGF-[beta] 1, 2, and 3 monoclonal antibody on wound healing and hypertrophic scar Formation. J Am Coll Surg 201: 391–397

[88] Tuan TL, Nichter LS (1998) The molecular basis of keloid and hypertrophic scar formation. Mol MedToday 4: 19–24

[89] Ladwig GP, Robson MC, Liu R, Kuhn M, Muir DF, Schultz GS (2002) Ratios of activated matrix metalloproteinasen9 to tissue inhibitor of matrix metalloproteinasen1 in wound fluids are inversely correlated with healing of pressure ulcers. Wound Repair Regen 10: 26–37

[90] Copcu E (2009) Marjolin's ulcer: a preventable complication of burns? Plast Reconst Surg 124: 156e

[91] Senarath-Yapa K, Enoch S (2009) Management of burns in the community. Wounds UK 5: 1–7

[92] Demling RH, DeSanti L (2010) Managing the burn wound. Burnsurgery.org. 11 December 2010 > http://burnsurgery.org >

Correspondence: Nicole S. Gibran, M.D., Director, UW Burn Center; Professor, Department of Surgery, Harborview Medical Center, Box 359 796, 325 Ninth Avenue, Seattle, WA 98 104, USA, E-mail: nicoleg@u.washington.edu

# Pain management after burn trauma

Richard Girtler, Burkhard Gustorff

Abteilung für Anästhesie und Intensivmedizin am Wilhelminenspital der Stadt Wien, Vienna, Austria

## Introduction

Pain after burn injuries is one of the most severe forms of acute pain. Although wound and pain management have gradually improved over the last years, a sufficient pain management after severe burn trauma is still a global problem and a major challenge for the health care personnel.

An adequate analgesia helps reducing complications and contributes to a faster healing.

Pain management is a vital part in the field of plastic surgery, anesthesia, psychology and physiotherapy.

## Significance of pain management

Severe pain causes a number of various problems in the acute phase after burn injury, during rehabilitation and in the following years.

Apart from that, the relationship between the patient and the health care personnel will be significantly disturbed and the patient's compliance with the therapy will be drastically influenced.

Uncontrolled or inadequately treated pain are associated with:

► Increased tonus of the sympathetic system: this results in declined hemodynamics with disturbed microcirculation and increased oxygen consumption

► Intensified catabolic metabolic status accompanied by weight loss, muscle loss, reduced immunologic resistance and increased risk of infection

► Suppressed breathing and immobility resulting in limited physiotherapy and longer recovery periods.

► Incidence of chronic pain: Persisting pain leads to sensitization in the peripheral and central nervous system an eventually results in a so called pain memory [1]. Up to 50% of the patients with burn injuries suffer from chronic pain [2].

► Incidence of stress disorder: uncontrolled pain and anxiety are high risk factors for acute stress disorder (for a maximum period of 4 weeks) or posttraumatic stress disorder (for a period of more than 6 months). Clinical symptoms include sleep disorders, increased nervousness, permanent psychic tension and depression. These symptoms affect all therapy phases negatively. A comparison of retrospective studies on surviving children after burn trauma from the years 1993–1994, 1998 and 2001 showed increased administration of opioids and benzodiazepines in this patient group whereas incidence of acute stress disorders decreased significantly during the same period [3].

► Economic problems caused by high costs.

# Pathophysiology of pain after burn injuries

Pain after burn injuries has various reasons and sources. Burn depth and pain intensity are not always directly related. Thus, a solid fundamental knowledge of physiology and pathogenesis of burn injury pain is an important prerequisite for an adequate therapy and medication.

## Nociceptive pain

Pain caused by stimulating the nociceptors play a vital role. Nociceptive pain has signal and warning functions for the human organism.

Nociceptors are situated at the free ends of the pain conducting nerve fibres. Depending on their localizations they are subdivided into somatic nociceptors (in the muscles, tendons, joints, bones and skin) and visceral nociceptors. A large proportion of them are sleeping nociceptors which can only be stimulated when inflammation occurs. Nociceptors are stimulated by chemical, thermal and mechanical noxa. This stimulation is conducted to the posterior horn of the spinal cord in the form of evoked potentials (translocation) via richly myelinated and fast conducting Aδ-fibers (giving sharp and terebrant pain that can be easily located) and unmyelinated and slowly conducting C-fibres (giving permanent dull pain that cannot be easily located). In the spinal cord stimulating amino acids, as for example aspartate and glutamate, and substance P and calcitonine gene related peptide (CGRP) are set free, which causes the transmission to second order neurons (nociceptive-specific neurons and wide dynamic range neurons). The second order neurons conduct the pain impulses via the tractus spinothalamicus and the tractus spinoreticularis to the thalamus and then to cortical areas. The somatosensoric pain processing is carried out in the lateral thalamocortical pain processing system whereas the medial thalamocortical pain processing system shows connections to the limbic system. Here affective nociception occurs.

Nociception can be treated well with opioids and non-opioids.

## Inflammation-related pain

Tissue trauma sets free inflammatory mediators (prostaglandines, cytokines, oxygen radicals. histamine, bradykinine and platelet activating factor). These cause a peripheral sensitization with decreasing the stimulus threshold of the nociceptors (primary hyperalgesia). Inflammation-related pain occurs within minutes and is reversible after wound healing.

Persistent and repeatedly occurring inflammation-related pain might be caused by wound infection [1].

Continuous nociceptive inflow from the periphery sensitizes secondary nociceptive neurons in the posterior horn of the spinal cord (central sensitization). Their reaction to stimuli is an increased discharging frequency. Thus a higher number of glutamate, substance P and CGRP are set free, glutamate receptors are depolarized (AMPA receptors, NMDA receptors) and calcium flows into central pain neurons. Via expression of immediate early genes, the receptive areas in the periphery, with an increased sensitivity to pain in the neighboring unaffected area of the primary lesion, are enlarged [4].

## Neuropathic pain

Neuropathic pain is caused by injury, deafferenciation, illness or functional disorders of the afferent nervous system. This kind of pain does not have any biological function and causes severe suffering and is often resistant to therapy.

The disorders in the afferent system can be accompanied by negative phenomena (hypesthesia and hypalgesia) and positive phenomena (paresthesia, dysesthesia, hyperalgesia, allodynia and burning, terebrant pain).

Neuropathic pain after burns can occur directly or after a period of time: on the one hand burns damage and partially destroy nerve structures. Some studies showed that neuropathic pain already occurred within 1 to 7 days after the burn injury happened [5]. On the other hand neuropathic sensation or pain can also occur a long time after the healing of a burn wound [6, 7]. It is assumed that this is due to an unsuccessful regeneration of the nerves with ingrowth of damaged neurons to neighboring healthy nerves or the formation of neurons.

Neuropathic pain occurs at the burn wound itself (especially IIb and III grade burns) as well as at donor sites for skin grafting.

Cyclooxygenasis-inhibitors are not effective in this case and the effective dose of opioids is increased.

## Special case: phantom-limb pain

Sensations of pain in a limb that has been amputated are called phantom-limb pain. Afferent fibers are cut at their axons and during regeneration an upregulation of sodium canals with an alteration of the sensoric afferences occurs. The uncontrolled sprouting of the ends of C- and demyelinised Aδ-fibres can generate neurons. On the peripheric level this results in spontaneous, ectopic impulses and an increased sensitivity to thermal and mechanic stimuli. Apart from that morphologic and biochemical alteration at the spinal cord and the cortical level (central plasticity) also play a role in the incidence of phantom-limb pain [4].

50 % of the relevant patients suffer from chronic pain after amputation of extremities (phantom-limb pain and stump pain) [8]. Phantom-limb pain occurs significantly more often after amputation due to an electrical burn injury than after amputation due to a flame burn injury [9]. A consequent multimodal treatment can minimize the incidence of chronic pain after burn injuries.

## *Sympathetically Maintained Pain (SMP)*

Sympathetically Maintained Pain occurs due to interaction or pathological linkage between sympathetical postganglionic neurons and primary afferent neurons after trauma with or without nerve injury.

Clinical indications are allodynia, hyperalgesia, autonomous disorders (sweating, perfusion and trophicity) and distal swelling of extremities.

A promising treatment is blocking the sympathetic nervous system. Depending on localization and risk factors, continuous sympathetic blockades with local anesthetics (e. g. ganglion stellatum) or neurolysis with alcohol or radio frequency thermolesions (e. g. thoracal trunk) are carried out. Neurolysis requires imaging diagnostics, sometimes accompanied by computertomographic checks.

## Complex regional pain syndrome (CRPS)

Complex regional pain syndrome is a disorder which occurs after injuries of the extremities. There are 2 forms of CRPS: type 1 (no injuries of the peripheral nerves) and type 2 (injured nerves). CRPS can occur anytime after sever flame burns or electrical burns [10–13].

# Pain rating and documentation

Patients with burn injuries suffer from various forms of pain to various times (chronic pain, breakthrough pain, pain caused by the treatment and postinterventional pain). These forms of pain require dynamic and flexible management. A regular and standardized documentation of the pain is the key to a successful pain management.

Sensation of pain is subjective and individual. Thus, sometimes the degree of the burn may be the same but the pain the patients suffer from may be different in each case.

Currently there are numerous ways to rate pain (one-dimensional scales, multi-dimensional scales and behavior-oriented scales). A one-dimensional scale is sufficient for the documentation of acute pain:

▶ Numerical analog scale (0–100; 0 = no pain, 100 worst possible pain)
▶ Visual analog scale (10 cm vertical scale, no subdivisions; bottom = no pain, top = worst possible pain)
▶ Verbal rating scale (no pain, mild pain, severe pain, very severe pain, extremely severe pain)

During rehabilitation pain can also be documented by multi-dimensional questionnaires, as for example the McGill Pain Questionnaire [14].

For children (approximately aged 4 to 10) it is recommended to use images to describe their pain as for example the faces pain rating scale.

Patients who cannot articulate their pain verbally need to be observed carefully and their pain can be rated due to behavior-oriented treatments:

In the intensive care unit, pain of patients who are analgo-sedated and are receiving artificial respiration, can be rated by means of the Behavioral Pain Scale (BPS), (see also Intensive care patient/Analgesia monitoring and Fig. 2) [15].

In older and cognitively limited persons it is recommended to use the Abbey Pain Scale [16]. In infants it is recommended to use the FLACC-Score [17] or the discomfort and pain scale for children [18].

In addition, fear and anxiety should also be rated in all burn patients. This can be done by applying the Burn Specific Pain Anxiety Scale [19].

Pain is measured at rest as well as on movement. Here, the pain quality (chronic pain, breakthrough pain, pain caused by the treatment) should be rated separately. Pain after the administration of analgesics must also be rated in regular intervals to document the efficacy or inefficacy of the analgesics.

In the early phase after the burn trauma, rating should be carried out every 2 to 4 hours. In pain-controlled patients it is sufficient to rate the pain twice a day. All collected data must be diligently documented. By visualizing the pain it is possible to identify the pain intensity in sufficient time and to evaluate the efficacy of the pain management correctly.

The rating procedures must be sufficiently explained to the patients. The nursing staff must also be trained and instructed regularly about the procedures. The patients' pain must not be evaluated based on the personal experiences of the health care professional. Studies have shown wide gaps between the self-assessment of the burn patient and the observational assessment done by the health care personnel [20].

A standardized pain rating contributes to a successful pain management: patients suffering from pain can be identified systematically and in due time. In addition it is possible to define an exact titration of opioids as well as target parameters with the health care personnel and the patient.

## Pain management and analgesics

### Pharmacokinetics in severe burns

Severe burns cause drastic alterations in the pharmacokinetics of numerous pharmaceuticals.

► Immediately after the burn trauma, burn patients might develop a systemic inflammatory response syndrome (SIRS) which causes massive hemodynamic alterations. The clearance of the pharmaceuticals is reduced due to a hypoperfusion of the

organs caused by macro and microcirculatory disorders. In the hypermetabolic phase that follows, the clearance of the pharmaceuticals is increased.

► In burns >20% body surface the incidence of a generalized capillary leak and high protein loss through the wound and into the interstitium is increased. Alterations in the overall protein content cause differences in the fraction of protein-bound and non- protein-bound free pharmaceuticals. That is the reason why the effect of pharmaceuticals with high protein binding (e. g. benzodiazepines) is difficult to manage.

► During the management of severe burns the total body water increases and the volume of distribution of numerous pharmaceuticals is increased. Especially in intensive care patients the alteration of the volume can come up to several liters, which can cause a redistribution of the active substances into the extracellular space within a few hours. There the pharmaceuticals can not be effective anymore. This apparent drug tolerance must not be confused with a pharmacodynamic drug tolerance.

► In large burns a considerable amount of pharmaceuticals is lost through the wound surface.

### Form of administration [21]

In the acute phase it is recommended to administer intravenously.

Intramuscular or subcutaneous injections must be avoided since the resorption ratio in the muscles and the skin vary, the action time is delayed (compared to an intravenous application) and the injection causes unnecessary pain. In the acute phase after the burn trauma, skin and muscles are constricted to a maximum. Thus this paper does not provide any information on the dosage for an intramuscular administration.

A peroral administration can start as soon as the patient is ready to receive it and if there are no contra-indications as for example gastrointestinal motility or resorption disorders.

Transdermal administration is only recommended if the skin is not damaged or already healed. Scarred areas do not give good indications of the resorption ratio. Furthermore, the patches might loosen from the wound during the numerous therapeutical measures and thus limit their efficacy.

## Modified WHO pain ladder (see Fig. 1)

Depending on pain intensity and pain history the application of the (modified) WHO pain ladder can be recommended: Therapy starts either on stage 1 and is increased until sufficient analgetics are administered or already begins on a higher stage, which is often necessary in burn injuries.

## Non-opioids (Table 1)

It is recommended to apply basic treatment with non-opioids. Side effects and possible complications as mentioned below should always be considered.

Non-opioids reduce the opioid requirement by 20% to 30% [22]. NSAID can reduce the side effects caused by opioids significantly [23]. By blocking the cyclooxygenasis or blocking the development of PG E2, a stimulation of the NMDA-receptor-NO system with development of an opioid tolerance and opioid-induced hyperalgesia can be reduced [24, 25].

### Paracetamol

Paracetamol is part of the non-acidic antipyretic analgesics. The exact mechanism of the analgentic and antipyretic effects has not been fully investigated yet. However, central and peripheral points of action might play a role in the efficacy of paracetamol. Influences to the serotonergic system have already been verified [26].

The maximum daily dose for adults of normal weight is 4 000 mg, maximum dose for children is 60 mg/kgBW. Daily doses of paracetamol above 100 mg/kgBW (6 g to 8 g daily) are hepatoxic. It has to be considered though that the administration of the normal daily dose can also cause liver cell necrosis and liver failure in case of pre-existing liver disorders and/or glutathione deficiency. N-acetycysteine is an efficient antidote and should be administered within 10 hours after the overdosage if possible.

A contra-indication for administering paracetamol is the presence of severe liver insufficiency.

| Step I | Step II | Step III |
|---|---|---|
| Non-opiod analgesics NSAID, Coxibe Metamizole Paracetamol | Weak/Moderate opioids Tramadol Pethidine + Step 1 | Strong opioids Morphine Hydromorphone Fentanyl Oxycodon Methadon +Step 1 |

Ketamin, anticonvulsants, antidepressants

Treatment without medication

Regional anesthetic

**Fig. 1.** Modified WHO pain ladder

Paracetamol should be administered carefully if the patient suffers from chronic alcoholism or chronic malnutrition as in these cases the reserves of hepatic glutathione are low. Paracetamol can be administered enterally, parenterally or rectally. The benefits of an intravenous administration is a rapid invasion of the active ingredients into the central nervous system. Compared to an oral administration, an intra-

**Table 1.** Pharmacological data of non-opioids

| Active Ingredient | HL (h) | Administration | Single dose in adults (mg) | Daily maximum dose (mg) |
|---|---|---|---|---|
| Diclofenac | 1–2 | p. o., i. v. | 50–75 | 150 |
| Ibuprofen | 1,5–2,5 | p. o. | 200–800 | 2400 |
| Lornoxicam | 3–4 | p. o., i. v. | 8 | 16 |
| Paracetamol | 1,5–2,5 | p. o. | 500–1000 | 4000 |
| | | i. v. | 1000 | 4000 |
| Metamizole | 2–4 | p. o. | 500–1000 | 4000 |
| | | i. v. | 1000–2500 | 5000 |
| Celecoxib | 11 | p. o. | 100–200 | 400 |
| Parecoxib | ~22 | i. v. | 40 | 80 |

venous administration takes effect faster and more effectively [27]. The analgesic effect of paracetamol administered intravenously occurs within 5 to 10 minutes and generally persists for 4 to 6 hours.

Among all non-opioids only paracetamol can be administered safely during pregnancy and lactation period.

## Metamizole

Metamizole belongs to the non-acidic antipyretic analgesics. It is one of the most efficient non-opioids and additionally has a spasmolytic effect.

The exact mechanism of metamizole is still unknown. Basically it is assumed that it has a central effect. An additional peripheral analgesic effect by inhibiting the prostaglandinesynthesis is described for pyrazolonederivates [28].

Metamizole does not combine in acidic tissue, does not have any pharmacologically active metabolites and is mostly egested renally. Compared to NSAID, the benefit of metamizole is few interaction with the thrombocyte function. Metamizole can be administered enterally, parenterally, intramuscularly, and rectally. Contrary to most of the NSAID, metamizole can be administered in any form to children of 3 months and older. A single dose for an adult is between 1 g and 2.5 g with a daily maximum dose of 5 g. In children it is recommended to administer 10 mg/kg/BW to 25 mg/kgBW orally or rectally and 10 mg/kgBW to 15 mg/kgBW intravenously every 4 to 6 hours.

The risk of agranulocytosis is described controversially, with incidences of 1 : 1,000,000 [29] to 1 : 1,451 in Sweden [30]. The risk of an agranulocytosis during a permanent therapy with metamizole can be minimized by regular blood counts. A rapid infusion of metamizole can cause severe hypotonia due to anaphylactoid reactions.

## Non-steroidal antirheumatics (NSAID)

NSAID have analgesic, antipyretic and antiphlogistic effects. They are nonselective inhibitors of the enzyme cyclooxygenasis, which plays a key role in the prostaglandine synthesis. They are bound with more than 90 % to plasmaproteins and enrich in tissue that has been altered by inflammation.

The mechanism relevant for an analgesic therapy might be the rise in the excitation threshold of nociceptors after inhibition of the prostaglandine synthesis. The anatomic area of action of the substances has not been fully explained yet, however central and peripheral points of action have been described so far.

NSAID have numerous side-effects. When administered only for a short-time, renal disorders and disorders in the thrombocyte function are most commonly observed. The risk of post-surgical bleeding under therapy with non-opioids is discussed controversially. The bleeding time is increased by approximately 30 % under the administration of NSAID. Thus, due to the inhibition of the thrombocyte aggregation, NSAID should only be administered when there is no more need for a bleeding intensive necrosectomy.

In a long-term administration, gastric, cardiac and renal effects are most commonly observed.

▶ Diclofenac: Approved for short-term administration (max. 2 weeks). No recommendation for children younger than 14 years. However, the administration is very common in numerous countries due to lack of alternatives. Dosage: 50 mg to 150 mg daily in 2 or 3 single doses.

▶ Lornoxicam: Not recommended for children and teenagers younger than 18 years. No special dosage instructions for older patients. Dosage: 8 mg to 16 mg daily in 2 or 3 single doses.

▶ Ibuprofen: Ibuprofen does not have many side-effects. It shows the lowest ulcerogenic potency of all NSAID. As syrup approved for children and infants from the age of 6 months.

## Selective cyclooxygenasis-2-inhibitors

The discovery of at least 2 cyclooxygenasis-isoenzymes has lead to the development of a cyclogenasis-2 selective group of analgesics, which differs from the other NSAID particularly because of their missing thrombocyte function disorder and the significantly reduced gastro-intestinal side-effects.

However, numerous large-scale randomized studies showed a cardiovascular toxicity [31–33]. According to the recommendation of the European Medicines Agency, selective cyclooxygenase-2-inhibitors are contra-indicated in the presence of clinically diagnosed coronary heart disorders, clinically diagnosed cerebrovascular disorders or heart diseases (NYHA II-IV). The risk of an acute renal failure is similar to when administering NSAID.

Selective cyclooxygenasis-2-inhibitors are not approved for persons under 18 years of age.

► Parecoxib: Approved for the short-term treatment (48 hours) of post-surgical pain. Recommended dosage is 40 mg and it is administered intravenously or intramuscularly. After a period of 12 hours, another 20 mg or 40 mg can be administered again. There are no special dosage recommendations for older patients. Due to the missing effect on the thrombocyte function, parecoxib is suitable for pain management after skin grafting or debridement.

► Celecoxib: Administered orally, daily dosage 200 mg in 1 or 2 single doses.

## Opioids (Table 2)

Opioids are the fundamental substances in pain management of severe burn injuries. Due to their various possibilities of application, opioids are suitable for all stages of the treatment.

Apart from the typical side effects as for example depressed breathing, bradycardia, obstipation, nausea and itching, the following facts have to be considered:

► After a short time of administration, opioids induce adaptation mechanisms and cause the development of functional antagonisms, which might lead to an opioid tolerance or an opioid-induced hyperalgesia [34, 35]. Whereas in an opioid tolerance the dosage of the analgesic has to be increased to have the same effect, in an opioid-induced hyperalgesia the sensation of pain is stronger. Although both phenomena have different pathophysiologic mechanisms, the activation of NMDA-receptors plays a key role in both cases [36–38]. It is recommended to combine opioids with NMDA-receptor antagonists.

► Liver and renal disorders cause an alteration of the pharmacokinetics of opioids. In the presence of liver insufficiency an increased bio-availability of morphine, hydromorphone and pethidine through reduction of the first-pass-metabolism has to be anticipated.

**Table 2.** Pharmacological data of opioids

| Active Ingredient | HL (h) | Administration | Single dose in adults (mg) | Action time (h) |
|---|---|---|---|---|
| Trama-dol* | 6–7 | p. o. | from 50 | 4–6 |
| | | p. o. (retard) | from 100 | 12 |
| | | i. v. | 100 | 4–6 |
| Morphine | 2–3 | p. o. | from 10 | 3–4 |
| | | p. o. (retard) | from 10 | 8–12 |
| | | i. v. (PCA-dose) | from 2 | lock out time 10–15 min |
| Fentanyl | 3–4 | TTS | from 0,6 mg/24h | 72 (48) |
| | | i. v. (PCA-dose) | 30–40 µg | lock out time 5 min |
| Hydro-morphone | 2–3 | p. o. | from 1,3 | 4–6 |
| | | p. o. (retard) | from 4 | 8–12 |
| | | i. v. | 1–1,5 | 3–4 |
| | | i. v. (PCA-dose) | from 0,2 | lock out time 5–10 min |
| Oxyco-done | 4–6 | p. o. | from 5 | 4–6 |
| | | p. o. (retard) | from 10 | 8–12 |
| | | i. v. | 1–10 | 4 |
| | | v. (PCA-dose) | 0.03 mg/kg | lock out time at least 5 min |
| Levo-metha-done | 20–55 | p. o. | from 2 | 6–12 |
| | | i. v. (PCA-dose) | from 0,5 | lock out time 5–10 min |
| Piritram-ide | 2–4 | i. v. | 15 | 6–8 |
| | | i. v. (PCA-dose) | 1–2 | lock out time 10–15 min |

* Max. Daily dosage: 400 mg–600 mg

- A renal insufficiency can cause the onset of active metabolites, e. g.:
- Morphine-6-glukuronid: little analgesic but significant sedating effect
- Morphine-3-glukuronid: pronociceptive, excitatoric effect [39]. A cumulation can be co-responsible for the development of an opioid tolerance [34].
- Norpethidine: neurotoxic effect

Thus the administration of opioids should always be embedded in a multimodal treatment. Due to different metabolites and different response rates to the opioid receptors, the opioid rotation is an important option. To administer the correct quantity during a change of opioids it is recommended to start with 50 % of the calculated equivalence dosage of the new opioid to be able to titrate as needed. This procedure is reasonable since the present equivalence tables are suited only for opioid naïve patients and due to a tolerance development the dosage equivalence varies greatly.

The genetic polymorphism with multiple isoforms for the μ-, κ-, and δ-receptors is the reason why the effects of opioids can interindividually be very different. Thus the dosage must be determined individually. In older or weak patients the initial dosage should be reduced and the effect of the initial dosage should be taken into consideration when further dosages are determined.

Any opioid-caused effect can be reversed immediately and entirely by administering a specific antagonist as for example Naloxon.

## Weak opioids

The daily dosage of weak opioids must be obeyed.

## Tramadol

Tramadol is an analgesic with a combination of opioid-antagonistic effects and re-uptake inhibition of serotonine and noradrenaline. It is available either as delayed-action preparation or non-delayed action preparation. In addition it is available as parenterally injectable pharmacon. It is suitable for the therapy of acute and chronic pain. Compared to morphine and other opioids, Tramadol's breathing depressing effect and its inhibition of the gastro-intestinal tract

are weaker. However, there is a higher incidence of vomiting and nausea. Due to genetic polymorphisms in the cytochrome oxydase system the analgesic effect of Tramadol is limited in some patients (appr. 10 % in Caucasians) [40].

Tramadol is also effective in the treatment of neuropathic pain [41]. Neuropathic pain might play a role in chronic pain after burn trauma (see III. Pathophysiology of pain after burn injuries/3. Neuropathic pain). However, the current literature does not provide any evaluation of the effects of Tramadol on neuropathic pain in burn patients.

## Pethidine

Although pethidine is slowly but steadily replaced by more modern preparations in numerous European countries, it still remains one of the most important analgesic medication throughout the world. Pethidine is a μ-receptor agonist with a 0.1–0.2 fold analgesic potence of morphine. Onset of action takes place after 5 minutes and lasts for 2 to 3 hours. During degradation the active neurotoxic metabolite norpethidine is produced which, when acculmulated, can cause convulsion and myoclonus. Thus pethidine is suitable for intravenous administration in acute cases but not as continuous treatment. Pethidine reduces the post operative shivering better than morphine. In addition it shows the least spasmogenicity of all opioids. Currently it is particularly used in the initial treatment of children with burn trauma.

## Strong opioids

There is no clinically relevant maximum dosage for strong opioids.

## Morphine

In pain management morphine is commonly used as reference opioid throughout the world. It can be administered orally or parenterally. Due to its high first-pass effect its bioavailability is only 20 %–40 %. When administered orally, the dosage needs to be 3-fold higher than when administered parenterally. Morphine is degraded in the liver to morphine-3-glucuronide (pronociceptive effect) and morphine-

6-glucuronide (sedating effect). These metabolites show a significantly higher elimination half-life (up to 72 hours) than morphine. In the presence of renal insufficiency both metabolites might accumulate. After intravenous administration the onset of maximum action takes place after 15 to 30 minutes. The action time of a single dosage is 3 to 5 hours. Possible side effects are a dosage-dependent respiratory depression and vasodilatoric effects as well as release of histamines with vasodilatation and bronchoconstriction.

## Piritramide

Piritramide is a μ-receptor agonist with a relative activity of 0.7 compared to morphine. It is very well suitable in post-operative intravenous pain management, in the intensive care unit and as patient-controlled analgesic. The onset of action takes place after 5 to 10 minutes and generally lasts for 4 to 6 hours. The sedative components are stronger than those of morphine. Piritramide acts hardly euphorizing and its spasmogenicity is low.

## Fentanyl

The potency of fentanyl is 100-fold higher than the potency of morphine (analgesic and side effects). A dosage of 100 μg equals approximately 10 mg morphine. It maintains the cardiac stability and has a high therapeutic index. Compared to morphine the histamine release remains low.

**Forms of administration:**
▶ Intravenous: The onset of maximum action takes place after 4 to 5 minutes and the time of action is 20 to 30 minutes. Fentanyl is officially approved for intraoperative analgesia (with artificial respiration) and for analgosedation in the intensive care unit. However, fentanyl is more and more used in awake patients not receiving artificial respiration: a successful administration of fentanyl in combination with propofol for the analgosedation of non-intubated children (5 to 60 months, ASA II-III, TBSA 5%-25%) during dressing change after skin grafting has been described [42]. Linneman et al. have investigated the effect of fentanyl in 55 burn patients (9 months to 75 years) in a

retrospective study. 31% of the patients developed a transient respiratory depression. However, additional oxygen or intubation have not been necessary for any patient. With adequate monitoring and in the presence of an anesthetist the administration of fentanyl during dressing change is described as effective and secure [43].
▶ Intravenous PCA: The patient-controlled analgesia with fentanyl during dressing change in burn patients is very effective. Signs of circulatory insufficiency or respiratory depression have not been described [44]. Recommended pump programming: bolus of 30 μg fentanyl with a lock-out time of 5 minutes after an initial loading dose of 1 μg/kg fentanyl.
▶ Transdermal: Only suitable for chronic pain management and in the presence of adequate resorption areas. Onset of action takes place after 12 to 24 hours.
▶ Oromucosal: Suitable in case of breakthrough pain despite of a permanent opioid therapy (see also breakthrough pain).

## Hydromorphone

Hydromorphone is a μ-receptor agonist and its analgesic potency is 6 to 7.5-fold higher than the analgesic potency of morphine. It can be administered orally (non-retarded, retarded) and parenterally injectably. Hydromorphone shows a favorable pharmacological profile due to its lack of active metabolites and its low plasma protein binding (appr. 8%). Thus it is particularly suitable, also for permanent treatment, for patients suffering from renal insufficiency.

## Oxycodone

Oxycodone acts at the μ-receptors and also at the κ- and δ-receptors. In case of decreasing analgesic effects of a permanent opioid treatment, the rotation to oxycodone may have positive effects. Apart from that, oxycodone has been described as particularly effective in neuropathic pain [45, 46].

It has a bioavailability of 70% to 87% and its analgesic potency is comparable to morphine. Metabolites of oxycodone are noroxycodone and oxymorphone, both showing only very low analgesic activity. The level of active metabolites in the blood is not significantly increased during a permanent oxycodone treatment. However, the plasma concentration can be increased in patients suffering from renal and liver insufficiency.

It can be administered in non-retarded (onset of action takes place after 15 to 25 minutes, action time 4 to 6 hours) and retarded (onset of action takes place after 60 minutes, action time 8 to 12 hours) form and is also available as parenterally injectable solution (rapid onset of action within 2 to 5 minutes, action time 4 hours). 2 mg orally administered oxycodone equals 1 mg parenterally administered oxycodone. However, due to individually different responses, a careful dosage titration is essential.

## L-Methadone

L-Methadone is a μ-receptor agonist with low addiction potential and a 2 to 3-fold higher potency than morphine. It is not suitable for acute pain management as its action time is relatively long and not clearly predictable. Apart from that there is a high risk of accumulation, particularly in the presence of liver insufficiency.

In addition to its action at the opioid receptors, methadone has also antagonistic properties at the NMDA receptors. During a permanent opioid treatment with tolerance development, a rotation to methadone can improve analgesia.

In a patient (TBSA 55%) with chronic neuropathic pain after wound healing, the rotation to methadone could reduce the pain by 70% and improve the quality of life significantly [47].

## Remifentanil

Remifentanil is an ultra short-acting, very well controllable opioid. Its potency is 200-fold higher than morphine. It is used intraoperatively during sedoanalgesia and in the intensive care unit (see IX. intensive care patients/6.2. analgesia). In single cases remifentanil is used with adequate monitoring for the treatment of burn pain in patients not receiving artificial respiration.

## Other analgesics

### Ketamine (see also intensive care unit and analgosedation)

Ketamine is used during sedoanalgesia in the intensive care unit and in the treatment of opioid-induced hyperalgesia and opioid tolerance as well as in chronic pain.

Literature provides numerous studies concerning the supplementation of an opioid therapy with ketamine in low, subanesthetic doses [48]. Psychomimetic side effects have only been reported in single cases.

Repeated surgical interventions as well as opioid therapy cause the activation of NMDA receptors. The effect of opioids is reduced due to a sensitization of the NMDA receptors through opioid induced hyperalgesia and opioid tolerance [49]. The application of NMDA receptor antagonists can lessen or inhibit these antinociceptive effects [50].

Weinbroum et al. showed that administering 250 μg/kg Ketamine in postoperative ineffectiveness of strong opioids could sufficiently relieve the pain [51].

Furthermore, an intraoperative intravenous administration of ketamine can reduce the postoperative demand for opioids and the opioid-induced side effects [52]. This effect should be taken advantage of after painful interventions with high demand for opioids (e.g. debridements in burn patients). Single studies show that a perioperative intravenous administration of ketamine can reduce the incidence of postoperative chronic pain [53, 54].

When administered for sedation during painful procedures stationary, ketamine is also effective and secure in children with burn trauma. An analysis of 347 sedations with administering ketamine according to a strict protocol and adequate monitoring showed a very low number (10 i.e. 2.9%) of complications that required interventions like oxygenation or volume substitution [55].

Compared to the racemate ketamine the analgesic potency of S(+)-ketamine is twice as high and has fewer psychomimetic side effects. Thus, when administering S(+)-ketamine half of the dosage of the racemate is sufficient.

## Anticonvulsants (Gabapentin and Pregabalin)

Gabapentin is important in numerous clinical settings: initially is was developed as an anticonvulsant for the treatment of epileptic partial seizures. However, nowadays gabapentin is a commonly used drug in the treatment of neuropathic pain of various causes. Additionally, several clinical studies have shown its effectiveness in the treatment of anxiety disorder [56–58]. Gabapentin also reduces the postoperative need for opioids and the opioid-induced side effects [59]. It is assumed that gabapentin has an antihyperalgetic component [60].

The exact mechanism of action remains unknown. The α2-δ-subunits of the voltage-dependent calcium channel were identified as binding spots. By inhibiting the calcium influx, the release of substance P, glutamate and calcitonin gene related peptide (CGRP) is suppressed.

In clinically relevant concentrations gabapentin does not bind to other receptors in the brain. In several in vitro test systems gabapentin decreased partially the effect on the glutamate agonist N-methyl-D-aspartic acid, however only in concentrations over 100 μg, which cannot be achieved in vivo.

Gabapentin does not bind to plasma proteins. There is no evidence of metabolism and it is only renally excreted. The dosage of gabapentin should thus be determined depending on the renal function of the patient (e.g. dependent on creatinine clearance).

To avoid side effects it is recommended to find the correct dosage by titrating: initially 300 mg once daily and after that depending on reaction and tolerance increase of the daily dosage in steps of 300 mg every second to third day until a maximum dosage of 3 600 mg daily is reached. In children of 6 years and older the initial daily total dosage is 10 mg/kg/day to 15 mg/kg/day dependent on the dosage of the onset therapy. The maximum daily dosage should be administered in three single doses as in adults. Dosages up to 40 mg/kg have proven well tolerated in clinical studies.

The usage of gabapentin in the management of burn injuries is still not sufficiently evaluated. A small study with burn patients (mean total burned surface area 25 %) showed that gabapentin could reduce significantly the opioid consumption and pain intensity. From day 3 to day 24 after the burn accident patients were administered 2 400 mg gabapentin in 3 single doses [61].

The neuropathic component of burn pain is often misinterpreted and has not been evaluated very extensively so far. Gabapentin could be administered successfully in a case series of 6 patients, who developed burning (neuropathic) pain in the area of the burned skin or the donor sites for skin grafting within 1 to 7 days after the burn accident [5].

Furthermore, a study in 35 children (6 months to 15 years of age) with severe itching of the healing burns showed that gabapentin could improve the symptoms significantly within 24 hours [62].

Pregabalin is a structure-related anticonvulsant and has the same mechanism of action as gabapentin. However, its pharmacological properties are better (oral bioavailability independent of the dosage, linear dose-effect relation). The initial dose is 150 mg in 2 single doses, the daily maximum dosage is 600 mg.

## Antidepressants with analgesic effects

Depression and pain are very often closely related and show several similarities in their psychopathology and pharmacology. A dysfunction of ascending and descending serotonergic and noradrenergic tracts not only can cause depressive syndromes but also maintain the pain syndromes.

Thus, antidepressants are a very important part of the multimodal general treatment of burn patients [63]. A study group from Texas showed that an early administration of antidepressants in children with burn trauma could treat acute stress reactions successfully [64]. An intensifying effect of descending and ascending serotonergic and noradrenergic tracts by antidepressants can inhibit the pain signals from the body's periphery and the intestines. The analgesic effect occurs mostly with a time lag of several days up to 3 weeks. Currently, the literature does not provide any studies concerning the analgesic effects of antidepressants in burn patients.

▸ Tricyclic antidepressant (TCA) as for example amitryptiline: For a long time the use of TCA was the golden standard in the coanalgesia with antidepressants. A downside of TCA is the high potential for anticholinergic side effects. Apart from disorders in the stimulus conduction of the heart and orthostatic hypotension, there may also occur weight gain, obstipation, retention of urine, dry mouth, impaired vision and cognitive limitation.

▶ Serotonin noradrenaline reuptake inhibitors (SNRI) as for example venlafaxine, milnacipran, duloxetine: In pain management, dually effective antidepressants are equally effective as TCA. However, they have significantly less severe side effects and a lower toxicity. Vomiting and nausea can be reduced by a slow dosage titration during the initial therapy phase. When administering venlafaxine the risk of arterial hypertonia must be considered. Furthermore the QTc-interval can be longer and arrythmia might occur. Milnycipran is recommended in patients with polypharmacy because it is not metabolized in the liver by cytochrome P450.

## Regional anesthesia

Regional anesthesia is an effective additional option in the analgesic therapy and can be applied if there are no objections concerning hygiene to a sterile catheterization. However in severe burns the increased bacterial colonization (e. g. pseudomonas aeruginosa) has to be considered. A precondition for a secure application is regular nursing and checking.

Potential benefits of regional anesthesia are the reduced vigilance impairment as a result of lower opioid administration and the possible preventive effects concerning chronic pain syndromes. Furthermore an epidural catheter improves perfusion and intestinal motility due to sympathicolysis (application of local anesthetics).

In any phase of the burn trauma management the indication to the following blockades should be examined:

▶ epidural anesthesia
▶ intercostal blockade
▶ blockade of the plexus brachialis (interscalenary, intraclaviculary and axillary)
▶ 3 in 1 block, fascia iliaca block, psoascompartment block
▶ single nerve blockades

Apart from the continuous supply of the local anesthetic or the opioid a patient-controlled analgesia with bolus administration is also possible. Due to the few data that exist for perineural PCA systems, no extensive recommendations concerning basal rates, gap intervals and bolus size can be given.

Some studies have already examined the topic application of local anesthetics with differing success.

## Pain management without analgesics

In awake, responsive and cooperative patients, various treatments without the use of analgesics can be additionally applied.

### Adequate communication

Lack of communication about diagnostic and therapeutic measures causes anxiety, frustration and rejection to the therapy in the patients. Burn patients need thoughtful support in all phases of the treatment. They need more information and more communication than any other patient group. A thorough explanation of the pain management concept to the patient (and the personnel) improves the compliance in the practical application.

### Psychological techniques [65]

Interventions in the field of behavior therapy have proven effective in the treatment of chronic pain. It has also been shown that behavior therapy is also effective in the treatment of acute pain.

Those interventions can only be carried out by professional psychologists. Psychological techniques are useful to relieve anxiety and worries. Patients should be given advice on how to cope with the treatment-induced pain and the rehabilitation phase.

In burn patients the psychological therapy must start as early as possible. In the initial phase it should be evaluated how susceptible the patient is to such a treatment.

For a perioperative treatment, techniques which are effective without a long training phase are recommended.

- Cognitive behavioral therapy (e.g. distraction techniques, cognitive revaluation, positive visualization): Pain reduction could be verified [66]
- Relaxation techniques (e.g. guided imagination with or without music): These techniques carried out before, during and after medical interventions could reduce postinterventional pain [67–70].
- Hypnosis: The effectiveness of hypnosis in pain and analgesics consumption is verified by meta analysis [71]. Furthermore it could be proven that preoperative anxiety could be reduced [72]. However, the success of this technique depends greatly on the individual susceptibility of the patient. Compared to stress reducing strategies, hypnosis has shown to relieve anxiety better in burn patients with frequent dressing change [73].

## Transcutaneous electrical nerve stimulation (TENS)

Electrical impulses are applied to the skin by electrodes. Generally, frequencies between 1Hz and 100Hz are used. The electrodes are placed in the vicinity of the painful areas. The stimulus itself does not cause any pain. Low-frequency stimulation (1Hz to 4Hz) releases autogenous endorphins. High-frequency stimulation (80Hz to 100Hz) stimulates the Aβ-fibers thus inhibiting the pain transmission in the spinal cord. TENS can be applied in all posttraumatic phases, also during painful interventions. The analgesic consumption is reduced and the patient learns how to influence the pain actively instead of just have to bear it passively. A meta analysis of 21 randomized studies with 1350 patients showed a significantly positive influence to the postoperative analgesics consumption. The average frequency in the studies with optimal treatment was 85Hz [74].

## Particularities of burn pain

### Wound pain

For the treatment of wound pain, a multimodal approach with the cooperation of plastic surgeons, anesthetists, physical therapists, psychologists and nursing personnel is recommended.

In most cases an opioid therapy is inevitable. In the initial phase and in the presence of gastrointestin-al motility and resorption disorders an intravenous dose of analgesics is often necessary to achieve a rapid pain control. In the intensive care unit this can be carried out as continuous intravenous infusion through a perfusor. Regarding a possible tolerance development an oral administration of long-term effective opioids is recommended after the initial phase. The administration of retard preparations according to a strict time schedule ensures an even activity of the medication. The dosage has to be adjusted until the patient feels no or only little pain (e. g. score > 4 according to the numeric analogous scale) at rest and in motion.

A combination of opioids and non-opioids has its benefits. Due to its few side effects paracetamol is the treatment of choice. NSAID are used only sparingly and in particular indications due to their effects on the renal and thrombocyte function.

The intravenous patient-controlled analgesia is a suitable treatment in burn patients with good compliance. However, its application can be limited in the presence of burn injuries on the hands.

In a multimodal treatment approach, the administration of other preparations (NMDA-receptor antagonists, anticonvulsants, antidepressants) should always be considered. In the acute phase of the treatment a general administration is not recommended to keep the pain management as simple as possible. With appropriate indication (e. g. burning or shooting pain) the therapy can be expanded gradually to be able to evaluate the effects and side effects of the additional analgesic.

### Breakthrough pain

Burn pain requires a dynamic and flexible pain management. In case of suddenly intensifying pain there must always be a place for an "emergency medication". These analgesics have to be effective in a very short time.

For this purpose the rapidly effective forms of opioid retard preparations are recommended. A very good option for the treatment of burn pain might be the oromucosal application of fentanyl (Actiq®: Fentanyl as throat lozenge with integrated applicator for dissolution of the preparation in the oral cavity). Currently, Actiq® is approved for the treatment of breakthrough pain during continuous opioid therapy in patients with chronic tumor pain. However it is increasingly administered in chronic pain (with breakthrough symptoms) of other reasons.

Generally the initial dosage is 200 µg. The dosage is increased as necessary in the available doses (200 µg, 400 µg, 600 µg, 800 µg, 1200 µg, and 1600 µg). In the oromucosal application the absorption kinetics is an interaction between a rapid absorption by the oral mucosa (25% of the total dosage) and a slower absorption by swallowed fentanyl by the gastrointestinal tract (75% of the total dosage). The action takes place within 15 minutes. Administration should be limited to 4 doses per day.

### Intervention-induced pain

Intervention-induced pain require a potent analgesia for a short period of time. An additional aim of the therapy should be to reduce anxiety and worries of the patients.

The therapeutic management needs to be carried out in accordance with the severity of the intervention [75].

## Necrosectomy and skin grafting

Necrosectomy can be more painful than wound pain after burn injuries. In such cases the method of choice is an intervention under surgical conditions with general anesthesia. However, long preoperative and postoperative nutrition gaps must be accepted.

## Dressing change of large burn wounds and removal of clamps in skin grafts

In an ideal case these interventions take place on a spontaneously breathing patient with good pain therapy directly in the burn unit. An intravenous administration of potent opioids in combination with sedatives is essential. The patient should be sedated to such an extent that an adequate pain evaluation is still possible. Sedating and anxiety relieving preparations must not be used as a replacement for analgesics.

An analgosedation of burn patients outside of the operating room has to be carried out by qualified personnel (generally anesthetists). A standard monitoring with pulse oxymetry, blood pressure measurement and continuous ECG recordings is a precondition for a secure process. Furthermore, oxygen should be supplied via mask or glasses [76].

Remifentanil is only approved for the administration in intensive care patients receiving artificial respiration. There are single reports about the administration of remifentanil in extubated intensive care patients. However, the increased rate of apnea or bradypnea has to be considered then [77].

In a study with spontaneously breathing, nonintubated burn patients, remifentanil could be administered successfully for analgesia and sedation during dressing change [78]. A randomized prospective study with 79 patients showed that the combination of opioids and Lorazepam could reduce the intervention-induced burn pain [79].

Patient-controlled therapies are very promising. Apart from the intravenous patient-controlled analgesia [44], the patient-controlled sedation has become a very well evaluated form of therapy in burn patients.

In a prospective study on a small number of burn patients (TBSA > 10%), a patient-controlled sedation with propofol/alfentanil showed a higher contentment among the patients during dressing change than when they were treated by an anesthetist during the interventions. Although there were no lockout times provided in the protocol, cardio-vascular complications did not occur in any case [80].

In another study on 44 patients in a burn unit, dressing changes were carried out under patient-controlled administration of midazolam/ketanest. Also in this case the contentedness among the patients as well as among the health care personnel was significantly higher than in the traditional treatment. In this study neither preoperative nor postoperative nutrition gaps were maintained. Side effects occurred rarely, the most common side effect was short-timed hallucinations [81]. For the application of patient-controlled analgesia relevant structural conditions must be present, so that in case of technical or medical problems a competent stand-by service (e. g. 24 hours acute pain service) is always available.

A limiting factor for the patient-controlled analgesia is that in severe burn injuries the upper extremities are very often affected and the patients cannot operate the pump sufficiently.

## Dressing change in smaller burn wounds, baths and physical therapy

It is mostly sufficient to administer a fast acting analgesic in due time before the scheduled intervention either as intravenous bolus of the opioid analgesic that is already in the perfusor or in non-retarded form of the retarded continuous opioid treatment.

In intervention-induced pain, treatments without medication are most effective. The susceptibility varies from patient to patient. However, this form of pain management should always be considered. In many cases the anxiety caused by the upcoming interventions is a bigger problem than the pain caused by these interventions.

## Postoperative pain

In the immediate postoperative phase pain must be measured more often to be able to react fast to increasing pain.

Donor sites for skin grafts can be much more painful than the burned skin areas themselves. Thus, most patients require an additional pain management for the days after skin grafting.

The postoperative pain management already starts intraoperatively. Analgesia by simple wound infiltration with a local anesthetic can be used as adjuvant measure if the wound healing of burned areas or donor sites is not inhibited.

The application of regional anesthetics can improve the intra and postoperative pain management in burn injuries [82].

Cuignet et al. examined the efficacy of an additionally administered continuous intra and postoperative fascia iliaca compartment block to the donor sites in skin grafting on 20 adult patients (mean TBSA 16%). This prospective randomized double blind study showed a significant postoperative reduction of opioid consumption and significantly reduced scores on the visual analogous scale [83].

Jellish et al. examined the topic application of local anesthetics on skin donor sites in skin grafting. It was shown that topic lidocaine (lidocaine 20% solution applied as aerosol) has an analgesic effect and that the narcotics consumption was reduced in comparison to the application of sodium chloride solu-

tion. A topic application of lidocaine does not affect the wound healing. Toxic blood concentrations were not detected [84].

The application of local anesthetics as cream does not influence local inflammation after burn trauma. A randomized double blind placebo-controlled study on 12 healthy patients showed that after induced burn injury (grade I and IIa), lidocaine-prilocaine cream (Emla®) applied under firm dressings immediately after the burn injury and for a period of 8 hours, did not have any effect on the development of primary or secondary hyperalgesia. Compared to the placebo group, alterations in wound healing were not detected either [85].

## Mental aspects

When making decisions concerning pain management, the psychosocial situation of the patient must always be considered. The sensation of pain is closely related to the overcoming of the burn trauma in the following therapy phase.

A small group of patients suffers, in particular after having spent several weeks in hospital, from depression. Depression is often linked with mood swings and varying sensations of pain.

Other factors that can intensify the sensation of pain are anxiety, worries, lack of orientation, loss of control, loneliness and insomnia. A prospective study on 28 stationary patients (TBSA 3.5 to 64%) showed a significant temporary correlation between the quality of sleep and the intensity of pain. A night without much sleep was followed by a day with significantly stronger pain [86].

These triggering factors should be avoided from the first day of the treatment on.

## Intensive care unit

Large area burns and inhalation trauma require intensive care. In the intensive care unit, several additional factors concerning pain management should be considered.

## Opioid-induced hyperalgesia and opioid tolerance

A continuous administration of highly effective opioids in the intensive care unit might lead even after a short time to the development of an opioid-induced hyperalgesia or opioid tolerance.

Schraag et al. showed that an administration of opioids adapted to the patient's needs is beneficial with regard to a tolerance development [87].

The additionally administered sedative/anxiolytic also plays a role in the development of an opioid tolerance. A simultaneous administration of high doses of benzodiazepine might foster a tolerance by causing a reduced stimulus of the opioid receptors [88, 89].

## Hypermetabolism

Severe burn injuries cause an extreme metabolism increase that can be 100% to 150% higher than the basal metabolic rate. In theses cases it is very important to reduce the catabolism by an early and sufficient nutrition and to avoid feelings of anxiety and stress, which are factors that increase the metabolic action.

A problematic aspect is the fact that a sedoanalgesia causes gastrointestinal dysfunction in several cases. Due to the high energy demand and the benefits of enteral nutrition compared to parenteral nutrition, an intact intestinal motility and avoiding opioid-induced obstipation is very important. Furthermore, the numerous surgical interventions and dressing changes cause longer nutrition gaps.

## Psychic stress factors

Severely burned patients are exposed to numerous additional stress factors during their stay in the intensive care unit. One stress factor is the intensive medical setting: loud and unfamiliar noises of the machines, bright light, care measures and numerous diagnostic and therapeutic measures disturb the day and night rhythm of the patient. Furthermore intensive care patients suffer from an enormous communication deficit. The invasive respiration limits their communication abilities and they can not participate actively in the visits of the medical personnel. All these stress factors cause anxiety and frustration in the patient and influence the sensitivity to pain and the coping with pain significantly [90].

## Risk of infection

Patients receiving artificial respiration and large burns have a greater risk for ventilation associated pneumonia. Particularly in such cases the artificial respiration should be kept as short as possible.

A general aim of the analgosedation for the patient should be an optimal sedation and an adequate pain management. The pain management should ensure an individually optimized artificial respiration, a problem-free weaning and a preferably scheduled extubation [91].

## Monitoring [92]

Individual and patient-specific aims and thus an adequate monitoring of the therapy effect is a precondition for the multimodal approach in an intensive treatment. Controlling the sedation depth and evaluating the pain level are very difficult in critically ill patients in the intensive care unit since very often they cannot articulate themselves verbally. An evaluation of indirect vegetative reactions as for example heart rate, blood pressure, breathing rate, lacrimation and pupil dilatation is not sufficient to securely avoid an overdose or underdose. The search for adequate means of control has lead to the development of numerous scoringsystems all of which having their benefits and shortcomings.

## Sedation monitoring

Today, the following scoring systems to determine the sedation level are most commonly used:
- RAMSAY-sedation-scale (RSS): very commonly used; patients are classified in 7 categories (Ramsay 0–6) [93]
- Sedation-agitation scale (SAS): first score which was evaluated for reliability and validity in intensive care patients, high concordance of the different evaluators and when compared to the Ramsay scale and the Harris scale; patients can be classified in 3 categories (anxious or agitated = SAS 5–7, calm = SAS 4, sedated = SAS 1–3) [94].
- Richmond agitation scale (RASS): score with 10 parameters to determine the level of sedation and agitation in intubated and non-intubated adult

patients; significant correlation with applied dosages of analgesics and sedatives [95].

▶ COMFORT-scale: Application in pediatric intensive care units; consists of 8 easily determinable parameters to evaluate the level of sedation during the daily nursing measures [96].

## Analgesia monitoring (see Fig. 2)

After evaluation of the level of sedation and analgesia, an individual aim for sedation and analgesia should be determined according to these scoring systems. The achievement of this aim should be verified on a regular basis (at least every 8 hours). A re-evaluation and re-defining of the level of sedation and analgesia should also be carried out regularly.

## Analgosedation (Table 3)

As there is a vast number of available preparations for an analgosedation, it is necessary to develop standard operating procedures [97]. It must not necessarily be decisive which concept is applied but that the concept is consequently and correctly applied.

Apart from an adequate sedation and analgesia, an adequate anxiolysis and vegetative protection are desirable. Modern concepts for analgosedation are based on a controlled sedation of the patient's state of awareness and an effective elimination of pain perception. They are not meant as a prolongation of a general anesthesia.

In severely burned patients a deeper sedation is often necessary. This holds true for patients with pronounced edema in the face and the upper respiratory tract. In such patients an accidental self-extubation can be a vital danger. A deeper analgosedation can also be necessary for a particular positioning of the patient due to the localization of the burn wound and to protect fresh skin grafts that are prone to shearing forces. However, this increases the risk for ventilator-induced pneumonia. In such cases the situation must be evaluated by the health care personnel depending on the patient's general condition and the surgical and pulmonary situation [98].

| Item | Description | Score |
| --- | --- | --- |
| Facial expression | Relaxed | 1 |
| | Partially tightened (e. g., brow lowering) | 2 |
| | Fully tightened (e. g., eyelid closing) | 3 |
| | Grimacing | 4 |
| Upper limbs | No movement | 1 |
| | Partially bent | 2 |
| | Fully bent with finger flexion | 3 |
| | Permanently retracted | 4 |
| Compliance with ventilation | Tolerating movement | 1 |
| | Coughing but tolerating ventilation for most of the time | 2 |

**Fig. 2.** Behavioral pain scale

## Sedation

Today there are various methods for the sedation of intensive care patients. The medication should not be ended abruptly after long-time sedation but slowly. Sedation and weaning protocols make this process easier and respiration time is reduced [99]. Sedatives must not be administered as a replacement for analgesics.

## Propofol

Propofol is approved for sedation in intensive care for a maximum of 7 days. It has sedative-hypnotic, but no analgesic effects. Due to its short and context-sensitive half-life and the production of inac-

**Table 3.** Sedoanalgesia in the intensive care unit

| | |
| --- | --- |
| Midazolam | 0,03–0,15 mg/kgBW/h |
| Propofol | 1–3 mg/kgBW/h |
| Clonidine | 0,03–0,15 mg/kgBW/h |
| S$_{(+)}$-Ketamine | 0,3–1,5 mg/kgBW/h |
| Sevoflurane* | endtidal Conc. 0,5–1,1 Vol% |
| Sufentanil | 0,5–1,5 mg/kgBW/min |
| Remifentanil | 0,05–2 mg/kgBW/min |

\* Calculation of the pumpfrequency (ml/h)
depending on breath volume per minute by nomogram

tive metabolites, the preparation is well controllable. Problems during application might occur through falling blood pressure and additional fat supply (1 ml = 0.1 g fat). A dosage limitation ( > 4 mg/kg/h) is required to minimize the risk of a propofol-infusion-syndrome. This is characterized by cardiac arrythmia, heart failure, rhabdomyolysis, severe metabolic acidosis and acute renal failure. Regular checks in the laboratory (in particular ph-value and lactate) facilitate an early detection of this syndrome. Propofol is approved for the sedation of children older than 16 years.

Fröhlich et al. evaluated in a randomized placebo-controlled study the effect of propofol to pain sensation with temperature stimulus (45°C, 47°C and 49°C). Propofol was administered as target-controlled infusion in 2 different concentrations (0.5 µ/ml and 1.0 µ/ml) to 18 test subjects. Pain intensity was measured by the visual analogous scale. Surprisingly, the authors could prove that propofol in mild and moderate doses increased the pain intensity and the patients' discontentment. Thus a sedation should always be combined with sufficient analgesia [100].

## Benzodiazepine

Benzodiazepine centrally enforces the inhibiting effect of δ-aminobutyric acid and has anxioloytic, sedative-hypnotic, centrally relaxing and anticonvulsant effects. It is administered during long-term sedation ( > 3 days). Compared to other benzodiazepines, midazolam has a shorter context-sensitive half-life and thus is very well suited. Another benefit is an anterograde amnesia caused by benzodiazepine. Liver and renal dysfunctions cause an extensively longer action time.

## Clonidine

Clonidin is a presynaptic α2-adrenoceptor antagonist with antihypertensive, analgesic, sedative and anxiolytic activity. It is administered as basic sedation (particularly in hypertensive patients), as prohylactic and in the therapy of withdrawal symptoms after long-time analgosedation and in preexisting alcoholism. Furthermore, clonidine causes a dosage reduction of sedatives and opioids and thus reduces the side effects induced by these preparations. However, complications as for example bradycardic arrhythmia, dropping blood pressure and inhibition of the gastro-intestinal motility have to be considered. After long-time application, the administration of clonidine must be stopped slowly and gradually to avoid a rapid increase of the blood pressure.

## Ketamine

Ketamine is a non-competitive NMDA-receptor-antagonist with dosage dependent activity. A higher dosage causes somnolence up to dissociate anesthesia (dissociation from the environment without sleeping). Due to the psychomimetic side-effects, ketamine should be administered in combination with propofol and benzodiazepine. Ketamine has proven beneficial in patients with bronchospasm or hypotensive circulation without cardiogenic reasons. However, ketamine stimulates the cardiovascular system by sensitizing the heart to catecholamines. A potential increase of the arterial blood pressure, tachycardia and increase of the myocardiac oxygen consumption have to be considered.

In subanesthetic dosages, ketamine acts exclusively as analgesic. Numerous studies have shown that ketamine can suppress effectively an opioid tolerance and an opioid-induced hyperalgesia [35, 38, 101]. The opioid-reducing property of ketamine could also be proven in intensive care patients [102].

## Volatile anesthetics

A long-term sedation by intravenous preparations is associated with respiratory depression, enteroparesis, renal and liver disorders and accumulation with retarded recovery. Volatile anesthetics can be an effective alternative. For this purpose special recirculation systems for inhalational anesthetics have been developed for the use in the intensive care unit (e. g. Anesthetic Conserving Device, suitable for isoflurane and sevoflurane). At present, however, there are no sufficient studies on the importance of volatile anesthetics in analgosedation in the intensive care unit. There are single case reports of a successful application in burn patients [103].

## Analgesia

A vital problem of pain management in the intensive care unit is the limited communication. A study by Whipple JK et al. (1995) showed that 74% of intensive care patients suffered from pain [104].

## Opioids

As in non-intensive care patients, opioids are a basic medication in the pain management in this case.

### Sufentanil

Sufentanil is the strongest opioid that is currently used (500 to 1000-fold higher analgesic potency than morphine) and has a high affinity to the μ-receptor. Compared to other opioids, its context-sensitive half-life is relatively low. Thus it is very well suited for a long-term sedation. Another benefit of sufentanil is its very good cardiovascular stability.

### Remifentanil

Remifentanil is a very well controllable analgesic with a context-sensitive half-life of 3 to 4 minutes, which remains constant even after a longer time of supply. Its degradation is carried out independently of liver and renal function by unspecific blood and tissue esterases. Thus its application is particularly beneficial in patients with liver and renal disorders. Remifentanil can only be administered as continuous infusion because a bolus application causes respiratory insufficiency and skeletal muscle rigidity, which can inhibit artificial respiration. Remifentanil does not cause release of histamines.

Literature describes the occurrence of an opioid-induced hyperalgesia and allodynia or the development of an opioid tolerance from a continuous supply of 0.1 μg/kg/min [35, 38, 101].

### Alfentanil

Alfentanil is a short-time effective, potent opioid with a maximum action time within one minute after administration. Its slow metabolic degradation makes it not very well suited for a long-term sedation. More effective is bolus application as on-top analgesia for care measures and short therapeutic interventions. When administered too fast, bradycardia and increased thoraxrigidity must be considered.

Other possible fields of application are during dressing change as patient-controlled analgesia with basic function and bolus application or as target-controlled infusion [105, 106]. In both studies, the patients were alert and cooperative without respiratory depression or haemodynamic instability.

### Non-opioids

In critic indication and consideration of the side effects, non-opioids are an important part of a multimodal therapy concept as well in the intensive care unit. Particular attention must be paid when treating older burn patients or burn patients with pre-existing cardiac and renal disorders. Furthermore interactions with other preparations must be considered (e. g. with diuretics, antihypertensives and corticosteroids).

## References

[1]   Kehlet H, Jensen TS, Woolf CJ (2006) Persistent post-surgical pain: risk factors and prevention. The Lancet 367: 1618–1625

[2]   Dauber A, Osgood PF, Breslau AJ et al (2002) Chronic persistent pain after severe burns: a survey of 358 burn survivors. Pain Med 3: 6–17

[3]   Ratcliff SL, Brown A, Rosenberg L et al (2006) The effectiveness of a pain and anxiety protocol to treat the acute pediatric burn patient. Burns 32(5): 554–562

[4]   Spacek A (2006) Der neuropathische Schmerz – aktuelle Therapiekonzepte. 1. Aufl. UNI-MED Verlag AG Bremen S. 20–23

[5]   Gray P, Williams B, Cramond T (2008) Successful use of Gabapentin in acute pain management following burn injury: a case series. Pain Med 9 (3): 371–376

[6]   Malenfant A, Forget R, Papillon J et al (1996) Prevalence and characteristics of chronic sensory problems in burn patients. Pain 67(2–3): 493–500

[7]   Choiniere M, Melzack R, Papillon J (1991) Pain and paresthesia in patients with healed burns: An exploratory study. J Pain Symptom Manage 6(7): 437–444

[8]   Macrae WA (2001) Chronic pain after surgery. Br J Anaesth 87: 88–98

[9]   Thomans CR, Brazeal BA, Rosenburg L et al (2003) Phantom limb pain in pediatric burns survivors. Burns 29(2): 139–142

[10]  Kumbhat S, Meyer N, Schurr MJ (2004) Complex regional pain syndrome as a complication of a chemical burn to the foot. J Burn Care Rehabil 25(2): 189–191

[11]  Van der Laan L, Goris RJA (1996) Reflex sympathetic dystrophy after burn injury. Burns 22(4): 303–306

[12]  Isakov E, Boduragin N, Korzets A, Susak Z (1995) Reflex sympathetic dystrophy of both patellae following burns. Burns 21(8): 616–618

[13] Kim CT, Bryant P (2001) Complex regional pain syndrome (type I) after electrical injury: A case report of treatment with continuous epidural block. Arch Phys Med Rehabil 82(7): 993–995

[14] Melzack R (1975) The McGill pain questionnaire: major properties and scoring methods. Pain 1: 277–299

[15] Payen JF, Bru O, Bosson JL et al (2001) Assessing pain in critically ill sedated patients by using a behavioral pain scale. Crit Care Med 29(12): 2258–2263

[16] Abbey J, Piller N, De Bellis A et al (2004) The Abbey Pain Scale: a 1-minute numerical indicator for people with end-stage dementia. Int J Palliative Nurs 10(1): 6–13

[17] Merkel SI, Voepel-Lewis T, Shayevitz JR, Malviya S (1997) The FLACC: a behavioral scale for scoring postoperative pain in young children. Paediatr Nurs 23(3): 293–297

[18] Büttner W et al (1998) Entwicklung eines Fremdbeobachtungsbogens zur Beurteilung des postoperativen Schmerzes bei Säuglingen. AINS 33: 353–361

[19] Taal LA, Faber AW, Van Loey NEE et al (1999) The abbreviated burn specific pain anxiety scale: a multicenter study. Burns 25(6): 493–497

[20] Rae CP, Gallagher D, Watson S, Kinsella J (2000) An audit of patient perception compared with medical and nursing staff estimation of pain during burn dressing changes. Eur J Anaesthesiol 17(1): 43–45

[21] Pallua N (2009) Kompendium der Schmerztherapie bei Verbrennungen. Deutsche Gesellschaft für Verbrennungsmedizin und Deutsche Gesellschaft zum Studium des Schmerzes. URL: http://www.dgss.org/filead min/pdf/Schmerz_KompendiumVerbrennung0901. pdf

[22] Barden J, Edwards J, Moore RA, MyQuay HJ (2004) Single dose oral diclofenac for postoperative pain. Cochrane Database Syst Rev(2): CD004 768

[23] Elia N, Lysakowski C, Tramer MR (2005) Does multimodal analgesia with acetaminophen, nonsteroidal anti-inflammatory drugs, or selective cyclooxygenase-2 inhibitors and patient- controlled analgesia morphine offer advantages over morphine alone? Anesthesiology 103: 1296–1304

[24] Koppert W, Wehrfritz A, Korber N et al (2004) The cyclooxygenase isoenzyme inhibitors parecoxib and paracetamol reduce central hyperalgesia in humans. Pain 108: 148–153

[25] Tröster A, Sittl R, Singer B et al (2006) Modulation of remifentanil-induced analgesia and postinfusion hyperalgesia by parecoxib in humans. Anesthesiology 105: 1016–1023

[26] Pelissier T, Alloui A, Caussade F et al (1996) Paracetamol exerts a spinal antinociceptive effect involving an indirect interaction with $_5$-hydroxytryptamine$_3$ receptors: in vivo and in vitro evidence. J Pharm Exp Ther 278: 8–14

[27] Beubler E (2009) Kompendium der medikamentösen Schmerztherapie, 4. Aufl. Springer Wien New York, S 19

[28] Larsen R (2001) Anästhesie, 7. Aufl. Urban und Fischer Verlag, München, S 806

[29] Kramer MS, Lane DA, Hutchinson TA (1988) The International Agranulocytosis and Aplastic Anemia Study (IAAAS). J Clin Epidemiol 41 (6): 613–616

[30] Hedenmalm K, Spigset O (2002) Agranulocytosis and other blood dyscrasias associated with dipyrone (metamizole). Eur J Clin Pharmacol 58(4): 265–274

[31] Ott E, Nussmeier NA, Dukie PC et al (2003) Efficacy and safety of the cyclooxygenase 2 inhibitors parecoxib and valdecoxib in patients undergoing coronary artery bypass surgery. J Thorac Cardiovasc Surg 125(6): 1481–192

[32] McGettigan P, Henry D (2006) Cardiovascular risk and inhibition of cyclooxygenase. A systematic review of the oberservational studies of selective and nonselective inhibitors of cyclooxygenase2. JAMA 296(13): 1633–1644

[33] Nussmeier NA, Whelton AA, Brown MT et al (2005) Complications of the COX-2 inhibitors parecoxib and valdecoxib after cardiac surgery. N Engl J Med 352: 1081–1091

[34] Freye E, Latasch L (2003) Development of opioid tolerance – molecular mechanisms and clinical consequences. AINS 38: 14–26

[35] Koppert W, Sittl R, Scheuber K et al (2003) Differential modulation of remifentanil-induced analgesia and postinfusion hyperalgesia by s-ketamine and clonidine in humans. Anesthesiology 99(1): 152–159

[36] Célèrier E, Rivat C, Jun Y et al (2000) Long-lasting hyperalgesia Induced by Fentanyl in rats. Anesthesiology 92(2): 465–472

[37] Xiangqi Li, Angst MS, Clark JD (2001) Opioid-induced hyperalgesia and incisional pain. Anesth Analg 93: 204–209

[38] Joly V, Richebe Ph, Guignard B et al (2005) Remifentanil-induced postoperative hyperalgesia and its prevention with small-dose ketamine. Anesthesiology 103(1): 147–155

[39] Smith MT, Watt JA et al (1990) Morphine-3-glucoronide – a potent antagonist of morphine analgesia. Life Sci 47: 579–585

[40] Stamer UM, Lehnen K, Höthker F et al (2003) Impact of CYP2D6 genotype on postoperative tramadol analgesia. Pain 105: 231–238

[41] Duhmke RM, Cornblath DD, Hollingshead JR (2004) Tramadol for neuropathic pain. Cochrane Database Syst Rev(2): CD003 726

[42] Tosun Z, Esmaoglu A, Coruh A (2008) Propofol-ketamine vs propofol-fentanyl combinations for deep sedation and analgesia in pediatric patients undergoing burn dressing changes. Pediatric Anesthesia 18: 43–47

[43] Linneman PK, Terry BE, Burd RS (2000) The efficacy and safety of fentanyl for the management of severe procedural pain in patients with burn injuries. J Burn Care Rehabil 21(6): 519–522

[44] Prakash S, Fatima T, Pawar M (2004) Patient-controlled analgesia with fentanyl for burns dressing changes. Anesth Analg 99(2): 552–555

[45] Ong EC (2008) Controlled-release oxycodone in the treatment of neuropathic pain of nonmalignant and malignant causes. Oncology 74(1): 72–75

[46] Gatti A, Sabato AF, Occhioni R et al (2009) Controlled-release oxycodone and pregabalin in the treatment of neuropathic pain: results of a multicenter Italian study. Eur Neurol 61(3): 129–137

[47] Altier N, Dion D, Boulanger A, Choiniere M (2001) Successful use of methadone in the treatment of chronic neuropathic pain arising from burn injuries: a case-study. Burns 27(7): 771–775

[48] Subramaniam K, Subramaniam B, Steinbrook RA (2004) Ketamine as adjuvant analgesic to opioids: a quantitative and qualitative systematic review. Anesth Analg 99: 482–495

[49] Mao J, Price DD, Mayer GJ (1995) Mechanisms of hyperalgesia and morphine tolerance: a current view of their possible interactions. Pain 62: 259–274

[50] Weinbroum AA, Gorodezky A, Niv D et al (2001) Dextromethorphan attenuation of postoperative pain and primary and secondary thermal hyperalgesia. Can J Anaesth 48: 167–174

[51] Weinbroum AA (2003) A single small dose of postoperative ketamine provides rapid and sustained improvement in morphine analgesia in the presence of morphine-resistant pain. Anesth Analg 96: 789–795

[52] Bell R, Dahl J, Moore R, Kalso E (2006) Perioperative ketamine for acute postoperative pain. Cochrane Database Syst Rev (1): CD004 603

[53] De Kock M, Lavand'homme P, Waterloos H (2001) Balanced analgesia in the perioperative period: is there a place for ketamine? Pain 92: 373–380

[54] Lavand'homme P, De Kock M, Waterloos H (2005) Intraoperative epidural analgesia combined with ketamine provides effective preventive analgesia in patients undergoing major digestive surgery. Anesthesiology 103: 813–820

[55] Owens VF, Palmieri TL, Comroe CM et al (2006) Ketamine: A safe and effective agent for painful procedures in the pediatric burn patient. J Burn Care Res 27(2): 211–216

[56] Menigaux C, Adam F, Guignard B et al (2005) Preoperative gabapentin decreases anxiety and improves early functional recovery from knee surgery. Anesth Analg 100: 1394–1399

[57] Pollack MH, Matthews J, Scott EL (1998) Gabapentin as a potential treatment for anxiety disorders. Am J Psychiatry 155: 992–993

[58] Chouinard G, Beauclair L, Belanger MC (1998) Gabapentin: long-term antianxiety and hypnotic effects in psychiatric patients with comorbid anxiety-related disorders. Can J Psychiatry 43: 305

[59] Eckhardt K, Ammon S, Hofmann U et al (2000) Gabapentin enhances the analgesic effect of morphine in healthy volunteers. Anesth Analg 91: 185–191

[60] Field MJ, Oles RJ, Lewis AS et al (1997) Gabapentin (neurontin) and S-(+)-3-isobutylgaba represent a novel class of selective antihyperalgesic agents. Br J Pharmacol 121(8): 1513–1522

[61] Cuignet O, Pirson J, Soudon O, Zizi M (2007) Effects of gabapentin on morphine consumption and pain in severely burned patients. Burns 33(1): 81–86

[62] Mendham JE et al (2004) Gabapentin for the treatment of itching produced by burns and wound healing in children: a pilot study. Burns 30: 851–853

[63] Pal SK, Cortiella J, Herndon D (1997) Adjunctive methods of pain control in burns. Burns 23(5): 404–412

[64] Tcheung WJ, Robert R, Rosenberg L et al (2006) Early treatment of acute stress disorder in children with major burn injury. Pediatr Crit Care Med 7(5): 498–499

[65] Deutsche Interdisziplinäre Vereinigung für Schmerztherapie, S3- Leitlinie "Behandlung akuter perioperativer und posttraumatischer Schmerzen", Stand: 21. 05. 2007, inkl. Änderungen vom 20. 04. 2009

[66] Cheung LH, Callaghan P, Chang AM (2003) A controlled trial of psycho-educational interventions preparing Chinese women for elective hysterectomy. Int J Stud 40(2): 207–216

[67] Good M, Anderson GC, Stanton-Hicks M et al (2002) Relaxation and music reduce pain after gynecologic surgery. Pain Manag Nurs 3(2): 61–70

[68] Good M, Anderson GC, Ahn S et al (2005) Relaxation and music reduce pain following intestinal surgery. Res Nurs Health 28(3): 240–251

[69] Huth MM, Broome ME, Good M (2004) Imagery reduces children's post-operative pain. Pain 110(1–2): 439–448

[70] Nilsson U, Rawal N, Unestahl LE et al (2001) Improved recovery after music and therapeutic suggestions during general anaesthesia: a double-blind randomised controlled trial. Acta Anaesthesiol Scand 45(7): 812–817

[71] Montgomery GH, David D, Winkel G et al (2002) The effectiveness of adjunctive hypnosis with surgical patients: a meta-analysis. Anesth Analg 94(6): 1639–45, table of contents

[72] Saadat H, Drummond-Lewis J, Maranets I et al (2006) Hypnosis reduces preoperative anxiety in adult patients. Anesth Analg 102(5): 1394–1396

[73] Frenay MC, Faymonville ME, Devlieger S et al (2001) Psychological approaches during dressing changes of burned patients: a prospective randomised study comparing hypnosis against stress reducing strategy. Burns 27(8): 793–799

[74] Bjordal JM, Johnson MI, Ljunggreen AE (2003) Transcutaneous electrical nerve stimulation (TENS) can reduce postoperative analgesic consumption. A meta-analysis with assessment of optimal treatment parameters for postoperative pain. Eur J Pain 7(2): 181–188

[75] Richardson P, Mustard L (2009) The management of pain in the burns unit. Burns 35(7): 921–936

[76] Gregoretti C, Decaroli D, Piacevoli Qu et al (2008) Analgo-sedation of patients with burns outside the operating room. Drugs 68(17): 2427–2443

[77] Wilhelm W, Wrobel M, Kreuer S, Larsen R (2003) Remifentanil – Eine Bestandsaufnahme. Anaesthesist 52: 473–494

[78] Le Floch R, Naux E, PilorgetA, Arnould J-F (2006) Use of remifentanil for analgesia during dressing changes in spontaneously breathing non-intubated burn patients. Ann Burns Fire Disasters XIX (3)

[79] Patterson DR, Ptacek JT, Carrougher GJ, Sharar SR (1997) Lorazepam as an adjunct to opioid analgesics in the treatment of burn pain. Pain 72(3): 367–374

[80] Nilsson A, Steinvall I, Bak Z, Sjoberg F (2008) Patient controlled sedation using a standard protocol for dressing changes in burns: patients preference, procedural details and a preliminary safety evaluation. Burns 34: 929–934

[81] MacPherson RD, Woods D, Penfold J (2008) Ketamine and midazolam delivered by patient-controlled analgesia in relieving pain associated with burns dressings. Clin J Pain 24(7)568–571

[82] Gupta A, Bhandari PS, Shrivastava P (2007) A study of regional nerve blocks and local anesthetic creams (Prilox) for donor sites in burn patients. Burns 33: 87–91

[83] Cuignet O, Pirson J, Boughrouph J, Duville D (2004) The efficacy of continuous fascia iliaca compartment block for pain management in burn patients undergoing skin grafting procedures. Anesth Analg 98: 1077–1081

[84] Jellis WS, Gamelli RL, Furry PA et al (1999) Effect of topical local anesthetic application to skin harvest sites for pain management in burn patients undergoing skin-grafting procedures. Ann Surg 229(1): 115–120

[85] Pedersen JL, Callesen S, Møiniche S, Kehlet H (1996) Analgesic and anti-inflammatory effects of lignocaine-prilocaine (EMLA) cream in human burn injury. Br J Anaesthesia 76: 806–810

[86] Raymond I, Nielsen TA, Lavigne G et al (2001) Quality of sleep and its daily relationship to pain intensity in hospitalized adult burn patients. Pain 92(3): 381–388

[87] Schraag S, Checketts M et al (1999) Lack of rapid development of opioid tolerance during alfentanil and remifentanil infusions for postoperative pain. Anesth Analg 89: 753-757

[88] Luger TJ, Hayashi T, Grabner Weiss C, Hill H (1995) The spinal potentiating effect and the supraspinal inhibitory effect of midazolam on opioid- induced analgesia in rats. European J Pharmacol 275(2): 153–162

[89] Palaoglu O, Ayhan IH (1986) The possible role of benzodiazepine receptors in morphine analgesia. Pharmacol Biochem Behav 25: 15–217

[90] Perkins FM, Kehlet H (2000) Chronic pain as an outcome of surgery. Anesthesiology 93: 1123–1133

[91] Kong R, Payen D (1994) Controlling sedation rather than sedation controlling you. Clin Intensive Care 5[5Suppl]:5–7

[92] Martin J, Bäsell K, Bürkle H et al (2005) Analgesie und Sedierung in der Intensivmedizin. S2-Leitlinien der deutschen Gesellschaft für Anästhesiologie und Intensivmedizin. Anaesthesiol Intensivmed 46 [Suppl 1: 1–20

[93] Ramsay MA, Savege TM, Simpson BR, Goodwin R (1974) Controlled sedation with alphaxalone-alphadolone. Br Med J 2(920): 656–659

[94] Riker R, Picard F, Fraser G (1999) Prospective evaluation of the sedation-agitation-scale for adult critically ill patients. Crit Care Med 27(7): 1325–1329

[95] Ely EW, Inouye SK, Bernard GR et al (2001) Delirium in mechanically ventilated patients: validity and reliability of the confusion assessment method for the intensive care unit (CAM-ICU). JAMA 286(21): 2703–2710

[96] Ambuel B, Hamlett KW, Marx CM, Blumer JL (1992) Assessing distress in pediatric intensive care enviroments: the COMFORT scale. J Pediatr Psychol 17(1): 95–109

[97] Weinert CR, Chlan L, Gross C (2001) Sedating critically ill patients: factors affecting nurses'delivery of sedative therapy. Am J Crit Care 10(3): 156–65; quiz 166–7

[98] Giessler GA, Mayer T, Trupkovic T (2009) Das Verbrennungstrauma. Anaesthesist 58: 474–484

[99] Costa J, Cabre L, Molina R Carrasco G (1994) Cost of ICU sedation: comparison of empirical and controlled sedation methods. Clin Intensive Care 5 [5Suppl.:17–21

[100] Frölich MA, Price DD, Robinson ME et al (2005) The effect of propofol on thermal pain perception. Anesth Analg 100: 481–486

[101] Guignard B, Coste C, Costes H et al (2002) Supplementing Desflurane-Remifentanil anesthesia with small-dose ketamine reduces perioperative opioid analgesic requirements. Anesth Analg 95: 103–108

[102] Edrich T, Friedrich AD, Eltzschig HK, Felbinger TW (2004) Ketamine for long-term sedation and analgesia of a burn patient. Anesth Analg 99: 893–895

[103] Jung C, Granados M, Marsol P (2008) Use of sevoflurane sedation by the AnaConDa® device as an adjunct to extubation in a pediatric burn patient. Burns 34: 136–138

[104] Whipple JK, Lewis KS, Quebbeman EJ et al (1995) Analysis of pain management in critically ill patients. Pharmacotherapy 15(5): 592–599

[105] Sim KM, Hwang NC, Chan YW, Seah CS (1996) Use of patient-controlled analgesia with alfentanil for burns dressing procedures: a preliminary report of five patients. Burns. 22(3): 238–241

[106] Gallagher G, Rae CP, Kenny GN, Kinsella J (2000) The use of a target-controlled infusion of alfentanil to provide analgesia for burn dressing changes: A dose finding study. Anaesthesia 55(12): 1159–1163

Correspondence: Dr. Richard Girtler, DEAA. Facharzt für Anästhesie und Intensivmedizin, Abteilung für Anästhesie und Intensivmedizin am Wilhelminenspital der Stadt Wien, Montleartstraße 37, 1160 Wien, Austria, E-mail: richard.girtler@wien kav.at

# Nutrition support for the burn patient

Amalia Cochran, Jeffrey R. Saffle, Caran Graves

Burn-Trauma Center, University of Utah Health Center, Salt Lake City, UT, USA

## Background

Nutrition support represents a critical component in the care of the acutely burned patient. Management of nutritional demands mandates attention to the unique hypermetabolic state that results from major burn injury; this pathophysiology results in loss of lean body mass, increased fat accretion and protein wasting, and impaired wound healing. Historically, failure to address these problems in victims of major burn injury often resulted in a fatal degree of inanition and death from infection and heart failure within a few weeks of injury [1, 2]. Current understanding and appreciation of burn hypermetabolism is still imperfect, but methods exist to support the patient throughout the critical period of muscle wasting and metabolic demand while healing occurs. Thus, the goal of nutrition support in the burn patient is to ameliorate- and hopefully optimize- the deranged metabolism resulting from burn injury and permit successful closure of the burn wound and resolution of the hypermetabolic state.

This chapter will review current knowledge of burn metabolism and nutrition with an emphasis on evidence-based literature. In doing so, it must be appreciated that much of our knowledge of nutritional support is extrapolated from studies in other patient populations, particularly trauma and critical care. The reader is referred to excellent recent reviews and practice guidelines on this subject [3, 4]; more limited guidelines have also been published specifically for burns [5, 6]. It is noteworthy that recommendations from North America regarding burn patient nutrition differ from those published in Europe [7], which illustrates the differences which can arise in interpreting the limited data available in this population. Thus, much of this information requires careful interpretation and leaves a number of important controversies in the care of burn patients unresolved.

## Case presentation

A 26-year-old healthy man (85 kg) was transferred to the burn center after he was injured in a propane gas flash explosion. He sustained approximately 48% TBSA burn injury, including face and neck, anterior arms and legs, and most of his anterior torso. His burn is a combination of full- and partial- thickness injury. Due to his facial burns and concern for inhalation injury, he was intubated prior to transport. His burn shock resuscitation proceeded normally; at 12 hours post-injury the clinician wished to determine what should be done about nutrition support for this patient.

## Patient selection: Timing and route of nutritional support

While all people require nutrition, not all patients require formal nutritional support. Patients with limited injuries who are anticipated to eat normally within 3–5 days will tolerate this short period of inadequate nutrition. However, these inferences can be wrong and more seriously injured patients should not be "permitted to fail" before beginning nutritional support. This case patient clearly fits this category: he was intubated and may be unable to take anything by mouth for many days. His major burn will unquestionably require more metabolic support than he could reasonably eat and even a few days of starvation would produce significant muscle wasting. Most experts would agree that nutrition should absolutely be started within the first three days of injury [8], and preferably within the first 24–48 hours [3].

**How early is early?** Debate continues over the value of "early" nutritional support, defined as that started within 24 hours of injury. Some studies have shown that intestinal feeding begun within 12 hours of injury – even in patients subjected to abdominal surgery – can be tolerated, and may reduce infectious complications [9]. However, providing this nutrition can be difficult; burn patients are prone to early ileus, and ongoing burn shock is associated with splanchnic hypoperfusion. Feedings are often poorly tolerated, leading to frequent interruptions, inadequate delivery of nutrients, and increasing the risks of serious complications such as aspiration and intestinal necrosis. Recent trials have confirmed these findings and found no major advantage to such early enteral nutrition in burn patients [10, 11]. A more reasonable goal is to institute nutrition by 48 hours post-burn with the goal of achieving full nutritional maintenance within 3–5 days.

**Enteral vs. Parenteral?** The superiority of enteral nutrition (EN) is universally acknowledged. Parenteral nutrition (PN) is expensive. Complications associated with intravenous access (pneumothorax, line sepsis) and major metabolic complications, including hypo- and hyper-glycemia, are both more common and more severe than those seen with enteral nutrition. Overall infections are also more common in ICU populations given PN [12]. In addition, EN directly nourishes bowel mucosa, preventing mucosal atrophy and preserving normal gut-associated immune and inflammatory status [13]. The enteral route is thus clearly preferred over PN for short- and long-term nutritional support for all critically-ill patients [3, 7].

There is less agreement, however, on the possible value of PN in two situations: as a supplement to "bridge" patients during the initial institution of EN or as "rescue" therapy in patients who cannot tolerate adequate (or sometimes any) enteral support. In some trials in burn patients, PN supplementation was associated with increased mortality compared to patients given even limited EN [14, 15], suggesting that PN should be avoided at all costs. However, this has not been supported in a meta-analysis of critically-ill patients [16]. Current guidelines restrict initial PN use to patients who are anticipated to be unable to tolerate EN for at least 7 days. However, once PN is begun, it should be maintained until patients can take at least 60% of required calories enterally [3]. Some burn authorities routinely use PN to supplement EN during the "ramp-in" phase of nutrition, and whenever tube feedings are interrupted by surgery, technical problems, or intolerance [5]. This can lead to smoother institution of enteral feedings, and fewer interruptions for distension, diarrhea, and other problems. With these few exceptions, however, EN should be the preferred – and usually the only-method of nutrition required for burn patients.

**Gastric vs. small bowel?** Another disagreement surrounds the best location for placement of enteral feeding tubes. Many patients tolerate feeding directly into the stomach. Large-diameter gastric tubes can be placed by nurses immediately and used for decompression and medications as well as nutrition. However, gastric ileus is common in burn patients, leading to distension and risking aspiration. Intestinal feeding is often better tolerated and may be continued to the time of and during surgery [17]. Enteric feeding tubes require skilled placement and are easily displaced; tubes also clog easily, and these technical complications can lead to delayed initiation and frequent interruptions in nourishment. There is some evidence that aspiration is more common with gastric feedings [18], but this is disputed [19]. In recent meta-analyses no differences in mortality or aspiration rates were found between gastric and small bowel feedings, but the latter took significantly longer to institute and experienced more frequent interruptions [20, 21]. Either route can be used successfully provided that this issue is incorporated into an overall plan for nutritional management.

**Application:** In the patient presented above, a naso-enteric feeding tube was placed on the morning following admission (24 hours after injury) under fluoroscopic guidance and carefully secured. Enteral nutrition (see below for a discussion of formulas) was started at a low rate, and increased gradually over the next 48 hours, so that the patient achieved goal-rate nutrition by 72 hours post-burn. We also elected to give a single enteral dose of erythromycin as a "pro motility" agent to help reduce gastric ileus and promote passage of the enteral tube into the small intestine [22].

## Determining nutritional demands

Initiation of nutritional support requires estimation of a caloric goal in ICU patients [3]. This estimation can prove particularly challenging in burns because of the profound hypermetabolic response that the body mounts in response to significant burn injury. Malnutrition is associated with the development of pneumonia in critically ill patients and is known to impair wound healing. Without appropriate management, the protein-calorie malnutrition that results from burn hypermetabolism may be life threatening.

Further, although adequate nutrition is desired, care must be taken not to provide calories in excess of the patient's needs. Overfeeding has been shown to result in fat accretion in burn patients and may contribute to difficulties with glycemic control and ventilator weaning. Estimated energy demands provide an appropriate starting point for nutritional support in major burns, with revision occurring based upon metabolic characteristics and patient tolerance of enteral feeds.

### What is an appropriate initial nutrition plan for this patient?

Energy expenditure in burn patients is a heterogeneous metabolic process and the protean manifestations of burn hypermetabolism make determination of energy and protein requirements particularly dif-

ficult. However, several algebraic formulas are widely used for determination of initial assessment of energy needs. Estimation of basal energy expenditure (BEE) using the Harris-Benedict equation or kcal/Kg formulas are used at most American Burn Association verified burn centers [23]. The baseline estimate acquired using the Harris-Benedict equation is usually multiplied by a factor of 1.2 to 1.4 to allow for the hypermetabolism associated with the burn injury. Although more varied methods are used in children, two methods are used most commonly to estimate caloric needs. The first of these is the recommended dietary allowances (RDA), recently revised and known as the Dietary Reference Index (DRI) [24]. This is a widely-used standard formula for estimating nutritional requirements. A burn-specific formula, the Galveston formula, is also widely used in pediatric burn care. Together, the RDA/DRI and/or Galveston formulas are the routine methods of estimating energy requirements used in over 70% of US burn centers [23]. Of note, the previously used Curreri formula appears to have fallen out of favor for both adult and pediatric burns, likely because of the marked overestimation of energy demands demonstrated by this formula [25, 26]. Table 1 shows each of the more commonly used formulas and includes additional comments on many of these formulas, including information on the accuracy of each formula versus measured energy demands using indirect calorimetry (IDC) when that data is available.

The primary pitfall of these commonly used formulas for caloric demands in burned adults and children is that they frequently overestimate patients' resting energy expenditure (REE) [3, 25, 26]. Feeding more than 1.2 times REE has been shown to increase fat accretion and does not improve maintenance of lean body mass in acute burn patients [27]. Therefore, although these formulas typically provide an appropriate method for initial estimates, measurement of energy expenditure by IDC provides a more precise representation of the burn patient's energy expenditure over time.

Estimation of caloric needs in the obese burn patient should use ideal body weight in any algebraic formula calculations; otherwise, these equations result in substantial overfeeding. Although the concept of "permissive underfeeding" in the obese currently predominates the ICU nutrition literature, the bene-

**Table 1.** Commonly used algebraic formulas for caloric needs in nutritional support

| ADULT FORMULAS | Formula | Daily caloric estimates for 25 year-old male, 85 kg, 180 cm, 48% TBSA | Comments |
|---|---|---|---|
| Harris-Benedict [111] | **Men:** 66.5 + 13.8 (Weight in Kg) + 5 (Height in cm) – 6.76 (Age in years) | Baseline = 1,946 kcal<br>If factor 1.5 = 2,918 kcal | Estimates basal energy expenditure (BEE). Best stress adjustment is a factor of 1.5; results in a % calorie variance of 19 ± 24% from measured REE (MREE) (p = NS). [26] |
| | **Women:** 655 + 9.6 (Weight in Kg) + 1.85 (Height in cm) – 4.68 (Age in years) | | |
| Kcal/Kg (Common use) [26] | 35 kcal/kg | 2,975 kcal | Variance of 23 ± 36% from MREE (p = NS) [26] |
| Curreri [112] | **Age 16–59:** 25 kcal/ kg/ day + 40 kcal/ %TBSA burn/ day | 4,045 kcal | Variance of 35 ± 35% from MREE (p = 0 001)[26] Now rarely used because of marked tendency to over-estimate calories. |
| | **Age ≥60:** 20 kcal/kg/day + 65 kcal/ %TBSA burn/ day | | |

| PEDIATRIC FORMULAS | Formula | Daily caloric estimates for a 15-month old male, 11 kg, 0.9 m² BSA | Comments |
|---|---|---|---|
| DRI [113] | On-line calculator | 899 kcal/day<br>If factor 1.2 = 1,078 kcal/ day<br>If factor 1.4 = 1,258 kcal/ day | Varies according to age, weight, and activity level. Includes allowances for growth and activity. |
| Galveston [114–116] | **0–1 Years:** 2 100 kcal/m²/day + 1 000 kcal/m² TBSA burn/day | | Like the Curreri formula, the Galveston formula was created with the goal of maintaining body weight. |
| | **1–11 Years:** 1 800 kcal/m²/day + 1 300 kcal/m² TBSA burn/day | 2,182 kcal/day | |
| | **12–18 Years:** 1 500 kcal/m²/day + 1 500 kcal/ m² TBSA burn/day | | |
| Curreri Junior [117] | **≤1 Year:** RDA + 15 kcal/ %TBSA burn | | Now rarely used because of marked tendency to over-estimate calories. |
| | **1–3 Years:** RDA + 25 kcal/ % TBSA burn | 2,099 kcal | |
| | **4–15 Years:** RDA + 40 kcal/ % TBSA burn | | |

fits and dangers of this practice have not yet been clearly established in patients with burn injury [28–30]. The physiologic principles of permissive underfeeding rely upon fat oxidation to mobilize peripheral energy stores in these patients, a pairing of metabolic processes that are known to be deranged in patients with significant burns.

Ratios for carbohydrate, protein, and fat intake must also be considered once a caloric goal has been established. Carbohydrates may limit loss of lean body mass by stimulation of protein synthesis, meaning that carbohydrates should be the primary energy source in the hypermetabolic burn patient [31]. In addition, glucose serves as the primary metabolic fuel for wound healing. However, glucose administration rates in excess of 7 mg/kg/min cause hyperglycemia with the attendant complications of impaired wound healing, conversion of excess calories to fat, and elevated rates of carbon dioxide production [32]. Optimal nutrition support in burns consists of at least 50% carbohydrate calories, with glucose administration occurring at rate of 5–7 mg/kg/min [33].

Protein requirements are also heterogeneous in burn patients and must be carefully considered in the development of a nutrition care plan. Protein demands in burn injury are increased due to the catabolic response to injury as well as the need for protein for wound healing and immune function. While healthy, uninjured individuals synthesize protein at a rate of 4 grams/ kg/ day, burn patients may induce protein synthesis rates of nearly twice that [34]. Administration of nutritional support with 1.5–2 grams/ kg/ day of protein balances protein synthesis and breakdown in the course of burn hypermetabolism [35]. The calories provided by protein are usually calculated as part of the total energy support of the patient. However, this protein should always be provided in addition to significant energy in the form of carbohydrate and fat calories; otherwise, the protein will be used entirely as an energy source rather than as a specific nutrient to provide substrate for wound healing and support of muscle mass. For that reason, the amount of protein contained in various nutrients is often expressed as the ratio of nonprotein calories to nitrogen (NPCal:N2). The optimal NPCal:N2 for burn patients has long been recognized to be a function of burn size [36], but is almost always a lower ratio than in unstressed patients.

Administration of nutrition support with lipid content in excess of 15% impairs immune function [37]. Lipids are necessary as a source of free fatty acids and for carriage of lipid-soluble vitamins, and some lipid calories are helpful in avoiding requirements for excessive quantities of glucose. Enhanced lipolysis occurs in burn hypermetabolism with the rate of free fatty acid oxidation being nearly double that measured in healthy volunteers [34]. This enhanced lipolysis may result in increased recycling of free fatty acids or increased total body fat stores. Optimal lipid content for burn nutrition support is therefore less than 15%, at least during the initial highly catabolic phase [33, 38, 39]. However, as will be shown below, few commercially-available enteral products fulfill this requirement. Patients given PN may be better off if fat is withheld entirely for short periods and given as little as once weekly [40], and this practice is recommended when instituting PN [3] even though this may contribute to aggravated glucose intolerance.

Demands for vitamins and trace minerals are increased in all critically ill patients, and this demand is marked in burn patients because of exudative losses that occur in the absence of the skin barrier. Use of micronutrient supplementation has increased remarkably over the last 20 years and now represents a widespread practice in burn nutrition. All centers that responded to a recent survey on nutrition care practices indicated daily use of a multivitamin supplement [23]. However, no evidence-based guidelines currently exist for additional micronutrient supplementation in burns [5].

Vitamins A and C are routinely supplemented in many burn centers and therefore merit consideration. Both of these vitamins show decreased levels following burn injury and demonstrate responsiveness to supplementation [41]. Vitamin A has multiple functions relevant to burn care, including prevention of free radical damage, maintenance of immune function, and assistance in wound epithelialization. Vitamin C also has antioxidant function and plays a critical role in collagen cross-linking and, therefore, wound healing. One group has recommended supplementation in burn patients with 1000 IU of Vitamin A and 500 mg of Vitamin C daily [42]. Clinicians should be mindful of the potential for toxicity with high doses of Vitamin A. High doses of Vitamin C, in contrast, seem to have no toxic effects with excess simply being excreted in urine.

Burned patients, especially children, are known to suffer bone demineralization, predisposing them to spontaneous fractures [43], and contributing to growth retardation. Reasons for this are multifactorial, including increased glucocorticoid production, reduced production of parathyroid hormone, and impaired synthesis of Vitamin D [44, 45].

Klein et al. have provided a detailed description of the events responsible for demineralization of bone following burn injury, the reduction in parathyroid hormone production, and the subsequent deficiency of 1,25 dihydroxyvitamin D. In addition, skin from burned patients cannot synthesize Vitamin D correctly and burn patients are encouraged to avoid sun exposure on the skin [46]. As a consequence, burn patients suffer chronic Vitamin D deficiency. This would imply that oral supplementation would be both necessary and helpful in enhancing Vitamin D levels in burn patients and improving bone metabolism. However, in one study oral Vitamin D supplementation did not improve serum levels in a group of burned children [47]. In addition, treatment of burned children with intravenous administration of the bisphosphonate pamidronate was associated with improved bone mineral content after six months, apparently by reducing the bone resorption in these patients [48]. As a result of this experience, it remains unknown whether vitamin D supplements are effective in burn patients and what the correct dose should be. Since all standard multivitamins contain substantial amounts of vitamin D, that is the only supplementation that is recommended at present.

Zinc is the antioxidant trace mineral that is most often routinely supplemented in burn centers. Zinc plays important roles in collagen cross-linking, wound healing, and immune function, and zinc levels have been shown to be depleted in burn patients due to the combination of urinary losses and exudative losses from wounds [49, 50]. Combined IV supplementation of zinc, selenium, and copper has demonstrated increased tissue levels and has resulted clinically in improved wound healing, decreased pulmonary infections, and diminished length of hospital stay [51–53]. However, this strategy has not been widely adopted outside of Europe; best current recommendation from a U.S. center has been for supplementation of zinc only with 200 mg of enteral zinc sulfate, recognizing that this dose may be associated with significant nausea and may interfere with the absorption of copper [42].

Trace mineral supplementation and its application to burn care is an area ripe for future research.

**Application:** *Calories and macronutrients:* The patient described in the case above weighed 85 kg and was 180 cm in height. If Harris-Benedict estimation of REE X 1.2 was used for initial calculation, his initial energy goal was 2 356 kcal/ day. If protein was set at 2 grams/ kg/day, the patient received 170 grams of protein, or 680 protein calories. Lipids should not exceed 350 kcal/day (39 grams) if they were to provide less than 15% of caloric demands. The balance of calories were supplied by carbohydrates, totaling 329 grams or 1 314 kcal (56% of estimated daily energy requirement).

*Micronutrients:* The patient was also given a daily adult multivitamin in the form of an enteral liquid preparation via nasoenteric tube. Administration of 1000 IU of Vitamin A, 500 mg of Vitamin C, and 220 mg of Zinc Sulfate on a daily basis were considered although none were administered. All micronutrient supplementation was enteral.

## Formulations for nutritional support

A variety of nutrient formulations are available for enteral nutrition of burn patients, as well as a number of pre-packaged supplements to standard products. While it is possible to prepare customized enteral formulations, this is extremely expensive and time-consuming, so clinicians should select a commercially available formula in feeding the patient presented in the case scenario. Parenteral nutrition, conversely, is made as needed from components and is easy to customize. Before beginning either type of nutrition the role of specific nutrients in critically-ill patients should be considered.

**Calorie considerations:** As discussed previously, estimates of total calories required for nutritional support are often used to guide the infusion rate of enteral or parenteral nutrient solutions. In planning this, however, clinicians should remember than other infusions can contain significant calories. In particular, dextrose-containing intravenous fluids given to provide adequate hydration contain significant calories; a liter of 5% dextrose contains 50 grams of dextrose, or almost 200 kcal. Because burn patients require large amounts of fluid to counteract evaporative losses, this can amount to a significant caloric load in itself. In addition, some medications may be given in dextrose-containing fluids. The sedative agent propofol is becoming increasingly popular in burn care, but propofol is a lipid emulsion that contains 1.1 kcal/mL. Use of these agents commonly leads to significant overfeeding unless these calories are calculated into the total requirements of the patient [54]. Also, because neither of these sources contains any protein, this increases the need to use high-protein nutrition to compensate for the effect of these "empty" calories.

**Dietary fat and fatty acids:** The potential benefits of low-fat diets have been discussed previously. Most common lipid sources contain mainly omega-6 fatty acids (ω-6 FFA's). These acids are metabolized through synthesis of arachadonic acid, a precursor of pro-inflammatory cytokines. Lipids such as fish oil (FO) contain mostly ω-3 FFA's, which are metabolized without creating pro-inflammatory compounds. Diets high in ω-3 FFA's have been associated with improved outcomes in a variety of clinical situations [55] and have been specifically recommended for use in patients with acute lung injury, in whom aggravated inflammation is thought to play an important pathophysiologic role [3]. Excessive inflammatory response from a pulmonary source may be an issue in some burn patients and use of diets high in ω-3 FFA's may have clinical advantages in this setting [56].

**Protein composition:** Glutamine (GLU): In addition to providing high-protein nutrition, the specific composition of the protein provided may be important in providing optimal nutrition to burn patients. The amino acids alanine and glutamine are important "transport" amino acids, elaborated in large quantities from skeletal muscle to supply energy to the liver and to healing wounds [57]. Glutamine performs other important roles, acting as a primary nutrient for gut enterocytes [58] and enhancing production of protective heat shock proteins [59]. Glutamine appears to reduce gut permeability and elaboration of inflammatory mediators and reduces infections in critically-ill patients [60]. Glutamine is almost entirely absent from standard PN solutions, which may partially explain the increased infections observed in association with PN use.

Glutamine may be of particular value to burn and trauma patients. Supplemental glutamine given either enterally [61, 62] or parenterally [63, 64] has been associated with reduced infectious complications and mortality in several small studies in burn patients. Because its effects are best seen when glutamine is given at high doses (≥ 0.25 gm/kg/day, or ≥ 18 gm/day in a 70-kg patient), specific supplementation of enteral formulations with glutamine is necessary to obtain its benefits and this supplementation should be used in addition to the high protein content recommended for all burn patients. Glutamine-containing enteral nutrition is recom-

mended for critically-ill populations, including burns [3], and many burn centers currently use it [23] in spite of the absence of conclusive data to support glutamine supplementation. A multicenter randomized trial to assess the benefits of glutamine supplementation in burns is currently underway.

**Arginine (ARG):** Arginine is another important amino acid in post-burn metabolism. Arginine stimulates T-lymphocytes and enhances synthesis of nitric oxide, both of which enhance immunity and inflammation [65]. Arginine-enhanced nutrition appears to be of value in reducing infections and improving wound healing, and stabilizing inflammation after burn injury [66]. However, there are reports of increased mortality in septic patients receiving arginine-containing formulas. Burn patients are at risk of this complication, making it difficult to advocate for the routine addition of arginine to the diets of burn patients.

**Immune-enhancing diets:** Because the potential value of the nutrients reviewed above appeared to be both clinically and commercially significant, few trials of individual compounds have been performed. Instead, they were quickly combined into "immune-enhancing" diets (IED's) containing GLU, ARG, ω-3 FFA's, and other compounds. In one early study, a customized low-fat diet supplemented with ω-3 FFA's, histidine, ARG, RNA, and vitamins was associated with reduced infections and mortality in a group of burned children [67]. IED's have been evaluated subsequently in a variety of clinical settings, with demonstration of reduced infections and hospital stay in some trauma and ICU populations [68, 69], but deleterious or no effects in patients with sepsis or pneumonia [70]. These inconsistent results have been attributed to the pro-inflammatory effects of ARG, which may be beneficial in preventing postoperative infections but harmful to patients with acute lung injury, possibly including burn patients [71].

This confusing experience serves to underscore the imperfect status of our knowledge of nutrition in various disease states. In addition, the rush to create commercially-available "cocktails" for clinical use has further obscured our understanding of the action of each of these specific nutrients. As a result, recommendations for use of these supplements are somewhat contradictory. In some publications standard multi-component IED's have been recommended for acutely injured patients, including burn victims, but not for patients with acute lung injury or severe sepsis, for whom ω-3-enhanced diets are suggested [3]. The benefits of these multi-component IED's have not been clearly demonstrated in burn patients [72, 73]; some reviews have not recommended IED's for this group [5, 74]. This appears to be one area of critical care in which data from one patient population CANNOT be safely extrapolated to others. As a result, there is little consistency in the nutritional regimens practiced among burn centers [75]. More conclusive recommendations will require the results of well-designed, large-scale clinical trials.

**Parenteral nutrition:** One advantage of PN is the ability (or necessity) to prepare customized formulas for each patient daily. Parenteral nutrition relies primarily on concentrated dextrose as an energy source. Protein is provided in the form of amino acids, but because glutamine is not stable in suspension it is almost entirely absent from PN formulations. Lipids can be provided as a soy-based lipid emulsion (Intralipid™ – Pharmacia/Upjohn). Vitamins, trace elements and some additional medications such as insulin or heparin can also be added. Also, because these solutions are hypertonic, free water can be added which reduces the need for additional dextrose-containing IV infusions. Parenteral formulations must be made by pharmacy professionals under strict sterile guidelines, and require central venous access for delivery.

Clinicians attempting to create the "ideal" PN solution encounter a paradox: data cited above suggests that nutrition should be low in fat, but that means providing most calories as dextrose with attendant problems of hyperglycemia. Supplemental insulin – which can be added directly to PN solutions – is very often necessary to help control blood sugar, but even with aggressive insulin infusions, hyperglycemia can become a critical problem. The challenge of hyperglycemia is addressed in more detail in the section on complications of nutrition.

**Enteral nutrition:** A bewildering array of commercial formulas is available for nutritional support. A selection of these is reviewed in Table 2. Before resorting to any of these, remember that many burn patients who tolerate oral intake may need only supplementation. Early diets using eggs, milk, and other inexpensive products were successful in many patients [76]. Patients often enjoy good-tasting milkshakes made with these products and powdered supplements (e. g., Instant Breakfast™, Nestle), or prepared supplements like Boost™ (Nestle). These formulations can also be infused into large-bore gastric tubes but are usually too thick for use in small enteral feeding tubes.

Reviewing Table 2 will reveal that the range of available commercial products is limited, restricting our ability to "mix and match" specific components. Based on the information reviewed previously, an "ideal" enteral formula might include the following: high-protein (NPCal:N2 of ≤ 100:1), low fat (> 15%), a high proportion of ω-3 FFA's, and a substantial dose (≥ 0.25 gm/Kg) of glutamine. Regardless, no commercial formula currently exists which combines all of these characteristics, leaving clinicians to select the components they think will be most helpful for particular situations. Complications such as diarrhea may limit the use of some formulas or require the addition of fiber. Cost and availability are also issues. Some of the formulas reviewed are intended for very specialized situations such as renal or respiratory failure. They are not well suited for general use in burn patients and are often far more expensive than "standard" formulas.

Clinicians can try to overcome the limitations of available formulas in two ways. First, formulas can be supplemented with protein, carbohydrates, fats, vitamins, fiber, or other specific components. Glutamine is now available as an additive for enteral nutrition but not for PN. Use of these agents can help make up for specific deficiencies of commercial formulas. Some standard additives are included in Table 3. Second, some units have resorted to use of elemental or semi-elemental diets. These diets contain simple carbohydrates, medium-chain triglycerides, and either free amino acids or short peptides. They require almost no digestion and are ideal for patients with short bowel or other absorptive problems. They can be also supplemented with additional nutrients in patients with the ability to digest them. They are relatively expensive, however, and because of increased osmolarity can be associated with diarrhea.

**Application:** For the patient presented previously, enteral nutrition was begun using Promote™ (Ab-

**Table 2.** Composition of a sampling of commercially-available adult and pediatric enteral nutrition products (contents are per 100 mL of feedings)

## I. ADULT FORMULAS

A. "Standard" formulas: These are relatively inexpensive formulas for general use. They provide complete balanced nutrition, including micronutrients, with moderate amounts of protein and fat primarily for non-stressed patients. Osmolarity varies; those intended for tube feedings are generally low. Only one (Boost©) is intended for oral use.

| Brand Name (Manufacturer) | Kcal1 | kcal to meet RDI | Osm | CARBS | | PROTEIN | | | FAT | | | Comment |
|---|---|---|---|---|---|---|---|---|---|---|---|---|
| | | | | Gm | %Kcal | Gm | %Kcal | NPCal: N2 | Gm | %Kcal | w6:w3 | |
| Boost™ (Nestle) | 100 | 1180 | 625 | 17 | 67 | 4.2 | 17 | 128:1 | 1.7 | 16 | 4.9:1 | These are both Inexpensive, good-tasting supplement for oral intake or gastrostomy feeds. Not for small bowel feeding. |
| Ensure™ (Abbott) | 106 | 1,000 | 620 | 17 | 64 | 3.8 | 14.4 | 149:1 | 2.5 | 22 | NA | |
| Osmolite (Abbott)2 | 106 | 1,321 | 300 | 14.4 | 54 | 4.4 | 17 | 125:1 | 3.5 | 35 | NS | Widely used relatively inexpensive formula for tube feedings. |
| Nutren 1.0 (Nestle) | 100 | 1,500 | 300–350 | 12.7 | 51 | 4.0 | 16 | 133:1 | 3.8 | 33 | 4.1:1 | Available with or without fiber; also available in 1.5 or 2.0 kcal/mL. |
| Isosource HN (Nestle)* | 120 | 1,400 | 490 | 16 | 53 | 5.3 | 18 | 115:1 | 3.9 | 29 | 2.7:1 | Relatively High-protein formula |

\* Similar products include Isocal-HN™ (Mead-Johnson) and Jevity™ (Ross) with and without fiber

B. High Calorie Standard Formulas: These are concentrated formulas for use in patients with fluid restrictions. Increased concentrations of fat and/or carbohydrates mean increased osmolarity, which can contribute to diarrhea.

| Brand Name (Manufacturer) | Kcal1 | kcal to meet RDI | Osm | CARBS | | PROTEIN | | | FAT | | | Comment |
|---|---|---|---|---|---|---|---|---|---|---|---|---|
| | | | | Gm | %Kcal | Gm | %Kcal | NPCal: N2 | Gm | %Kcal | w6:w3 | |
| Nutren 2.0© Nestle* | 200 | 1500 | 745 | 19.6 | 39 | 8 | 16 | 131:1 | 10 | 45 | 4.6:1 | |

\* Similar products include Isosource 1.5™ (Nestle), and TwoCalHN™ (Abbott)

C. High protein Critical Care and "Immune-Enhancing Adult Formulas: These are formulas to enhance healing in stressed patients. All have high nonprotein Cal:N2 ratios and provide part of fat as MCT oil for improved absorption. Many contain additional additives to enhance immune function or healing.

| Brand Name (Manufacturer) | Kcal1 | kcal to meet RDI | Osm | CARBS | | PROTEIN | | | FAT | | | Comment |
|---|---|---|---|---|---|---|---|---|---|---|---|---|
| | | | | Gm | %Kcal | Gm | %Kcal | NPCal: N2 | Gm | %Kcal | w6:w3 | |
| Impact™ (Nestle) | 100 | 1500 | 375 | 13 | 53 | 5.6 | 22 | 71:1 | 2.8 | 25 | 1.4:1 | Widely used "immune-enhancing" formula; supplemented with ARG, (12.5 gm/L), RNA; high in w-3 FFA's |
| Impact 1.5™ (Nestle) | 150 | 1500 | 550 | 14 | 38 | 8.4 | 22 | 71:1 | 6.9 | 40 | 1.4:1 | Concentrated formula, supplemented with ARG (18.7 gm/L); high in w-3 FFA's. Available with and without fiber |
| Impact Glutamine™ (Nestle) | 130 | 1300 | 630 | 15 | 46 | 7.8 | 24 | 62:1 | 4.3 | 30 | 1.4:1 | Concentrated. Supplemented with ARG (16.3g/L), GLU (15 gm/L), RNA, w-3 FFA's. Contains fiber 10g/L |
| Perative™ (Abbott) | 130 | 1500 | 460 | 18 | 55 | 6.7 | 20.5 | 97:1 | 3.7 | 25 | NA | Immune-enhancing formula supplemented with ARG (8gm/L), vitamins |
| Nutren™ Replete™ (Nestle) | 100 | 1000 | 300–350 | 11.3 | 45 | 6.2 | 25 | 75:1 | 3.4 | 30 | 2.3:1 | Inexpensive, High-protein formula. Available with or without fiber |
| Promote™ (Abbott) | 100 | 1000 | 340 | 13 | 52 | 6.2 | 25 | 75:1 | 2.6 | 23 | NA | High protein formula. Available with or without fiber |

D. "Specialty" Adult Formulas: These are examples of formulas for patients with unusual, specific nutritional requirements. None are well-suited for burn patients, and are generally much more expensive than more standard formulas.

| Brand Name (Manufacturer) | Kcal1 | kcal to meet RDI | Osm | CARBS | | PROTEIN | | | FAT | | | Comment |
|---|---|---|---|---|---|---|---|---|---|---|---|---|
| | | | | Gm | %Kcal | Gm | %Kcal | NPCal: N2 | Gm | %Kcal | w6:w3 | |
| Glucerna™ (Ross)* | 100 | 1420 | 355 | 11.2 | 34 | 4.2 | 17 | 125:1 | 2.3 | 30 | 11:1 | complex-carbohydrate formula for diabetics; Contains fiber. Used primarily as an oral nutrient/supplement |
| Pulmocare™ (Ross)** | 150 | 1420 | 470 | 10.5 | 28 | 6.2 | 17 | 125:1 | 9.3 | 55 | 4:1 | Customized formula for pulmonary failure relies on high fat content to avoid excessive $VCO_2$; limited efficacy in burn patients. For tube or oral feeding |

\* Similar products include Diabetisource AC™(Nestle), Nutren Glytrol Diet™ (Nestle)
\*\* Similar products include Oxepa™ (Abbott), Nutren Pulmonary™ (Nestle)

E. Elemental/Semi-elemental Diets: Nutritionally complete diets intended for patients with minimal digestive ability or absorption problems. Minimal residue, provide protein as peptides and/or free amino acids. Elemental diet are high osmolarity due to simple sugars and free amino acids; semi-elemental have lower osmolality, and some provide more balanced carbohydrate, fat, and protein composition.

| Brand Name (Manufacturer) | Kcal1 | kcal to meet RDI | Osm | CARBS | | PROTEIN | | | FAT | | | Comment |
|---|---|---|---|---|---|---|---|---|---|---|---|---|
| | | | | Gm | %Kcal | Gm | %Kcal | NPCal: N2 | Gm | %Kcal | w6:w3 | |
| Vital HN™ (Abbott)* | 100 | 1500 | 500 | 18.5 | 73.8 | 4.2 | 17 | 125:1 | 1.1 | 9.5 | NA | Basic semi-elemental diet, low in fat. |
| Optimental™ (Abbott) | 100 | 1422 | 585 | 13.9 | 54 | 5.1 | 21 | 97:1 | 2.8 | 25 | 1:1 | High-protein Immune-enhancing semi-elemental formula supplemented with Arginine (8 gm/L), vitamins |
| Peptamen AF™ (Nestle) | 120 | 1500 | 390 | 10.7 | 36 | 7.6 | 25 | 75:1 | 5.5 | 39 | 1.8:1 | High-protein semi-elemental diet, supplemented with w-3 FFA's, fiber |

\* Similar products include Tolerex™ (Nestle)

## II. PEDIATRIC FORMULAS

Nutritionally complete, intact protein products formulated to meet the nutrient needs of toddlers and children ( > 1 year). May be used as oral supplements or complete enteral nutrition. Not intended for use in infants

| Brand Name (Manufacturer) | Kcal1 | Kcal to meet RDI | Osm | CARBS | | PROTEIN | | | FAT | | | Comments |
|---|---|---|---|---|---|---|---|---|---|---|---|---|
| | | | | Gm | %Kcal | Gm | %Kcal | NPCal: N2 | Gm | %Kcal | w6:w3 | |
| Pediasure Enteral™ (Ross)* | 100 | 1000 | 535 | 13 | 53 | 3 | 12 | 180:1 | 4 | 35 | NA | Standard tube feeding. Available with or without fiber |
| Pediatric Vivonex™ (Nestle) | 80 | 1000 | 360 | 13 | 63 | 2.4 | 12 | 200:1 | 2.4 | 25 | 7.7:1 | Elemental formula supplemented with Arginine (1.5 gm/L), glutamine (3.1 gm/L) |

\* Similar products include Nutren Junior™ (Nestle)

**Table 3.** MODULAR PRODUCTS

These are incomplete products intended as supplements to tube feeding formulas for specific purposes

A. Carbohydrates: Polycose© Powder (Abbott): Glucose polymers, 95 gm (380 kcal)/100 gm powder.
B. Lipids:
  1. MCT Oil™ (Nestle): Medium-chain triglycerides from coconut oil, 85 gm MCT (767 kcal)/100 mL oil.
  2. Microlipid™ (Nestle): Safflower oil, 50.7 gm (456 Kcal)/100 mL.
C. Protein:
  1. ProPass© Protein Supplement (Hormel): Powdered whey protein concentrate. One scoop contains 6 gm protein,
    0.5 gm fat.
  2. Beneprotein™ (Nestle): Whey protein supplement. One scoop or packet (7gm) contains 6 gm whey protein.
D. Arginine and glutamine supplements
  1. Enterex Glutapac™ (Victus): 10g glutamine/pkt
  2. Sypmt-X™ (Baxter): Glutamina, 10g/pkt
  3. Glutasolve™ (Nestle): 90 kcal, 7g CHO 15g glutamine
  4. Arginaid™ (Nestle) 35 kcal, 4g CHO, 4.5g arginine, Vitamin C & E
  5. Juven™ (Abbott): powder contains 66 kcal, 4g CHO, 7g each arginine and glutamine

[1] Abbreviations: "mL" = milliliters of formula to contain; "Kcal to meet RDI"= Number of calories required to deliver 100 percent of recommended dietary intake of micronutrients (Includes micronutrients not listed); "Osm" = osmolarity, mOsm/kg H20; "gm" = grams; "%kcal": percentage of total calories; "NPCal:N2" = ratio of non-protein calories to nitrogen; "w6:w3" = ratio of w6 to w3 fatty acids. Information from manufacturers' websites as of April, 2010.

[2] Information from manufacturers' websites as of April, 2010. The composition of formulas marketed in different countries may be different. All values listed here are for US Products.

bott), a relatively inexpensive, high-protein formula. Infusion through the enteral tube was begun at 25 mL/hr and increased by 10 mL/hr increments every four hours, with a theoretical target rate of 100 mL hr (2,400 Kcal/day). However, at this time the patient was also receiving approximately 285 mL/hr of dextrose-containing maintenance IV fluid, which provided approximately 200 kcal/liter, or a total of 1,162 kcal/day. As the tube feedings were increased, this maintenance rate was reduced correspondingly. However, the problem of attempting to provide adequate amounts of fluid and protein while avoiding overfeeding total calories persisted. This required a compromise: tube feedings were increased to 90 mL/hr, plus a free water "flush" of 25 mL/hr, and IV fluid was reduced to 125 mL/hr. This provided 2,760 total calories (600 from intravenous dextrose, 2,160 from tube feedings) and 134 gm protein (1.6 gm/kg/D).

Any of the other "stress" formulas listed in the table would have been reasonable choices for this patient. ARG-supplemented formulas were not selected because of the patient's inhalation injury. The addition of supplemental glutamine could also be considered, but definitive support for this is pending the results of the ongoing randomized controlled trial. Finally, more free water could have been added to the tube feedings to increase fluid intake, which would have permitted reduction in IV fluids, but significant intake of oral/enteral free water is often associated with hyponatremia following burn injury.

This example indicates some of the issues which must be considered in providing optimal nourishment to severely burned patients. The value of a team-oriented nutrition protocol in this setting is apparent.

**Modulation of hypermetabolism:** Burn-related hormonal changes create tremendous problems in nutritional support, but also provide mechanisms by which hypermetabolism can be manipulated and at least partially controlled. Recent studies have suggested that manipulation of the metabolic response to injury can be beneficial in burn patients and other groups; this may become routine in the future. A variety of approaches have been utilized, including beta-blockade with propranolol, low-dose insulin infusions, use of counter-regulatory hormones such as insulin-like growth factor-1 (IGF-1), or anabolic agents such as testosterone and oxandrolone [77]. Use of propranolol appears to ameliorate both the cardiovascular response to acute burn injury, and reduce hypermetabolic muscle wasting during acute burn care [78]. Administration of the synthetic oral androgen oxandrolone has been shown to reduce muscle breakdown, speed rehabilitation, and lead to decreased length of stay in hospitalized patients [79,

80]. Although none of these therapies are now routine, they are becoming more widespread. Recommendations for their routine use will need to await larger controlled trials to demonstrate efficacy.

**Application:** The patient presented previously was started on oxandrolone oral supplementation, 10 mg twice daily, as an anabolic agent. He also received propranolol, 15 mg orally/enterally every 6 hours, with the dose titrated to achieve a 25 % reduction in heart rate from post-burn injury baseline.

## Monitoring nutrition support

Most patients with major burns who require nutrition support have a prolonged course, particularly because their metabolic demands remain above baseline even after wound coverage is complete. During the course of healing and convalescence from burn injury metabolic demands fluctuate significantly, displaying the classic "ebb and flow" pattern first described by Cuthbertson in 1930 [81], and also responding to changes in clinical status. Therefore, great importance is placed upon use of appropriate monitors of nutritional status.

Although a variety of methods exist for monitoring adequacy of nutritional support, validation of traditional tools used for monitoring nutritional status has not occurred in critically ill patients [3]. This lack of a "gold standard" is further complicated by the heterogeneity of burn patients' metabolic status and the associated variability in the findings from these methods. Therefore, employing a combination of clinical course, wound healing and objective measures, and an overall focus on trends optimizes monitoring [5]. Notably, neither the Canadian Clinical Practice guidelines nor the SCCM/ASPEN nutrition guidelines address monitoring of nutrition support once initiated [3, 82].

### Optimal monitoring of nutritional status

Various laboratory values have been suggested as potential surrogates for nutritional status, including the serum proteins transthyretin, c-reactive protein (CRP), retinol-binding protein (RBP), and transferrin. The relevance of measuring these proteins depends upon the extent of metabolic stress and alters with the patient's progression through injury recovery. Serum albumin levels become profoundly depressed with burn injury and are slow to recover even with provision of adequate nutrition. Further, serum albumin levels have no apparent correlation with nitrogen balance in burn patients, nor does supplementation of albumin to maintain serum levels have any evident clinical benefit [83, 84]. Transthyretin (prealbumin) has been considered as another surrogate, although levels also decrease precipitously following burn injury. Transthyretin levels do demonstrate consistent improvement as healing from burn injury occurs, as well as a weak association with nitrogen balance [83, 85]. However, no causality in those relationships has been established. Retinol-binding protein and transferrin have failed to demonstrate a relationship with nitrogen balance or any other indicator of nutritional adequacy [83]. Based upon the limited value of visceral proteins in monitoring nutritional status following burn injury, current recommendations consistently indicate that they should only be used in conjunction with other measures [25, 42, 83, 86]. Perhaps most importantly, none of these markers has demonstrated predictive capability for outcomes in burn patients, calling into question their validity as a surrogate for nutritional status; these may instead simply be a marker of severity of illness [87, 88].

The elevated protein demands associated with burn hypermetabolism imply relevance for nitrogen balance monitoring in assessing nutritional adequacy. Unfortunately, urinary urea nitrogen (UUN) has been best evaluated in children with major burns and has been demonstrated to be inaccurate [86]. This unreliability may be primarily present in patients with exceptional hypercatabolic responses [25]. Further, protein losses through wounds complicate the calculation of nitrogen balance. In spite of these limitations, measurement of UUN and calculation of nitrogen balance on a weekly basis allows estimation of nitrogen catabolism and modification of protein goals based upon trends [5, 25].

Indirect calorimetry (IDC) estimates energy expenditure by either oxygen consumption or carbon dioxide production; it also provides a means of estimating the composition of fuels that are being consumed to generate energy. IDC is often used to determine adequacy of nutrition support in critically ill patients, and has been posited as a necessary means of monitoring in complex patients [89]. Two-thirds of responding burn units in a recent survey indicated that they used IDC to monitor energy demands in adult patients [23]. IDC has been used as the "gold standard" for comparison of other methods of calculating energy demands in both adult and pediatric burn populations [26, 90]. Equipment for bedside performance of IDC has become more accessible over the last decade, and the associated technology has improved ease of use. However, IDC can be affected by a variety of factors including metabolic acid-base derangements, core temperature abnormalities, need for high levels of oxygen support, and even hyper- or hypoventilation. As any of these are commonly present in burn patients, particularly pediatric burn patients, the use of IDC as the sole monitor of nutritional adequacy has been called into question [91, 92]. In the absence of superior monitoring methods, weekly IDC used in conjunction with other means of monitoring nutritional status trends remains a cornerstone of nutrition management in burn patients [5, 90].

Fluctuations in weight can be helpful in healthy patients as they are associated with changes in lean body mass and fat accretion or loss. The fluid shifts resulting from the profound inflammatory response to burn injury as well as the massive fluid volumes required for resuscitation from burn shock confound the use of weight as a surrogate for lean body mass. Because of the complexities of the water component of total body weight, weights are best used in the context of long-term trends and with other nutritional markers [5]. As most fluid shifts have abated by the rehabilitative phase from burn injury, this stage of recovery may be when use of weights is most helpful and least complex.

**Application:** Monitoring of nutritional therapy in burn patients is complex and should be done using multiple methods and focusing on trends. This patient underwent weekly IDC determinations, as well as measurements of UUN and calculation of nitrogen balance. Alterations in feeding rates only occurred once weekly based upon the constellation of information available from IDC readings and UUN analyses.

## Problems and complications of nutritional support

Neither EN nor PN should be considered trouble-free. Both have significant complications that can range from mildly troublesome to life-threatening. Awareness and monitoring should detect most problems early, and help avert the worst consequences of nutritional support.

### Important complications include:

**Under/overfeeding:** Almost any disorder of electrolytes, fluids, or homeostasis can accompany prolonged nutritional support. Underfeeding is common in the early phases of burn treatment, when metabolic needs are highest and problems with administration of nutrition greatest. With increased emphasis on the importance of adequate nutrition and improved methods of delivering prolonged support, overfeeding is now more commonly encountered. As indicated previously, the additional caloric loads of IV fluids and some medications can contribute significantly to this problem. In addition to the obvious issue of weight gain and obesity, significant overfeeding of specific nutrients can produce three complications. First, excessive carbohydrate intake results in fat synthesis, elaboration of carbon dioxide, and increased respiratory quotient. In patients with ongoing respiratory failure, this can complicate weaning from respiratory support. This is a particular problem with PN [93]; switching patients to enteral nutrition may help resolve this issue. Use of low-carbohydrate diets may also help but such diets are typically high in fat, which may be harmful to burn patients in other ways. Regular monitoring of respiratory quotient (RQ) by IDC and adherence to calculated calorie guidelines based upon ideal body weight are also helpful.

Excess feeding of carbohydrates or fat to burn patients can also lead to deposition of fat in the liver parenchyma [94]. Hepatic enzyme elevation is common in burn patients regardless of nutrition, and this may be more pronounced with PN and with fluid overload. Hepatic enzymes should be followed regularly in all patients with major burn injuries. Finally, high-protein PN can contribute to azotemia, particularly when dehydration occurs [95]. Serum urea nitrogen and creatinine should be monitored frequently.

**Hyperglycemia:** Hyperglycemia occurs in up to 90% of all ICU patients during critical illness [96]. Burn patients are particularly prone to this problem, given their preponderance of catabolic hormones which cause relative insulin resistance – the "diabetes of injury". Both acute and chronic hyperglycemia is associated with immune deficiency and increased susceptibility to infection. Infection, in turn, exaggerates glucose intolerance, so the two problems often perpetuate each other.

Recent increased awareness of the value of glycemic control has led to several studies that attempted to maintain strict glucose control. In a widely-cited study, surgical ICU patients randomized to a regimen of "intensive" glucose control (maintaining levels at 80–110 mg/dL) had substantial reductions in mortality, organ failure, and other parameters, compared to patients given "traditional" treatment aimed at maintaining glucose at 180–200 mg/dL [97]. Additional evidence suggests that insulin may itself be beneficial by reducing circulating levels of C-reactive protein and other inflammatory mediators [98, 99]. These findings helped stimulate widespread recommendations for very rigorous glucose control in ICU populations [100]. However, use of these protocols has been called into question by other recent large studies suggesting that intensive insulin therapy is associated with increased mortality and a much higher incidence of critical hypoglycemia with attendant neuropsychiatric complications [101]. Although the value of blood sugar control is undisputed, the exact target level for blood sugar remains poorly defined; methodological differences and the ability of different ICU's to provide safe and effective glucose control appear to affect these results significantly [102]. Current recommendations are for "moderately strict" glucose control (target levels of 110–150 mg/dL), which would appear to offer many of the benefits of intensive therapy while minimizing the associated risks [3].

It is clear that hyperglycemia is both more severe and more common with PN as opposed to enteral nutrition, as are the extreme complications of catastrophic hypoglycemia and hyperosmolar coma. The nursing time and effort required for any aggressive regimen of blood sugar control is substantial, and this alone constitutes a strong argument for avoiding parenteral nutrition. Even with EN, blood sugar control can be a difficult task in the burn patient and complicates the care of most seriously burned individuals. Avoiding overfeeding is clearly beneficial in this regard and can help make glucose control more readily achievable. Use of oral hypoglycemic agents such as metformin and some anabolic hormones also help in blood sugar management [103].

**Bowel necrosis:** In recent years, reports have documented bowel necrosis and perforation in critically-ill patients given aggressive enteral nutrition [104, 105]. This problem may be increasing in frequency in burn patients [106]. A number of possible explanations for this phenomenon have been proposed, including occult abdominal compartment syndrome, use of vasopressors, bacterial overgrowth and stagnation of tube feedings, and bowel distension and ischemia caused by continued infusions in the face of narcotic-induced ileus. Regardless of the cause, mortality for this catastrophic complication is exceedingly high. This is one reason why enteral nutrition is not carefree and that patients must always be watched closely for subtle evidence of distension or distress. Tube feeding intolerance may be a harbinger of impending infection and feedings must sometimes be held in this situation.

**Diarrhea:** Tube feedings are also frequently associated with diarrhea, which can range from minor to a major source of morbidity, electrolyte losses, and even intestinal necrosis. Often the cause is multifactorial [107], including the osmotic effect of high glucose loads of tube feedings, enteral medications such as antacids and antibiotics, and infectious causes, including pseudomembraneous colitis caused by C. difficile [108]. Overfeeding can play a role here as well by overwhelming the gut's ability to absorb nutrients. A variety of compounds are used to control diarrhea, including opiates, bulk agents, and fiber-containing formulas [3]. None are entirely successful, and any of these agents can prolong intestinal transit and potentiate intestinal stasis and necrosis [109]. Often a short-term reduction or cessation of feedings will bring diarrhea under control. Diarrhea which persists in spite of optimal medical management should prompt a search for an infectious source inside or outside the bowel [110].

**Comprehensive nutritional regimen:** Providing adequate and safe nutritional support to a seriously burned patient can be a significant challenge to the burn team. The most successful approach to doing so is to develop a comprehensive, multidisciplinary regimen, involving physicians, nurses, dieticians, and pharmacists. Assessment of nutritional needs, the success of ongoing efforts to optimize nutrition, and careful monitoring for complications should be a routine part of the daily care of burn patients.

**Application:** The patient presented above was begun on a nutritional regimen developed by the interdisciplinary burn care team. Placement of the enteral feeding tube was ordered on admission as part of a standard order set. During multi-disciplinary rounds the next day, the dietician recommended the formula to be used and the target rate, and physicians ordered a standard protocol for increasing the infusion. The regimen was adjusted to include consideration of other sources of caloric intake, and the need to provide a high-protein formula, as discussed previously. Routine monitoring, also ordered at this time, included daily electrolytes and twice-weekly hepatic enzymes, indirect calorimetry (IDC), nitrogen balance determinations, and body weights. Blood glucose was monitored according to a protocol, beginning with determinations every 4 hours by nursing staff. When blood sugars remained high on a "sliding scale" regimen of subcutaneous insulin, he was switched to an intensive regimen of continuous insulin infusion and hourly blood sugar determinations. Nutritional status was reviewed on daily rounds with the entire team.

On hospital day 12, indirect calorimetry indicated that the patient's caloric expenditure had increased to 3,100 kcal/day and UUN was 22 gm in 24 hours. Because the patient was also receiving approximately 480 kcal/day in the form of dextrose-containing IV fluids (100 mL/hr) and 240 kcal/day from propofol for sedation (9 mL/hr), tube feedings were increased to a rate of 100 mL/hr for a total intake of 3,120 kcal and 148 gm protein per day (24 gm of nitrogen). Blood sugar control was better, so the continuous insulin infusion was stopped and the sliding scale restarted. Twelve days later, following three successful surgeries, IDC had dropped to 2,300 kcal/day; nitrogen balance was positive by 9 gm/day, and mild azotemia

(BUN 30 mg/dL, creatinine 1.6 gm/dL) was present despite good hydration. At this time propofol had been discontinued, and total IV fluid volume remained at 100 mL/hr (480 glucose kcal/day). Therefore, the enteral formula was changed to Osmolite™ providing 106 kcal and 4.4 gm protein/100 mL, and the rate was reduced to 72 mL/hr (1,831 kcal, 76 gm protein, 12.1 gm nitrogen per day).

On hospital day 21 the patient began to take oral fluids. He was started on high-calorie milkshakes, and tube feedings were held during waking hours to improve his appetite. Within 5 days he was able to take a normal diet, and the feeding tube was removed.

## Conclusion

Providing optimal nutritional support to the burn patient presents a number of unique challenges. Many of these can be solved with appropriate attention to specific nutritional requirements, careful monitoring, and a multi-disciplinary approach to nutrition that is integrated into the total program of burn care. Additional research into almost every aspect of burn-specific nutrition will be needed to resolve the controversies which still surround this important but imperfectly-understood aspect of burn care.

## References

[1]   Wilmore DW et al (1974) Catecholamines: Mediator of the hypermetabolic response to thermal injury. Ann Surg 180(4): 653–668

[2]   Newsome TW, Mason AD, Pruitt BA (1973) Weight loss following thermal injury. Ann Surg 178(2): 215–217

[3]   Martindale RG et al (2009) Guidelines for the provision and assessment of nutrition support therapy in the adult critically ill patient: Society of Critical Care Medicine and American Society for Parenteral and Enteral Nutrition: Executive Summary. Crit Care Med 37(5): 1757–1761

[4]   Heyland DK et al (2003) Canadian clinical practice guidelines for nutrition support in mechanically ventilated, critically ill adult patients. JPEN J Parenter Enteral Nutr 27(5): 355–373

[5]   Prelack K, Dylewski M, Sheridan RL (2007) Practical guidelines for nutritional management of burn injury and recovery. Burns 33(1): 14–24

[6] Saffle J (ed) (2001) Initial nutritional support of burn patients. J Burn Care Rehabil 22: 59S–66S

[7] Kreymann KG et al (2006) ESPEN Guidelines on Enteral Nutrition: Intensive care. Clin Nutr 25(2): 210–223

[8] Kreymann KG et al (2006) ESPEN Guidelines on Enteral Nutrition: Intensive Care. Clin Nutr 25(2): 210–223

[9] Moore EE, Jones TN (1986) Benefits of immediate jejunostomy feeding after major abdominal trauma – a prospective, randomized study. J Trauma 26(10): 874–881

[10] Gottschlich MM et al (2002) The 2002 Clinical Research Award. An evaluation of the safety of early vs delayed enteral support and effects on clinical, nutritional, and endocrine outcomes after severe burns. J Burn Care Rehabil 23(6): 401–415

[11] Wasiak, J., Cleland H, Jeffery R (2006) Early versus delayed enteral nutrition support for burn injuries. Cochrane Database Syst Rev 3: p. CD005 489

[12] Gramlich L et al (2004) Does enteral nutrition compared to parenteral nutrition result in better outcomes in critically ill adult patients? A systematic review of the literature. Nutrition 20(10): 843–848

[13] Alverdy J, Aoys E, Moss G (1988) Total parenteral nutrition promotes bacterial translocation from the gut. Surgery 104: p 185–190

[14] Herndon DN et al (1989) Increased mortality with intravenous supplemental feeding in severely burned patients. J Burn Care Rehabil 10(4): 309–313

[15] Herndon DN et al (1987) Failure of TPN supplementation to improve liver function, immunity, and mortality in thermally injured patients. J Trauma 27(2): 195–204

[16] Heyland DK et al (2001) Total parenteral nutrition in the surgical patient: a meta-analysis. Can J Surg 44(2): 102–111

[17] Jenkins M et al (1994) Enteral feeding during operative procedures. J Burn Care Rehabil 15: 199–205

[18] Mentec H et al (2001) Upper digestive intolerance during enteral nutrition in critically ill patients: frequency, risk factors, and complications. Crit Care Med 29(10): 1955–1961

[19] Kearns PJ et al (2000) The incidence of ventilator-associated pneumonia and success in nutrient delivery with gastric versus small intestinal feeding: a randomized clinical trial. Crit Care Med 28(6): 1742–1746

[20] Marik PE, Zaloga GP (2003) Gastric versus post-pyloric feeding: a systematic review. Crit Care 7(3): R46–51

[21] Ho KM, Dobb GJ, Webb SA (2006) A comparison of early gastric and post-pyloric feeding in critically ill patients: a meta-analysis. Intensive Care Med 32(5): 639–649

[22] Booth CM, Heyland DK, Paterson WG (2002) Gastrointestinal promotility drugs in the critical care setting: a systematic review of the evidence. Crit Care Med 30(7): 1429–1435

[23] Graves C, Saffle JR, Cochran A (2009) Actual burn nutrition care practices: An update. JBCR 30(1): 77–82

[24] Interactive DRI for Healthcare Professionals. [cited; Available from: http://fnic.nal.usda.gov

[25] Dickerson RN (2002) Estimating energy and protein requirements of thermally injured patients: Art or science? Nutrition 18(5): 439–442

[26] Dickerson RN et al (2002) Accuracy of predictive methods to estimate resting energy expenditure of thermally-injured patients. JPEN 26(1): 17–29

[27] Hart DW et al (2002) Energy expenditure and caloric balance after burn: Increased feeding leads to fat rather than lean mass accretion. Ann Surg 235(1): 152–161

[28] Choban PS et al (1997) Hypoenergetic nutrition support in hospitalized obese patients: a simplified method for clinical application. Am J Clin Nutr 66(3): 546–550

[29] Dickerson RN et al (2002) Hypocaloric enteral tube feeding in critically ill obese patients. Nutrition 18(3): 241–246

[30] Dickerson RN, Rosato EF, Mullen JL (1986) Net protein anabolism with hypocaloric parenteral nutrition in obese stressed patients. Am J Clin Nutr 44(6): 747–755

[31] Hart DW et al (2001) Efficacy of a high-carbohydrate diet in catabolic illness. Crit Care Med 29(7): 1318–1324

[32] Burke JF et al (1979) Glucose requirements following burn injury. Parameters of optimal glucose infusion and possible hepatic and respiratory abnormalities following excessive glucose intake. Ann Surg 190(3): 274–285

[33] Baytieh L et al: Nutrition and dietetics principles and guidelines for adult and pediatric burns patient management 2004, Sydney, Australia: New South Wales Severe Burn Injury Service

[34] Yu Y-M et al (1999) The metabolic basis of the increase of the increase in energy expenditure in severely burned patients. JPEN 23(3): 160–168

[35] Wolfe R et al (1983) Response of proteins and urea kinetics in burn patients to different levels of protein intake. Ann Surg 197: 163–171

[36] Matsuda T et al (1983) The importance of burn wound size in determining the optimal calorie:nitrogen ratio. Surgery 94: 562–568

[37] Garrel DR et al (1995) Improved clinical status and length of care with low-fat nutrition support in burn patients. JPEN 19(6): 482–491

[38] Gottschlich MM et al (1990) Differential effects of three enteral dietary regimens on selected outcome variables in burn patients. JPEN 14(3): 225–236

[39] Mochizuki H et al (1984) Optimal lipid content for enteral diets following thermal injury. JPEN 8(6): 638–646

[40] Battistella FD et al (1997) A prospective, randomized trial of intravenous fat emulsion administration in trauma victims requiring total parenteral nutrition. J Trauma 43(1): 52–8; discussion 58–60

[41] Rock CL et al (1997) Carotenoids and antioxidant vitamins in patients after burn injury. JBCR 18(3): 269–278

[42] Mayes T., Gottschlich MM, Warden GD (1997) Clinical nutrition protocols for continuous quality improve-

ments in the outcomes of patients with burns. JBCR 18(4): 365–368

[43] Mayes T et al (2003) Four-year review of burns as an etiologic factor in the development of long bone fractures in pediatric patients. J Burn Care Rehabil 24(5): 279–284

[44] Klein GL, Langman CB, Herndon DN (2002) Vitamin D depletion following burn injury in children: a possible factor in post-burn osteopenia. J Trauma 52(2): 346–350

[45] Gottschlich MM et al (2004) Hypovitaminosis D in acutely injured pediatric burn patients. J Am Diet Assoc 104(6): 931–941, quiz 1031

[46] Klein GL et al (2004) Synthesis of vitamin D in skin after burns. Lancet 363(9405): 291–292

[47] Klein GL et al (2009) Standard multivitamin supplementation does not improve vitamin D insufficiency after burns. J Bone Miner Metab 27(4): 502–506

[48] Klein GL (2006) Burn-induced bone loss: importance, mechanisms, and management. J Burns Wounds 5: e5

[49] Berger MM et al (1992) Cutaneous zinc and copper losses in burns. Burns 18: 373–380

[50] Voruganti VS et al (2005) Impaired zinc and copper status in children with burn injuries: Need to reassess nutritional requirements. Burns 31: 711–716

[51] Berger MM et al (2007) Trace element supplementation after major burns modulates antioxidant status and clinical course by way of increased tissue trace element concentrations. Am J Clin Nutr 85: 1293–1300

[52] Berger MM et al (2006) Reduction of nosocomial pneumonia after major burns by trace element supplementation: aggregation of two randomised trials. Crit Care 10(6): 153–161

[53] Berger MM et al (1998) Trace element supplementation modulates pulmonary infection rates after major burns: a double-blind, placebo-controlled trial. Am J Clin Nutr 68: 365–371

[54] Ravasco, P, Camilo ME (2003) The impact of fluid therapy on nutrient delivery: a prospective evaluation of practice in respiratory intensive care. Clin Nutr 22(1): 87–92

[55] Calder PC (2009) Hot topics in parenteral nutrition. Rationale for using new lipid emulsions in parenteral nutrition and a review of the trials performed in adults. Proc Nutr Soc 68(3): 252–260

[56] Mayes, T, Gottschlich MM, Kagan RJ (2008) An evaluation of the safety and efficacy of an anti-inflammatory, pulmonary enteral formula in the treatment of pediatric burn patients with respiratory failure. J Burn Care Res 29(1): 82–88

[57] Soeters PB et al (2004) Amino acid adequacy in pathophysiological states. J Nutr 134 [6 Suppl]: 575S–1582S

[58] Souba W (1991) Glutamine: a key substrate for the splanchnic bed. Ann Rev Nutr 11: 285–289

[59] Wischmeyer PE (2002) Glutamine and heat shock protein expression. Nutrition 18(3): 225–228

[60] De-Souza DA, Greene LJ (2005) Intestinal permeability and systemic infections in critically ill patients: effect of glutamine. Crit Care Med 33(5): 1125–1135

[61] Zhou YP et al (2003) The effect of supplemental enteral glutamine on plasma levels, gut function, and outcome in severe burns: a randomized, double-blind, controlled clinical trial. JPEN J Parenter Enteral Nutr 27(4): 241–245

[62] Garrel D et al (2003) Decreased mortality and infectious morbidity in adult burn patients given enteral glutamine supplements: a prospective, controlled, randomized clinical trial. Crit Care Med 31(10): 2444–2449

[63] Novak F et al (2002) Glutamine supplementation in serious illness: a systematic review of the evidence. Crit Care Med 30(9): 2022–2029

[64] Wischmeyer PE et al (2001) Glutamine administration reduces Gram-negative bacteremia in severely burned patients: a prospective, randomized, double-blind trial versus isonitrogenous control. Crit Care Med 29(11): 2075–2080

[65] Kirk S, Barbul A (1990) Role of arginine in trauma, sepsis, and immunity. J Parenter Enteral Nutr 14: 226S–229S

[66] Yan H et al (2007) Effects of early enteral arginine supplementation on resuscitation of severe burn patients. Burns 33(2): 179–184

[67] Gottschlich MM et al (1990) Differential effects of three enteral dietary regimens on selected outcome variables in burn patients. JPEN J Parenter Enteral Nutr 14(3): 225–236

[68] Bower RH et al (1995) Early enteral administration of a formula (Impact) supplemented with arginine, nucleotides, and fish oil in intensive care unit patients: results of a multicenter, prospective, randomized, clinical trial. Crit Care Med 23(3): 436–449

[69] Moore FA et al (1994) Clinical benefits of an immune-enhancing diet for early postinjury enteral feeding. J Trauma 37(4): 607–615

[70] Heyland DK, Samis A (2003) Does immunonutrition in patients with sepsis do more harm than good? Intensive Care Med 29(5): 669–671

[71] Wibbenmeyer LA et al (2006) Effect of a fish oil and arginine-fortified diet in thermally injured patients. J Burn Care Res 27(5): 694–702

[72] De-Souza DA, Greene LJ (1998) Pharmacological nutrition after burn injury. J Nutr 128(5): 797–803

[73] Saffle JR et al (1997) Randomized trial of immune-enhancing enteral nutrition in burn patients. J Trauma 42(5): 793–800; discussion 800–802

[74] Marik PE, Zaloga GP (2008) Immunonutrition in critically ill patients: a systematic review and analysis of the literature. Intensive Care Med 34(11): 1980–1990

[75] Masters, B, Wood F (2008) Nutrition support in burns – is there consistency in practice? J Burn Care Res 29(4): 561–571

[76] Ireton-Jones, C, Gottschlich M (1993) The evolution of nutrition support in burns. J Burn Care Rehabil 14: 272–280

[77] Pereira CT, Herndon DN (2005) The pharmacologic modulation of the hypermetabolic response to burns. Adv Surg 39: 245–261

[78] Herndon DN et al (2001) Reversal of catabolism by beta-blockade after severe burns. N Engl J Med 345(17): 1223–1229

[79] Wolf SE et al (2006) Effects of oxandrolone on outcome measures in the severely burned: a multicenter prospective randomized double-blind trial. J Burn Care Res 27(2): 131–139; discussion 140–141

[80] Demling RH, DeSanti L (2003) Oxandrolone induced lean mass gain during recovery from severe burns is maintained after discontinuation of the anabolic steroid. Burns 29(8): 793–797

[81] Cuthbertson, D (1930) The disturbance of metabolism produced by bony and nonbony injury with notes of certain abnormal conditions of bone. Biochemical Journal 24: 1244–1263

[82] Heyland DK et al (2003) Canadian Clinical Practice Guidelines for nutrition support in mechanically ventilated, critically ill adult patients. JPEN 27(5): 355–373

[83] Carlson DE et al (1991) Evaluation of serum visceral protein levels as indicators of nitrogen balance in thermally injured patients. JPEN 15(4): 440–444

[84] Greenhalgh DG et al (2005) Maintenance of serum albumin levels in pediatric burn patients: A prospective randomized trial. J Trauma 39(1): 67–73

[85] Moghazy AM et al (2009) Assessment of the relation between prealbumin serum level and healing of skin-grafted burn wounds. Burns 36(4): 495–500

[86] Prelack K et al (1997) Urinary urea nitrogen is imprecise as a predictor of protein balance in burned children. J Am Diet Assoc 97: 489–495

[87] Fuhrman MP, Charney P, Mueller CM (2004) Hepatic Proteins and Nutrition Assessment. J Am Diet Assoc 104: 1258–1264

[88] Seres DS (2005) Surrogate Nutrition Markers, Malnutrition, and Adequacy of Nutrition Support. Nutr Clin Prac 20(3): 308–313

[89] Boullatta J et al (2007) Accurate determination of energy needs in hospitalized patients. J Am Diet Assoc 107: 393–401

[90] Suman OE et al (2006) Resting energy expenditure in severely burned children: analysis of agreement between indirect calorimetry and prediction equations using the Bland-Altman method. Burns 32(3): 335–342

[91] Liusuwan RA et al (2005) Comparison of measured resting energy expenditure versus predictive equations in pediatric burn patients. JBCR 26(6): 464–470

[92] Manotok RA L, Palmieri TL, Greenhalgh DG (2008) The respiratory quotient has little value in evaluating the state of feeding in burn patients. JBCR 29: 655–659

[93] Askanazi J et al (1980) Respiratory changes induced by the large glucose loads of total parenteral nutrition. JAMA 243: 1444–1447

[94] Lowry, S, Brennan M (1979) Abnormal liver function during parenteral nutrition: relation to infusion excess. J Surg Res 26: 300–307

[95] Iapichino, G, Radrizzani D (1999) Parenteral Nutrition. In: Webb A et al (eds) Oxford Textbook of Critical Care. Oxford University Press, New York, pp 398–401

[96] Turina M, Fry DE, Polk, HC Jr (2005) Acute hyperglycemia and the innate immune system: clinical, cellular, and molecular aspects. Crit Care Med 33(7): 1624–1633

[97] van den Berghe G et al (2001) Intensive insulin therapy in the critically ill patients. N Engl J Med 345(19): 1359–1367

[98] Wu X et al (2004) Insulin decreases hepatic acute phase protein levels in severely burned children. Surgery 135(2): 196–202

[99] Solano, T, Totaro R (2004) Insulin therapy in critically ill patients. Curr Opin Clin Nutr Metab Care 7(2): 199–205

[100] Lewis KS et al (2004) Intensive insulin therapy for critically ill patients. Ann Pharmacother 38(7–8): 1243–1251

[101] Finfer S et al (2009) Intensive versus conventional glucose control in critically ill patients. N Engl J Med 360(13): 1283–1297

[102] Van den Berghe G et al (2009) Clinical review: Intensive insulin therapy in critically ill patients: NICE-SUGAR or Leuven blood glucose target? J Clin Endocrinol Metab 94(9): 3163–3170

[103] Gore DC et al (2005) Influence of metformin on glucose intolerance and muscle catabolism following severe burn injury. Ann Surg 241(2): 334–342

[104] Kowal-Vern A, McGill V, Gamelli R (1997) Ischemic necrotic bowel disease in thermal injury. Arch Surg 132: 440–443

[105] Marvin R et al (2000) Nonocclusive bowel necrosis occurring in critically-ill trauma patients receiving enteral nutrition manifests no reliable clinical signs for early detection. Am J Surg 179: 7–12

[106] Markell KW et al (2009) Abdominal complications after severe burns. J Am Coll Surg 208(5): 940–947; discussion 947–949

[107] Eisenberg P (1993) Causes of diarrhea in tube-fed patients: a comprehensive approach to diagnosis and management. Nutr Clin Pract 8: 119–123

[108] Grube BJ, Heimbach DM, Marvin JA (1987) Clostridium difficile diarrhea in critically ill burned patients. Arch Surg 122(6): 655–661

[109] Scaife CL, Saffle JR, Morris SE (1999) Intestinal obstruction secondary to enteral feedings in burn trauma patients. J Trauma 47(5): 859–863

[110] Wolf S et al (1997) Enteral feeding intolerance: an indicator of sepsis-associated mortality in burned children. Arch Surg 132: 310–313

[111] Harris, J, Benedict F (1919) A biometric study of basal metabolism in man. Carnegie Institute of Washington, Washington DC

[112] Curreri P et al (1974) Dietary requirements of patients with major burns. Journal of the American Dietetic Association 65: 415–417

[113] USDA National Agricultural Library. Interactive DRI for healthcare professionals (2010) [cited 10 April 2 [010]; Available from: http://fnic. nal. usda. gov/ interactiveDRI/

[114] Hildreth M et al (1993) Caloric requirements of patients with burns under one year of age. Journal of Burn Care and Rehabilitation 14(1): 108–112

[115] Hildreth M et al (1990) Current treatment reduces calories required to maintain weight in pediatric patients with burns. J Burn Care Rehabil 11(5): 405–409

[116] Hildreth M et al (1989) Caloric needs of adolescent patients with burns. J Burn Care Rehabil 10(6): 523–526

[117] Day, T, Dean P, Adams M (1986) Nutritional requirements of the burned child: The Curreri Junior formula. in Proceedings of the American Burn Association 1986

Correspondence: Amalia Cochran M.D., FACS, Dept. of Surgery, 3B-313, University of Utah Health Center, 50 N. Medical Dr., Salt Lake City, UT 84132, Tel: 801 581 7508, Facsimile: 801 587 9147, E-mail: Amalia.cochran@hsc.utah.edu
Jeffrey R. Saffle M.D., FACS, Dept of Surgery, 3B-306, University of Utah Health Center, 50 N. Medical Dr., Salt Lake City, UT 84132, Tel: 801 581 3595, Facsimile: 801 585 2435, E-mail: jeffrey.saffle@hsc.utah.edu

# HBO and burns

Harald Andel

Department of Anaesthesie and General Intensive Care, Medical University of Vienna, Vienna, Austria

## Historical development

The potential beneficial effects of HBO in the treatment of patients, who are suffering from burns, has been first recognized by Ikeda et al. [1] in1968 when he treated several patients after a coal-mining accident suffering from carbon monoxide poisoning (CO-intox) and thermal burns. Patients suffering from CO-intoxication and thermal burns where treated with adjunctive HBO treatment. Although they were basically more severely injured than the patients injured at the same accident but did not have a CO-intox the "HBO-group" had markedly faster wound healing and less length of hospital stay (LHOS). Several animal studies were carried out showing faster wound healing after HBO treatment than the controls. In 1960 Gruber et al. [2] could proof that the tissue around full thickness burns is hypoxic and that by administering HBO the oxygen partial pressure could be raised. In 1988, the Committee on Hyperbaric Oxygenation of the Undersea and Hyperbaric Medical Society removed thermal burn from a special considerations category and recommended that hyperbaric oxygen treatment of patients with thermal burns should be reimbursed by third-party carriers. Since then several case reports and cohort-studies have been published, most of them showing faster wound healing, less edema and less operations and shorter LHOS. However an adequately powered prospect-ive randomized controlled study as requested by EBM is still missing [3].

## Scientific background supporting the use of HBO in thermal burns

The mechanism of action of HBO is very simple. As the ambient pressure limits the maximal partial pressure of a gas the maximal $O_2$ pressure in normobaric conditions is 1 bar (760 mmHg). By increasing the ambient pressure up to a maximum of 3 bars (2 280 mmHg) the arterial $O_2$ partial is increased in a way that only every fourth capillary is needed to provide sufficient tissue oxygen partial pressure (Figs. 1 and 2).

Therefore the theoretical background for using hyperbaric oxygen in thermal burns is to provide the oxygen necessary to maintain viability in critically perfused zones. Moreover it has been assumed to maintain microvascular integrity and minimize edema. The mechanisms suggested include the preservation of ATP in cell membranes, as first demonstrated by Nylander et al. [4] and confirmed by Yamaguchi et al. [5].

In summary as traditional mechanism of action for HBO has been postulated that it improves the physiological state of hypoperfused, hypoxic tissues by providing metabolic substrate and by limiting edema formation due to hyperoxic vasoconstriction. These assumptions have been supported by controlled animal studies showing a reduction of 30 per-

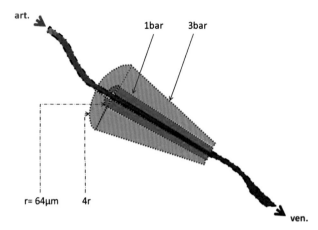

art.

1bar  3bar

r= 64µm    4r

ven.

**Fig. 1.** Due to the increase from 1 to 3bar the diffusion rate is increased and the diffusion distance within the tissue is xtended. The oxygen-diffusion distance in the tissue (Krogh cylinder model) increases through this up to the 4-fold radius and reaches a multiple of the normal tissue volume. Subsequently can also maintain areas with otherwise disturbed oxygen care, on the basis of lack blood circulation or increase of the diffusion opposition (e. g. desolate-conditioned), a normal oxygen care of the cells

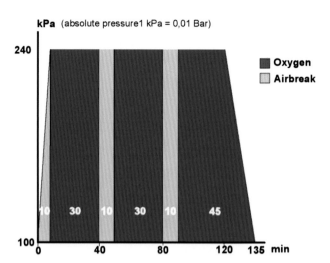

**kPa**  (absolute pressure1 kPa = 0,01 Bar)

240

■ Oxygen
□ Airbreak

10   30   10   30   10   45

100
0      40      80      120   135  min

**Fig. 2.** HBO Treatment Table for burn wounds

cent in the extravasations of fluid in the first 24 post-burn-hours. HBO was also able to reduce the generalized edema that occurs in burns [6]. Similarly biopsies of burned animals have shown progression to full-thickness injury in controls, while there is preservation of capillary patency and dermal elements in animals treated with HBO [6–8].

Main criticism has been that intermittent rise of $O_2$ offers in best-case only transient improvements. However, recent findings demonstrate a more sophisticated basis that is focused on oxidative stress. Whereas toxicity of $O_2$ is based on overshooting free radical formation appropriate intracellular levels of reactive oxygen species (ROS) and reactive nitrogen species (RNS) play a vital role in regulating many biological processes [9–11]. ROS are generated as natural by-products of metabolism and it is generally accepted that agents such as superoxide, hydrogen peroxide, and hydroxyl are elevated in tissues as a consequence of exposure to HBO. RNS such as nitric oxide ($\cdot$NO) and products generated by reactions between ROS and $\cdot$NO, or its oxidation products such as nitrite, are as well elevated by HBO. HBO is able to activate nitric oxide synthase enzymes and it can also increase pro-

duction of RNS capable of nitrosylation reactions through involvement of enzymes such as myeloperoxidase [12–14].

Moreover, HBO seems to have ideal properties for the treatment of burned patients as it reduces circulating levels of proinflammatory cytokines under stress conditions (e. g. endotoxin challenge), without altering circulating levels of insulin, insulin-like growth factors, or proinflammatory cytokines [15, 16]. Consequently HBO is reported to decrease the inflammatory response while significantly improving the microvasculature [7].

HBO therapy has been claimed to be effective in burn-wound sepsis in which the chief offending pathogen is Pseudomonas aeruginosa [17–19].

In a large non-randomized study Niu et al. found that in patients with 35 to 75 percent total body surface area burns, 6.8 percent of the 117 patients in the hyperbaric oxygen group died versus 14.8 percent deaths in the 169 controls (p = 0 028). The investigators also noted that fluid resuscitation could be achieved more rapidly, nasogastric feeding could be initiated in the second 24 hours or earlier, and there was an acceleration of reepithelialization. The average number of hospital days in the same high-risk group was 47 in the hyperbaric oxygen-treated group and 59 in the controls. However, this difference was not statistically significant [20].

In a small control study in humans, Hart et al. 61 found that using a two-way (air versus oxygen) factorial analysis of variance, the mean healing time in the controls was 43.8 days, whereas it was 19.7 days in a HBO group (p > 0 005) [21].

More recently, Cianci et al. [22] demonstrated that adjunctive hyperbaric oxygen therapy reduced the mean length of hospitalization in patients with 18 to 39 percent total body surface area bums from 33 to 20.8 days (p = 0 012). In another study published by Cianci et al., the average cost savings per patient was $10,850 when using hyperbaric oxygen. Hyperbaric oxygen costs averaged $8200, which is included in the total hospital charge [23].

Cianci et al. also looked into the effect of hyperbaric oxygen on the number of surgeries required in bum treatment. In patients burned over 40 to 80 percent of their total body surface area, matched for age and also percentage and thickness of burn, the number of surgeries required fell from 8 to 3.7 when hyperbaric oxygen was used (p = 0 041) [24].

In a negative clinical study by Waisbren et al. in which hyperbaric oxygen treatment of severe burns failed to reveal either a deleterious or salutary effect on mortality, grafting was reduced by 75 percent in the HBO group (p > 0.01) [25].

In a case series Baiba et al. published the course of ten patients suffering from burns and severe CO-intox showing major complications during the course of treatment:

two patients suffered from eustachian tube occlusion, two patients had episodes of aspiration, one patient had seizure activity, and severe hypocalcemia developed in another. Progressive hypovolemia was seen in three patients; respiratory acidosis was evident in four [26]. However in a letter to the editor Noble et al. explained the probable reason for these findings: "However, when critically ill patients are transported to a chamber outside the hospital and left without physician supervision for up to five hours as in the Heimbach series, these toxicities and complications are more likely co be experienced" [27].

## Contraindications for the use of HBO

Untreated pneumothorax is an absolute contraindication to hyperbaric oxygen, as is concurrent therapy with doxorubicin (Adriamycin), cis-platinum, and disulfiram (Antabuse). Doxorubicin has been shown to produce a high mortality when combined with hyperbaric oxygen in animals. Cis-Platinum given concomitantly with hyperbaric oxygen decreases the strength of healing incisions, while disulfiram blocks production of superoxide dismutase. Superoxide dismutase is protective against damage from high partial pressures of oxygen. All other contraindications are relative, such as upper respiratory infections, which make clearing the ears and sinuses difficult, low seizure threshold, which can be mitigated by anticonvulsants, emphysema with $CO_2$ retention, where low arterial $PO_2$ triggers breathing, high fevers, which lower seizure threshold, and congenital spherocytosis, which may provoke hemolysis [28].

Understanding the pathophysiology of burns and HBO is necessary to choose the right patient and the right time for treatment. In case both is available there is still the need for a team capable of providing the same level of care during the HBO treatment like on the intensive care unit (ICU). This limits the number of centers worldwide being currently able to provide a benefit for critically burned patients by administering adjuvant HBO therapy. However patients suffering from minor burns but having concomitant diseases like diabetes or other microvascular diseases leading to a delayed wound healing are likely to profit from adjuvant HBO therapy as they do not need special intensive care during the HBO treatment.

## Conclusion

Being aware of the small number of centers being able to maintain the level of treatment in critically burned patients during the HBO session and the large number of patients necessary to conduct a prospective randomized controlled study we must be aware that such a study will probably not be conducted within the next future. On the other hand HBO has been shown to promote wound healing and everybody treating burned patients is aware of the fact that the time until burn wounds are closed is critical – specially in patients with major burns (Figs. 3 and 4). Therefore burned patients will profit from every intervention shortening healing time. However it must be granted that the intervention itself does not put any harm to the patient. Therefore the right time for treatment and the right environment to ensure optimal transport-

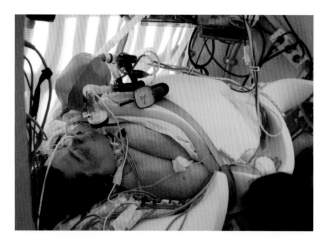

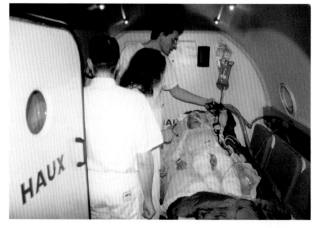

**Fig. 3.** Burn patient with additional inhalation injury treated in a HBO chamber

**Fig. 4.** Burn patient treated in multiplace HBO chamber

conditions and level of care during the HBO session is crucial – otherwise the overall effect will be similar to the Heimbachs series cited above.

As we had good results treating burned patients with HBO we can recommend adjunctive HBO therapy in patients with thermal injury.

At the burn center in Vienna the HBO program was initiated in 2003 starting with non-burned patients – mildly burned patients and finally after 1 year training severely burned patients. Assistant Professor Andrew Donner MD (+ 2005) who contributed substantially to the HBO-program also played an important role in the successful implementation of this therapeutic option – therefore we want to dedicate this chapter to him.

## References

[1]  Ikeda K et al (1968) [Hyperbaric oxygen therapy of burns]. Geka Chiryo 18(6): 689–693

[2]  Gruber RP et al (1970) Hyperbaric oxygen and pedicle flaps, skin grafts, and burns. Plast Reconstr Surg 45(1): 24–30

[3]  Villanueva E et al (2004) Hyperbaric oxygen therapy for thermal burns. Cochrane Database Syst Rev 2004(3): CD004 727

[4]  Nylander G (1986) Tissue ischemia and hyperbaric oxygen treatment: an experimental study. Acta Chir Scand Suppl 533: 1–109

[5]  Yamaguchi KT, Hoffman C, Stewart RJ, Cianci PA, Vierra M, Naito M (1990) Effect of oxygen on burn wound tissue levels of ATP and collagen (Abstract) Undersea Biomed Res 17[Suppl]: 65

[6]  Nylander G, Nordstrom H, Eriksson E (1984) Effects of hyperbaric oxygen on oedema formation after a scald burn. Burns Incl Therm Inj 10(3): 193–196

[7]  Boykin JV, Eriksson E, Pittman RN (1980) In vivo microcirculation of a scald burn and the progression of postburn dermal ischemia. Plast Reconstr Surg 66(2): 191–8

[8]  Germonpre P, Reper P, Vanderkelen A (1996) Hyperbaric oxygen therapy and piracetam decrease the early extension of deep partial-thickness burns. Burns 22(6): 468–473

[9]  Chandel NS et al (2000) Reactive oxygen species generated at mitochondrial complex III stabilize hypoxia-inducible factor-1alpha during hypoxia: a mechanism of $O_2$ sensing. J Biol Chem 275(33): 25 130–138

[10]  Kunsch C, Medford RM (1999) Oxidative stress as a regulator of gene expression in the vasculature. Circ Res 85(8): 753–766

[11]  Xia C et al (2007) Reactive oxygen species regulate angiogenesis and tumor growth through vascular endothelial growth factor. Cancer Res 67(22): 10 823–10830

[12]  Thom SR et al (2006) Stem cell mobilization by hyperbaric oxygen. Am J Physiol Heart Circ Physiol 290(4): H1378–1386

[13]  Thom SR et al (2003) Stimulation of perivascular nitric oxide synthesis by oxygen. Am J Physiol Heart Circ Physiol 284(4):H1230–1239

[14]  Gallagher KA et al (2007) Diabetic impairments in NO-mediated endothelial progenitor cell mobilization and homing are reversed by hyperoxia and SDF-1 alpha. J Clin Invest 117(5): 1249–1259

[15]  Chen SJ et al (2007) Effects of hyperbaric oxygen therapy on circulating interleukin-8, nitric oxide, and insulin-like growth factors in patients with type 2 diabetes mellitus. Clin Biochem 40(1–2): 30–36

[16]  Fildissis G et al (2004) Whole blood pro-inflammatory cytokines and adhesion molecules post-lipopolysaccharides exposure in hyperbaric conditions. Eur Cytokine Netw 15(3): 217–221

[17] Bartell PF, Orr TE, Garcia M (1968) The lethal events in experimental Pseudomonas aeruginosa infection of mice. J Infect Dis 118(2): 165–172

[18] Koehnlein HE, Lemperle G (1970) Experimental studies on local treatment of pseudomonas-infected burn wounds. Plast Reconstr Surg 45(6): 558–563

[19] Rittenbury MS, Hanback LD (1967) Phagocytic depression in thermal injuries. J Trauma 7(4): 523–540

[20] Niu AKC, Yang C, Lee H c, Chen SH, Chang LP (1987) Burns treated with adjunctive hyperbaric oxygen therapy: A comparative study in humans. J Hyperbar Med 2: 75

[21] Hart GB et al (1974) Treatment of burns with hyperbaric oxygen. Surg Gynecol Obstet 139(5): 693–696

[22] Cianci P et al (1989) Adjunctive hyperbaric oxygen therapy reduces length of hospitalization in thermal burns. J Burn Care Rehabil 10(5): 432–435

[23] Cianci P et al (1990) Adjunctive hyperbaric oxygen in the treatment of thermal burns. An economic analysis. J Burn Care Rehabil 11(2): 140–143

[24] Cianci P, Lueders HW, Lee H, Shapiro RL, Sexton J, Williams C, Green B (1988) Adjunctive hyperbaric oxygen reduces the need for surgery in 40–80 % burns. J Hyperbar Med 3: 97

[25] Waisbren BA et al (1982) Hyperbaric oxygen in severe burns. Burns Incl Therm Inj 8(3): 176–179

[26] Grube BJ, Marvin JA, Heimbach DM (1988) Therapeutic hyperbaric oxygen: help or hindrance in burn patients with carbon monoxide poisoning? J Burn Care Rehabil 9(3): 249–252

[27] Noble R, Grossman R (1988) Therapeutic HBO: help or hindrance in burn patients with CO poisoning? J Burn Care Rehabil 9(6): 581

[28] Kindwall EP, Gottlieb LJ, Larson DL (1991) Hyperbaric oxygen therapy in plastic surgery: a review article. Plast Reconstr Surg 88(5): 898–908

Correspondence: Harald Andel, M. D., Ph. D., M. Sc., Department of Anaesthesie and General Intensive Care, Medical University of Vienna, Währinger Gürtel 18–20, 1090 Vienna, Austria, E-mail: harald-lothar.andel@meduniwien.ac.at

# Nursing management of the burn-injured person

Judy Knighton[1], Mary Jako[2]

[1] Sunnybrook Health Sciences Centre, Ross Tilley Burn Centre, Toronto, ON, Canada
[2] Shriners Hospital for Children, Galveston, USA

## Introduction

Providing care to the burn-injured patient is a very challenging and, ultimately, rewarding profession for a nurse. The repertoire of skills needed is varied and includes comprehensive clinical assessment and monitoring, pain management, wound care and psychosocial support. The burn nurse cares for the burn survivor throughout the continuum of care, from entry into the hospital through to discharge home and reintegration into the community.

Further research into the practice of burn nursing is crucial to identify new knowledge to guide best practices. This chapter is written to assist the nurse in providing comprehensive care to the burn-injured person and his/her family.

## General definition and description

### Incidence

Each year, an estimated 500,000 people seek care for burns in the United States and approximately 40,000 require hospitalization, greater than half of whom require care in specialized burn units or centres [1,2]. Of those requiring hospital care, about 4500 die from their injuries. In Canada, about 50,000 people are injured and an estimated 4,000 are hospitalized, of whom about 450 die from their injuries. In both countries, children 4 years of age and younger and adults over the age of 55, about two-thirds of the total, form the largest group of fatalities.

### Prevention

Many burn injuries can be prevented and nurses have the opportunity to serve as advocates and educators in the area of burn and fire prevention. Worldwide, there has been a slow but steady decrease in the number of burns occurring annually. The focus of burn prevention programs has shifted from concentrating on individual blame and changing individual behaviours to include more legislative changes. There are several factors considered responsible for the steady decline in incidence. One factor is the raising of public awareness through fire department and burn centre-initiated burn education and fire prevention programs (Burn Awareness Week in February and Fire Prevention Week in October). Pamphlets and posters continue to be widely distributed though community mall displays, doctors' offices, public health departments, day care facilities and schools. Another factor involves those attempts aimed at having a positive impact upon government legislation for items, such as safe temperature levels for hot water heaters, childrens' flame-retardant sleepwear, self-extinguishing cigarettes and "child-proof" cigarette lighters. There is also increased awareness and use of fire sprinklers,

**Table 1.** American Burn Association Adult Burn Classification

| Classification | Assessment Criteria |
|---|---|
| Minor burn injury | < 15% TBSA burn in adults < 40 years age < 10% TBSA burn in adults > 40 years age < 2% TBSA full-thickness burn without risk of functional or esthetic impairment or disability |
| Moderate uncomplicated burn injury | 15–25% TBSA burn in adults < 40 years age<br>10–20% TBSA burn in adults > 40 years age<br>< 10% TBSA full-thickness burn without functional<br>or esthetic risk to burns involving the face, eyes, ears, hands, feet or perineum |
| Major burn injury | > 25% TBSA burn in adults < 40 years age<br>> 20% TBSA burn in adults > 40 years age<br>OR > 10% TBSA full-thickness burn (any age)<br>OR injuries involving the face, eyes, ears, hands, feet OR perineum likely to result in functional or esthetic disability<br>OR high-voltage electrical burn<br>OR all burns with inhalation injury or major trauma |

along with smoke and carbon monoxide detectors. Safer new home construction and stricter workplace safety standards are additional factors contributing to the decrease in burn injuries.

## Classification

Burn complexity can range from a relatively minor, uncomplicated injury to a life-threatening, multi-system trauma. The American Burn Association (ABA) has a useful classification system that rates burn injury magnitude from minor to moderate un-complicated to major (Table 1). This system takes into account the depth and extent of the injury, the location of the burns on the body and the person's overall medical history. With advances in burn care over the years and the establishment of specialized facilities staffed by skilled, multidisciplinary burn team members, more patients with severe injuries are surviving. However, survival is no longer enough. The ultimate challenge for the burn team is to support and guide the burned person and his/her family towards a complete and acceptable level of recovery, both physically and psychosocially.

## Etiology and risk factors

The causes of burn injuries are numerous and found in both the home, leisure and workplace settings (Table 2). At home, people are most frequently burned in the kitchen and bathroom, while involved in activities such as cooking, bathing or smoking. Campfires, trailers and boats serve as recreational sources for burn injuries, while industrial settings are common sites for workplace injuries, involving electricity, chemicals and explosions.

Burn injuries occur throughout the world, but predominantly to women in the developing world,

**Table 2.** Causes of burn injuries

| Home & Leisure | Workplace |
|---|---|
| ► Hot water heaters set too high (140 °F or 60 °C)<br>► Overloaded electrical outlets<br>► Frayed electrical wiring<br>► Carelessness with cigarettes, lighters, matches, candles<br>► Pressure cookers<br>► Microwaved foods and liquids<br>► Hot grease or cooking liquids<br>► Open space heaters<br>► Gas fireplace doors<br>► Radiators<br>► Hot sauna rocks<br>► Improper use of flammable liquids:<br>• starter fluids<br>• gasoline<br>• kerosene<br>► Electrical storms<br>► Overexposure to sun | ► Electricity:<br>• power lines<br>• outlet boxes<br>► Chemicals:<br>• acids<br>• alkalis<br>► Tar<br>► Hot steam sources:<br>• boilers<br>• pipes<br>• industrial cookers<br>► Hot industrial presses<br>► Flammable liquids:<br>• propane<br>• acetylene<br>• natural gas |

**Box 1.** Burn severity factors

1. Extent of body surface area burned
2. Depth of tissue damage
3. Age of person
4. Part of body burned
5. Past medical history

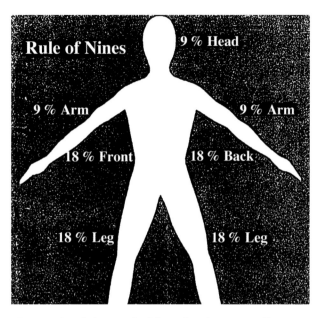

**Fig. 1.** Rule of Nines method for estimating extent of burn

amongst all cultures and across all age ranges. In the developed world, about two-thirds of those injured are male and about one-third are less than 16 years of age. A number of identifiable factors place someone at greater risk for sustaining a burn injury such as inattention, carelessness, lack of knowledge and resources, a sense of invincibility, and ingestion of alcohol, alone or in combination with drugs. Some incidents, however, are the result of unfortunate circumstances or medical illness, such as epilepsy or diabetes. Burn prevention programs aim to identify these risk factors, educate and heighten awareness of individual risk, and encourage people to practice safe strategies in order to decrease their level of risk at home, work or play.

## Pathophysiology

### Severity factors

There are five factors that need to be considered when determining the severity of a burn injury (Box 1).

**i) Extent** – The larger the area of the body burned, the more serious the injury. There are several methods available to accurately calculate the percentage of body surface area involved. The simplest and most easily recalled is the Rule of Nines (Fig. 1). *However, it is only for use with the adult burn population.* It cannot be used for persons under the age of 15 years. The Lund and Browder method (Fig. 2) is useful for all age groups, but is more complicated to use.

The chart assigns a certain percentage to various parts of the body and includes a table indicating adjustments necessary for different ages. For the pediatric population, there is a modified version of the Lund and Browder method (Fig. 3). If the burned areas are small and irregularly-shaped, the Rule of Palm can be used. One looks at the palmer surface of

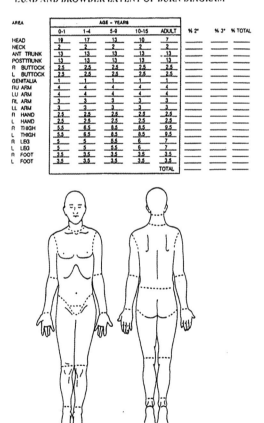

**Fig. 2.** Lund and Browder method for estimating extent of burn

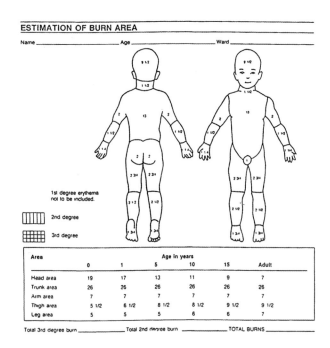

ESTIMATION OF BURN AREA

Name _____ Age _____ Ward _____

1st degree erythema
not to be included.

▥ 2nd degree

▤ 3rd degree

| Area | Age in years | | | | | |
|------|-----|-----|-----|-----|-----|-------|
| | 0 | 1 | 5 | 10 | 15 | Adult |
| Head area | 19 | 17 | 13 | 11 | 9 | 7 |
| Trunk area | 26 | 26 | 26 | 26 | 26 | 26 |
| Arm area | 7 | 7 | 7 | 7 | 7 | 7 |
| Thigh area | 5 1/2 | 6 1/2 | 8 1/2 | 8 1/2 | 9 1/2 | 9 1/2 |
| Leg area | 5 | 5 | 5 | 6 | 6 | 7 |

Total 3rd degree burn _____ Total 2nd degree burn _____ TOTAL BURNS _____

**Fig. 3.** Pediatric estimation of burn area using modified Lund and Browder

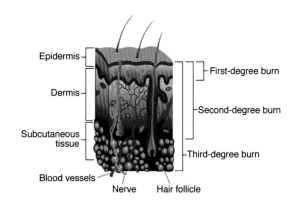

**Fig. 4.** Anatomy of burn tissue depth

the burned person's hand, which represents 1% body surface area, and uses that to calculate the scattered areas of burn. If approximately 10% or more of the body surface of a child or 15% or more of that of an adult is burned, the injury is considered serious. The person requires hospitalization and fluid replacement to prevent shock.

**ii) Depth** – Two factors determine the depth of a burn wound – temperature of the burning agent and duration of exposure time. In other words, the hotter the source and the longer it is in contact with the skin, the deeper the injury. Previously the terminology used to describe burn depth was first, second and third degree. In recent years, these terms have been replaced by those more descriptive in nature: superficial partial-thickness, deep partial-thickness and full-thickness. A description of each is included (Table 3).

Superficial burns, such as those produced by sunburn, are not taken into consideration when assessing extent and depth. The skin is divided into 3 layers, which include the epidermis, dermis and subcutaneous tissue (Fig. 4). The epidermis is the thin, outer, nonvascular layer. Its role is one of protection, heat regulation and fluid/electrolyte conservation. Below the epidermis lies the dermis, perhaps

the most important layer of skin, where the depth of burn has a profound impact. The dermis contains connective tissue, blood vessels, hair follicles, sweat and sebaceous glands. Skin-reproducing cells are located throughout the dermis and the sufficient presence or absence of these epidermal cells determines whether the wound will re-epithelialize or require skin grafting.

The subcutaneous tissue lies below the dermis and contains fat, lymphatics, nerves and vascular networks. Below the subcutaneous tissue is the muscle and bone, which may be affected by deep flame and major electrical injuries.

**iii) Age** – In patients less than 2 years of age and greater than 50, there is a higher incidence of morbidity and mortality. The severity of the burn increases with age. Infants, toddlers and the elderly have thinner skin, making the risk of a deeper burn greater in these age groups. Persons of this age also have weaker physical resources to mount a resistance against the debilitating effects brought on by a burn. Sadly, the infant, toddler and elderly are at increased risk for abuse by burning.

**iv) Part of the body burned** – Burn location is an important factor to consider. Patients with burns to the face, neck, hands, feet or perineum have greater challenges to overcome and require the specialized care offered by a burn centre. The challenges are both functional and esthetic in nature. Specialized care can minimize loss of permanent function, reduce infection and maximize esthetic outcomes.

**v) Past medical history** – A person's past medical history is an important variable to consider post-burn. Someone with pre-existing cardiovascular,

**390**

**Table 3.** Classification of burn injury depth

| Degree of Burn | Cause of Injury | Depth of Injury | Appearance | Treatment |
|---|---|---|---|---|
| First degree | Superficial sunburn Brief exposure to hot liquids or heat flash | Superficial damage to epithelium Tactile and pain sensations intact | Erythematous, blanching on pressure, no blisters | Complete healing within 3–5 days with no scarring |
| Superficial partial-thickness (2nd degree) | Brief exposure to flame, flash or hot liquids | Destruction of epidermis, superficial damage to upper layer of dermis, epidermal appendages intact | Moist, weepy, blanching on pressure, blisters, pink or red colour | Complete healing within 14–21 days with no scarring |
| Deep partial-thickness (deep 2nd degree) | Exposure to flame, scalding liquids or hot tar | Destruction of epidermis, damage to dermis, some epidermal appendages intact | Pale and less moist; no blanching or prolonged, deep pressure sensation intact, pinprick sensation absent | Prolonged healing time usually > 21 days with scarring. Skin grafting may be necessary for improved functional and esthetic outcome |
| Full-thickness (3rd degree) | Prolonged contact with flame, steam, scalding liquids, hot objects, chemicals or electrical current | Complete destruction of epidermis, dermis and epidermal appendages; injury through most of the dermis | Dry, leathery, pale, mottled brown or red in colour; visible thrombosed vessels insensitive to pain and pressure | Requires skin grafting |
| Full-thickness (4th degree) | Major electrical current, prolonged contact with heat source (i.e. unconscious patient) | Complete destruction of epidermis, dermis and epidermal appendages; injury involving connective tissue, muscle and bone | Dry, black, mottled brown, white or red; no sensation and limited movement of burned limbs or digits | Requires skin grafting and likely amputation |

pulmonary or renal disease will have a poorer predicted outcome than a previously healthy individual, since a burn injury will exacerbate pre-existing conditions. Persons with diabetes or peripheral vascular disease have a more difficult time with wound healing, a central factor in burn recovery, particularly if the burns are on the legs and/or feet. Burn patients with poor nutritional status pre-burn or with previous drug and/or alcohol abuse patterns have fewer physical reserves to draw from and, as such, require more resources for a prolonged period of time. Finally, burn patients, who have also sustained inhalation injuries, head trauma, fractures or internal damage, have a poorer prognosis overall.

## Local damage

Burn wounds are produced when there is contact between a source of energy, such as heat, chemicals, electricity or radiation, and body tissue. Local damage varies, depending upon the temperature of the agent, duration of contact time and the type of tissue involved. There are 3 zones of tissue damage in the burn wound. The deepest zone of *coagulation* (full-thickness) is the site of irreversible cell death, where blood vessels and re-epithelializing cells have been completely destroyed. These areas require skin grafting for permanent coverage. The middle layer, or zone of *stasis*, is the area of deep, partial-thickness injury where there are some skin-reproducing cells present in the dermis and circulation to the area is partially intact. Healing will occur generally within 14–21 days, as long as infection or desiccation are prevented. The outermost zone of *hyperemia* is the area of least damage. This superficial, partial-thickness wound has minimal cell involvement and will generally recover spontaneously within 7–10 days.

Coagulation necrosis occurring at the time of the injury damages or destroys tissues and vessels. During the inflammatory process post-burn, leukocytes and monocytes begin to appear at the site of the injury. Fibroblasts and collagen fibres gather within 6–12 hours after the burn to begin the task of wound repair. White blood cells begin the process of phagocytosis and necrotic burn tissue begins to slough. Fibroblasts and collagen fibres form granulation tissue. Areas of partial-thickness injury, devoid of infection and desiccation, will heal in by primary intention from the edges of the wound and from below. Full-thickness wounds require early excision and skin grafting. Over time, the collagen fibres and re-epithelializing cells continue to heal and add strength to the newly formed tissue. The healed areas initially look pale and flat. However, as the blood supply increases to those areas over the next month or so, they become red and raised. In addition to these scars forming, there is a natural tendency for burned tissue to shorten and contractures to develop. Over the next year to 18 months, the burn scars will fully mature and become less red and less raised.

## Fluid and electrolyte shifts

The immediate post-burn period is marked by dramatic circulation changes, producing what is known as "burn shock" (Fig. 5). Blood flow increases to the area surrounding the wound. The burned tissue then releases vasoactive substances, which results in increased capillary permeability. As early as 15 minutes post-injury, there is a shift of fluid from the intravascular compartment to the interstitial space, producing edema, decreased blood volume and hypovolemia. The hematocrit increases in response to the decrease in blood volume and the blood becomes more viscous. This increase in viscosity, coupled with a decreased blood volume, results in increased peripheral resistance. Hypovolemic or "burn" shock follows shortly thereafter. As the capillary walls continue to leak, water, sodium and plasma proteins (primarily albumin) move into the interstitial spaces in a phenomenon known as "second spacing". Potassium levels rise initially in the extracellular spaces due to release from injured cells and hemolyzed red blood cells. When the fluid begins to

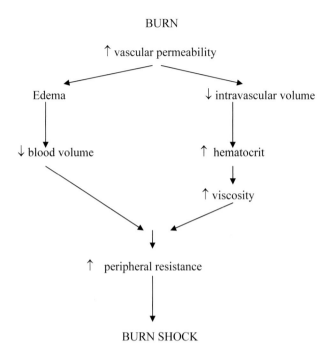

**Fig. 5.** Burn shock

accumulate in areas where there is normally minimal to no fluid, the term "third spacing" is used. This phenomenon is found in exudate and blister formation. As intravascular volumes are depleted, the edema increases and the body begins to respond to the hypovolemic shock (↑ pulse and ↓ blood pressure). There is also insensible fluid loss through evapouration from large, open body surfaces. A non-burned individual loses about 30–50 mL/hr. A severely burned patient may lose anywhere from 200 to 400 mL/hr.

Circulation is also impaired in the burn patient due to hemolysis of red blood cells. Hemolysis can be due to direct insult from the burn, circulating factors released post-injury and capillary thrombosis in burned tissue. The hematocrit is elevated secondary to hemoconcentration and returns to more normal levels once fluids shift back to the intravascular space. Following successful completion of the fluid resuscitation phase, capillary membrane permeability is restored. Fluids gradually shift back from the interstitial space to the intravascular space, bringing with them sodium to the vascular space and potassium to the cells. The patient is no longer grossly edematous and diuresis is ongoing.

## Cardiovascular, gastrointestinal and renal system manifestations

During the hypovolemic shock phase, only vital areas of circulation are maintained. As a result of decreased circulating volumes post-burn, the average cardiac output for a moderate to large burn is reduced by 30–50%. Patients with burns over 40% body surface area experience this drop as early as 15–30 minutes post-injury. Cardiac monitoring is essential and concerns are increased if the patient has a pre-burn history of cardiac problems. Electrical burn patients, who arrest at the scene or who experience cardiac arrhythmias post-injury, warrant particular vigilance. Hypovolemic shock and hypoxemia also produce the initial gastrointestinal complications seen post-burn. Lack of circulating blood volume to the splanchnic area results in decreased peristalsis and the development of abdominal paralytic ileus. The stress response post-burn releases catecholamines and may produce stress (Curling's) ulcers in burns >50% body surface area. Sepsis is primarily responsible for ulcers in patients with burns >50%. Renal complications are predominantly caused by hypovolemia and the lack of blood volume necessary to adequately perfuse the kidneys. If perfusion remains poor, high circulating levels of hemoglobin from damaged red blood cells and myoglobin from damaged muscle collect in the renal tubules and may clog them, causing acute tubular necrosis.

## Types of burn injuries

Burns can be grouped into numerous categories: thermal, chemical, electrical, smoke/inhalation and radiation. The causative agent does influence both the management and outcome of each injury.

### Thermal

Thermal injuries are caused by dry heat, such as flame and flash, moist heat, such as steam and hot liquids, and direct contact, such as hot surfaces and objects (Table 4). Thermal burns are a major source of morbidity and mortality across all age groups (Figs. 6 and 7).

**Table 4.** Causes of thermal burns

| Cause | Examples |
| --- | --- |
| Dry Heat – Flame | Clothing catches on fire<br>Skin exposed to direct flame |
| Dry Heat – Flash | Flame burn associated with explosion (combustible fuels) |
| Moist Heat – Hot liquids (scalds) | Bath water<br>Beverages – coffee, tea, soup<br>Cooking liquids or grease |
| Moist Heat – Steam | Pressure cooker<br>Microwaved food<br>Overheated car radiator |
| Contact – Hot surfaces | Oven burner and door<br>Barbecue grill |
| Contact – Hot objects | Tar<br>Curling iron<br>Cooking pots/pans |

### Chemical

The types of chemical injuries seen are usually related to the geography, industry and culture of the local population. There are more than 25,000 chemicals in the world and most can be divided into 2 major groups: acids and alkalis. Necrotizing substances in the chemicals cause tissue injury and destruction (Fig. 8). Acids, in general, cause coagulation necrosis with protein precipitation. Alkalis produce liquefaction necrosis with loosening of the tissue, which allows the alkali to diffuse more deeply into the tissues.

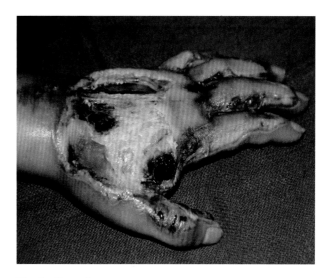

**Fig. 6.** Flame burn

393

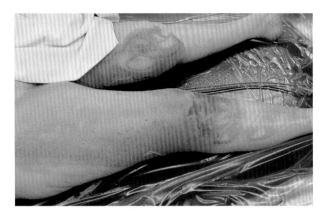

**Fig. 7.** Scald burn

Therefore, on a volume-to-volume basis, alkaline material can produce far more tissue damage than acids. The extent and depth of a chemical injury is directly proportional to the amount, type and strength of the agent, its concentration, extent of penetration, mechanism of action and length of contact time with the skin. Chemicals will continue to destroy tissue until they are inactivated by reaction with tissues, are neutralized or are diluted with water. The burning process may continue for variable and, often prolonged, periods of time (i. e. up to 72 hours) after the initial contact with the chemical agent. It is important to remove the person from the burning agent as soon as possible and to begin copiously flushing the area with water. Neutralizing agents should not be used as they may produce additional tissue damage through heat production. Dry chem-

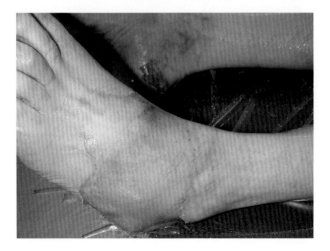

**Fig. 8.** Chemical burn

icals should be gently brushed off the skin before flushing begins. Most industries have detailed information on the chemicals their workers are exposed to and are required, by Occupational Health and Safety law, to have portable eyewash and shower stations for first aid use. Chemical burns to the eye require an ophthalmology consult, on admission, as late complications, such as corneal ulceration, secondary glaucoma and cataracts, are fairly common. Ingestion of caustic materials may cause chemical burns to the oropharynx, tongue, esophagus, stomach and duodenum. The patient should be given nothing by mouth, closely monitored and fluid resuscitated. Laryngeal edema may occur, producing upper airway obstruction. Endotracheal intubation or tracheostomy may be required to maintain airway patency.

## Electrical

Electrical injuries comprise a small portion of the burn population, but the outcomes can be devastating, including deep tissue damage and potential loss of one or more limbs (Fig. 9). Injuries occur mainly in males and are usually occupation-related. When electrical current passes through the body, intense heat is generated and coagulation necrosis results. Tissue anoxia and death are also the result of direct damage to nerves and vessels. The severity of the electrical injury is determined by the type and voltage of the circuit (whether alternating current –AC or direct current – DC), amperage of the current, resistance of the body, pathway of the current and duration of contact. Electrical current takes the path of least resistance through the body. Least resistance is offered by nerves and blood vessels, whereas bone and fat offer the most resistance. If major body organs, such as the heart, brain or kidneys are involved, the damage is more profound than if the current only passed through tissue. In some situations, electrical sparks may ignite the person's clothing, causing a flame burn, in addition to the electrical injury. If there is an explosion at an electrical panel and the clothing catches fire but no electricity passes through the body, it is termed an electrical flash burn, **not** an electrical burn. It is an important distinction to make in the early hours post-injury. The severity of an electrical injury can be difficult to

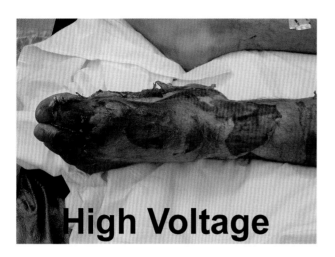

**Fig. 9.** Electrical burn

determine as most of the damage may be below the skin at the level of muscle, fat and bone. This phenomenon is referred to as the "iceberg" effect. Entry and exit points, produced at the time of the injury, may help determine the probable path of the current and potential areas of injury. The history of the event can provide valuable clues as to what actually transpired at the accident scene. Many electrical injuries occur when a worker is suspended from an aerial basket or ladder and makes contact with a live wire. If the person has fallen post-injury, precautions to protect the head and cervical spine must be taken during transport. Spinal x-rays and neurological assessment are necessary following admission to hospital. Contact with electrical current can cause tetanic muscle contractions that may produce long bone and vertebral fractures.

The person, who has sustained an electrical burn injury, may have also experienced cardiac arrhythmias or arrest post-injury. Immediate CPR is essential following cardiac arrest. He/she then continues to be at risk for cardiac arrhythmias for 24 hours post-burn, and must be monitored and have an electrocardiogram performed on admission to hospital.

Severe metabolic acidosis develops shortly after the injury occurs, because of extensive tissue destruction and cell rupture. Assessment includes arterial blood gas analysis and, if necessary to maintain normal serum pH levels, infusions of sodium bicarbonate. The kidneys also need to be closely monitored, because of potentially high circulating levels of hemoglobin from damaged red blood cells and myoglobin from damaged muscle. In small amounts, the kidney tubules can filter them sufficiently. In larger concentrations, however, there is a significant risk of developing acute tubular necrosis and possible renal failure. Treatment consists of the early initiation of Lactated Ringer's solution at a rate that maintains a good urinary output of between 75–100 mL/hour until the colour of the urine is sufficient to suggest adequate dilution. In addition, an osmotic diuretic (e.g. Mannitol) is usually given to establish and maintain acceptable urinary output.

*Smoke and inhalation injury*

Exposure to smoke and inhalation of hot air, steam or noxious products of combustion can seriously impair ventilatory function. Irritation of the mucosa can cause laryngeal edema and airway obstruction or pulmonary edema and severe respiratory insufficiency. In combination with a major burn, the presence of an inhalation injury can double or triple one's mortality rate.

Signs and symptoms of smoke inhalation include burns to the head and neck, singed nasal hairs, darkened oral and nasal membranes, carbonaceous sputum, stridor, hoarseness, difficulty swallowing, history of being burned in an enclosed space, and exposure to flame, including having clothing catch fire near the face out of doors (Fig. 10). The most critical period for patients with inhalation injuries is 24 to 48 hours post-burn. The airway becomes edematous and there is increased airway resistance. The respiratory mucosa sloughs, along with loss of ciliary function and poor diffusion of gases.

Smoke and inhalation injuries can be divided into 3 types:

*1. Inhalation injury above the glottis.* Most smoke/inhalation injury damage (60%) is limited to the upper airway (pharynx, larynx, vocal cords), since the vocal cords and glottis close quickly as a protective mechanism following exposure to smoke or thermal agents, such as hot air or steam. There is redness and blistering. Edema and the onset of rapid airway obstruction, resulting in a respiratory emergency, are the primary concerns with this type of inhalation injury.

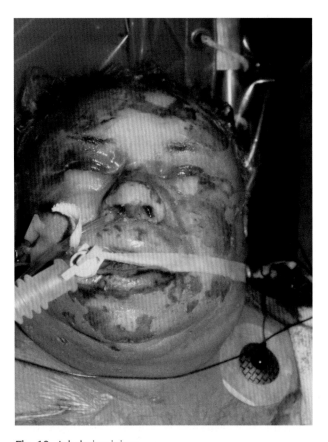

**Fig. 10.** Inhalation injury

**Table 5.** Signs and symptoms of carbon monoxide poisoning

| Carboxyhemoglobin Saturation (%) | Signs and Symptoms |
|---|---|
| 5–10 | Visual acuity impairment |
| 11–20 | Flushing, headache |
| 21–30 | Nausea, impaired dexterity |
| 31–40 | Vomiting, dizziness, syncope |
| 41–50 | Tachypnea, tachycardia |
| >50 | Coma, death |

2. *Inhalation injury below the glottis* – Most injuries below the glottis are chemically-produced through the inhalation of noxious products of combustion, resulting in tracheobronchitis. Major airway involvement (tracheobronchial tree) occurs about 30% of the time, with bronchopneumonia being the chief concern. Patients may not show symptoms until 12–24 hours post-burn. Since gases are usually cooled before they reach the lung parenchyma, there is only a 10% injury occurrence at the level of the terminal bronchioli and alveoli. Primary concerns here are pulmonary edema and adult respiratory distress syndrome (ARDS).

3. *Carbon monoxide poisoning.* Most fatalities at a fire scene are caused by carbon monoxide poisoning or asphyxiation. Carbon monoxide is produced by the incomplete combustion of burning materials. It then displaces the oxygen being carried by the hemoglobin molecules, resulting in less oxygen being delivered throughout the body. Carboxyhemoglobin levels should be measured following admission of the person to an emergency department or burn centre (Table 5). Treatment consists of the administration of 100% humidified oxygen until the carboxyhemoglobin falls to acceptable levels.

## Radiation

These burns involve overexposure to the sun or radiant heat sources, such as tanning lamps or tanning beds. Nuclear radiation burns require government intervention and specialized treatment.

## Clinical manifestations

Recovery from a burn injury involves successful passage through 3 phases of care: emergent, acute and rehabilitative. Principles of care for the emergent period involve resolution of the immediate problems resulting from the burn injury. The time required for this to occur is usually one to two days. The emergent phase ends with the onset of spontaneous diuresis. Principles of care for the acute period include the avoidance, detection and treatment of complications, and wound care. This second phase of care ends when the majority of burn wounds have healed. During the third, and final, phase of rehabilitative care, the goals are for the burn patient to return to an acceptable place in society and to accomplish functional and cosmetic reconstruction. This phase ends when there is complete resolution of any outstanding clinical problems resulting from the burn injury.

## Subjective symptoms

It is essential throughout all phases of a burn patient's recovery to seek out his/her perspective, when possible, and attempt to incorporate individual wishes into the plan of care. During the emergent period, patients and their families are in a state of physical and psychological shock. As a result of hypoxia, patients may also be disoriented or not able to recall what happened. Others remain very lucid throughout the ordeal and recall events with remarkable clarity. Some may not realize how serious their injuries are and be unrealistic about the care they require. Some may be intubated and sedated and not be aware for weeks to come. Pain may be a concern, while others experience little discomfort. Thirst may be a symptom, depending upon the degree of fluid loss. Some may complain of feeling cold or be seen to shiver as a result of heat loss, anxiety and pain. The combination of hypovolemic shock, facial edema, intubation and analgesics/sedative agents may alter a patient's sensory perception significantly over the first few days post-injury. If he/she is able to talk, common themes include "Will I die? What happened? Why me? I can't believe this is happening". In the acute phase, patients experience varying levels of pain during dressing changes and physical/occupational therapy, and may describe significant muscular discomfort, resulting from functional positioning and use of splinting materials. Unable to do any number of self-care activities, patients may become very frustrated about how dependent they have become on others. Concerns may be expressed regarding finances, family and work obligations. Adaptation to the hospital environment and necessary treatments may absorb a considerable amount of the patient's physical and emotional energy. Adjustment to a variety of losses (personal and property), feelings of grief, guilt and blame, a need for information about what to expect over the coming weeks, and a search for meaning behind the event, are also experienced. Patients may feel angry or depressed post-injury. Relationships with family may become strained as everyone seeks to readjust and cope with this unexpected and traumatic event. During the rehabilitative phase of care, patients come to realize they have completed the most difficult part of their recovery. However, they may experience impatience with the time required for complete healing and physical rehabilitation. There is usually a desire to resume as much independence as possible, sometimes coupled with slight fear and hesitation about

leaving the protective environment of the burn centre. Questions, such as "What will it be like when I leave the hospital? How will I manage when the nurses and therapists are no longer around to help?" reflect the primary concerns for patients and family members at this time. There may be concerns about resumed sexual intimacy with a partner and self-acceptance of an altered body image. A request may be made to speak with a recovered burn survivor, who can offer words of support and advice based on personal experience. Over time, burn patients express feelings of pride at having overcome such tremendous physical and emotional challenges, and begin to reflect on the path their lives will take post-burn as they move from burn "victim" to burn "survivor" and, perhaps, burn "thriver".

*Objective signs* The initial assessment of the burn patient is like that of any trauma patient and can best be remembered by the simple acronym "**ABCDEF**" (Box 2). During the emergent period, burn patients quickly begin to exhibit signs and symptoms of hypovolemic shock (Box 3). Lack of circulating fluid volumes will also result in minimal urinary output and absence of bowel sounds. The patient may also be shivering due to heat loss, pain and anxiety. If inhalation injury is a factor, the patient may demonstrate a number of physical findings upon visual assessment, laryngoscopy and fiberoptic bronchoscopy (Box 4). The patient may also experience pain, as exhibited by facial grimacing, withdrawing and moaning when touched, particularly if the injuries are partial-thickness in nature. Some areas of full-thickness burn may be anaesthetic to pain and touch if the nerve endings have been destroyed. The loss of sensation may be temporary if the nerves have been compressed by resulting edema in the hypovolemic shock phase. It is important to examine areas of cir-

**Box 2.** Primary survey assessment

| | |
|---|---|
| **A** | Airway |
| **B** | Breathing |
| **C** | Circulation |
| | – **C**-spine immobilization |
| | – **C**ardiac status |
| **D** | Disability |
| | – Neurological **D**eficit |
| **E** | Expose and evaluate |
| **F** | Fluid resuscitation |

**397**

**Box 3.** Signs and symptoms of hypovolemic shock

> ► Restlessness, anxiety
> ► Skin – pale, cold, clammy
> ► Temperature below 37 °C
> ► Pulse is weak, rapid, ↓ systolic BP
> ► Urinary output < 20 mL/hr
> ► Urine specific gravity > 1.025
> ► Thirst
> ► Hematocrit < 35; BUN ↑

**Box 5.** Signs and symptoms of vascular compromise

> ► Cyanosis
> ► Deep tissue pain
> ► Progressive paresthesias
> ► Diminished or absent pulses
> ► Sensation of cold extremities

cumferential full-thickness burn for signs and symptoms of vascular compromise, particularly the extremities (Box 5).

Areas of partial-thickness burn appear reddened, blistered and edematous. Full-thickness burns may be dark red, brown, charred black or white in colour. The texture is tough and leathery and no blisters are present.

If the patient is confused, one has to determine if it is the result of hypovolemic shock, inhalation injury, substance abuse, pre-existing history or, more rarely, head injury sustained at the time of the trauma. It is essential to immobilize the c-spines until a full assessment can be performed and the c-spines cleared. At this time, a secondary survey assessment is performed (Box 6). Additional objective data can then be collected, analyzed and a plan of care developed, which includes a set of Admission Orders. In the acute phase, the focus is on wound care and potential development of complications. At this point, the burn wounds should have declared themselves as being partial-thickness or full-thickness in nature. Eschar on partial-thickness wounds is thinner and, with dressing changes, it should be possible to see evidence of eschar separating from the viable wound bed. Healthy, granulation tissue is apparent on the clean wound bed and re-epithelializing cells are seen to migrate from the wound edges and the der-

mal bed to slowly close the wound within 10–14 days. Full-thickness wounds have a thicker, more leathery eschar, which does not separate easily from the viable wound bed. Those wounds require surgical excision and grafting.

Continuous assessment of the patient's systemic response to the burn injury is an essential part of an individualized plan of care. Subtle changes quickly identified by the burn team can prevent complications from occurring or worsening over time. Physical examination, laboratory tests and diagnostic procedures will assist in the rapid identification and treatment of complications.

During the final, rehabilitative phase, attention turns to scar maturation, contracture development and functional independence issues. The areas of burn, which heal either by primary intention or skin grafting, initially appear red or pink and are flat. Layers of re-epithelializing cells continue to form and collagen fibres in the lower scar tissue add strength to a fragile wound. Over the next month, the scars may become more red from increased blood supply and more raised from disorganized whorls of collagen and fibroblasts/myofibroblasts. The scars are referred to as hypertrophic in nature. If oppositional forces are not applied through splinting devices, exercises or stretching routines, this new tissue continues to heal by shortening and forming contractures. A certain amount of contracture development is unavoidable, but the impact can be lessened through prompt and aggressive interventions.

**Box 4.** Physical findings of inhalation injury

> ► Carbonaceous sputum
> ► Facial burns, singed nasal hairs
> ► Agitation, tachypnea, general signs of hypoxemia
> ► Signs of respiratory difficulty
> ► Hoarseness, brassy cough
> ► Rales, ronchi
> ► Erythema of oropharynx or nasopharynx

**Box 6.** Secondary survey assessment

> ► Head-to-toe examination
> ► Rule out associated injuries
> ► Pertinent history  – circumstances of injury
>                       – medical history

The scar maturation process takes anywhere from 6–18 months. During this time, the scars will progress from a dark pink/red to a pale pink/whitened appearance. The final colour is usually lighter than the surrounding unburned skin. For people with darkly pigmented skin, the process of colour return may be prolonged as the melanocytes work to produce pigment in the areas where it has been lost. Pressure may be necessary to gently and continually flatten the scars which, in turn, pushes the extra blood from the area, making them lighter in colour. Pressure is usually applied in increasing amounts as the fragile skin develops tolerance. Custom-fitted pressure garments and/or acrylic face masks apply constant pressure over a wearing period of 23 ½ hours a day. Extra pressure over concave and difficult-to-fit areas can be provided through elastomer inserts or silicone sheeting under the garments or face mask. The length of time a person might have to wear the garments varies, but is in the range of 1 to 1½ years, depending upon the intensity of the scarring and the body's response to pressure therapies. Patients will often experience itchiness and dry skin. One of the best ways to decrease the itchiness is to get at the source of the problem: the dry skin. However, burned skin is different from healthy skin. Once the skin has been damaged by a burn injury, there are less natural oils available since the oil-reproducing glands have been destroyed, in whole or in part. In other words, the skin is "internally" dry as opposed to "externally" dry, such as when hands get chapped in the cold weather. What burned skin needs is a product that will be absorbed through the outer layer of the epidermis into the dry, dermal tissues. Water-based products are needed in order to do this. The more predominant products available are oil-based and contain mineral oil, petrolatum or paraffin. These ingredients coat the surface of the skin and, in essence, block the pores. This prevents loss of natural oils from the dermis, oils which burned skin is lacking. These ingredients are not absorbed into the dry dermis and do not bring moisture back into the skin. Mineral oil also breaks down elastic fibres in pressure garments and should be avoided. Suggested water-based products include Vaseline( Intensive Rescue or Smith and Nephew's Professional Care®. Medications, such as diphenhydramine (Atarax®, Benadryl®), can also be ordered to help with moderate to severe itchiness on a short-term basis, as can massage therapy.

## Diagnostic findings

There are a number of baseline diagnostic studies that describe the patient's clinical condition at the time of the injury and monitor responses to care throughout the recovery period. They include laboratory tests, such as complete blood cell count (CBC), hemoglobin and hematocrit, group and screen, serum electrolyte levels, blood glucose, blood urea nitrogen (BUN), serum creatinine, calcium profile, serum lactate, liver function tests and coagulation studies (PT, PTT, INR). Drug and alcohol screens may be indicated, upon admission, if the circumstances of the accident and/or patient's clinical presentation warrant it. If inhalation injury is suspected, a serum carboxyhemoglobin, serum cyanide and arterial blood gas should be obtained, along with a chest x-ray. Laryngoscopy and/or fiberoptic bronchoscopy may also be indicated for inhalation-injured patients. Routine urinalysis, along with urine for hemoglobin and myoglobin in cases in electrical injury, also need to be collected. For patients with pre-existing cardiac disease or those sustaining electrical injuries, a 12-lead electrocardiogram (ECG) should be performed. For patients with suspected, head or spinal injury, fractures or internal trauma, x-rays or scans are indicated. Antibiotic resistant organism (MRSA and VRE) screening and wound swabs for culture and sensitivity (C + S) monitor the microbiological organisms present on admission. Blood cultures, along with urine and sputum for C + S, are also helpful when investigating patients who become febrile or who may be developing sepsis. As the patient's condition changes, medical specialists from various services may be consulted and they may order various diagnostic tests, such as ultrasound, magnetic resonance imaging (MRI) or computerized axial tomography (CAT) scans to rule out or confirm diagnoses. Placement and monitoring of transduced, invasive central and arterial lines provide the team with information on a patient's cardiac and pulmonary functioning. Access to this wide variety of diagnostic information allows for timely clinical interventions by members of the burn team.

## Possible complications

Complications can arise throughout all phases of burn care, although the potential for development is greater in the acute stage of recovery. Prompt identification and management are essential in order to effect the best possible patient outcome. The systems most commonly affected are cardiovascular, respiratory, gastrointestinal and renal.

**Cardiovascular system** – Cardiovascular system complications include hypovolemic shock and arrhythmias. When the intravascular volume is reduced immediately post-burn, the cardiac output decreases dramatically and blood flow through the tissues and coronary artery is reduced. Prompt and adequate fluid resuscitation can effectively address the decrease in circulating volumes. Circulation to the extremities can also be impaired by the decreased volumes, the presence of circumferential burns and the formation of edema. Incisions through the leathery, devitalized burned tissue may be necessary in order to restore circulation to these limbs. That procedure is called an **escharotomy** (Fig. 11). Deeper burns (severe electrical or prolonged flame exposure) may require a **fasciotomy**. Patients with pre-existing cardiac disease may be more prone to the development of arrhythmias, brought on by the stress of a major burn injury. Direct cardiac damage may have also occurred from the passage of electrical current through the heart. All moderate to major burns should be monitored, using an external cardiac monitor, and invasive lines transduced. Hemodynamic parameters, such as heart rate, central venous pressure and blood pressure/mean arterial pressure, are set within targeted ranges [3]. Attention should also be paid to electrolyte levels, especially sodium and potassium. Early post-burn, sodium shifts into the interstitial spaces, only to return at the end of the hypovolemic shock phase. Potassium is initially released into the extracellular spaces by hemolyzed red blood cells and those cells injured by the burn. As fluids are mobilized, potassium levels increase in the vascular spaces. As plasma leaks into the interstitial space, there is a temporary increase in blood viscosity. Appropriate fluid resuscitation can correct that situation satisfactorily. Arrhythmia management may require a collaborative consultation with Cardiology and medication on either a short-term or long-term basis. Evidence-based, venous thromboembolism prophylaxis should also be instituted and medications, such as enoxaparin, commenced as the incidence of DVT's in burns is estimated to be between 1 to 23 % [4].

**Respiratory system** – There are, generally, two ways in which the respiratory system can be affected by a burn injury. One involves mechanical, upper airway obstruction due to heat injury and edema formation and/or constricting circumferential burns to the neck and chest. The other involves inhalation of noxious products of combustion, which produces a chemical irritation reaction to the middle and lower airways. Early in the emergent phase of care, the upper airway can close off very quickly, because of massive facial and neck edema. Upon initial assessment, if there is any indication that the patient has a pharyngeal burn, is hoarse or has stridor, the patient should be nasally or, preferably, orally intubated with an *uncut* endotracheal tube. This action serves to splint the airway open and maintain patency. Arterial blood gases (ABG's) should then be drawn and oxygen saturation levels monitored. If necessary, the patient may need to be mechanically ventilated in order to maintain sufficient levels of oxygenation.

Mechanical ventilation protocols should be instituted and ventilator settings titrated to maintain desired PaCO2, PaO2 and SaO2 readings.

When the edema subsides and/or ventilation parameters improve, the patient can be appropriately assessed and extubated safely. In most clinical settings, tracheostomies are performed if the patient is intubated for longer than 3 weeks. Patients, who

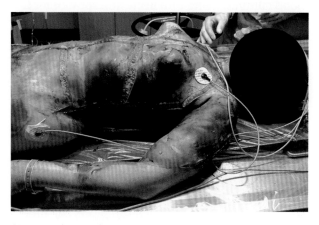

**Fig. 11.** Chest escharotomy

do not have inhalation injury, may benefit from a face mask or nasal cannula to maintain oxygen saturations >92%. If there are circumferential flame burns to the chest and back, escharotomies of the chest and/or abdomen may need to be performed in order to release the constricting eschar, decrease respiratory distress and improve chest expansion and ventilation. With an inhalation injury, it is not as obvious that there is damage to the middle or lower airways. At times, patients may present with bronchial and bronchiolar injury, such as bronchorrhea and/or expiratory wheezing. Examination of the lower respiratory tract, using fiberoptic bronchoscopy, should be performed. However, some may have an invisible injury at the level of respiratory gas exchange. This condition is often delayed and diagnosed by arterial blood gas analysis, rather than a chest x-ray. Impaired gas exchange may be related to carbon monoxide poisoning. Carboxyhemoglobin levels should be drawn on admission (Table 5). Treatment of inhalation injury includes aggressive chest physiotherapy, tracheobronchial suctioning, administration of nebulized heparin and acetylcysteine [5], use of bronchodilators (ipratropium) to treat severe bronchospasm and mechanical ventilation with positive end expiratory pressure (PEEP). PEEP prevents collapse of the alveoli and the development of progressive respiratory failure. If the patient's condition deteriorates and conventional ventilation strategies prove to be inadequate, newer forms of ventilation have been utilized in recent years and include strategies such as high frequency oscillation and implementation of prone positioning techniques. Patients, who have pre-existing respiratory problems, such as a history of frequent pneumonia or chronic obstructive pulmonary disease, are more likely to succumb to respiratory infection. Pneumonia is commonly seen in these patients since they are relatively immobile, may be debilitated and have an abundance of microbial organisms that can settle in the lungs and require aggressive therapy to eradicate. Older, more debilitated patients are also more prone to the development of pulmonary edema as a consequence of the fluid resuscitation required by inhalation-injured patients.

Maintaining the airway is crucial in these patients and frequent assessments of tube placement and stability are an essential part of care. Before patients are extubated, there is a weaning process which involves adjusting ventilator settings, so the machine is doing less of the work associated with breathing and patients are essentially breathing on their own. If they meet certain criteria, patients are extubated, placed in high Fowler's position and given 100% oxygen. In addition, they require chest physiotherapy, suctioning, frequent repositioning and deep breathing and coughing exercises. Mobilization at the bedside and in the hallways is also helpful in moving secretions from the upper and lower airways. Sometimes, patients tire too easily post-extubation and need to be reintubated. In situations where a patient cannot be weaned in the near distant future, a decision is made to perform a tracheostomy until such time as he/she can breathe unaided.

**Gastrointestinal system** – The gastrointestinal system is initially affected in the emergent phase by a lack of circulation to the splanchnic area. This hypoperfusion, secondary to hypovolemic shock, causes paralytic ileus and an absence of bowel sounds. The stress response post-burn causes a decrease in mucous production and an increase in gastric acid secretion, resulting in stress (Curling's) ulcers. Prompt and effective fluid resuscitation and a restoration of circulation to the gastrointestinal region result in a return of bowel sounds and indicate a functional gut. Bladder pressures should be measured q4h for 72 hours in body surface area burns >30% and pressures >20 mm Hg reported. Abdominal compartment syndrome is a life-threatening complication of high-volume fluid resuscitation [6,7]. Management includes keeping the patient NPO for a few hours post-admission until things stabilize and then, beginning early enteral feeds to address the profound hypermetabolic effects of a burn injury. Anti-catabolic, anabolic agents, such as oxandralone and propanolol, may also prove to be valuable adjuncts to therapy. Enteral feeding also maintains the integrity of the gut and avoids bacterial translocation. The hourly rate of feeds is advanced, in a timely manner, to the desired goal rate, usually arrived at in consultation with the burn centre dietitian. A nasogastric (NG) tube, connected to either straight drainage or wall suction, can be inserted for the purposes of gastric decompression and medication administration. Water flushes pre- and post-medication help ensure the tubes remain patent. Medications include

**401**

prophylactic use of intravenous $H_2$ antagonists (Ranitidine) to decrease hydrochloride secretion. During the acute phase of care, patients frequently become constipated as a result of codeine-containing pain medication received during their hospitalization and immobility. Prompt institution of a bowel regimen, upon admission, and attention to diet and/or choice of tube feedings can prevent or rectify the situation before it causes the patient unnecessary discomfort. Patients may also develop diarrhea, caused by certain tube feedings or antibiotics. Excessive diarrhea may warrant clostridium difficile testing. Recommendations from the dietitian or pharmacist should be sought to correct the problem. A bowel management system may need to be inserted if loose stools interfere with optimal wound care. Sepsis is the most common cause of gastric ileus occurring in the acute phase of care and should be monitored closely. Some burn centres are administering an anti-oxidant protocol, which includes selenium, acetylcysteine, ascorbic acid, vitamin E, zinc and a multivitamin. It is also important to monitor and, if necessary, institute potassium, calcium, magnesium and phosphate replacements, and administer thiamine and folic acid, particularly if the patient has a history of alcohol abuse. Blood glucose point-of-care testing should be performed and an insulin nomogram commenced, as per ICU protocol, in order to maintain strict glucose control of 80–110 mg/dL.

**Renal system** – With the renal system post-burn, an early warning sign of complications is an increase in the specific gravity, which usually occurs before the urinary output falls. Acute tubular necrosis is the most frequent emergent phase complication and is due to hypovolemic shock. Fluid resuscitation is usually sufficient to correct such problems. Careful attention to trends in urinary output and specific gravity is a more helpful strategy than haphazardly increasing or decreasing the intravenous fluids. Insertion of a urinary catheter should occur, upon admission, to allow for accurate intake/output. If the injury is deep to the tissue and/or muscle, there is the additional complication of high circulating levels of hemoglobin (red blood cell breakdown) or myoglobin (muscle cell breakdown) pigments blocking the renal tubules. This situation is so common in electrical burns that the fluid resuscitation formula

requires very aggressive resuscitation and the infusion of an osmotic diuretic (Mannitol). In the acute phase of care, a decrease in urinary output or the development of high output renal failure, with rising levels of BUN and creatinine, may be indicative of a septic episode. Consultation with the renal service is essential if the patient doesn't respond to fluid challenges or diuretics. In the most serious of situations, the patient may require dialysis as a life-saving measure. Rising glucose levels indicate stress response, due to catecholamine release, and sepsis. High levels lead to compensatory osmotic diuresis, which means the burn patient needs more fluid.

**Infection** – Burn patients are at risk for the development of infection due to both the high bacterial loads on their devitalized, burn eschar and the loss of their primary barrier against infection – the skin. Infection is the leading cause of morbidity and mortality in burn patients. The degree of risk is increased due to the presence of devitalized burn eschar, which serves as an excellent breeding ground for organisms, invasive catheters and tubes, and a state of immunosuppression that continues long after the wounds have healed. The larger the burn wound, the greater the risk of infection. However, the advent of early burn excision and prompt wound closure has decreased the overall incidence of burn wound infection and, consequently, the incidence of sepsis and death. Evidence-based procedures for the insertion of central lines have resulted in impressive reductions in central line blood stream infection rates. Ventilator-acquired pneumonia (VAP) rates have also declined since the advent of evidence-based practice bundles, such as chlorhexidine mouth rinse, head-of-bed elevation to $30^0$, gastrointestinal prophylaxis and turning patients, from side to side, q2h [8].

The primary sites for organisms are the burn wound, oral and pulmonary secretions, perineal and anal regions. Gram negative organisms, such as e. coli, klebsiella, pseudomonas and serratia, are largely responsible for more than 50% of all septic episodes. They release endotoxins, which serve as key triggers for the sepsis cascade. All burn wounds are colonized with bacteria, which can be identified through qualitative wound swabs. More specific determinations can be made using quantitative, burn wound biopsies. If the bacterial count on a wound rises above $1 \times 10^5$/gram of tissue, the wound is said to be infected, with the organisms having invaded into viable tissue. Local signs of burn wound infection include a change in wound exudate, alteration in wound appearance, increase in wound pain, erythema, edema, cellulitis and induration at the wound edges. In the presence of a burn wound infection, a partial-thickness wound can convert to a full-thickness wound. If the organisms enter the lymphatic system, the patient can develop septicemia. Sepsis accounts for about 70% of deaths post-burn. Multisystem organ failure, often secondary to sepsis, is a serious and frequently fatal consequence of septicemia. Signs and symptoms of sepsis include an elevated temperature, increased pulse and respiratory rate, and decreased blood pressure and urinary output. The patient may become confused, feel and look unwell, have a diminished appetite and experience chills. It is important to identify and treat the source of sepsis as quickly as possible before multiple organ systems begin to fail. Cultures should be obtained from the blood, urine, sputum, invasive device sites and wounds. Intravenous antibiotics may then be ordered by the burn centre physicians, in consultation with the Infectious Disease service in the hospital. Initially, antibiotics can be ordered on speculation, pending culture and sensitivity reports from the lab. If necessary, the antibiotics may be changed to provide coverage specific to the organisms cultured. If the burn wounds, grafted areas or donor sites appear infected, topical antimicrobial coverage on the burn wound may need to be changed or instituted in order to provide treatment at a local level.

## Clinical management

### Non-surgical care

Therapeutic management of the burned person is conducted within these same three phases of burn recovery – emergent, acute and rehabilitative.

The *emergent* phase priorities include airway management, fluid therapy and initial wound care. The goals of care are initial assessment, management and stabilization of the patient during the first 48 hours post-burn.

**Assessment**: During the rapid, primary survey, performed soon after admission, the airway and breathing assume top priority. Particularly with a large body surface area burn admission, some staff may feel a tendency to be overwhelmed by the sight and smell of the burn wound. The wounds are, however, a much lower priority than the airway. A compromised airway requires prompt attention and breath sounds verified in each lung field. If circumferential, full-thickness burns are present on the upper trunk and back, ventilation must be closely monitored as breathing might be impaired and releasing escharotomies necessary. The spine must be stabilized until c-spines are cleared. The circulation is assessed by examining skin colour, sensation, peripheral pulses and capillary filling. Circumferential, full-thickness burns to the arms or legs need to be assessed via palpation or doppler for evidence of adequate circulation. Escharotomies might be required. Typically, burn patients are alert and oriented during the first few hours post-burn. If that is not the case, consideration must be given to associated head injury, (including a complete neurological assessment), substance abuse, hypoxia or pre-existing medical conditions. All clothing and jewellery need to be removed in order to visualize the entire body and avoid the "tourniquet-like" effect of constricting items left in place as edema increases. Adherent clothing needs to be gently soaked off with normal saline to avoid further trauma and unnecessary pain. Attention then turns to prompt fluid resuscitation to combat the hypovolemic shock. The secondary, head-to-toe survey then rules out any associated injuries. A thorough assessment ensures all medical problems are identified and managed in a timely fashion. Circumstances of the injury should be explored as care can be influenced by the mechanism, duration and severity of the injury. The patient's pertinent medical history includes identification of pre-existing disease or associated illness (cardiac or renal disease, diabetes, hypertension), medication/alcohol/drug history, allergies and tetanus immunization status. A handy mnemonic can be used to remember this information (Box 7).

**Box 7.** Secondary survey highlights

| | |
|---|---|
| A | allergies |
| M | medications |
| P | previous illness, past medical history |
| L | last meal or drink |
| E | events preceding injury |

**Management**: The top priority of care is to *stop the burning process* (Box 8). During the initial first aid period at the scene, the patient must be removed from the heat source, chemicals should be brushed off and/or flushed from the skin, and the patient wrapped in a clean sheet and blanket ready for transport to the nearest hospital. Careful, local cooling of the burn wound with saline-moistened gauze can continue as long as the patient's core temperature is maintained and he/she does not become hypothermic. Upon arrival at the hospital, the burned areas can be cooled further with normal saline, followed by a complete assessment of the patient and initiation of emergency treatment (Box 9). In a burn centre, the cooling may take place, using a cart shower system, in a hydrotherapy room (Fig. 12). The temperature of the water is adjusted to the patient's comfort level, but tepid is usually best, while the wounds are quickly cleaned and dressings applied.

*Airway management* includes administration of 100% oxygen if burns are 20% body surface area or greater. Suctioning and ventilatory support may be necessary. If the patient is suspected of having or has an inhalation injury, intubation needs to be performed quickly. *Circulatory management* includes intravenous infusion of fluid to counteract the effects of hypovolemic shock for adult patients with burns >15% body surface area and children with burns >10% body surface area. Upon admission, 2 large bore, intravenous catheters should be in-

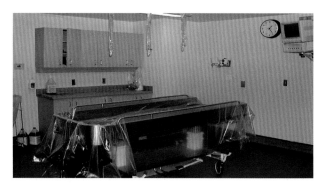

**Fig. 12.** Cart shower for hydrotherapy

serted, preferably into unburned tissue. However, if the only available veins are in a burned area, they should be used. Patients who have large burns, where intravenous access will be necessary for a number of days, benefit from a central venous access device inserted into either the subclavian, jugular or femoral

**Box 8.** First aid management at the scene

| STEPS | ACTION |
|---|---|
| Step 1 | Stop the burning process – remove patient from heat source. |
| Step 2 | Maintain airway – resuscitation measures may be necessary. |
| Step 3 | Assess for other injuries and check for any bleeding. |
| Step 4 | Flush chemical burns copiously with cool water. |
| Step 5 | Flush other burns with cool water to comfort. |
| Step 6 | Protect wounds from further trauma. |
| Step 7 | Provide emotional support and have someone remain with patient to explain help is on the way. |
| Step 8 | Transport the patient as soon as possible to nearby emergency department. |

**Box 9.** Treatment of the severely burned patient on admission

| STEPS | ACTION |
|---|---|
| Step 1 | Stop the burning process. |
| Step 2 | Establish and maintain an airway; inspect face and neck for singed nasal hair, soot in the mouth or nose, stridor or hoarseness. |
| Step 3 | Administer 100% high flow humidified oxygen by non-rebreather mask. Be prepared to intubate if respiratory distress increases. |
| Step 4 | Establish intravenous line(s) with large bore cannula(e) and initiate fluid replacement using Lactated Ringer's solution. |
| Step 5 | Insert an indwelling urinary catheter. |
| Step 6 | Insert a nasogastric tube. |
| Step 7 | Monitor vital signs including level of consciousness and oxygen saturation. |
| Step 8 | Assess and control pain. |
| Step 9 | Gently remove clothing and jewellery. |
| Step 10 | Examine and treat other associated injuries. |
| Step 11 | Assess extremities for pulses, especially with circumferential burns. |
| Step 12 | Determine depth and extent of the burn. |
| Step 13 | Provide initial wound care – cool the burn and cover with large, dry gauze dressings. |
| Step 14 | Prepare to transport to a burn centre as soon as possible. |

vein. The overall goal is to establish an access route that will accommodate large volumes of fluid for the first 48 hours post-burn. The aim of fluid resuscitation is to maintain vital organ function, while avoiding the complications of inadequate or excessive therapy. Fluid calculations are based on the extent of the burn, the weight and age of the patient, pre-burn conditions (dehydration) or pre-existing chronic illnesses (respiratory, renal). The most commonly used fluid resuscitation regimen is the Parkland (Baxter) formula (Box 10). It involves the use of crystalloid (Lactated Ringer's) solution. Fluids are calculated for the first 24 hours post-burn with "0" hours being the time of the burn, not the time of admission to hospital. One-half of the 24 hour total needs to be administered over the first 8 hours post-burn as this is the period during which extravasation of fluid into the interstitial space is greatest, along with the risk of renal tubule blockage from hemoglobin and myoglobin pigments. The remaining half of the estimated resuscitation volume should be administered over the subsequent 16 hours of the first post-burn day. It is important to remember that the formula is only a guideline. The infusion needs to be adjusted based on the patient's clinical response, which includes vital signs, sensorium and urinary output. For adults, 30–50 mL urine per hour is the goal and 1 mL/kg/hr in children weighing less than 30 kg. An indwelling urinary catheter needs to be inserted at the same time as the IV's are established in order to reliably measure the adequacy of the fluid resuscitation [9]. Vital signs should be trending around a systolic BP of ≥ 90 to 100 mg Hg, a pulse rate of < 120

for the older child/adult, < 140 bpm in the child between 2–5 years of age and < 160 bpm in the child under 2 years of age, with respirations at 16–20 breaths/minute. The patient's sensorium should be such that he/she is alert and oriented to time, person and place. An exception is made regarding the sensorium assessment for the intubated patient. During the second 24 hours post-burn, the need for aggressive fluid resuscitation is generally less as capillary permeability begins to return to normal. Colloids, such as albumin, can be given as volume expanders to replace lost protein and minimize ongoing fluid requirements. Earlier administration of colloid would result in leakage out of the vascular space because of the increased capillary permeability. Some patients require extra fluid above and beyond the formula guidelines in order to produce satisfactory urinary output, stable vital signs and an adequate sensorium. They include those with a) high voltage injury, b) inhalation injury, c) delayed resuscitation, or d) prior dehydration. Those patients with a high voltage injury require administration of a diuretic to produce a urinary output of 75–100 mL/hour in order to clear the tubules of hemoglobin and myoglobin pigments. The usual choice is Mannitol 12.5 gram/litre of fluid. Since the heme pigments are more soluble in an alkaline medium, sodium bicarbonate can be added to the resuscitation fluid as needed to maintain a slightly alkaline urine. Patients with severe inhalation injury and body surface area burns may require 40–50% more fluid in order to achieve adequate tissue perfusion. The need for extra fluid must be balanced against the risk of pulmonary ede-

**Box 10.** Fluid resuscitation using the Parkland (Baxter) formula

| Formula | Administration | Example |
|---|---|---|
| 4 mL Lactated Ringer's solution per kg body weight per % total body surface area (TBSA) burn<br>=<br>total fluid requirements for the first 24 hours post-burn (0 hours = time of injury) | ½ total in first 8 hours<br>¼ total in second 8 hours<br>¼ total in third 8 hours | For a 65 kg patient with a 40 % burn injured at 1000 hours:<br>4 mL x 65 kg x 40% burn = 10,400 mL in first 24 hours<br>½ total in first 8 hours (1000-1800 hours)<br>= 5200 mL (650 mL/hr)<br>¼ total in second 8 hours (1800-0200 hours)<br>= 2600 mL (325 mL/hr)<br>¼ total in third 8 hours (0200-1000 hours)<br>= 2600 mL (325 mL/hr) |

**N.B. Remember that the formula is only a guideline. Titrate to maintain urinary output at 30–50 mL/hr, stable vital signs and adequate sensorium.**

ma and "fluid creep"/overload[10]. There are others who are considered "volume sensitive". They are a) ≥ 50 years of age, b) ≤ 2 years of age, or c) have pre-existing cardiopulmonary or renal disease. Particular caution must be exercised with these patients.

*Wound care.* Once a patent airway, adequate circulation and fluid replacement have been established, attention can turn to wound care and the ultimate long-term goal of wound closure. Such closure will halt or reverse the various fluid/electrolyte, metabolic and infectious processes associated with an open burn wound. The burns are gently cleansed with normal saline, if the care is being provided on a stretcher or bed. If a hydrotherapy cart shower or immersion tank are used, tepid water cleans the wounds of soot and loose debris (Fig. 13).

Sterile water is not necessary. Chemical burns should be flushed copiously for at least 20 minutes, preferably longer. Tar cannot be washed off the wound. It requires numerous applications of an emulsifying agent, such as Tween 80®, Medisol® or Polysporin® ointment. After several applications, the tar will have been removed without unnecessary trauma to healthy tissue. During hydrotherapy, loose, necrotic tissue (eschar) may be gently removed (debrided) using sterile scissors and forceps. Hair-bearing areas that are burned should be carefully shaved, with the exception of the eyebrows. This serves to minimize the accumulation of organisms. Showering or bathing should be limited to 20 minutes in

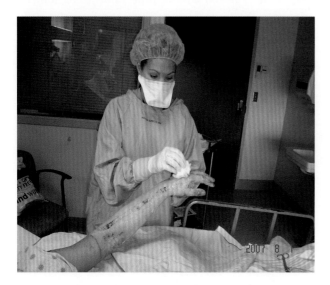

**Fig. 13.** Initial wound care post-admission

order to minimize patient heat loss and physical/emotional exhaustion. More aggressive debridement should be reserved for the operating room, unless the patient receives conscious sedation. After the initial bath or shower, further decisions are made regarding wound care. There are three methods of treatment used in caring for burn wounds. In the *open method*, the wound remains exposed, with only a thin layer (2.0 mm to 4.0 mm) of topical antimicrobial ointment spread on the wound surface using a sterile gloved hand or applicator. With the closed method, a dressing is left intact for two to seven days. The most common approach is to make multiple dressing changes, usually twice a day. The frequency depends on the condition of the wound and the properties of the dressing employed. The choice of treatment method varies among institutions and also according to the severity of the burn wound. All treatment approaches have certain objectives in common (Table 6). In the emergent phase, wounds are generally treated with a thin layer of topical antimicrobial cream. Topical coverage is selected according to the condition of the wound, desired results, and properties of the topical agent (Table 7). Assessment criteria have been established for choosing the most appropriate agent (Box 11). The most commonly selected topical antimicrobial agent is silver sulphadiazene, which can be applied directly to saline-moistened gauze, placed on the wound, covered with additional dry gauze or a burn pad, and secured with gauze wrap or flexible netting (Fig. 14). These dressings are usually changed twice a day. If the hydrotherapy room is used for the morning dressing change, the evening dressing is done in the patient's room as it is too physically and emotionally exhausting to shower the burned person twice daily. It is preferred that the antimicrobial be applied directly to the gauze as opposed to being spread on the wound for two reasons: it is less likely that you will spread organisms from one part of a burn wound to another and it is generally less painful for the patient. Patients lose a lot of body heat during dressing changes, so it is advised that the temperature of the room be elevated slightly and that only small to moderate-sized areas of the body be exposed at any one time. Cartilagenous areas, such as the nose and ears, are usually covered with mafenide acetate (Sulfamylon®), which has greater eschar penetration

**Table 6.** Objectives of burn wound care

| Objective | Rationale |
|---|---|
| Prevention of conversion | Wounds that dry out or develop an infection can become deeper. A partial-thickness wound could then convert to full-thickness and require skin grafting. |
| Removal of devitalized tissue | Debridement, either through dressing changes or surgery, is necessary to clean the wounds and prepare for spontaneous healing or grafting. |
| Preparation of healthy granulation tissue | Healthy tissue, free of eschar and nourished by a good blood supply, is essential for new skin formation. |
| Minimization of systemic infection | Eschar contains many organisms. Removal is essential in order to decrease the bacterial load and reduce the risk of burn wound infection. |
| Completion of the autografting process | Full-thickness wounds require the application of autologous skin grafts from available donor sites. |
| Limitation of scars and contractures | Wounds that heal well the first time tend to have fewer scars and contractures. Some degree of scar and contracture formation are, however, part of the healing process and cannot be entirely prevented. |

ability. Face care includes the application of warmed, saline-moistened gauze to the face for 20 minutes, followed by a gentle cleansing and reapplication of a thin layer of ointment, such as polymyxin B sulphate (Polysporin®) (Fig. 15). A number of silver-impregnated dressings (Acticoat®/Acticoat®Flex, AQUACEL® Ag) have also been commonly used in the emergent phase of burn wound care. These dressings are moistened with sterile water, placed on a burn wound and left intact anywhere from 3–4 days to as long as 21 days, depending on the patient's individual clinical status and particular product.

Infection may develop under the eschar as a result of organisms that were present deep in ducts or on adjacent areas which were not destroyed at the time of the burn. Topical antimicrobial coverage is

**Table 7.** Topical antimicrobial agents used on burn wounds

| Product | Preparation | Antimicrobial Action | Applications |
|---|---|---|---|
| Silver sulphadiazene (SSD®, Silvadene®, Flamazine®) | 1% water-soluble cream | Broad-spectrum antimicrobial activity<br>Poor solubility with limited diffusion into eschar. | *Burn wound:*<br>Applied using the open or closed dressing method of wound care. |
| Mafenide acetate (Sulfamylon®) | 8.5% water-soluble cream | Bacteriostatic for gram-positive and gram-negative organisms. Highly soluble and diffuses through the eschar. | *Deep partial-thickness and full-thickness burns:*<br>Applied using either the open (exposure) or closed (occlusive) dressing method.<br>*Graft site:*<br>Saturated dressings are applied. |
| | 5% solution | Same as above | |
| Silver Nitrate | 0.5% solution | Broad-spectrum antimicrobial activity<br>Hypotonic solution | *Burn wound or graft site:*<br>Saturated, multi-layered dressings are applied to the wound or grafted surface. |
| Petroleum and mineral oil-based antimicrobial ointments (e.g. Neosporin®, Bacitracin®, Polysporin®) | Neosporin® (neomycin, bacitracin, polymyxin B); Bacitracin® (bacitracin zinc); Polysporin® (bacitracin, polymyxin B) | Bactericidal for a variety of gram-positive and gram-negative organisms.<br>Ointments have limited ability to penetrate eschar. | *Superficial burn wound:*<br>Applied to wound in a thin (1 mm) layer. Should be reapplied as needed to keep ointment in contact with wound. |

**Box 11.** Properties of topical antimicrobial agents

- ► Readily available
- ► Pharmacologic stability
- ► Sensitivity to specific organisms
- ► Non-toxic
- ► Cost effective
- ► Non-painful on application
- ► Capability of eschar penetration

**Box 12.** Criteria for burn wound coverings

- ► Absence of antigenicity
- ► Tissue compatibility
- ► Absence of local and systemic toxicity
- ► Water vapour transmission similar to normal skin
- ► Impermeability to exogenous micro-organisms
- ► Rapid and sustained adherence to wound surface
- ► Inner surface structure that permits in-growth of fibrovascular tissue
- ► Flexibility and pliability to permit conformation to irregular wound surface; elasticity to permit motion of underlying body tissue
- ► Resistance to linear and shear stresses
- ► Prevention of proliferation of wound surface flora and reduction of bacterial density of the wound
- ► Tensile strength to resist fragmentation and retention of membrane fragments when removed
- ► Biodegradability (important for "permanently" implanted membranes)
- ► Low cost
- ► Indefinite shelf life
- ► Minimal storage requirements and easy delivery

selected according to the condition of the wound and desired results and properties of the topical agent. Whatever topical and dressing strategies are chosen, basic aseptic wound management techniques must be followed. Personnel need to wear isolation gowns over scrub suits, masks, head covers and clean, disposable gloves to remove soiled dressings or cleanse wounds. Sterile gloves should be used when applying inner dressings or ointment to the face. The choice of dressings should take into consideration the condition of the wound, desired clinical results, the properties of the particular dressing, physician preference and availability in each burn centre. There are currently a number of biologic, biosynthetic and synthetic wound coverings available. The ideal dressing should possess particular criteria (Box 12). During the first few days post-burn, the wounds are examined to determine actual depth. It usually takes a few days for deep, partial-thickness wounds to "declare" themselves. Some wounds are deeper than they initially appear on admission. Scald

injuries are almost always deeper than they appear on admission and need to be closely monitored. A treatment plan is then developed to ultimately close the burn wound, either through surgical or non-surgical means.

The focus of therapy in the *acute* phase is the management of any complications which might arise during the recovery period and closure of the burn wound. This phase can have a duration of anywhere from a week to several months. Com-

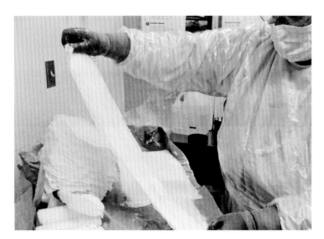

**Fig. 14.** Applying silver sulphadiazene cream to saline-moistened gauze

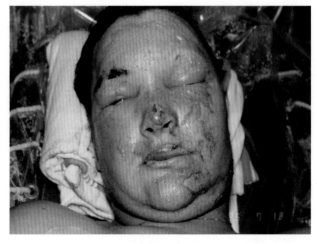

**Fig. 15.** Facial burn wound care

mencement of this phase begins with the onset of spontaneous diuresis and return of fluid to the intravascular space.

**Assessment:** The focus of attention is on the continued need for fluid therapy, wound care, physiotherapy and occupational therapy, pain and anxiety management. *Fluid therapy* is administered in accordance with the patient's fluid losses and medication administration. *Wounds* are examined on a daily basis and adjustments made to the plan of care. The colour, drainage, odour, appearance and amount of pain are noted on a wound assessment and treatment record. If a wound is full-thickness, arrangements need to be made to take the patient to the operating room for surgical excision and grafting.

The *physiotherapist and occupational therapist* will see the patients daily and revise their plan of care accordingly. The plan of care is understandably different if the patient is critically ill versus acutely ill but ambulatory. Efforts are made to adapt the care around major treatments, such as O. R.'s, when the patient will be on bed-rest for a number of days. The patient's level of *pain and anxiety* need to be measured and responded to on a daily basis. A variety of pharmacologic strategies are available (Table 8) and require the full commitment of the burn team in order to be most effective. It is helpful to have multiple modalities of medications to handle both the background discomfort from burn injury itself and the intense pain inflicted during procedural and rehabilitative activities.

**Table 8.** Sample burn pain management protocol

| RECOVERY PHASE | TREATMENT | CONSIDERATIONS |
|---|---|---|
| Critical/acute with mild to moderate pain experience | – IV morphine continuous infusion i.e. 2–4 mg q 1h<br>– bolus for breakthrough i.e. 1/3 continuous infusion hourly dose.<br>– Bolus for acutely painful episodes/ mobilization, i.e. 3 x continuous infusion hourly dose; consider hydromorphone or fentanyl if morphine ineffective. | – Assess patient's level of pain q 1h using VAS (0–10)<br>– Assess patient's response to medication and adjust as necessary<br>– Assess need for anti-anxiety agents i.e. Ativan®, Versed®<br>– Relaxation exercises<br>– Music distraction |
| Critical/acute with severe pain experience | 1. IV Morphine<br>– continuous infusion for background pain i.e. 2–4 mg q 1h<br>– bolus for breakthrough<br>2. IV fentanyl<br>– bolus for painful dressing changes/ mobilization<br>3. IV Versed®<br>– bolus for extremely painful dressing change/mobilization<br>4. Propofol Infusion<br>– consult with Department of Anaesthesia for prolonged and extremely painful procedures i.e. major staple/ dressing removal | – Consider fentayl infusion for short-term management of severe pain<br>– Assess level of pain q1h using VAS<br>– Assess level of sedation using SASS score<br>– Relaxation exercises<br>– Music distraction<br>– Assess need for anti-anxiety/sedation agents i.e. Ativan®, Versed®. |
| Later acute/rehab with mild to moderate pain experience | – Oral continuous release morphine or hydromorphone – for background pain BID<br>– Oral morphine or hydromorphone for breakthrough pain and dressing change/ mobilization<br>– Consider adjuvant analgesics such as gabapentin, ketoprofen, ibuprofen, acetaminophen | – Assess level of pain q1h using VAS<br>– Consult equianalgesic table for conversion from I.V. to P.O.<br>– Assess for pruritis |

**Management:** Selecting the most appropriate method to close the burn wound is by far the most important task in the acute period. However, the team needs to be able to respond quickly to a patient's change in clinical status as he/she can become very sick despite an improvement in wound status. Common *fluid replacement* choices include intravenous normal saline, glucose in saline or water, or Lactated Ringer's solution. On occasion, albumin, plasma and packed red blood cells might be given. Central lines, with multiple lumens, are essential when administering fluids and multiple medications simultaneously.

*Wound care* is performed daily and treatments adjusted according to the changing condition of the wounds (Table 9). During the dressing changes, nurses debride small amounts of loose tissue for a short period of time, ensuring that the patient is receiving adequate analgesia and sedation. A constant dialogue needs to take place between the nursing and medical staff to ensure the right medication in the right amount is available for each and every patient to avoid needless suffering by patients who live in fear of each dressing change. That preoccupation interferes with their ability to perform self-care and reduces their existence to a state of misery, both of which are unacceptable and unnecessary in the world of burn care today. As the eschar is removed from the areas of partial-thickness burn, the type of dressing selected is based on its ability to promote moist wound healing. There are biologic, biosynthetic and synthetic dressings and skin substitutes available today (Table 10). Areas of full-thickness damage require surgical excision and skin grafting. There are specific dressings appropriate for grafted areas and donor sites.

*Physiotherapy and occupational therapy* are an important part of a patient's daily plan of care. Depending on the patient's particular needs and stage of recovery, there are certain range-of-motion exercises, ambulation activities, chest physiotherapy, stretching and splinting routines to follow. The program adjusts on a daily/weekly basis as the patient makes progress towards particular goals and as his/her clinical condition improves or worsens. *Pain and anxiety management* are critical in the acute period of care. Many of the activities a patient is required to do in order to get well cause him/her a degree of dis-

comfort. The ongoing nature of the pain and the unfamiliar world of burn care can quickly exhaust a patient's pre-burn coping strategies. Establishment of unit-based protocols that can be adjusted to meet each patient's individual needs assists greatly in managing the pain and anxiety so often associated with burn care.

The focus of therapy during the *rehabilitative* phase is directed towards working with the patient to return him/her to a state of optimal physical and psychosocial functioning. The clinical focus in on ensuring all open wounds eventually close, observing and responding to the development of scars and contractures, and ensuring that there is a plan for future reconstructive surgical care, if the need exists. The transition from hospital to home or to a rehabilitation facility is a difficult one for most burn survivors and their family members to make. Although they are given information as to what to expect on a number of occasions by various members of the burn team and reassured that things will be fine, pre-discharge anxiety levels can run high. Wound care is generally fairly simple at this time. Dressings should be minimal or non-existent. Most of the wounds should have healed or be very small. Frustration may result, however, when the patient realizes that his healed skin in still quite fragile and can break down with very little provocation. The need to moisturize the skin with water-based creams is emphasized in order to keep the skin supple and to decrease the itchiness that may be present. As the burn patient prepares to leave the protective environment of the burn centre, numerous feelings may be experienced. Burn team members need to be sensitive to and encourage patients to verbalize concerns and questions. The burned person may experience feelings of uncertainty, fear and anxiety about what lies ahead, decreased confidence following weeks and, perhaps, months of dependence on hospital staff, along with concerns about coping with treatment protocols and impaired physical mobility. Some may have to re-enter society with an altered body image and decreased sense of self-esteem. Ongoing counselling to assist with adjusting to an altered appearance and a dramatic change in one's life plan is a very necessary part of post-discharge care. Nervousness about returning home after a prolonged absence and concerns about resumption of previous roles and re-

**Table 9.** Sample burn wound management protocol

| WOUND STATUS | TREATMENT | CONSIDERATIONS |
|---|---|---|
| Early acute; partial or full – thickness; eschar/blisters present | – Silver Sulphadiazene – impregnated gauze <br> → saline-moistened gauze <br> → dry gauze – outer wrap <br> – Mafenide acetate (Sulfamylon®) to cartilagenous areas of face i.e. nose, ears polymyxin B sulphate (Polysporin®) ointment to face <br> – Change BID to body; face care q4h | – Apply thin layer (2-3mm) of Silver Sulphadiazene to avoid excessive build up. <br> – Monitor for local signs of infection i.e. purulent drainage, odour and notify M.D. re. potential need for alternative topical agents i.e. acetic acid, mafenide acetate. |
| Mid-acute; partial or full-thickness; leathery or cheesy eschar remaining | – Saline – moistened gauze → dry gauze – outer wrap <br> – Change BID <br> – Full-thickness wounds to be excised surgically | – Saline dressings to be applied to a relatively small area due to potentially painful nature of treatment <br> – Potential use of enzymatic debriding agents (Collagenase Santyl®, Elase®, Accuzyme®) <br> – Monitor for local signs of infection and notify M.D. |
| Late acute; clean partial-thickness wound bed | – Non-adherent greasy gauze dressing (Jelonet®, Adaptic®) <br> → Saline-moistened gauze → dry gauze – outer wrap <br> – Change once daily | – Monitor for local signs of infection and notify M.D. |
| Post-op graft site | – Non-adherent greasy gauze dressing (Jelonet®, Adaptic®) <br> → Saline–moistened gauze → dry gauze → outer wrap <br> – Leave intact x4 days <br> – Post-op day 4, gently debulk to non-adherent gauze layer <br> → redress once daily <br> – Post-op day 5, gently debulk to grafted area <br> → redress once daily | – Select appropriate pressure-relieving sleep surface <br> – Monitor for local signs of infection and notify M.D. |
| Early rehab; healed partial-thickness or graft site | – polymyxin B sulphate (Polysporin®) ointment until wound stable BID <br> – When stable, moisturizing cream applied BID and prn | – Apply thin layer (2mm) of polymyxin B sulphate (Polysporin®) ointment to avoid excessive build-up <br> – Avoid lanolin and mineral-oil containing creams which clog epidermal pores and don't reach dry, dermal layer |
| Post-op donor site | – Hydrophilic foam dressing (i.e. Allevyn®, Mepilex®) or medicated greasy gauze dressing (i.e. Xeroform®) <br> – Cover foam with transparent film dressing and pressure wrap x 24 hrs <br> – Remove wrap and leave dressing intact until day 4; replace on day 4 and leave intact until day 8. Remove and inspect <br> – If wound unhealed, reapply a second foam dressing <br> – If healed, apply polymyxin B suphate (Polysporin®) ointment BID <br> – When stable, apply moisturizing cream BID and prn <br> – Cover Xeroform® with dry gauze and secure. Leave intact for 5 days. <br> – Remove outer gauze on day 5 and leave open to air. Apply light layer of polymyxin B sulphate (Polysporin®)ointment. If moist, reapply gauze dressing for 2–3 more days. <br> – When Xeroform® dressing lifts up as donor site heals, trim excess and apply polymyxin B sulphate (Polysporin®) ointment | – Monitor for local signs of infection and notify M.D. |
| Face | – Normal saline-moistened gauze soaks applied to face x15 minutes <br> – Remove debris gently using gauze <br> – Apply thin layer of polymyxin B sulphate (Polysporin®) ointment <br> – Repeat soaks q 4–6 h <br> – Apply light layer of mafenide acetate (Sulfamylon®) cream to burned ears and nose cartilage | – For male patients, carefully shave beard area on admission and as necessary to avoid build-up of debris. Scalp hair may also need to be clipped carefully on admission to inspect for any burn wounds. |

**Table 10.** Temporary and permanent skin substitutes

| BIOLOGICAL | BIOSYNTHETIC | SYNTHETIC |
|---|---|---|
| **Temporary** | **Temporary** | **Temporary** |
| ▶ Allograft/Homograft (cadaver skin)<br>– clean, partial and full-thickness burns<br>▶ Amniotic membrane<br>– clean, partial thickness burns<br>▶ Xenograft (pigskin)<br>– clean partial and full-thickness burns | ▶ Nylon polymer bonded to silicone membrane with collagenous porcine peptides (BioBrane®)<br>– Clean, partial-thickness burns, donor sites<br>▶ Calcium alginate from brown seaweed (Curasorb®, Kalginate®)<br>– exudative wounds, donor sites<br>▶ Human dermal fibroblasts cultured onto BioBrane® (TransCyte®)<br>– clean, partial-thickness burns<br>▶ Mesh matrix of oat beta-glucan and collagen attached to gas-permeable polymer (BGC Matrix®)<br>– clean, partial-thickness burns, donor sites | ▶ Polyurethane and polyethylene thin film (OpSite®, Tegaderm®, Omiderm®, Bioclusive®<br>▶ Composite polymeric foam (Allevyn®, Mepilex® , Curafoam® , Lyofoam® )<br>– clean, partial-thickness burns, donor sites<br>▶ Nonadherent gauze (Jelonet®, Xeroform®, Adaptic®)<br>– clean partial-thickness burns, skin grafts, donor sites |
| **Semi-permanent** | **Semi-permanent** | |
| ▶ Mixed allograft seeded onto widely-meshed autograft<br>– clean, full-thickness burns | ▶ Bilaminar membrane of bovine collagen and glycosaminoglycan attached to Silastic layer (Integra®)<br>– clean, full-thickness burns | |
| **Permanent** | | |
| ▶ Cultured epithelial autografts (CEA) grown from patient's own keratinocytes (Epicel®)<br>– clean, full-thickness burns<br>▶ Allograft dermis decellularized, freeze-dried and covered with thin autograft or cultured keratinocytes (AlloDerm®)<br>– clean, full-thickness burns | | |

sponsibilities may also be experienced. If the burn survivor is being transferred to a rehabilitation facility, concerns are often expressed about adjusting to a new environment where one is unfamiliar with staff and routines. Anticipating these concerns and talking with patients and families before the transition occurs is an important part of the plan of care. Support to family is also important as they will assume the primary caretaker role once held by members of the burn team. Home care may need to be arranged and those health team members can bear some of the burden of care until the patient is more self-sufficient. Community-based caregivers can also alleviate some of the anxieties of family members. Visits to the outpatient burn clinic serve as important connections for staff, patients and family and provide an opportunity to have questions and concerns answered, to receive feedback on progress to date, and to talk about changes in the treatment plan. The occupational therapist plays an important role in the rehabilitation period for this is the time when scar maturation begins and contractures may worsen. Scar management techniques, including pressure garments, inserts, massage and stretching exercises, need to be taught to patients and their importance reinforced with each and every visit. Encouragement is also essential in order to keep patients and families motivated, particularly during the times when progress is slow and there seems to be no end in sight to the months of therapy. The burn surgeon can also plan future reconstructive surgeries for the patient, taking into consideration what improvements the burn patient wishes to see first. For many, the wish is for functional improvements first before the esthetic procedures.

## Surgical care

Full-thickness burn wounds do not have sufficient numbers of skin-reproducing cells in the dermal appendages to satisfactorily heal on their own. The area may slowly fill in with granulation and fibrous scar tissues, migrating in from the wound margins and underlying connective tissue. However, the process is very slow and the results unacceptable from a functional wound closure and esthetic outcome perspective. Common practice in surgical burn management is to begin surgically removing (excising) full-thickness burn wounds within a week of admission. This technique of early excision has had a significant positive impact on survival, especially for those patients with moderate to large-sized burn wounds. In the past, patients with extensive burns frequently died of overwhelming sepsis and/or malnutrition while awaiting surgery to remove the devitalized burn tissue (eschar). Most patients undergo excision and grafting in the same operative procedure. In some instances, if there is concern the wound bed may not be ready for a graft, the wounds are excised and covered with topical antimicrobials, followed by a temporary biologic or synthetic dressing. The donor skin (skin graft), which is harvested in this first O. R., is then wrapped up in sterile fashion and placed in a skin fridge for later application. Two days later, if the the recipient bed is clean, the patient returns to the OR to have the donor skin laid as a skin graft on the clean recipient bed. With large burn areas, it is necessary to serially excise and graft over a period of days to several weeks. Concern over blood loss and lack of sufficient donor sites are the two limiting factors when attempting to excise and graft patients with extensive wounds.

Burn surgery involves excision of the non-viable eschar down to the point of punctate bleeding at the level of subcutaneous tissue or fascia (Fig. 16). Harvesting of donor sites for skin grafts is performed using a dermatome (Fig. 17). Hemostasis of both surgical sites must then be achieved and the donor skin placed onto the freshly excised recipient bed. Attempts are made to match skin thickness and colour

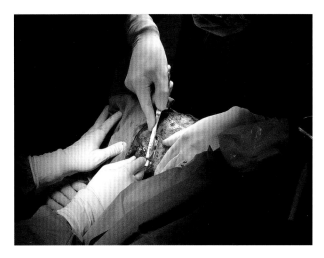

**Fig. 16.** Surgical excision of full-thickness burn wound

as closely as possible between donor sites and recipient sites. Grafts can be split-thickness or full-thickness in depth, meshed or unmeshed in appearance, temporary or permanent in nature (Table 11). The skin grafts are very thin (about.017 of an inch thick), but may be thicker, depending on the location of the recipient bed. For example, skin for an upper eyelid site would be much thinner than that intended for the back or a leg. Grafts should be left as unmeshed sheets for application to highly visible areas, such as the face, neck or back of the hand (Fig. 18). Sheet grafts are generally left open and frequently observed for evidence of serosanguinous exudate under the skin. In order to encourage a good blood supply from the recipient site to the donor site, the exudate needs to be removed. Two strategies fre-

- Adrenalin/saline soaks may be applied to donor sites to control bleeding before the donor dressing is applied

- Electrocautery may also be used

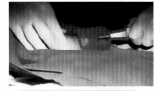

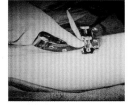

**Fig. 17.** Harvesting a split-thickness skin graft

**Table 11.** Sources of skin grafts

| Type | Source | Coverage |
|------|--------|----------|
| Autograft | Patient's own skin | Permanent |
| Isograft | Identical twin's skin | Permanent |
| Allograft/Homograft | Cadaver skin | Temporary |
| Xenograft/Heterograft | Pigskin, amnion | Temporary |

- Once harvested, graft is placed on a plastic dermatome carrier and run through a meshing machine

- Mesh ratio pattern from 1.5 :1 (most common) to 12:1
- If donor sites are few and area to cover is large, meshing ratio will increase to 3:1 or 6:1
- Exudate can come up through the holes in the mesh pattern to be wicked into the intact dressing

- Grafts to the face and hands are not meshed for optimal cosmetic results
- These sheet grafts are nursed open

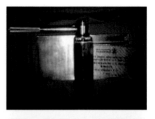
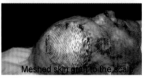

Meshed skin graft to the scalp

**Fig. 19.** Putting a skin graft through a dermatome mesher

quently recommended include aspirating the exudate using a small gauge needle and syringe, or creating a small slit in the blister and gently using normal-saline soaked, cotton-tipped applicators to roll the fluid from the centre of the "bleb" to the opening. On other parts of the body, grafts can be meshed using a dermatome mesher (Fig. 19). The mesher is set to an expansion ratio chosen by the surgeon. If there are sufficient donor sites to cover the excised areas, a 1½: 1 ratio is selected. This expansion ratio allows for exudate to come through and be wicked into a protective dressing, while at the same time be cosmetically acceptable (Fig. 20). Wider expansion ratios (3:1, 6:1) allow for increased coverage when there are limited donor sites. However, the long-term appearance is less acceptable as the mesh pattern is more visible after healing and scar maturation are complete. Meshed skin grafts are generally covered with one of a number of possible options, including silver-impregnated, vacuum-assisted closure, greasy gauze, or cotton gauze dressings. Most are left intact for 5 days to allow for good vascularization between the recipient bed and the skin graft. Following the initial "take- down" at post-op day 5, the dressings are changed every day until the graft has become adherent and stable, usually around day 8. It is possible to gradually determine the percentage of "graft take" during these dressing changes. If necessary, "touch-up" surgeries can be arranged over the next few weeks. For the next year or so post-burn, the skin grafts mature and their appearance improves (Fig. 21). In the Operating Room, once hemostasis has been assured through the application of pressure and thrombin/adrenalin soaks, the donor site can be dressed with either a transparent occlusive, hydrophilic foam or greasy gauze dressing (Fig. 22). To encourage moist wound healing, the dressing should be left intact for several days, inspected and reapplied if indicated. Donor sites generally heal in 10–14 days and can be reharvested, if necessary, at subsequent operative procedures (Fig. 23).

Blood loss during burn excisions poses significant concerns from an operative point of view. The burn surgeon must carefully gauge how much excision and grafting can be performed in a single opera-

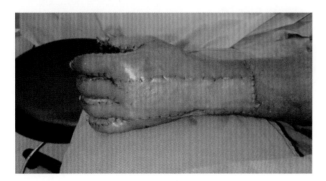

**Fig. 18.** Unmeshed split-thickness sheet graft

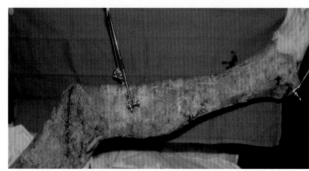

**Fig. 20.** Meshed split-thickness skin graft

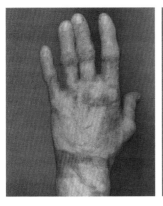
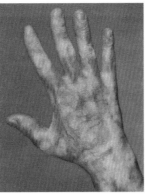

**Fig. 21.** Mature split-thickness skin graft

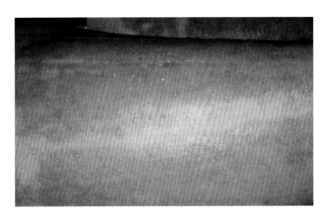

**Fig. 23.** Healed donor site

tion and be prepared to conclude earlier if the blood loss is too great. From the anaesthetist's perspective, it is a challenge to estimate blood loss during a burn excision and then to know what blood replacement to give intraoperatively. From the patient's point of view, he/she may not wish to receive donated blood unless it is absolutely necessary. Today, with modern operative techniques, blood loss is less of a problem. The application of pressure, thrombin/adrenalin soaks, use of surgical tourniquets and the newer tumescent technique have decreased blood loss significantly for burn excision procedures.

Over the past 10 years, there have been major advancements in the development, manufacture and clinical application of a number of temporary and permanent, biologic skin substitutes. Most of these products were initially developed in response to the

problems faced when grafting the massive (i. e. > 70%) burn wound where donor sites are limited (Table 12). As experience increases with these products, alternate applications are also being explored in both the burn patient and wound care populations. The search for a permanent skin substitute continues.

**Table 12.** Biologic skin replacements

| Source | Product | Description |
|---|---|---|
| Cultured epithelial autograft (CEA) | Epicel® (Genzyme Corporation, Massachusetts) | – cultured, autologous keratinocytes grown from patient's donated skin cells<br>– 6–8 cells thick, 2–3 weeks culture time<br>– lacks dermal component; susceptible to infection<br>– lacks epidermal cell-to-connective tissue attachment and is, therefore, very fragile |
| Dermal replacement | Integra® (Johnson & Johnson, Texas) | – synthetic, dermal substitute<br>– neodermis formed by fibrovascular ingrowth of wound bed into 2 mm thick glycosaminoglycan matrix dermal analog<br>– epidermal component, Silastic, removed in 2–3 weeks and replaced with ultrathin<br>– autograft<br>– functional burn wound cover<br>– requires 2 O.R.'s: 1 for dermal placement, 1 for epidermal graft |
| Dermal replacement | AlloDerm® (LifeCell Corporation, Texas) | – cadaver allograft dermis rendered acellular and nonimmunogenic<br>– covered with autograft in same O.R. procedure |

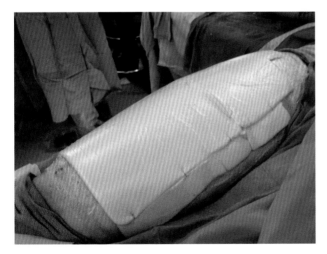

**Fig. 22.** Harvested donor site

## Coordination of care: Burn nursing's unique role

Burn nursing offers many challenges and rewards. To be burned is to sustain one of the worst injuries possible. The complex physical and psychosocial demands challenge patients for weeks to months. The one constant health care professional through all stages of recovery is the burn nurse. While the patient and family are the central focus of care around which all activities of the burn team revolve, it is the burn nurse who serves as the central coordinator of patient care (Table 13).

### Nursing interventions: Emergent phase

During the *emergent phase* of care, the nurse is present for the admission procedure and is a participant-observer during the head-to-toe assessment and stabilization procedures. In collaboration with the burn physician, a wound care plan is decided upon and implemented by the nurse. The bedside nurse closely monitors the patient, which includes maintaining effective airway clearance and gas exchange, assessing the adequacy of fluid resuscitation, and monitoring adequate perfusion to vital organs and extremities. Supportive care to the patient and family are key features of the nursing role at this time.

Thorough assessments and prompt interventions are important as the patient's clinical condition can change quite rapidly. Documenting and interpreting trends in objective patient data, along with keen subjective observations and guided clinical intuition alert the nurse to subtle changes in the patient's condition that might require intervention. Interpreting the complex environment and required treatments to patients and families is very important. Preparing the family for their first glimpse of the patient since admission requires careful thought and sensitivity. If the patient's face is burned, edema from the injury, compounded by the fluid resuscitation, may change the appearance dramatically. The eyes may swell shut and the head become enormously swollen. Reassuring the patient that the edema is only temporary and that his/her eyesight will return to normal is very important during the first 24 hours or so post-injury. If there is concern about the eyesight, the patient should be reassured that ophthalmology

will conduct a thorough examination as soon as the swelling subsides. Concerns about disfigurement are often high at this time, particularly with family members who can see the patient's edematous, burned face. It is so very helpful if the nurse can instill in the family the importance of taking one day at a time and cautioning them that circumstances can change quickly and often in the first days post-burn.

Burn wounds are not uniform in depth and may need various wound care techniques. During the first few dressing changes, the nurse may notice changes in the wound appearance, indicating a deeper or lesser injury than initially diagnosed. Wounds should be assessed for their colour, size, odour, depth, drainage, bleeding, edema, eschar separation, possible infection, cellulitis, epithelial budding, and altered sensation. Clean technique can be utilized for dressing removal and wound cleansing, with sterile technique reserved for the inner, sterile cream/ointment/dressing application [11]. Loose, necrotic and broken blister tissue can be removed with scissors and forceps as bacteria proliferate in burned tissue. Burn wounds can be cleansed using tap water, such as in a Home Care or Burn Clinic setting, or when using a cart shower system in a burn centre.

Normal saline can be used for dressing changes at the bedside on a nursing unit. Some burn centres utilize a mild soap solution to cleanse the wound of debris and reduce the microbial count. Consultation with the burn surgeon may result in an alteration in wound care or plan for surgery. Nursing's role would include informing and explaining the change in care to the patient and family, and appropriate documentation in the nursing plan of care. Face care is conducted about every 6 hours with special attention paid to cartilagenous areas. Tie tapes used to secure endotracheal and/or nasogastric tubes should be inspected every hour to ensure they are not pressing into the burned skin or nose/ear cartilage, cutting off circulation and deepening the tissue damage. Eye drops or lubricating ointments are gently administered to protect the eye from further damage. Pulses to circumferentially-burned extremities need to be monitored closely, in the event the patient needs a releasing escharotomy or fasciotomy to restore circulation. Peripheral pulses should be palpated hourly in the emergent phase, when the onset of edema is profound. A hand-held audible, doppler may also be

**Table 13.** Nursing process for burns

### Emergent phase

**Assessment**

**Subjective**

► Obtain a thorough history of how the burn occurred along with the patient's pre-burn health status, with attention given to the presence or symptoms of other dieseas or co-morbid conditions.

**Objective**

► Assess patient's neurological status – alert, oriented, cooperative, confused, disoriented, combative, restless
► Assess patient's airway for patency, speaking voice, symmetrical chest expansion, normal breath sounds and adequate control of secretions
► Assess respiratory rate and rhythm
► Assess face, nose and mouth for signs of soot, singed hairs/eyebrows, carbonaceous sputum, darkened oral and nasal membranes
► Ensure a chest x-ray is obtained
► Assess for presence/absence of tachypnea, stridor or severe wheezing
► Assess chest expansion in presence of circumferential, full-thickness chest and back burns
► Assess level of oxygenation by measuring SpO2 via pulse oximetry and sending off arterial blood gases.
► Assess for presence of carbon monoxide poisoning by sending off a blood sample for carboxyhemoglobin levels
► Assess peripheral extremities for circulation – pulses, temperature, colour, sensation, pain
► Assess urinary output and send off a sample for serum electrolytes, hematocrit and osmolality
► Assess blood pressure and pulse
► Assess mucous membranes and unburned skin for colour and moistness
► Assess intravenous sites for patency, secure positioning and absence of infection
► Assess for presence of cardiac dysrhythmias
► Assess patient's level of fear, anxiety and pain
► Assess patient's level of understanding about circumstances of his hospitalization and treatments being performed

**Nursing Diagnoses**

► Impaired gas exchange related to tissue hypoxia secondary to upper airway, middle airway and lower airway inhalation injury
► Ineffective airway clearance related to airway obstruction associated with upper airway edema, laryngoedema, bronchospasm and ineffective breathing patterns secondary to injury from chemicals, heat or steam
► Fluid and electrolyte inbalance related to inadequate fluid resuscitation and hypovolemia secondary to evapourative loss, plasma loss and fluid shift into the interstitium
► Altered tissue perfusion related to decreased circulation to all extremities, hypovolemic shock and decreased blood pressure secondary to thermal injury.
► Anxiety related to new surroundings and experiences, separation from family, painful treatments related to burn injury, fear of death and uncertain future

**Expected Outcomes**

► The patient will maintain and regain optimal pulmonary/airway status as manifested by:
– patent airway – alert and oriented behaviour
– respiratory rate appropriate for age, injury and pre-burn status if known
– arterial blood gases within 10% of normal limits for PaO2 and PCO2
– SpO2 > 90% per oximeter (with inspired O2 of < 50%)
– carboxyhemoglobin < 10% within 3 hours after admission
– absence of tachypnea, stridor or severe wheezing
– chest x-ray shows evidence of progressive improvement of pulmonary infiltrate, atelectasis and pneumonia
– patient tolerates physical activity without SpO2 desaturation
– mucous membranes and skin in unburned areas are usual colour (pink) and adequate level of moistness
– absence of cyanosis
► The patient will experience normal electrolyte values and fluid balance as manifested by:
– electrolyte levels within acceptable range
  i.e. Na+     135–145 mEq/L
  K+          3.5–5.5 mEq/L
  CL–         94–108 mEq/L
– hematocrit levels within acceptable range (normal limits 32–42%)
– urinary output (in the absence of glycosuria) is maintained at :
  30–50 mL/hr or 0.5 mL/kg/hr
  75–100 mL/hr for hemoglobinuria/myoglobinuria until urine clears
– blood pressure within acceptable range for age and stage of recovery
– CVP between 1–6 mm Hg
– absence of cardiac dysrhythmia
– balanced intake and output
– serum osmolality within acceptable range (280–290 mOsm/kg)
– no additional tissue loss secondary to restrictive circumferential eschar or hypovolemia
► The patient will achieve normal tissue perfusion and hemodynamic stability as manifested by:
– presence or return of extremity pulses
– minimal tissue edema in burned and unburned areas
– normal acid/base balance
– body temperature warm to touch
► The patient will demonstrate increased physical and psychological comfort as manifested by:
– verbalization of needs, concerns, feelings and anxieties
– participation in treatment
– achievement of a degree of control over care
– coping in an effective manner with the present situation and feeling a decreased sense of anxiety

**Implementation**

► Assess and monitor hourly and PRN for signs and symptoms of altered respiratory function: respiratory rate, dyspnea, stridor, wheeziness, symmetry of chest expansion, use of accessory muscles, adventitious breath sounds, restlessness, confusion, irritability and cyanosis

417

▶ Assess and monitor hourly and PRN for signs of airway obstruction: dyspnea, stridor, tachycardia, use of accessory muscles, respiratory effort, limited chest expansion

▶ Assess for signs and symptoms of smoke inhalation injury: burns of the head, neck, face and chest, singed nasal hairs, eyebrows and eyelashes, darkened oral and nasal membranes, carbonaceous sputum, hoarseness, dyspnea, cough, headache, dizziness and irritability

▶ Monitor arterial blood gases and carboxyhemoglobin results and report significant changes to physician

▶ Elevate head of bed 30 degrees, if not contraindicated

▶ Administer oxygen as ordered

▶ If necessary, assist with chest escharotomies

▶ Be prepared to intubate

▶ If patient mechanically ventilated, monitor inspiratory pressures, tidal volume and minute volume hourly; report changes to respiratory therapist and physician

▶ Suction patient down endotracheal or nasotracheal tube every hour and PRN

▶ Establish 2 large-bore IV access lines for prompt IV fluid resuscitation

▶ Insert indwelling urinary catheter

▶ Assess and monitor urinary output every hour and PRN

▶ Maintain accurate intake and output records from admission, including ambulance and emergency department volumes

▶ Monitor serum electrolytes, osmolality and hematocrit

▶ Titrate IV fluids as necessary to maintain urinary output between 30–50 mL/hr and a CVP between 1–6 mm Hg

▶ Monitor blood pressure and pulse hourly and PRN

▶ Assess and monitor for signs and symptoms of hypovolemic shock : ↓BP, ↑HR, ↓urinary output, ↓cardiac output, ↓CVP

▶ Monitor peripheral pulses on all burned extremities hourly and PRN, obseving for capillary refill and skin temperature

▶ Assist physician with escharotomies and/or fasciotomies to extremities and/or chest if indicated

▶ Monitor acid/base balance

▶ Regulate IV resuscitation to maintain adequate BP, pulse, urinary output and level of sensorium

▶ Provide frequent and repeated explanations and information about care, procedures and new surroundings/personnel

▶ Reunite patient and family as soon as possible following admission

▶ Offer repeated explanations, information and support to family

▶ Familiarize them with burn centre facilities and hospital layout

▶ Describe burn care routines and visiting policies

▶ Establish contract between family and social worker PRN

▶ Assess and monitor mental status to determine level of anxiety

▶ Assess how anxiety may interfere with sleep or activity

▶ Demonstrate willingness to listen and talk to patient and family at frequent intervals in order to encourage ventilation of feelings

▶ Identify previous methods of coping with stressful situations

▶ Encourage and reinforce individual/family participation in care

**Evaluation**

▶ The patient, without inhalation injury, will maintain optimal pulmonary/airway status.

▶ The patient, with inhalation injury, will regain optimal pulmonary/airway status.

▶ The patient will regain an appropriate fluid and electrolyte balance and recover completely from the burn-induced hypovolemia.

▶ The patient will maintain optimal cardiac and circulatory status.

▶ The patient will freely discuss ongoing fears, concerns and anxieties related to being burned.

▶ The patient will begin to verbalize a reduction in fears, concerns and anxieties.

▶ The patient will communicate that anxiety does not interfere with sleep or activity.

## Acute Phase

### Assessment

#### Subjective

▶ Ask the patient whether his grafted donor site areas are causing him any discomfort. Inquire as to the overall assessment of pain.

▶ Discuss the patient's assessment of his ability to participate in self-care activities

#### Objective

▶ Assess mesh graft donor site areas post-op for intact dressings and absence of bleeding

▶ Assess sheet grafts open to air for any accumulated secretions or blood clots

▶ Assess need for specialty low-air loss or air fluidized bed to reduce pressure, friction or shear to grafted sites

▶ Assess need for bed cradles to keep linen off grafted sites

▶ Assess patient's level of pain at the graft site(s), donor site(s) and in general

▶ Assess physician's post-operative orders and intraoperative notes to determine what burn wounds were debrided and grafted, what type of grafts were used, location of donor site(s)

and dressing orders for wounds, grafted sites and donor sites

▶ Perform post-op blood work i.e. CBC and electrolytes

▶ Assess and document patient's level of pain every 4 hours and PRN using a visual analog scale

▶ Assess and document effectiveness of administered pain medications one hour post-administration

▶ Assess patient's range of motion and level of strength in all areas not involved in the burn injury

▶ Assess patient's range of motion and level of strength in areas affected by the burn injury

▶ Gather data from physiotherapist and occupational therapist regarding patient's level of functioning and their plan of care

▶ Assess patient's ability to ambulate

#### Nursing Diagnosis

▶ Altered skin integrity related to skin graft donor sites secondary to full-thickness burn injury

▶ Alteration in comfort: acute pain related to burn injury and associated treatments and interventions

▶ Impaired physical mobility related to pain, dressings and joint contractures

**Expected Outcomes**
► The patient will have a graft take of >90% as manifested by:
- intact, adherent, vascularized graft
- progressive re-epithelialization of interstices of meshed grafts
- no signs of infection
- no signs of graft breakdown due to pressure, shear or friction

► The patient will verbalize satisfaction with level of pain control and demonstrate a tolerable level of pain as evidenced by:
- verbal reports of an acceptable level of comfort based on a measurable scale after pain intervention
- asking for pain intervention in the presence of pain
- improved mobility and ability to participate in self-care
- relaxed facial expression and body posture
- absence of crying, moaning or stoic behaviour during dressing changes, positioning, rehabilitation exercises or treatments
- non-communicative patients exhibiting signs of comfort during rest periods and after comfort interventions i.e. vital signs within acceptable range, absence of facial grimacing, resistance, withdrawal, triggering ventilator alarm, biting down on endotracheal tube
- verbal reports that pain does not interfere with physical activity, self-care or sleep
- successful use of non-pharmacological techniques, such as relaxation, distraction, self-hypnosis, and assistive devices, such as patient-controlled analgesia or therapeutic touch, to manage discomfort
► The patient will maintain or attain an optimal level of function as manifested by:
- normal range of motion in all areas not involved in the burn injury
- range of motion in areas affected by the burn injury show progressive signs of improvement
- muscle strength in unburned areas remains same as on admission
- muscle strength in burn-involved muscle groups shows progressive improvement
- demonstration of functional ambulation
- demonstration of physiotherapy routines and occupational therapy program with and without assistance
- demonstration of appropriate application, care and use of splints
- participation in activities of daily living
► The patient will be as free from complications associated with immobility as possible.

**Implementation**
► Protect grafted areas from excess pressure, friction and shear by using low-air loss or air fluidized specialty beds
► Protect open sheet grafts from bedding through use of overbed cradles
► If protective bolster dressings or plaster casts are utilized, inspect every shift for intactness or excessive pressure
► Reduce incidence of infection by washing hands well before and after patient contact, changing gloves after removing soiled dressings and before applying clean dressings, and following aseptic technique during dressing changes
► If grafted donor areas are in the perineal region, keep area clean and dry following bladder and bowel movements
► Culture graft donor sites if purulent drainage is noted, and commence topical or IV antibiotic therapy, if indicated, to minimize graft loss

► Gently aspirate or roll accumulated hematomas and drainage from centre of sheet graft to slit made in "bleb" using saline-moistened cotton-tipped applicators
► Notify physician for management of excessive accumulations or signs of infection
► Apply topical treatments and dressings as ordered to grafted areas to prevent infection and enhance graft "take"
► When grafted donor sites areas are healed and stable, gently apply water-based moisturizers to prevent dry skin and reduce itchiness
► Observe grafts donor sites for signs of hypertrophic scarring and need for pressure therapies i.e. silicone sheeting, pressure garments
► Resume therapy program under guidance of physiotherapist and/or occupational therapist to preserve functional status and prevent/reduce contractures
► Assess the patient's level of pain by using a verbal, subjective response. If non-communicative, observe vital signs, facial grimacing, withdrawal or biting down on the endotracheal tube and triggering the ventilator alarm
► Administer IV analgesia at a level that keeps the pain tolerable, such as continuous infusions for background pain and bolus doses for treatment-specific pain
► Consider a range of IV and po medications, and opioid and non-opioid drugs
► Ensure increasing fluids and fibre in diet to prevent constipation due to immobility and use of codeine-containing medications
► Document patient ratings of pain intensity and effectiveness of medications
► Consult with a pain service for suggestions if usual practices are not optimal
► Explore use of non-pharmacologic pain management strategies, such as relaxation, distraction, music therapy, therapeutic touch
► Ask patient what he/she has found helpful in the past to manage previous painful experiences
► Evaluate patient's response to pain medications every 4 hours or PRN and notify physician if strategies are ineffective in managing the patient's suffering
► Administer analgesics about 30 minutes before painful treatments, such as dressing changes or exercises
► Provide procedural and sensory information prior to and during painful interventions
► Elevate burned arms on pillows to reduce swelling and decrease pain
► Provide emotional support to patient and ensure he knows you believe he has pain and you will do whatever you can to alleviate the discomfort
► Provide age and condition-appropriate diversional activities, such as television, radio, music, reading, videos
► Provide knowledge to patient/family regarding pharmacologic and non-pharmacologic strategies and the overall plan of care to manage the pain during the difficult wound healing phase, in particular
► Provide adequate opportunities for the patient to rest between dressing changes and therapy sessions. Consider hydrotherapy once a day and any second dressing changes to be performed at the bedside. Consider negotiating for "time outs" during dressing changes to make them more tolerable. Limit debridement to 20 minutes/session.
► Discuss rehabilitation plan with physiotherapist and occupational therapist

▶ Maintain burned areas in position of physiological function
▶ Assess burned areas prone to develop contractures for range of motion and strength
▶ Explain rationale for exercise program, functional activities and proper positioning.
▶ Encourage patient involvement, wherever possible, in selecting meaningful activities and varied selection of exercise routines to avoid monotony and disinterest
▶ Provide assistive devices as necessary to promote independence with self-care activities
▶ Assess, teach and observe patient performing active and passive range of motion exercises during hydrotherapy and in the patient's room
▶ Reinforce rationale behind splints and pressure therapies, and observe appropriate application by patient/family
▶ Encourage ambulation as tolerated
▶ Encourage out-of-bed activities and general conditioning exercises
▶ Apply elastic bandages to legs when ambulating if grafts, donors, burn wounds or edema are present

▶ Provide encouragement to keep motivation high and celebrate small, steady signs of progress
▶ Wrap digits individually and use minimal bulk when applying dressings over joints to facilitate movement
▶ Ensure patient has uninterrupted periods of sleep for restorative purposes

**Evaluation**
▶ The patient will achieve and maintain healed grafted donor areas of full-thickness burn.
▶ The patient will experience a decrease in hypertrophic scarring and contracture development due to pressure therapies, splinting, positioning and therapy routines.
▶ The patient will verbalize a general feeling of well-being with less frequent and less intense periods of pain.
▶ The patient will eventually require little to no analgesic medication on a daily basis.
▶ The patient will continue to maintain or attain an optimal level of functioning.
▶ The patient will experience few to no areas of permanent contraction.

## Rehabilitative Phase

### Assessment
#### Subjective
▶ Obtain the patient's perspective on how the burn has impacted upon his body image, self-esteem and ability to return home and/or to work/school. Explore what the patient expects will occur during the next few weeks and months of rehabilitation.

#### Objective
▶ Assess patient's feelings about his altered appearance
▶ Determine if the patient has seen his burn wound, particularly if the face in involved
▶ Explore with the patient the importance of his appearance to his self-esteem and self-concept pre-burn
▶ Identify patient's current support systems
▶ Assess patient's previous coping strategies
▶ Identify patient's needs for rehabilitation and whether he/she requires inpatient or outpatient management
▶ Assess patient's desire/readiness to return home
▶ Assess patient's desire/readiness to return to work/school
▶ Determine if patient requires vocational education for job retraining

### Nursing Diagnosis
▶ Potential disturbance in self-concept related to potential or actual change in body image, and potential or actual change in role responsibilities
▶ Knowledge deficit related to rehabilitation process including home care and long-term rehabilitation program

### Expected Outcomes
▶ The patient will grieve over the loss of the pre-burn self in an adaptive and therapeutic manner.
▶ The patient will be able to discuss the meaning of the loss and specific feelings over the altered appearance and interruption in roles and responsibilities.
▶ The patient will develop effective coping strategies to handle the alteration in appearance and lifestyle, and the lengthy rehabilitation process.

▶ The patient will resume activities of daily living and be able to socialize with others in the community aside from family and close friends.
▶ The patient will incorporate his altered appearance into a positive sense of self-esteem.
▶ The patient will acknowledge that his appearance will continue to change for the next year to two years post-burn, and that improvements are slow and somewhat unpredictable.
▶ The patient will display hope and verbalize goals regarding home/school/work, which are realistic.
▶ The patient will be able to identify and utilize available support systems and resources, and be open to suggestions of additional resources as the need arises.
▶ The patient will be able to identify and utilize strategies to handle problems as they might arise with respect to altered self-concept and role responsibilities.
▶ The patient will return to work/school/job retraining when medically fit to do so.
▶ The patient will demonstrate an understanding of post-hospital care and the rehabilitation process as manifested by:
- knowledge regarding wound care performed at home by home care nurses
- knowledge regarding wound care performed by patient/family
- ability to perform a return demonstration of self-care activities - appropriate care of healed skin, signs and symptoms of wound infection
- knowledge about scar formation and the role of pressure therapies
- knowledge about exercise routines and participation in activities of daily living - ability to apply and care for pressure therapy products
- realistic understanding of the time required for complete rehabilitation post-burn
- understanding the importance of follow-up care in the Burn Clinic
- having the number of the burn centre if questions or problems arise

**Implementation**

► Encourage patient to discuss meaning of loss to him as they pertain to an altered appearance and disruption of roles and responsibilities at home/school/work

► Provide patient/family with information on scar maturation process

► Reassure patient that the burn wound appearance will continue to improve slowly over the next one to two years

► Encourage sharing of patient's feelings with family to foster understanding and ongoing support

► Encourage family to be supportive to patient and assist them with expression of their feelings and concerns

► Provide family with concrete examples of how to be helpful and supportive to the patient

► Discuss impact of body image and roles/responsibilities changes on patient and on family system

► Provide support to patient and family as they adjust to these various changes

► Provide patient with a nonjudgemental atmosphere in which to share fears/concerns/grief

► Encourage a feeling of hope for a meaningful future for the patient

► For patient with a facial burn re-entering society, role play possible communication and socialization techniques to assist with community reintegration

► Help patient to identify helpful coping strategies that might be effective in working through adjustments to appearance, roles and responsibilities

► Assist patient in setting realistic expectations during rehabilitation process

► Reinforce individual nature of grieving and adjustment process and the importance of adopting a hopeful, one-day-at-a-time philosophy

► In conjunction with physician, physiotherapist and occupational therapist, identify long-term rehabilitation needs and options for achieving long-term goals

► If long-term rehabilitation involves transfer to an inpatient facility, familiarize patient and family with new facility, personnel and services to assist in the transition from the familiar surroundings of the burn centre to a new environment

► Communicate with rehabilitation facility about patient's current status to foster a seamless continuum of care

► Set up home care referral if indicated

► Explain role of home care personnel prior to discharge

► Distribute discharge planning literature to patient and family, if available

► Discuss importance of follow-up burn clinic appointments and schedule one following discharge

► Provide patient/family with burn centre telephone number if questions arise at home

► Consider formal referral to a burn survivors' support group, if the patient/family are interested

► Consider informal introductions of one patient to another during burn clinic and following discharge through the mutual exchange of telephone numbers for mutual support and information-sharing, if appropriate

► When/if appropriate, discuss supportive self-esteem enhancement strategies, such as  paramedical cosmetic camouflage, communication techniques, wardrobe and colour analysis

► Encourage questions and discussion of anxieties regarding discharge

► Review care activities/procedures required at home with patient/family

► Have patient/family perform a return demonstration of skills required at home

► Prepare patient/family for adjustments that will take place upon the return home

► Discuss the return home and any problems/concerns that arose when patient/family return to burn clinic

**Evaluation**

► The patient will continue to experience positive self-esteem and be able to incorporate his altered appearance into his self-concept.

► The patient will continue to participate in meaningful activities in society related to home, family, friends and work/school.

► The patient will verbalize satisfaction with his life post-burn.

► The patient will express satisfaction with his recovery during return-to-clinic appointments and begin to discuss future reconstructive surgeries, if applicable.

© Copyright Judy Knighton, Reg.N., M.Sc.N. November 2010

needed, if palpation is ineffective. Signs of impaired circulation include progressive decrease or absence of pulses, progressive paresthesias, pallor and deep tissue pain. Burned arms and hands should be elevated, above the heart, on pillows or wedges to minimize edema. Patients with neck burns should not have pillows in order to prevent contractures. Burned ears must also be protected from external pressure as the blood supply to the cartilage is poor and infection can occur quite quickly. Patients should be positioned appropriately i. e. anti-contracture positioning, and assessed regularly for comfort and warmth. Moist dressings and prolonged dressing changes can increase the incidence of hypothermia. Care must be taken to continually monitor the patient's temperature and hypothermia avoided or minimized by increasing the ambient temperature of the room, using overbed heat lamps and covering the patient with a hypothermia blanket. Intravenous fluids can also be warmed using a specially designed infusion device. In concert with the rehabilitation staff, the patient's range of motion should be assessed at least twice a day. Rehabilitative or orthopedic devices should be inspected for appropriate application and specific instructions written in the patient's plan of care or posted in the patient's room for easy visibility and reference. The patient should also be turned frequently i. e. q2h, assessed for his/her susceptibility to pressure sores and appropriate preventive or therapeutic interventions.

For the critically ill, ventilated patient, the nurse pays close attention to the security of the airway – that the endotracheal tube is placed correctly, secured adequately to prevent accidental dislodgement during care or transport, and providing appropriate ventilation to the patient. The respiratory rhythm and character need to be monitored closely, along with signs of respiratory distress including nasal flaring, wheezes, stridor, intracostal/sternal retraction, tachypnea, and triggering the ventilator. When suctioning the patient, attention should be focussed on the colour (especially if there is soot from an inhalation injury), odour and amount of sputum. For non-intubated patients, the same assessment takes place when the patient coughs up sputum on his/her own. Chest excursion needs also to be monitored to ensure good expansion and quality of respirations and, whether or not a releasing escharotomy is needed or requires revision. The nurse also ensures the patient is receiving adequate amounts of analgesia to control pain and anxiolytics/sedating agents to minimize anxiety and agitation. Background pain (pain that is continuously present) and procedural pain (intermittent pain related to activity or procedures) must be continually assessed, through the use of evidence-based pain scales. Unrelieved pain can have long lasting effects, including stress-related immunosuppression, increased potential for infection, delayed wound healing and depression [11]. The patient's level of responsiveness to his/her surroundings, family members and stimuli in the room should also be assessed each hour. The use of neuromuscular agents and sedatives also needs to be documented, along with the use of an evidence-based sedation scale.

Peripheral and central lines must be inspected frequently to ensure they are patent and secure as access is usually very limited in burn patients and so very necessary during the emergent phase. Fluid resuscitation, vasoactive drugs, pain and anxiety medications, along with numerous other intravenous drugs, require this method of access. Great care is taken not to pull them out during the admission procedure, dressing changes or transport. The urinary catheter should also be examined routinely for pa-

tency and the perineal area kept clean and dry. The bladder should be palpated for distention. Hourly urinary output is a crucial indicator of the success of emergent period fluid resuscitation, in addition to colour, clarity, odour and sediment.

## Nursing interventions: Acute phase

As the patient progresses to the *acute phase* of care, the focus of nursing expertise is on *wound management*, *psychosocial interventions*, *pain management* and *physical/occupational therapy*. Wound care focuses on time-limited debridement of loose tissue, evacuation of blisters and gentle removal of exudate from the wound surface. A variety of dressings and/or biological/biosynthetic/synthetic skin substitutes are available and may be incorporated into the patient's plan of care. If the patient requires surgery, the nurse can explain the procedures and care required. Patients are frequently too overwhelmed to remember the burn surgeon's explanations pre-operatively.

Patient and family education about wound care procedures, rationale for particular dressings and pre and post-op care can be provided verbally and enhanced through booklets, articles and videos. Incorporating cultural and learning styles into the educational process increases the likelihood the knowledge will be retained by the patient and family. Burn patients continue to be hypermetabolic long after their wounds have healed. Proper nutrition plays a key role in their recovery. Increased caloric and protein requirements are usually met through nasogastric or nasojejunal tube feeding to maintain mucosal integrity. Nursing assessment includes frequent inspection of tube placement and patency. Placement is initially confirmed through radiographic confirmation. If gastric residuals are greater than the desired parameters stated in the patient's care plan, modifications need to be made in a timely fashion. The involved nare should be assessed for pressure necrosis and the feeding tube secured to avoid premature removal. The tube may also be used for free water flushes, if the patient has high sodium levels, and for medication administration. The patient should also be assessed for a daily bowel movement. Progress during the acute phase can be slow. It may be a very frustrating time for patients and families when the efforts being put forward seem to result in such small, daily gains. The nurse can play an important role as coach and cheerleader, bringing to the patient's attention the progress that he/she notices. Nursing can also reinforce the rehabilitation therapists' plans of care by ensuring exercises are performed and splints are worn according to schedule. Encouraging the patient to sit up in a chair for periods at a time and to ambulate to/from hydrotherapy and around the nursing unit, not only brings physical benefit, but emotional rewards as well. Staff and visitors alike comment on how well the patient is doing and how much improvement they see.

Families may need to be encouraged to take care of themselves now that their loved one is out of immediate danger. For some, that may mean spending more time taking care of things at home and less time at the hospital. Out-of-town families may return home for a few days. Upon their return, they may also be encouraged to participate in their loved one's care, to the extent they feel comfortable. Activities include assisting with hygiene and skin care, helping apply splints, and coaching through the exercise routines. As the patient is able to demonstrate increasing levels of self-care, family may need to be advised when to help and when to stand back and offer encouragement. Emotional support may be needed as the patient can verbally lash out in frustrated anger when he/she is having difficulty doing something and family don't intervene. It may also be helpful for family to see the patient's wounds, from time to time, as it helps to put the recovery process into perspective. From then on, they have a reference point to compare how far the patient has come and what might lie ahead in the next phase.

## Nursing interventions: Rehabilitative phase

Patients and families alike eagerly anticipate the final, *rehabilitative phase* of care. The focus for nursing is on *psychosocial interventions* and *discharge planning*. But for some, the reality is harder to accept than they had imagined. Some patients have magical expectations about how things will be once they return home. Others express frustration at not being able to go home just yet and of the need to be transferred to a rehabilitation facility. Some patients may not want to participate in their exercise routines or wear their pressure garments and splints as often as

is really necessary. Nursing staff can play an important role of supportive listener/coach, acknowledging how hard it must be to keep going, day after day, knowing all the patient has been through and how long and difficult the journey back can be. Short-term compromises can be negotiated to a full recovery in order to get the patient back on track towards optimal recovery. Every patient can benefit from a day off to recharge one's energy and renew one's commitment to the plan of care.

Wound care during the rehabilitation period is usually minimal. The healed skin, fresh grafts and donor sites are fragile and require a thin layer of polymyxin B sulphate (Polysporin®) ointment until they have "toughened" up a bit. At that point, water-based moisturizers are applied to reduce the dryness, flakiness and itchiness. The gentle act of applying the cream serves as a form of beneficial massage during the scar maturation process. Nursing staff can also point out to patients that the act of applying creams is a useful, non-threatening way to both desensitize the skin and to familiarize oneself with the parts of one's body that are burned. It can be a helpful strategy for family members also. For couples, it may be a helpful adjunct to restoring intimacy back into their relationship, as the spouse makes the slow transition from care-giver to lover. The time that nurses spend with patients performing wound care can be very therapeutic if the nurse takes cues from the patient and uses the opportunity to explore how the patient views his/her altered appearance.

During this final phase of care, patients are encouraged by their nurses to perform as many self-care activities as possible. Rehabilitation routines are adjusted as the patient's abilities improve. There may be periods, however, when patients are depressed, frustrated and angry, and don't want to participate in care. Those very normal feelings need to be acknowledged and worked through in order to be able to move forward. Perhaps for the first time, patients are able to acknowledge the losses they have experienced since the burn injury. Now that physical survival is ensured, the body seems to shift its energies to the psychological impact of the trauma. Some of this realization begins in the acute phase, but the majority of the work begins now. Nurses can provide patients with opportunities to verbalize their feelings in a non-judgemental atmosphere. Talking about their fears and anxieties is an important first step in overcoming them. Many therapeutic conversations take place between nurses and patients if the nurse is responsive to the sometimes subtle cues the patient gives out indicating a readiness to talk. In general, patients need someone to listen, to acknowledge what they are feeling, and to validate that other burn patients have felt the same things and successfully returned to a productive life. Burn nurses can see the possibility of a new and rewarding life at a time when the burn patient sees nothing but endless adjustments, physical and emotional. The leap from seeing oneself not as a "burn victim" but as a "burn survivor" takes time and helpful encouragement from people who know that things will get better. Nurses can encourage patients to link up with burn survivor support groups and seek support from a social worker, clinical nurse specialist, psychologist or psychiatrist. Family therapy may be helpful if there are issues between husband and wife, parents and children. Couple therapy may assist in overcoming difficulties with sexuality post-burn. In most instances, these problems correct themselves, with love and patience, as both partners need time to adjust to the burn survivor's altered body image, fragile tissues and stiff joints.

Adapting to a facial difference can be a very difficult journey for patients and families. The biggest challenge is posed by the social response they experience. They can no longer blend into the crowd anonymously. Preparing the burn survivor to see him/herself for the first time requires careful thought and preparation. Nurses can assist patients to iden-

tify their pre-burn coping strategies and help apply them to the present situation. Social re-entry and communication skills need to be learned and practiced in order for patients to be able to move about in public with as much self-confidence as possible. Burn survivor, Barbara Kammerer Quayle [12] has developed the BEST program that teaches simple, effective ways to improve communication and create positive relationships, using STEPS to Self-Esteem (Fig. 24). REACH OUT is based on "Changing Faces" founder, James Partridge's work [13] on how communication skills can be used to help people cope with feelings of self-consciousness and others' reactions (Fig. 25). More recently, his "3-2-1-GO" [14] program has given burn survivors another useful skill to develop, while navigating through the challenges of communicating and interacting with the public when you have a facial difference.

Nurses can begin to explore such opportunities with patients before and after discharge. Post-discharge, nursing care is provided in a burn clinic setting that may be staffed by burn centre nurses, a clinic nurse and/or a clinical nurse specialist. Follow-up during this time is extremely important as the transitions from hospital to home are difficult and complex. The need for support and guidance continues for several years post-burn. From a professional nursing perspective, the opportunity to work among the burned through months and years of recovery is a privilege. The courage and perseverance displayed by burned people and their families is truly a testament to the resilience of the human spirit.

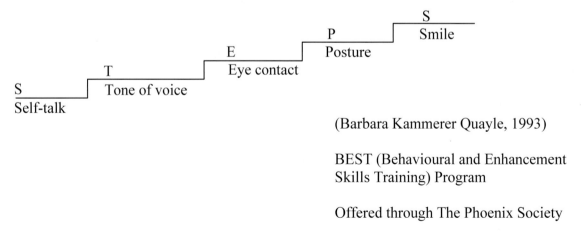

(Barbara Kammerer Quayle, 1993)

BEST (Behavioural and Enhancement Skills Training) Program

Offered through The Phoenix Society

**Fig. 24.** STEPS to Self-Esteem

R  **R**eassurance
E  **E**nergy and effort
A  **A**ssertive
C  **C**ourage
H  **H**umour

O  **O**ut
U  **U**nderstanding
T  **T**ry again

(James Partridge, 1998)

**Fig. 25.** REACH OUT Communication Skills

## "3 – 2 –1 GO" Program

▶  3  things to do when someone stares at you
▶  2  things to say when someone asks what caused your scars/facial difference
▶  1  thing to think if someone turns away from you

(James Partridge in Blakeney, 2008)

## Ongoing care

In addition to the care already discussed, there are a number of areas that require ongoing attention. They include infection prevention and control, rehabilitation medicine, nutrition, pharmacology and psychosocial supports.

### Infection prevention and control

Infection prevention and control is a major focus in burn care and multifactorial in nature. Since 70% of patients who die do so from sepsis, the onus lies with all members of the burn team to eliminate potential reservoirs and prevent transfer wherever possible. Broad strategies include suppression of infection transfer, elimination of reservoirs of infection, use of antimicrobials and support of immune mechanisms.

*Suppression of infection transfer.* In simple terms, all burn patients have organisms on their contaminated burn wounds. Some organisms are located in the gut and can migrate to other areas of the body, such as the lungs. If one considers that everything in a patient's room becomes contaminated to him/her, then the focus can be on controlling that environment. Activities would include reducing items in that environment to those strictly essential, scrupulously cleaning those items that come in and out of the room, such as unused equipment, x-ray and ECG machines, wearing isolation gowns before entering a patient's room and scrupulous hand washing technique by all those entering and leaving the room. These techniques can dramatically reduce the po-

tential for spread of infection from one patient to another by a variety of vectors, the most frequent source being hands of caregivers. Common patient-care areas, such as hydrotherapy, dressing and operating rooms, need to be scrupulously cleaned after each patient use and swabbed every few months for the presence of organisms. Those patients, who have been identified as carriers of resistant or "difficult-to-treat" organisms, should be placed in strict isolation and not taken to the common areas. Particular concern centres around hydrotherapy rooms and the risk that water-borne resistant organisms could reside in the hose system or water supply.

*Elimination of reservoirs of infection.* Such practices include frequent dressing changes and surgical excision of eschar to reduce the bacterial load at the wound site. This also decreases the opportunity for invasive burn wound infections and systemic sepsis to develop. Another important practice is the physical handling and removal of soiled dressings and linen, and rapid, effective cleanup of body substance spills, such as urine and blood.

*Use of antimicrobials.* Most burn wounds are covered with a broad-spectrum antimicrobial in either a cream format (silver sulphadiazene or mafenide acetate) soaks (sodium hypochlorite – Dakin's; mafenide acetate, acetic acid) or silver-impregnated dressings (Acticoat®/Acticoat® Flex/Aquacel®Ag).

The bacterial load is, therefore, controlled until such time as the eschar is physically debrided through dressing changes or through surgical excision. As the bacterial load is reduced, the patient's clinical condition is more likely to improve.

*Support of immune mechanisms.* Burn patients are immunosuppressed until such time as their burn wounds have completely healed and sometimes longer. The immune system can be enhanced by maintaining the integrity of unburned skin, proper nutrition, including antioxidants, and administration of fresh frozen plasma albumin.

## Rehabilitation medicine

Although the formal rehabilitative phase of burn care begins when the wounds have closed, rehabilitation begins shortly after the patient is admitted to hospital. The physiotherapist and occupational therapist are key members of the burn team and work hard to engage the patient's participation in a long-term plan of care. The focus of this plan is aimed at regaining and maintaining function and independence. Interventions include edema management, positioning, splinting, passive/active-assisted/active range-of-motion (ROM) exercises, and ambulation. Attention is also directed towards functional activities, including activities of daily living (ADL's), stretching, strengthening and endurance exercises, work hardening and conditioning activities, and burn scar management. Particular areas of the body pose greater rehabilitation challenges and require care in specialized burn treatment facilities. They include the face, neck, axillae, feet, hands and burns across joints.

***Physical therapy:*** The main goals are to: a) *regain and maintain normal range of motion to all the joints.* Range can be achieved through passive, active or active-assisted means; b) *prevent/reduce contractures.* Wounds heal by the process of contraction and vigourous efforts must be made to position and/or splint patients into positions of function as opposed to comfort (anti-function). Joints and limbs must be moved and stretched numerous times a day to overcome the powerful forces attempting to reduce full range; c) *increase muscle strength.* Patients need to continue to use muscles unaffected by the burn to avoid muscle wasting. In addition, a program to learn to reuse and regain strength and endurance of those muscles affected by the burn needs to be set up for each patient; and finally, d) *restore/maintain cardiorespiratory function.* Chest physiotherapy, suctioning, deep breathing and coughing, and early ambulation are essential to the plan of care. Physiotherapy

can take place in the patient's room, during hydrotherapy, in the operating room while the patient is under anaesthesia, and in a burn centre rehabilitation room. The patient then receives the benefits of a varied and intensive program. Progress can be evaluated and activities altered to meet the patient's changing needs.

***Occupational therapy.*** The primary goals of occupational therapy are to assist the patient in returning to as functional an ability level as possible, to maximize his/her independence and to assist with burn scar management. In order to enhance personal motivation and to encourage active participation, the occupational therapist helps the patient to record and celebrate progress through wall charts and personal diaries. Encouraging participation in activities that are meaningful to the patient and journaling as a means of personal reflection are two strategies to engage a patient in long-term and often painful therapy. Early active involvement in activities of daily living is very important both from a physical and psychological perspective. Making a conscious effort to maximize independence is one of the major keys to successful rehabilitation. Use of adaptive devices, such as padded handles for cutlery and button hooks, should be restricted to such time as the patient can perform the activities unassisted.

The occupational therapist also fabricates custom-fitted splints to maintain appropriate positioning for burned hands, feet, neck and axillae. These splints are essential during the early post-burn period (for antideformity/anticontracture positioning), immediately post-op (to preserve function) and during rehabilitation/post-burn reconstructive surgery periods (to maintain or increase elongation of scar tissue). Splints need to be reassessed and remolded frequently as the patient's edema increases or decreases, the contours of the wound change or range of motion improves. A very important part of the occupational therapist's role is the application of pressure devices to flatten burn scars. Conventional goals for the treatment of burn scars include minimizing hypertrophy, increasing pliability, preventing or minimizing contracture, maximizing the formation of scar to normal anatomic contours, and optimizing cosmetic outcomes. Application of pressure during the early to mid-phases of wound healing is useful in treating edema. Products include elastic bandages, self-adherent wraps, such as Coban® (and tubular, cotton elasticized bandages like Tubigrip®). Later, when the skin is less fragile, patients are measured for custom-fitted pressure garments to be worn 23½ hours a day for anywhere from 1–1½ years. It is essential to provide patients with much support and encouragement during this difficult period of adapting to these garments. It is exceptionally difficult for patients to adjust to facial masks, whether they be fabric or rigid, transparent plastic in nature. In order to provide extra support to contoured areas on the central face, in finger/toe web spaces, on the palm of the hand or interscapular area, inserts made from a variety of foam, rubberized materials or thermoplastic splinting materials can be used. Silicone gel sheets have recently been used to treat smaller areas of the body where adequate pressure cannot be achieved, such as the face, arm or hand.

Other physical agents commonly used as part of occupational therapy include hydrotherapy, paraffin, ultrasound, electrical stimulation and continuous passive motion machines.

## Nutrition

During the early hypovolemic shock phase, there is decreased perfusion to the gastrointestinal system, resulting in temporary paralytic ileus. Patients are generally kept NPO until their bowel sounds return. In recent years, there has been some movement towards feeding patients enterally soon after admission in order to preserve gut function and prevent stress ulcers. A nasogastric tube is inserted and connected to low intermittent suction to decompress the area. Intravenous fluid replacement is begun and the patient assessed for nutritional/metabolic needs by the burn centre dietitian. When bowel sounds return in about 48–72 hours post-burn, the patient can be fed using the most appropriate route, based on stage of recovery and size of burn. Nutrition plays an important role in burn recovery. Patients require a diet high in calories and protein to counteract the hypermetabolic response noted post-burn and to support the growth of healthy tissue. A burn patient's metabolic rate increases in proportion to the size of the injury. Burns are considered the most extreme example of hypermetabolic stress. Inadequate nutrition can negatively impact upon an individual's im-

mune response, wound healing, metabolic function and survival. Metabolic expenditures can be calculated using a metabolic cart. Most caloric requirements now are based on a formula of $1.4 \times$ basal energy expenditure (BEE).

After the burn injury occurs, catecholamines are released and there is an increase in the patient's metabolic rate. In fact, there is a direct relationship between the size of the burn, the increase in metabolic rate and urinary catecholamine excretion. The metabolic rate returns to normal, but it may be several years after the burn wounds have completely healed. In addition to hypermetabolism, the patient experiences a state of hypercatabolism in which lean body mass is broken down to provide amino acids for gluconeogenesis. Nitrogen loss through urine and wounds is a concern, as are the heightened requirements for protein necessary for anabolism, wound repair and improved immune response. Burn patients require fat in the form of lipids, vitamins and trace minerals.

In order to determine each patient's caloric needs, the dietitian assesses his/her energy requirements using indirect calorimetry. A decision in then made as to what product should be given at what rate and by which route of enteral access. For burns less than 20%, many patients are well enough to consume sufficient calories and protein by mouth in the form of diet trays and oral supplements. If the oral intake doesn't meet metabolic demands, supplementation is required. The enteral route is preferred in order to maintain the functional integrity of the gut. If patients don't receive food early enough in their post-burn recovery period, it can result in intolerance to later feeding, diarrhea, greater likelihood bacteria will translocate from the gut to another part of the body, and increased risk of infectious complications. Patients can be fed enterally by both noninvasive and invasive procedures. The least complex method is nasogastric feeding, which can be administered continuously or by bolus feeds. Critically ill patients may have a gastric ileus and can't be fed by the gastric route. A small-bore, feeding tube, with a weighted end to facilitate passage, can then be passed beyond the pylorus into the small intestine. This approach is also safer for patients with altered levels of consciousness, artificial airways, ineffective cough reflexes and altered swallowing ability.

Duodenal feeding tubes can be placed, endoscopically or via fluoroscopy, if the specialized equipment and staff are available. This allows for quicker absorption of nutrients and a decrease in the nausea and vomiting that may occur with large volume tube feedings into the stomach. If long-term placement is required, percutaneous endoscopic gastrostomy (PEG) or percutaneous endoscopic jejunostomy (PEJ) tubes are available. The position of any feeding tube must be checked at frequent intervals and attempts made to secure it safely into position. The measurement of gastric residuals to monitor gastric motility and the addition of blue dye to enteral feeds to monitor gastric and pulmonary secretions for these feeds are two safety precautions that should be followed. Some disadvantages associated with these tubes include displacement and blockage. The feeds may also give patients diarrhea, although that may have more to do with medications, particularly antibiotics. Less common nutrition-related complications include abdominal distention and delayed gastric emptying, both of which can be assessed by a general surgery or internal medicine consultant. Patients also require monitoring for hyperglycemia and electrolyte imbalances associated with enteral feeding. As the patient's wounds heal, the metabolic demands are decreased and a reassessment is performed at least weekly by the dietitian to determine the optimal nutritional plan of care. Tube feedings are generally reduced, then tapered, as oral intake increases. Adaptive devices to feeding utensils, such as padded handles, can assist patients with burned hands to feed themselves. Families are also encouraged to bring in favourite foods from home to stimulate their loved one's appetite. Before discharge, the burn patient is advised on dietary requirements at home by the dietitian to avoid unnecessary weight gain once the burn injury has completely healed.

## Pharmacology

Throughout burn recovery, patients require a number of medications. Some are admitted with a past medical history that includes drugs for pre-existing conditions. A number of patients have a drug and/or alcohol abuse history. The role of the pharmacist in burn care is an important one in order to ensure patients receive the most appropriate medications in the correct amounts for the most appropriate period of time.

When burn patients are first admitted, they are assessed for tetanus toxoid, because of the risk of anaerobic burn wound contamination. Tetanus immunoglobulin is given to those patients who have not been actively immunized within the previous 10 years. They are also given pain medication, which should always be administered intravenously during the hypovolemic shock phase as gastrointestinal function is impaired and intramuscular (IM) medications would not be absorbed adequately. There is a risk that the IM medications would pool in the edematous tissue and the patient would be overdosed when fluid mobilization begins. The medication of choice for moderate to severe pain management is an opioid, such as morphine or hydromorphone, as they are generally quite effective for most patients, can be given intravenously and orally, and are available in fast-acting and slow-release forms. There are a number of other analgesics that have been identified as very effective with the burn patient population (Table 8). It is essential that burn patients' pain be acknowledged and treated from the time of admission until that point in their rehabilitation when the physical discomforts have lessened to the extent they don't require medication. A combination of analgesics for background pain (resting) and acute episodes (dressing changes, therapy) is most effective and gives team members flexibility to use the medication that is best for a variety of painful situations. As the burn wounds close and the patient's pain level decreases, reductions in analgesic therapy should occur by careful taper, rather than abrupt discontinuation, of opioids. If tapering does not occur, acute opioid withdrawal syndrome can occur. Burn patients, understandably, may be highly anxious and agitated. Sedative agents, along with analgesics, are necessary and can be very effective (Table 14). Non-pharmacologic approaches to pain management (hypnosis, relaxation, imagery) can serve as useful adjuncts to opioid-based approaches.

Topical antimicrobial therapy is an important part of burn wound care (Table 7). Most centres have one agent of choice and add others if a resistance pattern emerges. The most widely used, broad-spec-

**Table 14.** Anxiolytics commonly used in burn care

| Generalized Anxiety | Situational Anxiety (dressing changes, major procedures) | Delirium |
|---|---|---|
| Lorazepam (Ativan®) I.V | Midazolam (Versed®) I.V. | Haloperidol (Haldol®) I.V. |
| ▶ works nicely in combination with analgesics for routine dressing changes and care | ▶ works nicely in combination with analgesics when very painful and prolonged procedures are performed | ▶ works nicely for patients who appear agitated or disoriented |

trum antimicrobial agent is silver sulphadiazene. Its role is to reduce the bacterial load on the burn wound until the eschar can be removed. Local application on the burn wound is necessary, as systemic antibiotics would not be able to reach the avascular burn wound. Mafenide acetate is indicated for burned ears and noses as it has a greater ability to penetrate through cartilage. It is, however, more painful upon application than silver sulphadiazene and its use to restricted to small areas of the body. Systemic antibiotics are indicated when a burn wound infection has been clinically diagnosed or other indicators of sepsis are present, such as pneumonia or uncontrolled fever.

Additional medications are generally prescribed to manage gastrointestinal complications, treat antiobiotic-induced superinfections and boost the patient's metabolic and nutritional status (Table 15). Because they receive pain medications that are constipating, patients should be placed on a bowel routine upon admission. Attention must also be paid to reviewing and ordering those medications the patient was on before the burn injury, and possibly arranging follow-up with a family physician upon discharge.

## Psychosocial supports

Psychosocial support to burn survivors and their family members is an essential part of their ongoing care. Concern for family provides them with necessary comfort so they, in turn, can be the patient's single most important social support. Family frequently keep vigil by their loved one's bedside throughout a potentially lengthy recovery period and become primary caregivers once the patient returns home. The social worker in a burn centre can provide ongoing counselling and emotional support to patients and family members. Assistance in coping with difficult or stressful matters, such as financial concerns, finding accommodation, questions about hospital insurance coverage or ongoing problems at work or home, is also available. Chaplains offer spiritual support during times of crisis and at various points along the road to recovery. For some, the burn injury is a tremendous test of spiritual faith and brings forward troubling questions for which there are no easy answers, such as "Why did this happen to me? to my husband? to my daughter?" Coming to terms with this traumatic event does much to free up a patient's energies to move forward

**Table 15.** Medications commonly used in burn care

| Types and Names | Rationale |
|---|---|
| **Gastrointestinal Care** | |
| Ranitidine (Zantac®) | Decreases incidence of stress (Curling's) ulcers |
| Nystatin (Mycostatin®) | Prevents overgrowth of *Candida albicans* in oral mucosa |
| Milk of Magnesia, Lactulose, Docusate sodium, Sennosides, Glycerin or Bisacodyl suppository | Prevents/corrects opioid-induced constipation |
| **Nutritional Care** | |
| Vitamins A,C,E and multivitamins | Promotes wound healing, immune function, |
| Minerals: selenium, zinc sulfate, iron (ferrous gluconate and sulfate), folic acid, thiamine | hemoglobin formation and cellular integrity |

in a positive way. Some burn patients are troubled psychologically pre-burn. They may have formal psychiatric diagnoses and/or histories of drug and/or alcohol abuse. For others, the psychological trauma begins with the burn injury. Referral to a psychiatrist or psychologist for supportive psychotherapy and/or medication can make a positive difference in those situations. It is important, however, before such referrals are made, to discuss the situation with the patient (if he/she is considered mentally competent). This disclosure provides the team with an opportunity to share their interpretation of the patient's behaviours and to listen to how the patient views his/her coping abilities and behaviours. The burn patient and his family need to feel supported and not stigmatized by the recommendation to seek psychological support.

In recent years, the role of patient and family support groups has been examined and encouraged by burn team members. The power of the lived experience is profound. The advice and caring that comes from one who truly knows what it is like to survive a burn injury or the family member of one who has been burned are valuable beyond measure. Many burn centres are fortunate to have a burn survivors support group affiliated with them. Based in the United States, but with members from around the world, The Phoenix Society has hundreds of area coordinators and volunteers, through the SOAR (Survivors Offering Assistance in Recovery), who meet with burn survivors in their communities and help however they can http://www.phoenix-society.org or email info@phoenix-society.org or call 1–800–888–2876 (BURN). In Canada, each province has either a formalized support group to call upon or a group of former patients and/or family members, who can be contacted to support an inpatient or follow up with one who has been recently discharged into the community. School re-entry programs and burn camps are also widely available through most pediatric burn centres. Additional information can be obtained from The Phoenix Society.

## Conclusion

Few injuries require the full repertoire of skills possessed by nurses of today as much as the burn-injured person, child or adult. The demands are challenging, both intellectually and emotionally, but the rewards are immeasurable. This chapter has been written to provide those working among the burned with a comprehensive review of theoretical and practical knowledge, aimed at promoting the delivery of evidence-based nursing practice to this most deserving of patient populations.

## References

[1] Centers for Disease Control and Prevention: Burns – injury fact sheet, Atlanta, 2005, the Centers. Available at www.bt.cdc.gov.

[2] American Burn Association: Burn incidence fact sheet – 2002. Available at www.ameriburn.org.

[3] Mansfield MD, Kinsella J (1996) Use of invasive cardiovascular monitoring in patients with burns > 30 % BSA: a survey of 251 centers. Burns 22: 349

[4] Faucher LD, Conlon KM (2007) Practice guidelines for deep venous thrombosis prophylaxis in burns. J Burn Care & Res 28: 661

[5] Holt J et al (2008) Use of inhaled heparin/N-acetylcysteine in inhalation injury: does it help? J Burn Care & Res 29: 192

[6] Cheatam ML et al (2007) Results from the International Conference of Experts on intra-abdominal hypertension and ACS II recommendations. Intensive Care Med 33: 951

[7] Berger MM et al (2001) Resuscitation, anaesthesia and analgesia of the burned patient. Curr. Opin Anaesthesiol 14: 431

[8] Latenser BA (2009) Critical care of the burn patient: the first 48 hours. Crit Care Med 37: 2819

[9] Ahrns KS (2004) Fluid resuscitation in burns. Crit Care Nurs Clin North Am 16: 75

[10] Saffle JR (2007) The phenomenon of "fluid creep" in cute burn resuscitation. J Burn Care & Res 28: 382

[11] Helvig EI (2005) Burn wound care. In: Lynn-McHale Wiegand DJ, Carlson KK (eds) AACN Procedure Manual for Critical Care, ed 5. Elsevier, St. Louis

[12] Kammerer-Quayle BJ (1993) Helping burn survivors face the future. Progressions 5: 11

[13] Partridge J (1998) Taking up MacGregor's challenge. J Burn Care & Rehabil 19: 174

[14] Blakeney P et al (2008) Psychosocial care of persons with severe burns. Burns 4: 433

Correspondence: Judy Knighton, Reg. N., M. Sc. N., Sunnybrook Health Sciences Centre, Ross Tilley Burn Centre, Rm D7-38, 2075 Bayview Ave. Toronto, ON M4N 3M5, Canada, E-mail: Judy.Knighton@sunnybrook.ca

# Outpatient burn care

Bernd Hartmann[1], Christian Ottomann[2]

[1]Zentrum für Schwerbrandverletzte mit Plastischer Chirurgie, Unfallkrankenhaus Berlin, Germany
[2]Plastische Chirurgie und Handchirurgie, Intensiveinheit für Schwerbrandverletzte, Universitätsklinikum Schleswig Holstein
 Campus Lübeck, Germany

## Introduction

### Epidemiology

Burns are one of the most frequently-occurring types of injuries. Estimates place the number of burn victims in the United States at 1.25 million annually, 40,000 of which require inpatient treatment at a hospital [1]. Other sources write that the US has 700,000 burn victims annually, with 35,000 hospital visits. Both sources show that the percentage of victims with severe injuries requiring inpatient care is around 5%. The figures are similar in Germany. With a total of 350,000 burn victims and 15,000 inpatient cases, the ratio here is 4.3% [2].

### Accident causes

The most frequent cause of all injuries from scald burns and burns resulting from contact with flames and hot objects are accidents around the home. The number of such injuries which occur in the workplace has dropped significantly. In this context, most injuries occur in the food service industry as a result of scald burns and contact burns [3].

### Care structures

The care structures in highly-developed industrialized nations are, to a large extent, the same. Patients are offered both outpatient as well as inpatient treatment. In Germany, hospitals' emergency departments and doctors in private practice are the first point of contact for burn victims. In addition to correctly assessing and evaluating the wound, this is where the patients' further course of treatment is determined.

The goal of the following chapters is to explain the indications for inpatient burn treatment as well identify the most important care principles. If, in the course of providing inpatient care, complications such as an infection or delayed wound healing should arise, the approach to inpatient treatment must but reconsidered and the patient must be submitted to a specialized burn care facility. In the cooperation between specialized outpatient and inpatient care structures, this is the only way to achieve ideal treatment results for the patient while simultaneously cutting healthcare costs [4].

## Indications for inpatient treatment

Upon receiving a patient with a burn injury, the physician first treating the patient at a hospital's emergency department or in their own practice must determine whether an indication for inpatient treatment exists. In doing so, the physician must initially determine whether the indication for transferring the patient to a specialized center for severe burn treatment exists as set forth in the guidelines published by the German Association of Burn Medicine (Deutsche Gesellschaft für Verbrennungsmedizin). These indications (Table 1) must be adhered to in order to begin providing the patient with burn treatment in a timely and professional manner. In addition to the indications set forth in these guidelines which govern whether a patient must be transferred to a specialized burn care center, other indications exist which determine whether a patient should be provided inpatient treatment and forgo outpatient care [5]. The following chapters discuss in detail the most important criteria for making this determination in a professional manner. These include the patient's age, the depth of the burn, the surface area of the body which has been burned, as well as special burn cases. In this context, correctly evaluating the depth of the burn plays a crucial role. In particular, superficial second degree burns represent an area of conservative treatment. In special cases, they are suitable for outpatient care [6].

In this context, physicians must pursue the following goals:

▶ An optimal functional and aesthetic result for the patient when receiving treatment outside of specialized centers
▶ Palliation of physical and mental discomfort
▶ Adequate follow-up care
▶ Changing the treatment regimen in a timely fashion should complications arise

## Patient age

The elderly above the age of 70 as well as small children are particularly at risk for injuries from burns. The group of patients between 5 and 20 years of age has the best prospects for recovery, as this group's 50% mortality rate now applies to cases where 94.5% of the body's surface area is burned [7]. In contrast, patients over 70 have a 50% mortality rate in cases where burns cover 29.5% of their body [8]. This age-related risk is also reflected in the aforementioned guidelines governing indications for transferring patients to specialized burn centers. Patients under the age of 8 as well as those over the age of 60 require special care, which includes hospitalization in spe-

**Table 1.** Partial and full thickness burn ointments

| Dressing agent | Active substance | Presentation | Main use | Advantages | Disadvantages |
|---|---|---|---|---|---|
| Bacitracin | Bacitracin | Ointment | Superficial burns, skin grafts | Gram (+) coverage | No G(−) or fungal coverage |
| Polymyxin | Polymyxin B | Ointment | Superficial burns, skin grafts | Gram (−) coverage | No G(+) or fungal coverage |
| Mycostatin | Nystatin | Ointment | Superficial burns, skin grafts | Good fungal coverage | No bacterial coverage |
| Silvadene | Silver sulfadiazine | Ointment | Deep burns | Good bacterial and fungal coverage, painless | Poor eschar penetration, sulfa moiety, leucopenia, pseudoeschar formation |
| Sulfamylon | Mafenide acetate | Ointment and liquid solution | Deep burns | Good bacterial coverage, good eschar penetration | Painful, poor fungal coverage, metabolic acidosis |
| Dakin's | Sodium hypochlorite | Liquid solution | Superficial and deep burns | Good bacterial coverage, inexpensive and readily available | Very short half life |
| Silver | Silver nitrate, silver ion | Liquid solution, dressing sheets | Superficial burns | Good bacterial coverage, painless | Hyponatremia, dark staining of wounds and linens |

cialized centers. Patients above the age of 60 particularly exhibit a slowed biological wound healing process. This must be taken into consideration when making the necessary plans for outpatient treatment. Similarly, small children and the elderly also often have thinner skin [9].

Age represents an important factor for deciding whether a person requires conservative outpatient treatment or inpatient care.

## Total burned body surface area (TBSA)

Ultimately, the extent of the surface of the body affected is the deciding factor which determines whether a person can be offered outpatient treatment. When making this estimation, Wallace's well-known "Rule of Nines" as well as the "Rule of Palms", which is particularly suited for estimating the size of smaller injuries, are both used. This rule states that the surface of the patient's palm represents 1% of their body surface area. When initially evaluating a patient's burns, one must always estimate the size of the affected area [10].

Depending on the location of the burns, patients with superficial burns covering up to 10% of the body can be given outpatient treatment. The location of the burn is extremely important, however. A completely burned hand or a 1% burn in the face, covering large joints, in the genital area, or near the feet is enough to cause numerous complications, and such burns can heal badly. In such a case, inpatient treatment for patients with smaller wounds in these areas must be considered, and the patients should be transferred to a specialized center pursuant to the aforementioned guidelines [11].

## Depth of the burn

Under conservative treatment, individual superficial burns heal with a positive aesthetic and functional result within a maximum period of three weeks. The different burn depths from first to third degree have already been explained in one of this book's earlier chapters. It is important to note that when dealing with second-degree (partial-thickness) burns, one must differentiate between superficial and deep partial-thickness burns. Similar to third-degree burns, deep partial-thickness burns usually also require

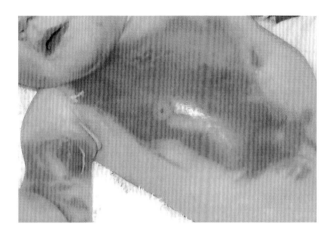

**Fig. 1.** Shows a significantly reddened superficial partial-thickness burn

surgery, which means that outpatient treatment is not suitable for patients with such burns [12].

In order to differentiate between the two types of wounds outside of a specialized environment, the following rule can be applied:

Second-degree burns are moist, painful, associated with the formation of blisters and have a coloration from white to pink or red, while third-degree burns are dry, painless, and have a coloration running from grey-white to brown. Superficial partial-thickness burns exhibit significant capillary regrowth, which means that the skin's dermal plexus has survived and is enlarged similar to an inflammation. This capillary regrowth is one of the most important signs used to differentiate between superficial and deep partial-thickness burns. At this point however, we must once again refer to the special locations which can also complicate superficial burns, and as such to these zones (see indications for transfer to a burn center). Physicians should select inpatient treatment for those affected by these cases [13,14].

## Pre-existing conditions

The burn victim's pre-existing health condition has both an influence on the healing process as well as on the results which can be expected. Burn patients in reduced states of consciousness, with neurological diseases with paresthesia, as well as those with mental health illnesses should receive inpatient

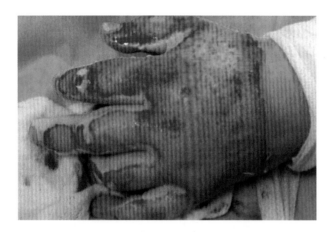

**Fig. 2** Shows a deep partial-thickness burn, which from its outward appearance looks similar to a third-degree burn

treatment. The same applies to those taking sedative medications and/or drugs and alcohol [15].

When it comes to internal diseases the focus is on renal insufficiency as well as cardiovascular disorders such as cardiac defects, arrhythmia, high blood pressure and also pulmonary diseases. In addition, this also includes diseases that have an effect on wound healing, such as diabetes mellitus, chronic alcoholism and chronic steroid use. Furthermore, this also includes autoimmune disorders and malignant tumors [16].

When determining a patient's medical history, these individual diseases must be analyzed and their impact on the entire burned area as well as the patient's overall condition must be estimated. A person can only receive inpatient treatment after a reliable estimation and risk analysis has been carried out. Frequently analyzing such a patient's overall health condition may also be necessary during the course of providing inpatient treatment.

## Accompanying injuries

The most frequent injury accompanying burns is damage to the pulmonary system as a result of smoke and carbon monoxide. This is known as inhalation trauma and can always occur alongside burns from flames. In this case, the physician providing initial treatment must determine whether the patient has suffered a smoke inhalation injury, and if so, the ex-

tent of the damage [17]. An examination of the patient using auscultation as well as a blood gas analysis are obligatory. Carbon monoxide poisoning can particularly cause the patient to appear disoriented, tired, or exhibit signs of other psychological or mental impairments. Determining the level of carbon monoxide in the patient's blood is also necessary. It is not enough to simply measure the oxygenation of the patient's hemoglobin.

If there is reason to suspect that the patient's upper respiratory tract has been injured through heat or a relevant smoke inhalation injury, they must receive inpatient treatment, and if they only exhibit signs of inhalation trauma, they should at least be kept in the hospital for observation [18].

An additional point of interest are accident-related accompanying injuries. The physician providing initial treatment must always search for additional injuries that may have been caused by falling, jumping from significant heights or trauma caused by the force of explosions. If findings are inconclusive or the mechanics of the accident require it, this case also requires clarification by a team specialized in dealing with such trauma [19].

## Special injuries

Finally, one must respond to special types of injuries which are also known to lead to complications during the wound healing process, and as a result, require the injured person to receive inpatient care. This includes electrical burns, chemical burns, as well as self-inflicted injuries or those caused by third parties [20].

### Electricity

In day-to-day life, we usually deal with high-voltage electricity of over 1,000 volts or regular household electricity which has between 110 and 220 volts. While injuries from high-voltage electricity or electric arcs can cause significant tissue damage, contact with household electricity often causes heart conditions from arrhythmia to ventricular fibrillation [21].

Since the electrical resistance of the skin is relatively high, the electrical current often looks for other paths through the body. It flows under the skin through neurovascular bundles as well as muscles and can leave the skin relatively unharmed between the point of entry and exit. Evaluating electrical injuries and in particular, differentiating between them and injuries from electric arcs (which only cause heat) is extremely difficult, and as a result, should only be carried out in a specialized center. Patients should only receive outpatient treatment in exceptional cases for tiny burns from sparks. Contact with household electricity should always result in short-term observation of the patient's heart and circulatory functions in order to detect any resulting complications. The electricity's entry and exit points are usually deep lesions with a poor prognosis for healing. In this case, inpatient treatment is usually also indicated.

## Chemical burns

The effect of corrosive chemicals to our skin causes coagulative necrosis if the chemical is an acid. Depending on the length of exposure, these chemicals can cause different degrees of damage similar to burns [22]. On the other hand, bases more often cause liquefactive necrosis, which causes the tissue to liquefy. Similar to acid, this can also result in varying degrees of damage. Chemical burns caused by hydrofluoric acid represent a special case, since after penetrating the skin, the acid often causes necrosis which stretches deep into the tissue and even destroys bone.

The first main step when treating such injuries is to rinse them with copious amounts of water. This dilutes the damaging substance while at the same time washing it out. Antidotes are also used in special cases, for example when treating chemical burns caused by hydrofluoric acid. In this case, the affected area is coated with calcium gluconate and if the extremities are injured, calcium gluconate is also administered intra-arterially [22]. When providing initial treatment it is often difficult to evaluate the effects of a chemical burn as well as its progression, which means that in this case the injured person must be monitored at close intervals after receiving inpatient treatment, even if injuries appear to be minor. People with chemical burns caused by hydrofluoric acid must always be transferred to a specialist clinic to receive inpatient treatment.

## Self-inflicted or externally-inflicted injuries

If the burn or scald is the result of a self-inflicted injury or one inflicted by a third party, the person must receive inpatient treatment regardless of the extent of the local damage. Even when dealing with small injuries, this is an important step as it serves to remove the patient from the dangerous place and determine the exact cause of the trauma. In these cases it can sometimes be necessary to get family members, caretakers, and even the police involved. Offering the injured person outpatient treatment is not indicated, because in these types of cases further injuries to the patient are to be expected [23].

## Treatment

### Initial treatment

There is no question that immediately cooling the tissue to under 44 degrees Celsius after a trauma is sensible, since allowing the tissue to remain at a high temperature would lead to even more extensive tissue necrosis. The method used to cool the tissue as well as the length of time the tissue should be cooled are the subjects of much debate, however.

It is generally recommended to use cool tap water for a period of up to 30 minutes. However, when doing so one must take care of not to cool too large of an area due to the risk of hypothermia. Cooling the area not only reduces tissue temperature to more normal levels but further stabilizes mast cells. As a result, the release of inflammatory mediators is decreased, pain is alleviated, and edema is reduced [24]. Using extremely cold water and/or ice packs or ice should be avoided, since the resulting reduction in capillary circulation can actually increase the amount of tissue damage.

Based on the aforementioned, cooling a burn wound is more of an immediate emergency procedure to be carried out at the location of the accident, and as a result, represents a method of first aid which one can carry out themselves or can be provided by a layperson. On the other hand, in the scope of initial medical treatment by a physician, cooling the burn wound is only recommended when tissue is severely overheated [25].

## Pain therapy

Burns are extremely painful, especially superficial burns affecting the dermis. This strong burning pain can continue for several hours and can also reappear due to sticking dressings and/or repeatedly manipulating the burn wound while providing treatment or changing bandages. Deep burn wounds are often less sensitive and are associated with reduced pain due to the destruction of the skin's nerve receptors. Providing sufficient pain therapy represents an important first step in treating all burns [26].

Providing non-steroidal anti-inflammatory drugs (NSAID) at an early stage should be considered. Drugs containing acetylsalicylic acid should not be used due to coagulopathy resulting from platelet function disorders.

When treating kids, the use of an age-appropriate and weight-appropriate dose of acetaminophen is recommended. If this first stage of pain therapy is not sufficient, a combination using codeine or metamizole or an orally-administered opiate should be considered. Significantly agitated patients benefit from the use of a fast-acting benzodiazepine, which will have a sedative effect. For the first few days a sufficient number of analgesics should prescribed as the standard medication. Prescribing an increased dose for bandage changing procedures, physical therapy, and/or for nights may be necessary. When it comes to the use of analgesics, one must always consider the patient's additional alcohol intake or, if applicable, factor other addictive disorders into a calculated pain therapy program.

If a patient has significant and/or uncontrollable pain, they should not receive outpatient treatment but rather be transferred to an inpatient setting. Once there, pain medication should be administered intravenously. The use of local anesthetics, or rather injecting local anesthetics into the area of the burn wound should not be carried out within the course of burn treatment.

## Local treatment

### Burn blisters

Particularly in the case of dermal burns, part of the epidermis rises up in the form of a thin blister. In deeper burns, the necrotic area is thicker, which means that these blisters usually do not form. The substance inside the blister shows the disruptive effect on wound healing [27]. Nevertheless, an intact blister represents a closed wound, which reduces the risk of infection. As a result, the proper method of handling blisters is a subject of much debate. In our own procedures, with the exception of extremely tiny blisters and thick blisters located on the palms of the hands or the soles of the feet, we completely remove all blisters. It is imperative that all blisters in the area to be treated are completely removed, particularly when planning to use modern wound dressings. Since torn blisters do not offer any protection against infection, the wound needs to be treated with topical substances anyway. Similarly, in order to prevent the hair from sticking to the wet wound, any body hair remaining in the wound area must also be removed, with the exception of the eyebrows.

## Debridement

As previously mentioned, all burn wounds must be debrided. Removal of the blisters is carried out either using scissors and tweezers, with a moist compress, or a soft brush. Manipulating the wound in this way requires the patient's pain to be sufficiently numbed, and as a result, such procedures are often carried out while the patient is anesthetized. The goal of this procedure should always be to thoroughly clean the wound bed. This is the only way to properly evaluate the depth of the burn as well as initiate proper wound treatment procedures. Mild liquid soap, or better yet, Lavasept or octenide solution are perfectly suitable for cleaning contaminated wounds. In our procedures, we completely refrain from using products which contain iodine to avoid contaminating our waste water [28]. Extremely adhesive substances such as tar, asphalt, or lubricants can be removed using baby oil or butter.

## Surface treatment/Topical substances

The rationale for using topical substances in the treatment of burns is primarily to reduce superinfection of the burn wound. In addition, particularly when it comes to the superficial wounds which are usually the focus of outpatient treatment, these substances should not slow down reepithelialization. Furthermore, priority is given to the patient's comfort with an almost painless or truly painless application [29].

A number of substances more or less fulfill these criteria and as a result, are suitable for use when treating superficial burn wounds.

### Povidone-Iodine

Povidone-Iodine (PVP-I) is effective against most germs which are relevant to the treatment of burn wounds. However, it is important to take note of the substance's considerable cytotoxicity, which can slow down the wound healing process [30]. Furthermore, its absorption toxicity must also be considered. A contraindication exists in case of hyperthyroidism, dermatitis herpetiformis, hypersensitivity to iodine, as well as use before and after radioiodine therapy (Kramer). In our procedures, ointments containing iodine are only used for deep burn wounds under consideration of the contraindications, since the iodine also has an drying effect on the skin which makes it easier to operate on later. Liposome capsules filled with PVP-I in hydrogel form are an affordable galenical which have a reduced iodine content and are more gentle on the wound. As a result, this iodine preparation (Repithel, Mundipharma GmbH, Limburg, Germany) is also suitable for follow-up treatment of transplanted wounds.

### Silver sulfadiazine (Flamazine®) and other silver products

Dressings containing silver have been used to cover wounds since ancient times. The free silver ions can damage bacteria cell walls, and silver sulfadiazine bonds with bacterial DNA. This means Flamazine has a bacteriostatic and bactericidal effect, and is suitable for all burn wounds [31]. However, when using Flamazine, as is the case with all silver ion applications, one must always take its cytotoxic effect (with slowed wound healing) into consideration. In addition, Flamazine forms a residue on the wound ("Flamazine eschar") which makes evaluating the wound after several days significantly more difficult. Due to these drawbacks, we completely refrain from using Flamazine in our own procedures. New products are currently offered like Acticoat® and

Mepilex Ag®. There benefit is that do not require daily dressing changes like Flammazine, but the use of silver products are more and more under discussion.

### Polyhexanide (PHMB)

In the past few years, a new topical antiseptic has gained popularity in burn wound treatment thanks to it also having a wide range of effects and extremely low cytotoxicity when it comes to keratinocytes and fibroblasts. Polyhexanide was primarily sold as a raw material under the name Lavasept® by the company Fresenius, and customers had to prepare ready-to-use gels and solutions themselves. But since then a number of manufacturers have created such ready-to-use solutions or gel forms of polyhexanide which, as a result, are now available for use in burn wound treatment. The advantage of the limpid gel or limpid solution is that it doesn't change the color of the wound, which means the wound can be evaluated at any time while providing treatment. Because it is highly diluted, Lavasept gels can be used in the wound area not only in short-term but also long-term applications. The applied solutions or gels do not cause any pain, which means children can tolerate them as well. Polyhexanide is the first known wound antiseptic with a selective mechanism of action. This is due to a strong effect on the acidic phospholipid bacterial cell membranes but only a slight effect on neutral phospholipid human cell membranes. This explains polyhexanide's extremely minimal cytotoxicity. Due to its molecule size, based on the current state of knowledge we can assume that polyhexanide is not absorbed by the body and as a result, only has an effect on the area of application [32].

In day-to-day clinical practice, gel preparations which use polyhexanide have proved to be of great value in the moist treatment of superficial burn wounds. We use the solutions both as a gentle method of disinfecting wounds when providing initial treatment and as part of subsequent dressing changes.

### Obsolete and unnecessary substances

Dyes and organic mercury compounds should be viewed as obsolete and unnecessary for use as burn wound antiseptics. In addition, hydrogen peroxide is another substance which should not be used for disinfecting wounds.

## Wound dressings/Bandages

Currently, the market is flooded with an almost unlimited number of high-quality wound dressings. When providing outpatient burn treatment, products should be used that simultaneously fulfill several criteria. The products should have the proper structure and absorbency to allow patients to keep the dressings on the wound for a number of days. Ideally, they should be suited for use in combination with topical therapeutic agents (polyhexanide gel) within the scope of moist wound treatment. We prefer silicon-coated wound coverings, which prevent the dressing from sticking to the newly-grown epithelium in the wound bed. Ideally, such dressings can be left on the wound until the wound is completely healed. In this context, one must only change the absorbent outer bandages and apply new polyhexanide gel, if necessary.

When treating superficial burn wounds, paraffin gauze dressings should not be used, as they can dry out relatively quickly and stick to the wound bed. This can cause wound healing problems when removing the dressing [33].

When appropriate, biosynthetic membranes such as Suprathel® or Biobrane® can also be used on superficial burn wounds. However, the use of these products requires the treating physician to be especially good at evaluating wounds, and also calls for primary radical debridement of the wound surface. In addition, these products are fairly expensive. Due to these reasons, they are only used in outpatient wound treatment in individual cases and under the supervision of trained specialists.

As a matter of principle, dressings should be sufficiently thick, absorb moisture, and be padded. When burns cover joints, certain cases might call for a splint to be used to immobilize the area for a short period time.

### Course of treatment

After providing initial treatment, primary debridement, and dressing and bandaging the wound, the further course of treatment calls for follow-up examinations. Depending on the selected dressing regime, dressings must be examined and changed regularly. As mentioned above, treatment strategies should be pursued which offer the greatest possibility for the dressing to remain on the wound, as doing so prevents complications during wound healing. Clinical examinations deal with clear signs of infection such as reappearing pain, redness around the wound, fever, and the patient complaining of feeling sick. Laboratory tests of the inflammatory parameters may also be required in certain cases. Without wound healing complications, grade IIa° burns, which fall under the domain of outpatient treatment, completely heal without any scarring within a period of one to three weeks [34].

## Complications

Both infections and/or the failure of the wound to heal represent complications which can occur during the aforementioned course of treatment. Both of these cases are serious and should lead to the patient being admitted to a specialize burn treatment facility.

### Infections

Burn wounds are usually colonized by germs, and topical treatment should prevent the occurrence of relevant wound infections [28].

The occurrence of pain, fever, exudation, redness, smells, and illness should always lead to the patient's admittance to a specialized facility. In addition to the danger of a systemic infection (sepsis), infections of the wound surface also cause delayed wound healing and as a result, ultimately lead to a worse healing result.

If an infection occurs, conducting a swab examination to determine the pathogen makes sense. In most cases, the treatment regime should be changed, regardless of the diagnosis. As previously explained, an infected burn wound represents an indication for admittance to a burn center for treatment. Whether the use of systemic antibiotics is required must be viewed as dependant on the patient's general condition.

## Delayed wound healing

In most cases, superficial wounds usually heal within a period of up to three weeks without any further consequences. If healing occurs without any complications, one should not expect the formation of excessive scars and the resulting functional and aesthetic effects. If during the course of treatment, the physician ascertains that the wound is healing slowly or not at all without any epithelialization, and instead discovers the formation of granulation tissue, the patient should be admitted to a specialized facility. Incorrect diagnoses during the primary evaluation, the wound deepening due to toxic substances in the dressing, and an infection can all cause the aforementioned to occur. Depending on the location and extent of the wound, the selected treatment regime should be changed. It may be necessary to remove the granulation tissue and/or remaining necrotic tissue once again, with subsequent skin grafting. In individual cases, the use of a keratinocyte cell spray to close the wound has proven to be successful, particularly when dealing with partial-thickness wounds [35].

It is important to know that if the wound does not heal, the treatment regime must be changed in order to achieve the best healing results for the patient.

## Follow-up care

Patients with burn wounds that receive outpatient treatment still require adequate follow-up care after the epithelialization process is complete. This includes providing the patient with extensive information regarding the further course of action [36]. The patient should avoid applying shear force to the area of the former wound, since this could result in the formation of new tension blisters. In addition, depending on the type and dryness of the patient's skin, it is recommended that they apply lubricant to the formerly burned area [37]. Systematically protecting the area from UV rays should also be recommended to the patient. Besides avoiding exposure, this can be achieved through the use of suntan lotion with an SPF around 30.

Since the focus of outpatient burn care is on superficial burn wounds, additional follow-up care

methods using silicone gel sheets and/or compression bandages will not be discussed here in detail. However, if hypertrophic scars do form after a burn victim receives outpatient care, these products should be used as described in another section of this book.

## References

[1] Brigham PA, McLoughlin E (1996) Burn incidence and medical care use in the United States: estimates, trends and data sources. J Burn Care Rehabil 17: 169–171

[2] Burd A, Yuen C (2005) A global study of hospitalized burn patients. Burns 31(4): 432–438

[3] Statistisches Bundesamt. Todesursachen in Deutschland 2004 (Fachserie 12/ Reihe 4) Wiesbaden 2006

[4] Blome-Eberwein S, Jester A, Küntscher M, Germann G (2001) Besonderheiten in der Erstversorgung von Brandverletzten. Akt Traumatol 31: 201–204

[5] Germann G, Barthold U, Lefering R, Raff T, Hartmann B (1997) The impact of risk factors and pre-existing conditions on the mortality of burn patients and the precision of predictive admission-scoring systems. Burns 23(3): 195–203

[6] Hartford CE, Kealy GP (2007) Care of outpatient burns. In: Herndon DN (ed) Total burne care, 3rd edn. Saunders Elsevier

[7] Tobiasen J, Hiebert JH, Edlich RF (1982) Prediction of burn mortality. Surg Gynecol Obstet 154(5): 711–714

[8] Smith DL, Cairns BA, Ramadan F, Rutledge R et al (1994) Effect of inhalation injury, burn size and age on mortality: a study of 1447 consecutive burn patients. J Trauma 37(4): 655–659

[9] O'Keefe GE, Hunt JL, Purdue GF (2001) An evaluation of risk factors for mortality after burn trauma and the identification of gender-dependent differences in outcomes. J Am Coll 192(2): 153–160

[10] Raff T, Germann G, Barthold U (1996) Factors influencing the early prediction of outcome from burns. Acta Chir Plast 38(4): 122–127

[11] Muller MJ, Pegg SP, Rule MR (2001) Determinants of death following burn injury. Br J Surg 88(4): 583–587

[12] Wachtel TL et al (1986) B-mode ultrasonic echo determination of depth of thermal injury. Burns 12: 432–437

[13] Groeneveld AB (1990) Septic shock and multiple organ failure. Int Care Med 16: 489–490

[14] Lavrentieva A, Kontakiotis T Lazaridis L et al (2008) Inflammatory markers in patients with severe burn injury. What is the best indicator of sepsis? Burns 33(2): 1 89–94

[15] Atiyeh BS, Gunn SW, Hayek SN (2005) State of the art in burn treatment. World J Surg 29(2): 131–148

[16] Brusselaers N, Hoste EA, Monstrey S et al (2006) Outcome and changes over time in survival following severe burns from 1985 to 2004. Intensive Care Med 31(12): 1648–1653

[17] Artuson MG (1985) The pathophysiology of severe thermal injury. J Burn Care Rehabil 6: 129

[18] Wittram C, Kenny JB (1994) The admission chest radiograph after acute inhalation injury and burns. Br J Radiol 67: 751–754

[19] Schultz JH, Schmidt HG, Queitsch C et al (1995) Die Behandlung schwerer Begleitverletzungen beim Verbrennungspatienten. Unfallchirurg (98): 224–228

[20] Kildal M, Willebrand M, Andersson G et al (2005) Coping strategics, injury characteristics and long-term outcome after burn injury. Injury 36(4): 511–518

[21] Dokov W (2009) Assessment of risk factors for death in electrical injury. Burns 35: 114–117

[22] Burd A, Ahmed K (2010) The acute management of acid assault burns. Ind J Plast Surg 43(1): 29–33

[23] Theodorou P, Phan V, Weinand C et al (2011) Suicide by Burning: Epidemiological and Clinical Profile. Ann Surg 10: 204

[24] Cross KM, Leonardi L, Fish JS et al (2009) Noninvasive measurement of edema in partial thickness burn wounds. J Burn Care Res 30(5): 807–817

[25] Lund T, Onarheim H, Reed RK (1992) Pathogenesis of endema formation in burn injuries. World J Surg 16: 2

[26] Browne Al, Andrews R, Wood F (2011) Persistant pain outcomes and patient satisfaction with pain management after burn injury. Clin J Pain 27(2): 136–145

[27] Burton F (2004) An evaluation of non-adherent wound-contact layers for acute traumatic and surgical wounds. J Wound Care 13(9): 371–373

[28] Mozingo DW, McManus AT, Kim SH, Pruitt BA (1997) Incidence of bacteremia after burn wound manipulation in the early postburn period. J Trauma 42: 1006–1010

[29] Sörensen R, Fisker NP, Steensen JP (1984) Acuta excision of exposure treatment? Final results of a three-year randomised controlled clinical trial. Scan J Plast Reconstr Surg 8: 87–93

[30] Pallua N, von Bülow S (2006) Behandlungskonzepte bei Verbrennungen. Teil II: Technische Aspekte. Chirurg 77(2): 179–186

[31] Costagliola M, Agrosi M (2005) Second-degree burns: a comparative, multicenter, randomized trial of hyaluronic acid plus silver sulfadiazine vs. silver sulfadiazine alone. Curr Med Res Opin 21(8): 1235–1240

[32] Daeschlein G, Assadian O, Koch S et al (2007) Feasibility and clinical applicability of polihexanide for treatment of second-degree burn wounds. Skin Pharm Phys 20(6): 292–296

[33] Wilder D, Rennekampff HO (2007) Debridement of burn wounds – rationale and options. Hamipla 39(5): 302–307

[34] Philipp K, Gazyakan E, Germann G, Öhlbauer M (2005) Von der Erstversorgung bis zur Plastischen Chirurgie – Spezielle Behandlungsaspekte bei Verbrennungen. Klinikarzt 34: 249–254

[35] Enoch S, Grey JE, Harding KG (2006) ABC of wound healing: Recent advances and emerging treatments. BMJ 332(7547): 962–965

[36] Acton A, Mounsey E, Gilyard C (2007) The burn survivor perspective. J Burn C Res 28(4): 615–620

[37] Chapman TT (2007) Burn scar and contracture management. J Trauma 62(6): 8

Correspondence: Dr. med. Bernd Hartmann, Zentrum für Schwerbrandverletzte mit Plastischer Chirurgie, Unfallkrankenhaus Berlin, Warener Straße 7, 12683 Berlin, Germany, E-mail: bernd.hartmann@ukb.de

# Non-thermal burns

# Electrical injury

Brett D. Arnoldo, John L. Hunt, Gary F. Purdue

UT Southwestern Medical Center, Dallas, TX, USA

## Introduction

Electricity is a ubiquitous, indispensable, and invisible part of modern civilization. We often take it for granted until a natural disaster renders it and us nearly useless. Another instance when an individual is reminded of its presence unfortunately and all too commonly is the severe electrical burn injury. Electrical burns are the most devastating of all thermal injuries on a size by size basis. They affect primarily young, working males, and often lead to legal entanglements. They are the most frequent cause of amputation on the burn service [1]. Cutaneous manifestations of high voltage electrical injuries have been equated to the *tip of the iceberg*. Index of suspicion must be high, as deep tissue injury is often hidden yet common. Long term morbidity and disability is often the end result of these injuries and this has led to the recommendation for their evaluation and treatment in qualified burn centers.

Electricity causes more than 400 unintentional-injury fatalities per year in the United States according to the Centers for Disease Control (CDC) data. It is estimated that 10% of all admissions to burn units worldwide are from burns caused by electrical injuries [61]. In 1999 the impact of electrical injuries was estimated to be in excess of $1 billion annually and is the leading cause of work related injury [10, 32, 39].

## Pathophysiology

Some experts have described electrical trauma as a severe form of thermal injury while others more accurately liken it to a crush injury [3]. Electrical burn injury severity is related to voltage, current (amperage), type of current (alternating or direct), path of current flow, duration of contact, resistance at the point of contact, and "individual susceptibility" for lack of a better term. Electrical burns are most simply classified as either low-voltage ( < 1000 volts) or high-voltage (≥ 1000 volts). Low voltage injuries are generally localized to the area immediately surrounding the injury and subsequently are less destructive and easier to manage. Nearly all injuries occurring indoors with the exception of some industrial settings are low voltage. High-voltage injuries are typically deceptive and hide a significant amount of destruction beneath the cutaneous burn. While voltage is generally known or relatively simple to surmise, the amount of current is unknown. Current flow is related to voltage by Ohm's Law:

Current (I) = Voltage (E)/Resistance (R)

Electrical injury experiments in a canine model have shown a three-phase response of amperage due to tissue resistance [25]. The initial slow rise in amperage represents a progressive decrease in skin resistance. The second phase is characterized by an abrupt rapid increase in amperage which coincides with the complete breakdown of skin resistance and unimpeded flow of current. The third phase is characterized by the abrupt fall in amperage, representing tissue dessication and carbonization. The charred skin then acts an insulator and current flow ceases [25]. Tissue temperature, the critical factor in the severity of these injuries increases parallel with amperage. Older articles and discussion of electrical injury often emphasize the different resistances of internal tissue (i. e. R: Bone > Fat > Tendon > Skin > Muscle > Blood > Nerve). For all practical purposes however, once the skin resistance is overcome, the internal milieu of the body acts as volume conductor, resistance being averaged. The severity of injury is then inversely proportional to the cross-sectional area of the tissue able to carry current. Clinically this is evident with the most severe injuries typically at the wrist and ankle. An interesting finding in the experimental model was the lack of tissue injury distal to the contact points. Deep tissue tends to retain heat so that peri-osseous tissue especially between two bones (tibia-fibula; radius-ulna) often sustains worse injury. This accounts for the clinical occurrence of a central "core" of necrotic muscle in association with relative sparing of superficial muscle. There is a slower dissipation of heat in deeper tissue around the bone and often then more severe injury [26]. Tissue temperature is of utmost importance and for all practical purposes tissue obeys Joule's Law:

Power (J-Joule) = $I^2$ (Current) × R (Resistance)

Electrical current can flow in one of two types of circuits: direct current (DC) or alternating current (AC). Current type plays a role in tissue injury with alternating current being more hazardous than direct [59]. More than 90% of all electrical burns in the United States are caused by 60 cycle-per-second (60 Hertz) commercial alternating current, which reverses its polarity 120 times per second. This leads to the terminology of 'contact points' as opposed to the inaccuracy of entrance and exit wound verbiage. The cyclic flow of electrons also causes muscle tetany that generally prolongs the victim's contact with the source. If the source of contact is the hand, the strength of the forearm flexors causes the victim to grasp and the "no-let-go" phenomenon is seen. Direct current is seen in some industrial settings, medical appliances, batteries, and battery powered devices. Most DC cir-

cuits are relatively low voltage. A car battery is approximately 12 volts and is as high a DC voltage as most people will ever use. Direct current is more likely to cause a single convulsive contraction and push the victim away from the current source.

Resistance of the skin is varied. The moist sweaty palm in summer compared to a dry calloused hand in the winter months will exhibit significant differences in resistance. The path of the current relates to injury. Current path is difficult to interpret clinically and predictions of potential injury may be inaccurate. If current passes across the chest for example this may result in cardiac or respiratory arrest. The mere presence of contact points on both upper extremities however is not proof positive of current flow across the chest. Individual susceptibility is another term like "idiopathic". There are likely other factors that render one patient more susceptible than another, we simply do not understand them as such.

Progressive muscle necrosis is an often described clinical phenomenon in electrical injuries. Arteriographic studies would suggest that this is in fact the natural progression of the injury. Microvascular thrombosis may occur in marginally injured adjacent muscle accounting for a small portion of muscle necrosis. The bulk of involved muscle appears to sustain irreversible damage at the time of injury. Care must be taken that progression does not occur as a result of inadequately released muscle compartments.

Direct and indirect electrical destruction of cells also plays a role in tissue injury. This is particularly important in the nervous system as injury there is not entirely explained by heating alone. Cell membrane disruption is a potential explanation given that membrane integrity is maintained by the sodium-potassium-ATPase pump operating at -90millivolts direct current. Breakdown of cell membranes via the process of electroporation may also explain injury not apparently caused by heat [37, 38].

## Initial assessment and acute care

The first priority is protection of the field team and initial responders. Patients should not be handled until electrical power has been disconnected. Initial evaluation follows Advanced Trauma Life Support (ATLS) and the American Burn Association Advanced Burn Life Support (ABLS) protocols. Electrical injuries are associated with trauma in approximately 15% of cases, double the rate of other burns. Most commonly this is due to a fall from a height or the victim being thrown. Tetanic muscle contraction may also generate enough force to cause compression fractures [35]. After the initial assessment is completed several complex management decisions need to be addressed. These are the issues that make the electrical injury somewhat unique. They include: (1) how to proceed with resuscitation given that there is likely a deep unquantifiable component to the injury, (2) when and how to treat pigmented urine, and what is its implication (3) who needs cardiac monitoring and for how long (4) who needs emergent operative intervention. These unique acute care issues often overlap and will be addressed together in the next section.

Resuscitation should be kept simple. The deep tissue injury makes the use of resuscitation formulas based on body surface area burned inaccurate. The goal of resuscitation should be the maintenance of normal vital signs and a urine output of approximately 30–50 mL/h (or 0.5 ml/kg) with Ringer's lactate. This rate is adjusted on an hourly basis to achieve goal.

This becomes more difficult in complex circumstances such as glucosuria. Urine output becomes less reliable in the face of this finding. Unreliable urine output may necessitate the monitoring of central venous pressure (CVP) from a subclavian or internal jugular central line. In this instance a goal CVP of 8–10 mmHg is reasonable. Some would also consider monitoring central venous saturations (Scv02) with a goal of 60–65%, or even the placement of a pulmonary artery catheter, although this has not generally been required in our experience.

The presence of pigmented (darker than light pink) urine in this patient population indicates significant muscle damage. This should alert the clinician to be aggressive in efforts to clear the urine and thus prevent renal failure, and also vigilant for compartment syndromes. Myoglobin and hemoglobin pigments present significant risk of acute tubular necrosis (ATN). Dark urine must be cleared promptly to minimize precipitation into the renal tubules.

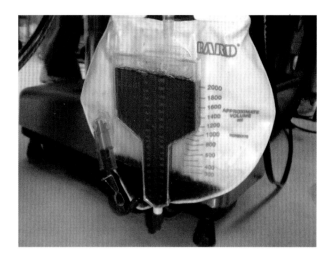

**Fig. 1.** Pigmented urine

Gross pigmenturia is diagnosed visually (Fig. 1) and confirmed positive on dipstick test for blood and negative on microscopy for red blood cells. Confirmatory urine myoglobin is unnecessary and may lead to over treatment and over resuscitation. The most important component of treatment is adequate fluid resuscitation with Ringer's in an effort to more or less double the urine output. Typically the urine output goal is approximately 100 mL/hr until the urine visually appears clear. Treating to a negative myoglobin level in the urine can lead to volume overload. Several methods to enhance this process have been recommended, including osmotic diuresis with mannitol and alkalinization of the urine with bicarbonate. These adjuncts while seemingly affective are not supported by level I evidence [23, 52, 62]. The authors however have had success treating grossly pigmented urine with 2 ampules of sodium bicarbonate and 25 grams of mannitol, both given as an IV push, as an adjunct to increased IV fluid infusion. Patients who do not clear their urine are candidates for repeat doses. These patients however require careful evaluation for ongoing ischemia and muscle necrosis. They will very likely need surgical intervention requiring either fasciotomy or amputation. Additional evidence of muscle necrosis is confirmed by checking serial serum creatine kinase isoenzymes. This is generally not required however and are often too sensitive to to be used as a guide for therapy. Diagnosis can most commonly be made by physical exam.

Both low- and high-voltage electrical can interfere with the conducting system of the heart. Ventricular fibrillation is the most common cause of death at the scene, however any cardiac dysrhythmia may be encountered in the setting of electrical injury. Dysrhythmias are treated as per Advanced Cardiac Life Support (ACLS) algorithms, similar to those of medical etiology. All electrical injured patients require a twelve lead electrocardiogram (ECG). This should occur as soon as is practical in the emergency department. Cardiac monitoring is recommended for: (1) ECG abnormality, (2) cardiac dysrhythmia during transport or in the emergency department, (3) documented cardiac arrest, (4) loss of consciousness, and (5) patients with other standard indications for monitoring. The duration of monitoring is generally between 24 and 48 hours, however this is based on scant data. [2]. Most patients with low voltage injuries and no indications for monitoring can generally be discharged from the emergency department. The authors have applied this same criteria to high-voltage injuries based on their own published data, however this is not universally accepted in all institutions [4, 54]. Direct myocardial injury may also occur. This injury presents more like a myocardial contusion rather than myocardial infarction. Creatine kinase (CK) and MB-creatine kinase in these patients are poor indicators of myocardial damage especially in the presence of muscle injury [8, 24, 42]. Utility of troponin levels in these patients has yet to be determined.

Patients with high voltage electrical injuries may harbor deep tissue injury (Fig. 2) and may require immediate operative exploration for compartment syndrome, and/or debridement. Damaged muscle, swelling within the investing fascia of the extremity, may increase pressures to the point where muscle blood flow is impaired. Loss of pulses is one of the last findings of compartment syndrome unlike early loss of pulses occurring in circumferential burns requiring escharotomy. Conventional wisdom states that compartment syndromes may develop over the first 48 hours. While this is true the author's experience has been that the decision to operate can generally be made with confidence at initial evaluation in the emergency department. These are not subtle injuries. Those patients who were operated on in the subsequent 24–48 hours

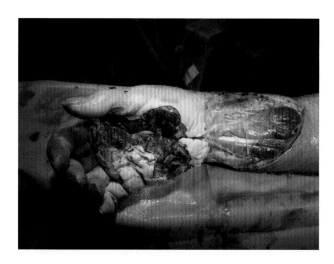

**Fig. 2.** High voltage injury with deep tissue necrosis

after admission generally had findings at admission or else had larger total body surface area (TBSA) burns and required generous resuscitation volumes. A good teaching point here is that these patients either have normal extremities on physical exam or they have significant findings, and if they have significant findings they generally need to be explored. Having said that, ABA guidelines recommend extremity exploration for: (1) progressive neurologic dysfunction, (2) vascular compromise, (3) increased compartment pressure, (4) systemic clinical deterioration from suspected ongoing myonecrosis [2]. If compartment pressures are measured as an adjunct to diagnosis, a pressure greater than 30 mmHg is considered significant. Patients not meeting indications for exploration may be debrided on the third to fifth postinjury day [41]. Elevated CK levels have been correlated to the extent of muscle damage and the requirement for surgical intervention [34]. Four compartment fasciotomies of the lower leg and anterior/posterior fasciotomies of the upper extremity done in the operating room under general anesthesia is standard of care. Upper extremity decompression will generally require carpal tunnel release and may in some cases require release of intrinsic muscles of the hand. The carpal tunnel release which is challenging in elective settings is made simpler by the significant underlying edema. By inserting the open jaw of the straight scissors under the proximal end of the transverse carpal ligament (while remaining ulnar to the Palmaris longus ten-

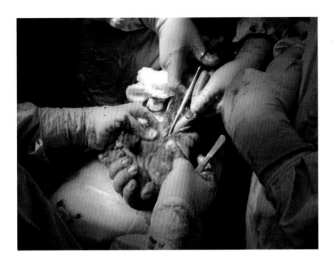

**Fig. 3.** Carpal tunnel release

don), and then simply pushing distally across the ligament, the carpal tunnel release is performed with relative ease (Fig. 3). A second look operation should be performed at 48–72 hours post op.

Serial debridement may be required before the patient is ready for closure or skin grafting. Care must be taken to prevent dessication of the open wound prior to closure. Moist dressings soaked every four hours with 5% mefanide acetate (sulfamylon) solution is one option. The wound vacuum assisted closure (VAC®) device may also be used in this setting.

The one instance when immediate amputation is contemplated is in the setting of mummified and contracted tissue. This occasionally occurs and most commonly involves the upper extremities. In this instance an aggressive approach can be undertaken which may include proximal disarticulation such as at the shoulder joint. These are infrequently performed operations however are relatively simple in that one must only differentiate viable from nonviable tissue (this is not a cancer operation). This is most easily accomplished with electrocautery working judiciously through muscle bundles in a deliberate fashion. Once the neurovascular structures are controlled the operative pace can be accelerated.

## Wound care

Wound care follows the recommendations outlined in ABLS. Full thickness contact points are best treated with mefanide acetate ointment (sulfamylon®). The excellent eschar penetration of sulfamylon makes this a good treatment option in these deep wounds. Silver sulfadiazine for flash and flame burn areas provides good broad spectrum coverage at low cost with few side effects. Physical Medicine and Rehabilitation (PM&R) consultation should occur at admission and ongoing involvement is required to minimize scar complications. Physical therapy and functional splinting is begun on the day of admission and continued throughout the hospital stay. Meticulous neuromuscular examination is performed and careful documentation of neurologic status is required. This should be performed on admission and prior to discharge. Many of these cases end up in the court system and careful documentation is a must.

Operative debridement can begin on post burn day two or three either as a second look operation following fasciotomy or as the first procedure. All necrotic tissue should be excised while tissue of questionable viability retained and re-evaluated every 2–3 days until wound closure is achieved.

## Diagnosis

There are several modalities that have been investigated in an effort to definitively differentiate viable from nonviable tissue. Radionuclide scanning with xenon-133 [6] and technetium pyrophosphate [27] have been shown to be accurate but not shown to decrease hospital length of stay or number of operations Hammod. Gadolinium enhanced MR imaging demonstrates potential viability in zones of tissue edema and good correlation with histopathology [11, 47, 39]. While these adjuncts can be sensitive and specific they add very little other than expense and we have refrained from their use in our institution.

## Low voltage injuries

Low voltage injuries are generally localized to the contact points (Fig. 4). A careful evaluation for contact points including the scalp must be included in the physical examination. Contact point can be deep injuries with significant local tissue destruction however they do not generally extend laterally. These may require amputation of digits but can usually be treated with local debridement and coverage. Oral commissure burns in children are more complex injuries. These oral cavity burns occur when a child chews on an electric cord. The child's saliva completes the circuit between positive and neutral leads; the resulting resulting electrical short may cause significant local tissue destruction of the lips and or tongue [16]. These injuries are initially treated conservatively as the extent of injury is difficult to predict. Acutely these injuries should be evaluated and managed by a qualified burn surgeon. These children require admission for pain control and nutrition however outpatient management is possible once parents are comfortable with wound care and overall management [9, 36]. Parents should be warned that the eschar may separate and result in serious bleeding from the labial artery, which typically occurs at 10–14 days postburn. They should be instructed to hold pressure in this event and return immediately to the emergency department for suture ligation. Stretching and oral splinting gives good result in many and others may need reconstructive surgery. Plastic surgery consult is often required for complications and burns in the mid-portions of the mouth. These heal poorly and may require more aggressive surgical intervention [50, 57].

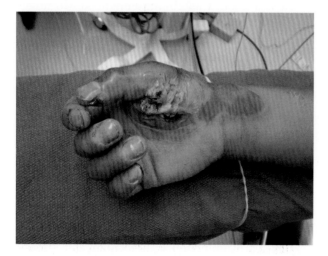

**Fig. 4.** Low voltage contact point

## Lightning injuries

Lightning strikes cause 50–80 fatalities per year in the United States with Florida and Texas having the most deaths (Lightning-Associated deaths 1998) [22, 60]. Estimates of fatalities and overall injuries may be low however due to underreporting [7]. No outdoor location is safe from lightning strike. Lightning may strike as much as 10 miles in any direction from a thunderstorm even before the rain starts and while the sky is still clear. Risk factors are height of an object, isolation, and narrowness of the tip of the object. One must be indoors to be safe. Hard-wired telephones and television sets may become conduits for the charge however. Cell phones pose no inherent risk although they may be a risk factor due to the users inattentiveness to weather conditions.

Lightning strikes are high voltage injuries with the potential of reaching into the millions of volts. They are however brief, on the order of milliseconds. Current often flows around the victim in what is known as a flash-over-phenomenon which accounts for survival in a majority of individuals [12, 43, 48]. The most common cause of death is cardiac standstill and paralysis of the respiratory center. Cardio pulmonary resuscitation (CPR) is particularly effective when promptly initiated [45]. The pathognomonic cutaneous sign of a lightning strike is a dendritic fern-like branching erythematous pattern on the skin (Lichtenberg figure). This pattern on the skin fades rapidly much like a wheal and flare reaction. Major cutaneous injury is rare unless a nearby object is turned incandescent, causing a flash/flame injury, such as when a bag of golf clubs on a victims is struck. A rare and interesting complication is keraunoparalysis, which is a transient paralysis associated with extreme vasoconstriction and sensory disturbances of one or more extremity. This usually lasts only an hour but may be as long as twenty-four. Ruptured tympanic membrane is common and may be complicated by vertigo [31]. Neurologic complications ranging from loss of consciousness, seizures and traumatic brain injuries should prompt a high index of suspicion and consideration of head CT scan. Systemic effects of these injuries are managed in a fashion similar to high-voltage injuries.

## Complications

Early complications are related to critical care issues such as cardiac, renal failure, sepsis. Neurologic complications may present at any time from admission to months after injury [33, 55, 58]. Neuromuscular defects include paresis, paralysis, Guillain-Barre syndrome, transverse myelitis or amyotrophic lateral sclerosis [51]. In a key paper by Grube of 90 patients with electrical injuires 64 had high-voltage injury [13]. Two-thirds of the 64 patients had immediate central or peripheral neurologic symptoms with twenty-nine patients having loss of consciousness of whom 6 remained comatose. Three of these 6 ultimately died, and three awoke but had neurologic sequelae. One-third of the high-voltage group had one or more acute peripheral neuropathies, approximately two-thirds of these resolved or improved. The late onset peripheral neuropathies had a propensity to be more permanent. The most common clinical finding in electrically injured patients with peripheral neuropathy is weakness [15]. Reflex sympathetic dystrophy (now more commonly known as complex regional pain syndrome), is also seen in these patients and is often difficult to manage. These patients present with neuropathic pain, edema, and skin changes that may be disabling. Patients with chronic pain are also at high risk for depression [19, 20]. Depression occurs in 77% of patients with chronic pain although 89% of these patients never had been depressed before the onset of their pain [18]. Not only do survivors of electrical injury and lightning strikes have problems with depression but a whole spectrum of neuropsychological issues may be present. These range from cognitive dysfunction, memory impairment, attention disturbances, affective problems, anxiety, irritability and poor frustration tolerances, to physically aggressive outbursts [21, 29, 49, 53] Post traumatic stress disorder is also more common after electrical burns than after thermal burns [40].

Cataract formation is the most common ocular complication in electrical injury, although ocular manifestations may affect all portions of the eye [5, 30]. Ocular changes may affect 5–20% of patients with electrical injury. Saffle reported seven patients with 13 cataracts, noting a high degree of bilaterality with little association to voltage. Associated contact points were more commonly on the head, neck, and upper trunk [56]. Seventy-seven percent of these ultimately progressed to where surgical intervention was required. This complication may present rarely within months or as late as many years after injury [46].

Heterotopic ossification (HO) occurs at the cut ends of amputation sites in this patient population. This may occur in about 80% of patients with long bone amputations but not those with disarticulations or small bone amputation [17]. In a recent report of one center's experience over 21-years 42 patients were identified with HO and of these 7% were high-voltage electrical burns. Those patients requiring surgery can be managed by the burn team without need of orthopaedic consultation. Work-up includes plain films of the involved bodypart and PM&R consultation for postoperative care.

Electrical burn patients make up a relatively small number of overall injured patients in large burn and trauma centers. They do however consume large amounts of resources in these centers. The definitive care of these patients should be delivered in specialized centers in order to maximize good long-term outcomes and properly utilize scare resources.

## References

[1]  Arnoldo BA, GF Purdue, Kowalske K, Helm PA, Burris A, Hunt JL (2004) Elecrical injuries: A 20-year review. J Burn Care Rehabil 25: 479–484

[2]  Arnoldo BA, Klein M, Gibran NS (2006) Practice guidelines for the management of electrical injuries. J Burn Care Res 27: 439–447

[3]  Artz CP (1967) Electrical injury simulates crush injury. Surg Gynecol Obstet 125: 1316

[4]  Bailey B, Guadreault P, Thiviege RL (2000) Experience with guidelines for cardiac monitoring after electric injury in children. Am J Emerg Med 18: 671–675

[5]  Boozalis GT, Purdue GF, Hunt JL et al (1991) Ocular changes from electrical burn injuries: a literature review and report of cases. J Burn Care Rehabil 5: 458–462

[6]  Clayton JM, Hayes AC, Hammel J et al (1977) Xenon-133 determination of muscle blood flow in electrical injury. J Trauma 17: 293–298

[7]  Cooper MA, Andrews CJ, Holle RL (2006) Lightning injuries. In: Auerbach PS (ed) Wilderness emergencies, chapter 3. CV Mosby, Elsevier

[8]  Dilworth D, Hasan D, Alford P et al (1998) Evaluation of myocardial injury in electrical burn patients. J Burn Care Rehabil 19(Pt2):S239

[9] D'Italia JG, Hulnick SJ (1984) Outpatient management of electrical burns of the lip. J Burn Care Rehabil. 5: 465–466

[10] Esselman PC, Thombs BD, Magyar-Russell G, Fauerbach JA (2006) Burn rehabilitation: state of the science. Am J Phys Med Rehabil 4: 383–413

[11] Fleckenstein JL, Chason DP, Bonte FJ et al (1993) High-voltage electric injury: assessment of muscle viability with MR imaging and Tc-99 m pyrophosphate scintigraphy. Radiology 195: 205–210

[12] Graber J, Ummenhofer W, Herion H (1996) Lightning accident with eight victims: case report and brief review of literature. J Trauma 40: 288

[13] Grube B, Heimbach D, Engrav L et al (1990) Neurologic consequences of electrical injury. J Trauma 30: 254–258

[14] Hammod J, Ward CG (1994) The use of technetium-99 pyrophosphate scanning in management of high voltage electrical injuries. Am Surg 68: 886–888

[15] Haberal MA, Gureu S, Akman N et al (1996) Persistent peripheral nerve pathologies in patients with electrical burns. J Burn Care Rehabil 17: 147–149

[16] Heimbach DM, Gibran NS (2007) ACS Surgery Principles & Practice, 6th edn. Miscellaneous burns and cold injuries. WebMD Professional Pub, New York, NY, pp 1437–1448

[17] Helm PA, Walker SC (1987) New bone formation at amputation in electrically burn-injured patients. Arch Phys Med Rehabil 68: 284–286

[18] Hendler N (1982) Diagnosis and treatment of chronic pain. The four stages of pain. Editors: Hendler N, Long DM, Wise T. John Wright-PAG, Inc, Boston

[19] Hendler N (1984) Depression caused by chronic pain. J Clin Psychiatry 45: 30–36

[20] Hendler N (1989) Validating and treating the complaint of chronic pain: Mensana clinic approach. Clin Neurosurg 35: 385–397

[21] Hendler N (2005) Overlooked diagnosis in chronic pain: Analysis of survivors of electric shock and lightning strike. J Occup Environ Med 47: 796–805

[22] Hiestand D, Colice GL (1988) Lightning injury. J Intensive Care 3: 303–314

[23] Holt SG, Moore KP (2001) Pathogenesis and treatment of renal dysfunction in rhabdomyolysis. Intensive Care Med 27: 803–811

[24] Housinger TA, Green L, Shahangian S et al (1985) A prospective study of myocardial damage in electrical injuries. J Trauma 25: 122–124

[25] Hunt JL, Mason AD, Masterson TS, Pruitt BA (1976) The pathophysiology of acute electric injuries. J Trauma 16: 335–340

[26] Hunt JL, McManus WF, Haney WP, Pruitt BA (1974) Vascular lesions in acute electrical injuries. J Trauma 14: 461–473

[27] Hunt JL, Lewis S, Baxter C (1979) The use of technetium-99 stannous pyrophosphate scintigraphy to identify muscle damage in acute electrical burns. J Trauma 19: 409–413

[28] Hunt JL, Sato RM, Baxter CR (1980) Acute electric burns. Arch Surg 115: 434–438

[29] Janus TJ, Barrash J (1996) Neurologic and neurobehavioral effects of electric and lightning injuries. J Burn Care Rehabil 17: 409–415

[30] Johnson EV, Klein LB, Skalka HW (1987) l Electrical cataracts: a case report and review of the literature. Ophthalmic Surg 18: 283–285

[31] Jones D, Ogren F, Rot L et al (1991) Lightning and its effects on the auditory system. Laryngoscope 101: 830

[32] Kidd M, Hultman CS, Van Aalst J, Calvert C, Peck MD, Cairns BA (2007) The contemporary management of electrical injuries, resuscitation, reconstruction, rehabilitation. Ann Plast Surg 3: 273–278

[33] Ko SH, Chun W, Kim HC (2004) Delayed spinal cord injury following electrical burns: A 7-year experience. Burns 30: 691

[34] Koop J, Loos B, Spilker G et al (2004) Correlation between serum creatinine kinase levels and extent of muscle damage in electrical burns. Burns 30: 680–683

[35] Layton TR, McMurty JM, McClain EJ et al (1984) Multiple spine fractures from electric injury. J Burn Care Rehabil 5: 373–375

[36] Leake JE, Curtin JW (1984) Electrical burns of the mouth in children. Clin Plast Surg 11: 669–683

[37] Lee RC, Kolodney SB (1987) Electrical injury mechanisms: Dynamics of the thermal injury. Plast Reconstr Surg 80: 663–671

[38] Lee RC, Kolodney SB (1987) Electrical injury mechanisms: Electrical breakdown of cell membranes. Plast Reconstr Surg 80: 672–680

[39] Lee RC (1997) Injury by electrical forces: pathophysiology, manifestations, and therapy. Curr Probl Surg 9: 677–764

[40] Mancusi-Ungar HR Jr, Tarbox AR, Wainwright DJ (1986) Posttraumatic stress disorder in electric burn patients. J Burn Care Rehabil 7: 521

[41] Mann R, Gibran N, Engrav L et al (1996) Is immediate decompression of high voltage electrical injuries to the upper extremity always necessary. J Trauma 40(4): 584–589

[42] McBride JW, Labrosse KR, McCoy HG et al (1986) Is serum creatine kinase-MB in electrically injured patients predictive of myocardial injury? JAMA 255: 764–768

[43] Milzmann DP, Moskowitz L, Hardel M (1999) Lightning strike at a mass gathering. South Med J 92: 708

[44] MMWR (1998) Lightning-associated deaths–United States, 1980–1995. 19: 391–394

[45] Moran KT, Thupari JN, Munster AM (1986) Electric and lightning induced cardiac arrest reversed by prompt cardiopulmonary resuscitation. JAMA 255: 2157

[46] Mutlu FM, Duman H, Chi Y (2004) Early-onset electrical-cataract: a rare clinical entity. J Burn Care Rehabil 25: 363–365

[47] Ohashi M, Koizumi J, Hosoda Y et al (1998) Correlation between magnetic resonance imaging and histo-

pathology of an amputated forearm after electrical injury. Burns 24: 362–368

[48] O'Keefe Gatewood M, Zane RD (2004) Lightning injuries. Emerg Med Clin North Am 22: 369

[49] Patten BM (1992) Lightning and electrical injuries. Neurol Clin 10: 1047–1058

[50] Pensler JM, Rosenthal A (1990) Reconstruction of the oral commissure after electrical burns. J Burn Care Rehabil 11: 50–53

[51] Petty PG, Parkin G (1986) Electrical injury to the central nervous system. Neurosurgery 19: 282–284

[52] Pham TM, Gibran NS (2007) Thermal and electrical injuries. Surg Clin North Am 87: 185–206

[53] Primeau M, Engelstatter GH, Bares KK (1995) Behavioral consequences of lightning and electrical injury. Semin Neurol 15: 279–285

[54] Purdue GF, Hunt JL (1986) Electrocardiographic monitoring after electrical injury; necessity or luxury. J Trauma 26: 166–167

[55] Ratnayake B, Emmanuel ER, Walker CC (1996) Neurological sequelae following high voltage electrical burn. Burns 22: 578

[56] Saffle JR, Crandall A. Warden GD (1985) Cataracts: a long-term complication of electrical injury. J Trauma 25: 17–21

[57] Sadove AM, Jones JE, Lynch TR et al (1988) Appliance therapy for perioral electrical burns: conservative approach. J Burn Care Rehabil 9: 391–395

[58] Singerman J, Gomez M, Fish JS (2008) Long-term sequelae of low-voltage electrical injury. J Burn Care Res 29: 773–777

[59] Solem L, Fisher RP, Strate RG (1977) The natural history of electrical injury. J Trauma 17: 487

[60] Tribble CG, Persing JA, Morgan RF et al (1984) Lightning Injury. Curr Concept Trauma Care. Spring: 5–10

[61] Tomkins KL, Holland AF (2008) Electrical burn injuries in children. J Paediatr Child Health 44: 727–730

[62] Yowler CJ, Fratianne RB (2000) Current status of burn resuscitation. Clin Plast Surg 27: 1–10

Correspondence: Brett D. Arnoldo, M.D., UT Southwestern Medical Center, 5323 Harry Hines Blvd., Dallas, TX 75390–9158, USA, E-mail: Brett.arnoldo@utsouthwestern.edu

# Symptoms, diagnosis and treatment of chemical burns

Leila Kolios[1], Günter Germann[2]

[1] Clinic for Hand-, Plastic & Reconstructive Surgery – Burn Center – Clinic for Plastic & Hand Surgery at Heidelberg University Hospital, BG Trauma Center Ludwigshafen, Germany
[2] ETHIANUM, Clinic for Plastic, Aesthetic & Preventive Medicine at Heidelberg University Hospital, Heidelberg, Germany

## Chemical burns

Injuries from caustic substances usually occur in chemical industry, during transportation and handling of hazardous materials, at home, during job training and at school.

Chemical burns are described as injuries to the skin or mucous membranes caused by chemical substances. Usually, strong acids or bases cause protein denaturation in tissues, resulting in cell damage and apoptosis with subsequent necrosis. In addition some substances may cause toxic as well as thermal damage. The extent of cutaneous damage depends on type, amount, and concentration of the caustic substances, but also on the duration of exposure. Disrupting the pathophysiological mechanism of the chemical reaction at an early stage is therefore the foremost goal of any medical treatment, before treating the actual damage.

### Decontamination

As an initial procedure, decontamination of the affected patient is of utmost importance to reduce the contact time between the caustic substance and the tissue. The decontamination process has to be divided into specific procedures:

► unspecific decontamination: mechanical removal of toxic agents, when indicated extensive rinsing additionally provides for a desired diluting effect

► specific decontamination: transformation of the acid into its salt, cleavage/hydrolysis of toxic compounds, application of antidotes, etc.
► natural decontamination: vaporization of volatile substances

First aid treatment, which has to be initiated immediately after exposure, should ensure in particular the protection of those providing first aid. The effects of hazardous substances must be reduced for the individual involved, for others at risk, and for rescue personnel. In this regard, caustic substances are labeled in the chemical industry with specific hazardous material declarations and accompanied by accident procedure sheets from which instructions can be gathered for administering first aid.

Contamination with caustic substances in solid, liquid or gas form affects several organ systems in different ways depending on the concentration, the way of contact with the body, and the duration of exposure.

## Affection of different organ systems

### Respiratory tract

Odor and irritation of breathing such as coughing following inhalation have a significant warning effect. If vapors are inhaled, symptoms such as burning, dryness of the nose and throat, coughing, dyspnoea, and angina pectoris symptoms may appear [4]. Increased production of secretion, raised capillary permeability, surfactant destruction, bronchoconstriction, and pulmonary hypertension are possible sequelae [12]. Inhalation of higher concentrations can lead to laryngospasm and complete obstruction of the respiratory tract due to a direct caustic toxic effect. All symptoms can occur in two phases. After a transient stimulation phase and a symptom-free interval, toxic pulmonary edema can occur up to 72 hours post exposure [25, 31].

Emergency treatment of inhalation trauma is still a subject of controversy. After first aid such as rescue of the victim, avoiding further exposure and supplying oxygen, has been provided, the question of administering of steroids is still under vehement discussion. In particular, efforts are directed to attain a rapid, unspecific anti-inflammatory effect by inhibiting the biosynthesis of prostaglandins and leukotrienes [12]. In case of doubt, inhalation administration is therefore recommended in various dosages and intervals [4, 26, 31] as well as intravenous administration for prophylactic and anti-edematous treatment [4, 19]. On the other hand, the anti-inflammatory effect that occurs especially with high-dose intravenous administration is viewed critically, since the immunosuppressive effect of corticoids has to be considered at the same time. This should be avoided at all costs, particularly in the case of more severely injured persons and/ or patients with extensive thermal burns [12, 26]. For bronchial spasm, ß2-mimetics are indicated, such as those approved for the treatment of bronchial asthma [15]. Initially, X-ray images of the thorax typically appear normal. Clear signs of pulmonary edema, such as hilus enlargement or centrally accentuated and patchy shadows, are late radiological signs that often cannot be recognized until the second phase of the injury [25]. For monitoring purposes, an initial chest X-ray should be made, particularly in patients with concomitant cardiopulmonary medical conditions.

## Eye

In the eye, the exposure to fumes and vapors leads to painful paresthesias with spasmic eyelid closure, redness, lacrimation, and conjunctivitis. Due to protein denaturation, severe corneal ulcers and necroses

are to be expected, as well as clouding of the cornea and lens through direct contact with acid components. Complete loss of vision and subsequent blindness are possible in severe cases.

In the case that vapors or liquid components come into direct contact with the eyes, they must be flushed immediately with plenty of water or neutral saline solution, if possible while everting the eyelids [19]. The therapeutic aim is the normalization of the conjunctival pH value (7.0). Any possible eyelid spasms can be resolved by applying locally anesthetizing eye drops [8]. Rinsing with chelating agents such as diphoterine is discussed for decontamination purposes. Due to their broad buffering capacity (neutralizing capacity from pH 1 to 13), they can be used for eye-contaminations with acids as well as bases [2, 20].

## Gastrointestinal tract

Oral ingestion of diluted concentrations leads to nausea and gastroenteritic symptoms. Retrosternal burning and bloody vomiting have been described [4, 19, 31]. Higher concentrations cause severe damage to the mucous membranes especially of the larynx ant the esophagus. Constrictions and perforations have been described [35].

If caustic substances are ingested orally, inducing emesis is contraindicated. Repeated contact of the esophageal mucosa with the substance raises the risk of perforations. In addition, neutralization and administration of charcoal is not necessary [4, 19, 31]. Administering water by mouth with the aim of rinsing the esophageal tissue and achieving a diluting effect is recommended. The administration of proton pump inhibitors in analogy to gastroesophageal reflux disease (GERD) is recommended, as chemical burns cause dysmotility of the esophagus with gastroesophageal reflux, consequently impairing recovery [1, 19]. In animal experiments it could be shown that omeprazole and vitamin E prevent inflammatory changes of the affected esophagus and can thereby reduce the development of strictures [30].

In case of ingestion or suspected chemical burns, gastroduodenoscopy should be taken into consideration to determine the extent of intra-gastral damage and, if necessary, should be combined with surgical intervention [4, 19, 31].

The primary administration of antibiotics is indicated for deep burns (deep second-degree and third-degree burns) and perforations and should cover a broad spectrum [17]. Treatment with steroids is a subject of controversy, because an advantage for preventing strictures could not yet be clearly proven [3, 17, 19, 22]. In the case of difficulties of swallowing and when there is no risk of perforation, the use of a nasogastric tube placed under visualization is recommended [19]. Parenteral nutrition is necessary at least in the acute phase (up to 7 days), but in some cases also until healing is completed, to prevent infection and strictures [17].

## Hematological signs

Following extensive exposures, methemoglobinemia, hemolysis and methemoglobinuria can develop due to the formation of nitrous gases ($NO_x$) [4, 8, 31]. Depending on the concentration, typical clinical signs consist of gray-blue skin color (15–30% MetHb), headache, fatigue, dizziness, tachycardia, dyspnea (30–50% MetHb), stupor, bradycardia, cardiac arrhythmia, respiratory depression (50–70%), cardiac arrest, unconsciousness, or coma (60–70%). If the MetHb level exceeds 90%, a fatal outcome is to be expected.

Routine laboratory tests should include a complete blood count as well as glucose and electrolyte levels. In symptomatic patients, an arterial blood gas analysis should be carried out with determination of the methemoglobin concentration [7].

It is recommended that toluidine blue, methylene blue or thionine, as well as vitamin C should be given to accelerate the reduction of MetHb to hemoglobin [4, 16]. Therapy with positive end-expiratory pressure (PEEP) and an exchange transfusion should be taken into consideration in life-threatening situations.

## Nephrologic symptoms

Acute kidney failure can occur in the form of tubular necrosis due to disturbances of the acid-base balance (metabolic acidosis) and due to hemolytic products [8].

If renal involvement is suspected, all efforts should be directed towards the induction of an in-

creased diuresis. The addition of mannitol to the infusion regimen supports this process with its osmotic diuretic effect. Consequences of acute tubular, necrotic tissue change can be treated symptomatically with the body-weight adapted administration of bicarbonate and fluids [8].

## Skin

Tissue damage from contamination is due to protein denaturation. Interaction with acids causes coagulation necroses that in most cases keep the acids from penetrating into deeper-lying tissue. Only those tissue areas are damaged that, depending on duration and concentration, were in direct contact with the acting acid (exception: hydrofluoric acid, see below).

In contrast, bases cause colliquative necroses that permit progression of the corrosive effect into deeper layers of the skin and thus more extensive damage. The results are diffusion and penetration into underlying tissues with a subsequent more extensive corrosive effect [31].

Skin contact with less concentrated fumes or vapors of caustic substances can lead to burning pain, redness, and inflammation. First- to third-degree burns with their respective subsequent scarring result from direct contact with the concentrated substance [31]. The classification of chemical burn injuries and their signs and symptoms follows that of thermal burn injuries.

As initial treatment, decontamination and extensive flushing of the affected skin areas are certainly of critical importance to reduce the duration of contact between the substance and the skin as much as possible. In addition, unspecific anti-inflammatory, analgesic and skin care ointments for first-degree injuries are well established. Dermal chemical burns, however, require more specific therapy. Particularly during the exudative and proliferative phase, treatment regimens must allow protection against dehydration and microbial colonization [27]. Both goals can be accomplished using the commonly used therapy with silver sulfadiazine [23], which is effective against a broad spectrum of germs including gram-negative ones and Candida albicans. Silver sulfadiazine, however, carries the risk of leukopenias and disturbances of the acid-base balance when applied to large areas [32]. Likewise, top-

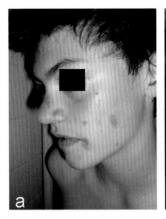 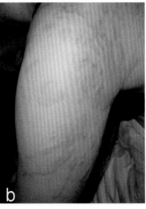 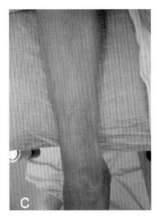

**Fig. 1.** Different forms of appearance of nitric acid induced skin lesions 1 hour after trauma
a superficial, brown-stained lesions of the face.
b II° splash-formed chemical burn of the shoulder.
c IIb-III° laminar chemical burn of the lower leg

ically effective antiseptics such as polyhexanide combined with polyethylene glycol in Ringer's solution or octenidine with phenoxyethanol in gel form can be used. In their main indication as surface antiseptics, such substances permit a better clinical assessment of the injury compared to sulfadiazines [32].

Depending on the state of the wound, enzymatic conditioning with plant and bacterial proteases may also be applied. If the wounds are in the process of normal healing but are still secreting fluid, absorbent foam bandages can be used that can be left in place for up to 3 days but which still permit assessment of the wound at all times. The silver sulfadiazine dressings used at the beginning should be changed to the procedure described above to ensure a reliable clinical assessment of the wounds. Later in the healing process, they can be changed to simple cremes with a high fatty component. Until healing and possible scarring are complete, sunblocker should be applied before the wound is exposed to UV and sunlight.

The role of modern methods of semi-permanent wound dressings (for example Acticoat®, Biobrane®, Suprathel® and Matriderm®) widely used in he treatment of superficial and partial thickness thermal burns is not yet defined in the treatment of acid burns at the present time. Since clinical experience with such injuries is much lower than that with thermal burns, it is our opinion that procedures using permanent wound dressings should not be recommended for chemical burns. Clinical monitoring of such wounds should be possible at all times.

## Specific agents

### Nitric acid

Nitric acid, also called hydrogen nitrate and having the chemical formula $HNO_3$, is an inorganic oxoacid of nitrogen. At room temperature, concentrated nitric acid (65 % $HNO_3$) is a colorless to yellow or brown liquid with a pungent odor. Its corrosiveness is due to both its acidic effect and an oxidation reaction [31]. Contact with metal has an explosive effect. It is used in the production of fertilizers, explosives and dyes, and in metal processing [4].

The maximum allowable concentration (MAC value) of nitric acid at which no health risks can be expected is 2.6 mg/m³ or 1 ml/m³ [11]. According to the German Ordinance on Hazardous Materials (GefStoffV), it is classified depending on its concentration as Xi (irritant) to C/O (corrosive, oxidizing agent) and carries the risk phrase R 35 [6]. There is no known antidote.

Due to the so-called xanthoproteic reaction, in which nitration takes place on the benzene ring of aromatic amino acids, contact between the skin and nitric acid results in coagulative tissue damage with specific, partially persisting neon-like yellowing of the wound areas (Figs. 1, 2) [8, 31]. Overall, the typically yellow nitric acid burns demarcate more slowly than thermally damaged areas (Fig. 2) [18]. Plastic surgical procedures and follow-up treatment of nitric acid burns follow the same principles as in thermal burn injuries.

Attention must be paid to possible involvement of the eyes, ingestion trauma, kidney function, and the development of MetHb.

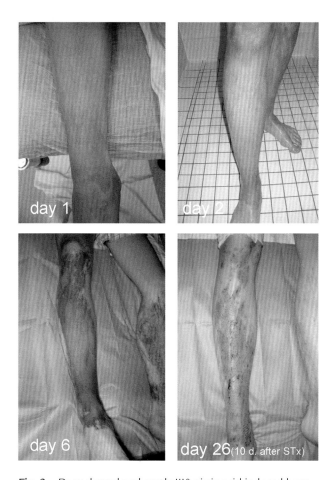

**Fig. 2.** Deep dermal and partly III° nitric acid induced burn 1 hour after trauma, with intensified yellow staining on the second day and beginning demarcation from the 6th day under enzymatic therapy. The healing situation on day 26, 10 days after mesh-graft transplantation

## Sulfuric acid

Sulfuric acid, also called dihydrogen sulfate according to IUPAC nomenclature [International Union of Pure and Applied Chemistry], is a compound of sulfur with the chemical formula $H_2SO_4$. It is a colorless, oily, nonflammable, very viscous and hygroscopic liquid with a penetrating odor. Sulfuric acid is one of the strongest acids and has a very corrosive effect. It finds wide application in the production of fertilizers, synthetic materials, paints, and paper. It is also used as an electrolyte in car batteries as well as in metal processing and in the preparation of food [4].

The mechanism of action of sulfuric acid depends on its concentration. In the case of diluted sul-

furic acid, the raised proton concentration has a caustic effect, similar to that of other diluted acids. Its effect upon contact with the skin mainly consists of local irritation and is therefore less hazardous than concentrated sulfuric acid [9]. The latter, even in small amounts, severely damages the skin and eyes and affects organic substances by dehydration under carbonization. Painful wounds develop that heal only very slowly. Surgical treatment i. e. excision and possible grafting, as well as conservative wound care is identical with protocols in thermal burns.

The inhalation of vapors of sulfuric acid can also result in inhalation trauma. The mists of concentrated sulfuric acid have a carcinogenic effect (IARC Group 1) [14]. Dose-effect relationships show the odor threshold at a concentration of $1 \text{ mg/m}^3$, a concentration of $5 \text{ mg/m}^3$ is subjectively intolerable and triggers the urge to cough, and the immediately life-threatening concentration is $80 \text{ mg/m}^3$. The MAC value is $0.1 \text{ mg/m}^3$ [4, 11]. Sulfuric acid is likewise assigned to the hazard class C (caustic) and carries the risk phrase R35.

## Hydrofluoric acid

The aqueous solution of hydrogen fluoride (HF) is called hydrofluoric acid. Hydrofluoric acid is a colorless, pungent-smelling liquid that as a strong acid generates heat upon reaction with many compounds and is thereby inflammable and explosive. It corrodes metal, glass and rock and is also used in a diluted form in the electronic and semiconductor industry as well as a detergent. A solution of 38.2% HF in water forms an azeotropic boiling mixture with a boiling point of 112 °C [4].

Hydrofluoric acid is a strong contact poison. Due to its quick resorption, the destruction of deeper tissue layers including bone is possible without the skin being visibly injured. A latent period of up to 24 hours until the appearance of first symptoms has been described for lower concentrations [4]. Excruciating pain following dermal exposure is a significant diagnostic feature. At higher concentrations, contact between hydrofluoric acid and the skin results in whitening of the skin, blisters, and colliquative necroses. A burn the size of a hand with 40% hydrofluoric acid is fatal due to the resorptive poisonous action. The IDLH value (Immediately Dan-

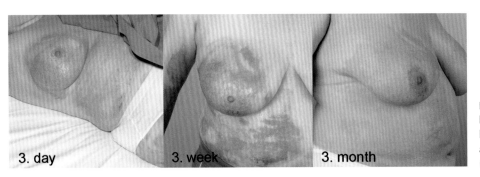

3. day      3. week      3. month

**Fig. 3.** Superficial chemical burns caused by sodium hydroxide at 3 days, 3 weeks and 3 months after trauma under conservative wound care

gerous to Life or Health) has been established at 25 mg/m$^3$ (30 ppm) [9]. The MAC value is 1 ml/m$^3$ or 0.83 mg/m$^3$ [11].

Deeper skin penetration can be counteracted by repeatedly injecting the surrounding of the damaged tissue areas with 5–10% calcium gluconate solution. The distinct reduction of pain is an indicator for the amount to be injected and the frequency of injections. Therefore, local anesthetics should not be used. Upon contact with lower concentrations of hydrofluoric acid, the affected skin areas can also be treated with 2.5% calcium gluconate gel. The use of calcium chloride instead of calcium gluconate should be strictly avoided if calcium gluconate is not available, ice-cold 0.13% benzalkonium chloride compresses can be applied as an alternative. 2.5% aqueous calcium gluconate aerosols can be applied with 100% oxygen in the case of inhalation [4].

Fluoride ions are absorbed rapidly through the skin and eyes and thereby cause systemic involvement. The electrolyte balance is severely disturbed by the binding of calcium and magnesium; cardiac arrhythmias, ventricular fibrillation, and asystoly can result. Hydrofluoric acid also has neurotoxic effects. The warning effect of pain can therefore often occur with a delay of several hours. Involvement of the CNS can lead to coma and respiratory failure. Metabolic acidosis, acute kidney failure, and coagulation disorders can occur.

## Caustic soda

Caustic soda is the term used for solutions of sodium hydroxide (NaOH) in water. Sodium hydroxide dissolves in water, thereby releasing heat, and forms an alkaline solution. Unimolar caustic soda (1 Mol NaOH (40 g) in 1 liter) has a pH value of 14. It is one of the most frequently used laboratory and industry chemicals [4].

Upon contact with concentrated caustic soda, the local caustic effect stands out, characterized by necrosis that quickly progresses to deeper layers of tissue. The tissue-damaging effect of caustic soda is due to its basic pH which causes protein compounds to dissolve. The specific picture of colliquative necrosis is attributed to the formation of hydrophilic alkali albuminates and saponification [9] (Fig. 3). Eschar formation does not take place. The extent of tissue damage depends to a large degree upon duration of exposure, concentration, pH value, dose, and the introduction of treatment measures. It should be noted that contact with the substance can remain unnoticed or underestimated at the beginning due to the delayed sensation of pain. The IDLH value (Immediately Dangerous to Life or Health) has been established at 10 mg/m$^3$.

Quantitative data on skin resorption are not available. The absorption of systemically effective doses is not expected for concentrations that are not damaging to the skin. Numerous reports have been made about serious poisoning through ingestion of formulations containing sodium hydroxide (i. e. paint strippers, drain pipe cleaners). In case of resorption, the main systemic reaction consists of an influence on the blood pH value due to the release of hydroxyl ions. Homeostatic mechanisms can counteract an excess of sodium through increased excretion. Upon inhalation of sodium hydroxide, significant amounts may also become systemically effective [9].

Depending on the reaction conditions, serious eye irritation with swelling of the eyelid and mild corneal damage to severest damage to the conjunctiva, cornea, and sclera (clouding, perforation/ulceration, vascularization, symblepharon), and less often of the inner eye (retinitis) have been described.

## Phenol

Phenol, also known as carbolic acid, hydroxybenzene or phenylic acid is a toxic, white crystalline solid with the chemical formula $C_6H_5OH$. Its structure is that of a hydroxyl group (-OH) bonded to a phenyl ring, making it an aromatic compound. The boiling and melting points are 182 and 41 °C respectively [21]. Nowadays it is used in the manufacture of plastics, explosives, fertilizers, paint or textiles [24], but its disinfectant properties were investigated and used already 1867 by Lister in aseptic surgery. Since that time, phenol is used widely in medical and pharmaceutical properties.

Phenol is corrosive to human skin, but due to its local anesthetic properties, extensive damage may occur before pain is recognized. Dependent on its concentration, dermal contact with phenolic compunds result in irritation, dermatitis, abnormal pigmentation and burns. Up to second- or third degree burns may be caused by the concentrated phenol because of its caustic and defatting (hydrophobic effect of phenol) properties [21]. Prolonged contact elicits denaturation, necrosis and gangrene. However, systemic toxicity and poisoning usually occur by skin absorption with a possibly lethal result. It is reported that the application of a 1% lotion for 7–17 days will result in seizures and coma [33]. Chemical burns from skin exposures with phenol must be decontaminated by washing with polyethylene glycol 300 or 400 [5] isopropyl alcohol [13] or water [28]. Removal of contaminated clothing is required, as well as immediate hospital treatment for large splashes. This is particularly important if the phenol is mixed with chloroform (commonly used mixture in molecular biology for DNA & RNA purification from proteins). It is essential to obtain blood count, electrolytes, urinanalysis and baseline renal and liver measurements after phenol exposure. The acid-base balance of blood should be monitored closely. The normal blood concentration of total phenol is 0.15–7.96 mg/100 mL. The normal range of phenol in urine is 0.5–81.5 mg/L. The highest level of phenol is detected in urine 8–10 h after initial exposure [21].

In case of pulmonary exposure, tachypnea, stridor, pulmonary edema and bronchospasm may occur. However, phenol is not considered a serious respiratory hazard in the workplace because of its low volatility [21]. In case of inhalation a cardio-vascular monitoring and administration of symptomatic treatment is necessary. Endotracheal intubation and assisted ventilation should be provided as required, as phenol-induced pulmonary trauma being consistent with adult respiratory distress syndrome.

Phenol and its vapor are irritating and corrosive to the eyes with resulting tearing, conjunctivitis and corneal/conjunctival edema. Severe corneal injury may result in white and hypesthetic corneas or corneal necrosis [29]. Again, irrigation of the eyes with copious amounts of water or 0.9% saline solution, local anesthesia application and ophthalmologic examination should be performed.

The substance can cause harmful effects on the central nervous system and heart, such as dysrhythmia, seizures, and coma [33]. In cases of long-term or repeated exposure of phenol effects on the liver and kidneys are reported [34]. Exposure may result in death and the effects can be delayed. The substance is a suspected carcinogen. Besides its hydrophobic effects, another mechanism for the toxicity of phenol may be the formation of phenoxyl radicals [10].

## Summary

Chemical burn traumata usually occur in chemical industry, during transportation and handling of hazardous materials or at home. The acids or bases cause protein denaturation in tissues, resulting in cell damage and apoptosis with subsequent necrosis. The extent of damage depends on the type, amount, and concentration of the caustic substances, but also on the duration of exposure. Disrupting the pathophysiological mechanism of the chemical reaction at an early stage is therefore the foremost goal of any medical treatment. In the skin, acids causes coagulation necroses that in most cases keep the acids from penetrating into deeper-lying tissue. Bases cause colliquative necroses that permit diffusion and penetration into underlying tissues with a subsequent more extensive corrosive effect. First- to third-degree burns with their respective subsequent scarring result and treatment can occur according to thermal burns. All other possibly affected organ systems must be examined. Pulmonary emergency diagnostics and therapy are preeminent: monitoring of peripheral oxygenation, thoracic x-rays, oxygen donation and periodical steroid application. Inoculation traumata are to be rinsed out extensively, decontaminated with diphoterines / chelates and treated with panthenol-containing gel after ophthalmologic consultation. In the case of oral ingestion regurgitation is contraindicated to avoid another contact of the acid with the oesophageal mucosa. Application of any liquid for dilution and of proton pump inhibitors to prevent inflammation and strictures is necessary as well as a gastroduodenoscopy. To reduct Met-Hb in case of a methemoglobinaemia application of toluidin-blue, methylen-blue, thionine or ascorbic acid is recommended. A renal affection requires forced diuresis, if necessary supported by mannitol and bicarbonate.

# References

[1]   Abdülkadir G, Oktay M (2002) Esophageal motility changes in acute and late periods of caustic esophageal burns and their relation to prognosis in children. J Pediatr Surg 37: 1526–1528

[2]   Alan H, Hall MD (2002) Diphoterine zur Notfallbehandlung zur Dekontamination von chemischen Augen/Hautspritzern: Ein Überblick. Vet Human Toxicol 44 (4)

[3]   Anderson KD, Rouse TM, Randolph JG (1990) A controlled trial of corticosteroids in children with corrosive injury of the esophagus. N Engl J Med 323: 637–640

[4]   BASF Medical Guidelines for Acute Exposure of Chemical Substances, R1. State 2006. Codes D015–001, D018–002, D026–002, D023–001

[5]   Brown VKH, Box VL, Simpson BJ (1975) Decontamination procedures for skin exposed to phenolic substances. Arch Environ Health 30: 1–6

[6]   Canadian Centre for Occupational Health and Safety (CCOHS). Nitric acid, Cheminfo 2007

[7]   Desel H, Neurath H, Behrens A (2004) Toxikologische Labordiagnostik und Bedside-Tests bei Vergiftungen. Monatsschrift Kinderheilkd 152: 1062–1068

[8]   Gabilondo Zubizarreta FJ, Melendez Baltanas J (1999) The management of chemical burns. Eur J Plast Surg 22: 157–161

[9]   GESTIS-database on hazardous substances (2010) www.dguv.de/ifa/gestis-database

[10]  Hanscha Corwin, McKarnsb Susan C, Smith Carr J, Doolittle David J (2000) Comparative QSAR evidence for a free-radical mechanism of phenol-induced toxicity. Chemico-Biological Interactions 127: 61–72

[11]  Health and Safety Executive (HSE) (2005) EH40/2005 Workplace Exposure Limits

[12]  Hoppe U, Klose R (2005) Das Inhalationstrauma bei Verbrennungspatienten: Diagnostik und Therapie. Intensivmed 42: 425–439

[13]  Hunter DM, Timerding BL, Leonard RB, McCalmont TH, Schwartz E (1992) Effects of isopropyl alcohol, ethanol, and polyethylene glycol/industrial methylated spirits in the treatment of acute phenol burns. Ann Emerg Med 21: 1303–1307

[14]  International Agency for Research in Cancer (2010) IARC Monographs on the evaluation of Carcinogenic Risks to Humans. http://monographs.iarc.fr

[15]  Kafka G, Maybauer DM, Traber DL, Maybauer MO (2007) Das Rauchgasinhalationstrauma in der präklinischen Versorgung. Notfall Rettungsmed 10: 529–540

[16]  Karow T (2002) Allgemeine und Spezielle Pharmakologie und Toxikologie, 10th edn. Karow, Pulheim

[17]  Katzka DA (2001) Caustic injury to the esophagus. Curr Treat Options Gastroenterol 4: 59–66

[18]  Kolios L, Striepling E, Kolios G, Rudolf KD, Dresing K, Dörges J, Stürmer KM, Stürmer EK (2009) The Nitric acid burn trauma of the skin. J Plast Reconstr Aesthet Surg [Epub ahead of print]

[19]  Kurzai M, Köhler H (2005) Gastrointestinale Verätzung und Fremdkörperingestion. Monatsschrift Kinderheilkd 153: 1197–1208

[20]  Langefeld S, Press UP, Frentz M, Kompa S, Schrage N (2003) Verätzungen des Auges, Diphoterinhaltige Augenspüllösung in der Erste-Hilfe-Therapie. Ophthalmologe 100: 727–731

[21]  Lin TM, Lee SS, Lai CS, Lin SD (2006) Phenol burn. Burns 32: 517–521

[22]  Mamede RCM, De Mello Filho FV (2002) Treatment of caustic ingestion: an analysis of 239 cases. Dis Esophagus 15: 210–213

[23]  Monafa WW, Bessey PQ (1997) Wound care. In: Herndon DN (ed) Total burn care. WB Saunders, pp 88–97

[24]  Monteiro-Riviere NA, Inman AO, Jackson H, Dunn B, Dimond S (2001) Efficacy of topical phenol decontamination strategies on severity of acute phenol chemical burns and dermal absorption: in vitro and in vivo studies in pig skin. Toxicol Ind Health 17: 95–104

[25]  Mutschler E, Geisslinger G (2008) Lehrbuch der Pharmakologie und Toxikologie, Arzneimittelwirkungen, 9. Aufl., Wissensch. Verlagsgesellschaft mbH, Stuttgart

[26]  Pallua N, Noah EM, Radke K (2000) Inhalationstrauma bei Verbrennungen. Intensivmed 37: 284–292

[27]  Pallua N, von Bülow S (2006) Behandlungskonzepte bei Verbrennungen. Der Chirurg 77: 179–192

[28]  Pullin TG, Pinkerton MN, Johnson RV, Kilian DJ (1978) Decontamination of the skin of swine following phenol exposure: a comparison of the relative efficacy of water versus polyethylene glycol/industrial methylated spirits. Toxicol Appl Pharmacol 43: 199–206

[29]  Saydjari R, Abston S, Desai MH, Herndon DN (1986) Chemical burns. J Burn Care Rehabil 7: 404–408

[30]  Topaloglu B, Bicakci U, Tander B (2008) Biochemical and histopathologic effects of omeprazol and vitamin E in rats with corrosive esophageal burns. Pediatr Surg Int 24: 555–560

[31]  Toxin Information Centre of Rheinland-Pfalz and Hessen (2008) Clinical toxicology of the II. Medical Clinic. Johannes-Gutenberg University Mainz

[32]  Vogt PM, Kolokythas P (2007) Innovative Wundtherapie und Hautersatz bei Verbrennungen. Chirurg 78: 335–342

[33]  Warner MA, Harper JV (1985) Cardiac dysrhythmias associated with chemical peeling with phenol. Anesthesiology 62: 366–367

[34]  World Health Organization/International Labour Organization: International Chemical Safety Cards, http://www.ilo.org/public/english/protection/safework/cis/products/icsc/dtasht/_icsc00/icsc0070.htm

[35]  Zargar SA, Kochhar, Metha S (1991) The role of fiberoptic endoscopy in the management of corrosive ingestion and modified endoscopic classification of burns. Gastrointest Endosc 37: 165–167

Correspondence: Leila Kolios, M.D., Clinic for Hand-, Plastic & Reconstructive Surgery – Burn Center – Clinic for Plastic & Hand Surgery at Heidelberg University Hospital, BG Trauma Center Ludwigshafen, Ludwig-Guttmann-Straße 13, 67071 Ludwigshafen, Germany, E-mail: lkolios@bgu-ludwigshafen.de

# Necrotizing and exfoliative diseases of the skin

David A. Sieber, Gerard J. Abood, Richard L. Gamelli

Loyola University Medical Center, Stritch School of Medicine, Chicago, IL, USA

## Introduction

Diseases of the skin are a common problem seen in burn units internationally. These common disorders can be generally classified into two categories: necrotizing soft tissue disorders and exfoliative soft tissue disorders. Oftentimes patients present initially to primary medical centers but ultimately require transfer to tertiary burn centers due to the physiologic derangements associated with the large amount of total body surface area (TBSA) involved as well as for complex dressing care and wound management. As is the case with extensive thermal injuries, patients presenting with exfoliative and necrotizing diseases of the skin present unique challenges to the burn surgeon This chapter will address the relevant pathophysiology, as well as how to promptly diagnose and adequately treat each disease process.

## Necrotizing diseases of the skin

The necrotizing skin disorders include a variety of disorders ranging from severe cellulitis to necrotizing fascitis. If these disorders are not treated properly in a prompt manner, severe disfigurement or even death may be the end result. Prompt transfer of these patients to a burn center is necessary to ensure maximal medical care to the patient.

## Cellulitis

Local cutaneous soft tissue infections commonly occur in what appear to be otherwise healthy patients. These infections may be propagated through minor trauma and are commonly caused by gram-positive organisms such as Staphylococcal and Streptococcal species [1]. These infections may become more severe with major trauma or in patients with compromised immune functions. If not controlled early with adequate antibiotics, these infections may propagate systemically leading to severe sepsis and possibly death [2–4].

Upon presentation, differentiating cellulitis and impetigo from something more serious like necrotizing fascitis is of utmost importance. However, this can often times be a very difficult task [5]. The mainstay of initial treatment for patients presenting with severe cellulitis is the initiation of antibiotic therapy such high dose penicillins [6]. Additional antibiotic coverage is also warranted with Clindamycin, Vancomycin, or another B-lactam antibiotics due to a recent increase in community acquired methicillin resistant Staphylococcus aureus (MRSA) seen in patients presenting with soft tissue infections [7]. Daily wound checks should be instituted as standard of care to ensure improvement in wound appearance and to assess for progression of infection.

## Staphylococcal scalded skin syndrome

Staphylococcal scalded skin syndrome (SSSS, pemphigus neonatorum or Ritter's disease) is used to described a specific skin disorder characterized by a range of blistering skin disorders incited by specific exfoliative toxins from Staphylococcus aureus (S. aureus)[8, 9]. This disorder is most commonly seen in patients lacking the necessary antibodies to S. aureus [10], namely neonates, infants, and toddlers.. The majority of cases are seen in neonates, infants, and toddlers >5 years old, and carries with it overall low mortality rates of approximately 4% [10–15]. While there are reported cases of SSSS in adults it is exceedingly rare. However, it does have a much higher mortality when present, approaching 60%–70% in some reports [13, 15–17].

S. Aureus contains a variety of properties that confer a high degree of virulence. These include: disruption of epithelial barriers, use of antibodies and complement to inhibit opsonization, interference with neutrophil chemotaxis, neutrophil cytolysis, and inactivation of antimicrobial peptides. The exfoliative toxins, more specifically exfoliative toxin-A, released by S. aureus disrupt cell-to-cell adhesions by cleaving desmoglein-1, leading rapid intraepithelial spread of the organism [18–20]. Through the expression of exotoxins, which act as superantigens, the bacteria is also able to induce T-cell activation resulting in ultimate immunosuppression from T-cell anergy. This rapid onset, life-threatening illness is seen is toxic shock syndrome (TSS) and has been shown to be caused by S. aureus toxin-1 (TSST-1) [13, 21].

### Clinical presentation

The clinical course in patients often begins with a prodrome of generalized erythema and fever followed by formation of large, friable blisters within 48 hours of onset of symptoms. Once these blisters rupture, the patient is left with large areas of partial thickness skin loss leading to severe pain, hypothermia, hypoproteinemia, hypovolemia, electrolyte imbalances, and secondary infections (Fig. 1) [8, 15, 22].

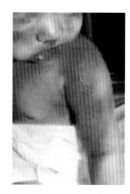

**Fig. 1.** Patient with Staphylococcal scalded skin syndrome (SSSS) with partial thickness skin loss over head, chest, and upper extremity

### Treatment

Initial evaluation of any patient presenting with a skin disorder should include determination of depth of infection as well as whether or not the infection appears to be rapidly spreading [23]. Often times fluid may be culture from ruptured blisters to help in directing further antibiotic therapy [14]. After the initial evaluation is complete, appropriate intravenous antibiotics should be started for empiric coverage of all possible inciting organisms [24]. Children carry more challenge in antibiotic selection, as certain antibiotics have known side effects resulting in growth deformities. Appropriate initial antibiotics include: penicillins, macrolides, and second- and third-generation cephalosporins as most of these may be initiated in an inpatient setting and continued once patient is ready for discharge as an oral alternative [23].

## Autoimmune blistering diseases

This group of heterogenous autoimmune bullous diseases is characterized by autoantibody-mediated desquamation leading to significant morbidity and possible mortality. This class of diseases may be further divided according to the subclass of autoantibodies involved as well as the dermal level affected. Each antibody targets specific structural proteins within the epidermis, basement membrane, and dermis leading to intra- or subdermal blistering.

Subtle differences are present within each subclass of disease that is readily detectable using direct immunofluorescence, immunoblotting, and ELISA [25–31].

## Epidermolysis bullosa acquisita

This is a subclass of the autoimmune blistering diseases which is an IgG mediated process against type VII collagen. One of the major components of the anchoring fibrils which help to form bonds along epithelial basement membrane cells is type VII collagen. The autoantibodies in epidermolysis bullosa acquisita specifically attack the amino-terminal non-collagenous (NC1) domain of the basement membrane leading to formation of tense vesicles and bullae primarily on extensor surfaces and areas of local trauma. A more severe form of the disease may also occur causing generalized erythema, with rapid formation of widespread vesicles and bullae not related to traumatized areas. At times these vesicles and bullae may be hemorrhagic in nature [32, 33]. A rare congenital form of epidermolysis bullosa, with variable severity of disease, is also present in which patients have an inherited defect in basement membrane structural proteins [34]. Treatment should be directed at controlling the autoimmune response through the use of corticosteroids or other immunosuppressants.

## Linear IgA bullous dermatosis

This disease process is driven by either IgA autoantibodies or antibodies formed from drug reactions which act against specific proteins in the basement membrane along the dermal-epidermal junction [35–37]. Any portion of the skin may be involved, most commonly seen over the extensor surfaces and the buttocks, including mucous membranes of the aerodigestive and reproductive tracts [26, 38]. The acquired drug induced form of the disease has been reportedly caused most commonly by exposure to vancomycin, but phenytoin and other medications have also been implicated [39–41]. Initial treatment should begin with dapsone, but due to its ability to cause hemolytic anemia, alternative agents such as sulfapyridine or prednisone may need to be started [26].

## Bullous pemphigoid

Bullous pemphigoid (BP) IgG autoantibodies associate with the basal membrane hemidesmosomes and lead to a separation at the dermal-epidermal junction causing subepidermal desquamation. BP usually is seen in older individuals with onset usually occurring between 60 and 80 years of age. Symptoms begin as a urticarial eruption and gradually progresses over the course of weeks to months into large, tense bullae. Discrete lesions are scattered in the axilla, medial thighs and groin, abdomen, flexor surface of forearm and lower legs (Fig. 2a and 2b). There have been reports of mucosal surface involvement in 10–25% of patients. Pemphigoid usually has a more prolonged course and often times spontaneous remission. Histologically, BP is characterized by the presence of IgG autoantibodies against specific hemidesmosome autoantigens, BP230 and BP180 [26, 30, 42].

## Pemphigus vulgaris/Pemphigus foliaceus

In pemphigus vulgaris (PV) IgG autoantibodies bind to autoantigens located on keratinocyte desmosomes, causing intraepidermal blistering. PV almost always displays mucosal involvement, with the disease beginning in the oral mucosa, soon followed by painful blistering of the skin. Pem-

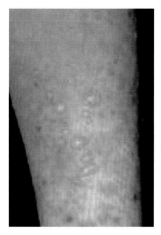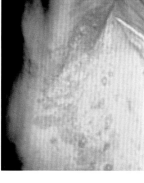

**Fig. 2a and 2b.** Forearm of patient with bullous pemphigoid demonstrating characteristic lesions. Axilla of patient with bullous pemphigoid

phigus foliaceus (PF) has a similar presentation to PV except that it does not display mucosal involvement. These diseases differ in that PF autoantibodies bind to only desmoglein 1 (Dsg1), while PV autoantibodies bind to desmoglein 3 (Dsg3) or both Dsg1 and Dsg3 [43].

Commonly affected areas of these diseases include: conjunctiva, esophagus, labia, vagina, cervix, penis, urethra, and anus. There are two tests which are suggestive of, but not diagnostic of PV/PF. The first is Nikolsky's sign in which when pressure is applied to seemingly normal skin, it induces epidermal detachment. The second is the Asboe-Hansen sign where, when vertical pressure is applied to a blister, it causes lateral extension of epidermal detachment into normal skin [27]. There is believed to be a genetic predisposition to PV due to the identification of common major histocompatibility complexes (MHC) class II molecules, DR4 and DRw6. Likewise, PV has been found to be associated with other autoimmune diseases such as myasthenia gravis and the presence of thymomas. If not treated promptly, the loss of natural mucosal barriers often times leads to sepsis with high mortality rates [26, 30, 42].

## Diagnosis

For diagnosis of these diseases a tissue biopsy is needed for immuno testing. Two punch biopsies should be taken, the first involving the margin of a bullae with the biopsy containing half normal and half affected tissue. The second biopsy should be taken of normal skin located approximately 2 cm from the edge of a bullae. These samples should then be sent immediately to pathology for further examination.

## Treatment

The mainstay treatment of both diseases is through corticosteroids alone or in combination with other immunosuppressants. In patients with BP, remission of disease has been demonstrated to occur within 1.5–5 years of beginning treatment. For those patients who have contraindications to corticosteroids or for those whom conventional therapy has been unsuccessful, plasmapheresis has been shown to be an effective treatment option [26, 44, 45].

## Necrotizing fasciitis

Necrotizing fasciitis (NF) is a severe, rapidly progressing soft tissue infection involving the superficial fascial layers of the extremities, abdomen, and/or perineum, which if not identified and treated rapidly may have fatal outcomes. Estimated survival rates in the literature range from 50–96% [46–48]. Higher survival rates are directly dependent on immediate diagnosis, swift surgical debridement, and intensive critical care. However, if a patient is able to survive the acute illness, there is evidence to suggest that these same patients have a decreased long-term survival due to various infectious processes [49]. Other factors shown to significantly increase mortality are age >1 or >60 years old, history of intravenous drug use, presence of cancer, renal insufficiency/failure, heart failure, positive blood cultures, trunk or perineal involvement, peripheral vascular disease, and positive wound cultures for β-Streptococcus or anaerobes [50].

Group A Streptococcus is the mostly commonly isolated bacteria cultured from patients with NF, however the majority (>70%) of cases are polymicrobial in nature, containing Gram-positive, Gram-negative, aerobic, and anaerobic bacteria [5, 51, 52]. The pathogenesis of NF is still not completely understood, but it is believed that the initial inciting infection produces local toxins that subsequently damage local fascia by causing vasoconstriction of blood vessels supplying the cutaneous fascial spaces [50, 51]. This now avascular tissue serves as an ideal medium to support further bacterial growth and propagation leading to additional vascular thrombosis and tissue destruction. It is believed that these rapidly spreading infections occur due to a synergist effect between β-hemolytic Streptococcus and the other microbes present in the tissue [53].

## Clinical presentation

The inciting event leading to NF may be traumatic in nature or seemingly otherwise harmless events such as minor ecchymosis or erythema, with rapid progression of disease along superficial facial planes [5, 51]. When a patient presents with cellulitis or impetigo, it is imperative to closely monitor erythema and induration with a high index of suspicion for advancement of disease. One of the main symptoms that is able to differentiate NF from simple cellulitis is pain out of proportion to degree of injury [50, 51]. The patients will present early with erythema, few blisters and intense pain on palpation of involved areas. Other non-specific symptoms may also be present on initial exam such as malaise, GI distress, and fevers. If lesions are observed and the patient does have NF, they will quickly transform from erythematous lesions into larger blisters, then to large areas of edematous, cellulitic tissue with central areas of dusky, necrotic tissue (Fig. 3.) [50, 51].

Initial evaluation should begin with a thorough history and physical, focusing on predisposing factors to NF such as: immunocompromise, vascular disease, and systemic diseases such as diabetes [51]. Laboratory data is oftentimes unspecific in diagnosis of NF, although one study states that serum Na >135 mmol/L and white blood cell count (WBC) >15,400 may be suggestive of active NF on initial presentation [54]. If a patient presents later in the disease course they are likely to have findings more consistent with sepsis: high fevers, hypotension, tachycardia, mental status changes, and WBC >25,000 [50]. Diagnostic imaging such as CT or MRI may be considered looking for edema or air but must be weighed against the time delay needed to complete the testing. A quick bedside maneuver that has been described is the "finger test". This is performed by anesthetizing the skin overlying the tissue in question. A 2 cm incision is then made and carried down to the deep fascia. In the presence of NF there is usually a lack of bleeding with dissection and an expression of "dishwater" fluid. A finger is then inserted down to the deep fascia and if one is able to dissect free the overlaying subcutaneous tissue from the deep fascia with little to no resistance, this is considered a positive "finger test" and that patient should be taken to the operating immediately for surgical debridement [50].

## Management

Surgical debridement is the primary mode of definitive management in NF. Patients presenting to non burn centers for initial care will likely need eventual transfer to a burn center for definitive management. One study reported that 87% of patients who pres-

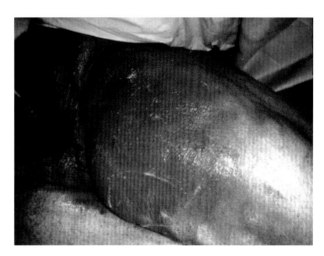

**Fig. 3.** Patient with necrotizing fasciitis of the lower extremity on presentation

ented with a diagnosis of NF were definitively treated at a burn center most likely due to severity of illness and acuity of care [55]. It has been shown that through early referral to burn centers for care, patients have increased rates of survival with improved patient outcomes [56, 57]. With rapid diagnosis, wide surgical debridement, and intensive critical care management survival rates may be as high as 83% with 54% of survivors able to return home with no further rehabilitation needs [58].

Once the diagnosis is made, patients should be started on broad-spectrum antibiotics and taken to the operating room. In the operating room wide debridement must be carried out until the skin and soft tissue can no longer be separated off of the underlying deep fascia and until healthy bleeding occurs along wound margins. Even if undermined skin appears to be macroscopically healthy, one study found that microscopically this tissue was still found to have early thrombosis which would lead to eventual full thickness necrosis [50]. It is better to perform an initial wide debridement then leave thrombotic tissue behind, allowing for further spread of disease (Fig. 4a and 4b). Wounds should be check daily on rounds to assess for the need for further surgical debridement. Patients should return to the operating room as often as needed to ensure no additional progression of disease. One report estimated that patients require approximately 4 operative procedures before wounds are able to be definitively closed [59].

467

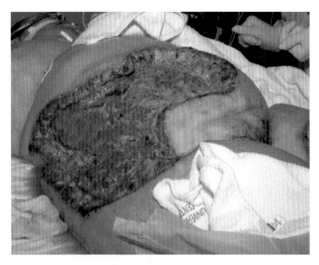

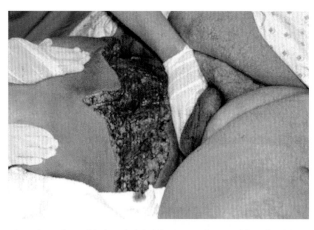

**Fig. 4b.** After wide local debridement of necrotizing fascitis, tissue appears healthy at wound edges with no signs of necrosis, but still with good active bleeding

**Fig. 4a.** Postoperative photo of patient with necrotizing fasciitis after wide surgical debridement of abdominal wall

Equally important as the initial management of these patients is their postoperative care and nutrition. The main post-operative principles are continued resuscitation and critical care, management of the wound, continued therapeutic coverage with broad-spectrum antibiotics, and initiation of aggressive nutritional management. Multiple daily dressing changes should be performed until the wound bed is clean and free of debris. If at any time there is question about the viability of tissue, the patient should be taken back down to the operating room for further surgical debridement. Once dressing changes are completed, wound vacuum assisted closure (VAC) devices assist in formation of granulation tissue and prepare the wound bed for eventual skin grafting (Fig. 5) [60]. Antibiotics should be continued for a complete course of treatment and until signs of systemic and local infection have resolved. There is some debate regarding the efficacy of hyperbaric oxygen in these patients. Recent studies have shown hyperbaric oxygen to not be beneficial in treatment of NF [61].

As long as there are no contraindications to enteral feedings, a feeding tube should be inserted with feeds initiated as soon as possible. For patients who would not tolerate enteral feedings due to an ileus, obstruction, or other mechanical cause, a central venous line should be inserted and total parenteral nutrition (TPN) started. These patients have profoundly accelerated metabolic demands due to the stress of sepsis and surgery. It is estimated that their basal energy expenditure (BEE) is approximately 60%–200% above normal, requiring an increase in caloric feedings of up to 124% basal rate [62]. Weekly nutritional labs should be followed and feedings adjusted as needed to improve protein calorie malnutrition caused by the disease process.

## Fournier's Gangrene

Fournier's Gangrene (FG) is a subclass of necrotizing soft tissue infections with similar etiology to NF involving the soft tissue of the genitals and perineum. Treatment for this disease is the same as it is with NF; rapid diagnosis with wide surgical debridement and broad-spectrum antibiotics. Predisposing factors identified in patients presenting with FG are the presence of diabetes, immunosuppression, and morbid obesity (BMI >40)[63]. Poor prognostic factors associated with FG are chronic renal failure, length of duration of symptoms prior to presentation, TBSA involvement >6%, presence of shock on admission, and female gender [63, 64]. Postoperative care for patients with FG is very similar to those patients with NF. One main difference however is that patients with FG may require fecal or urinary diversion through the placement of a suprapubic catheter or an ostomy in order to allow for wound healing. These patients also require aggressive wound care, nutritional management, and critical care usually best provided at a burn center.

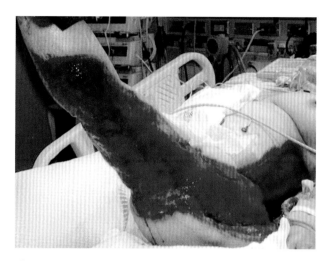

**Fig. 5.** After wound VAC therapy, a patient with necrotizing fasciitis demonstrates healthy granulation tissue reading for skin grafting

## Synergistic necrotizing cellulitis

Synergistic necrotizing cellulitis (SNC) is a variant of necrotizing fasciitis that extends beyond the fascial borders causing myonecrosis and is most commonly seen in immunocompromised patients or those with chronic diseases [65]. This disease process is perpetuated through a symbiotic relationship between aerobic Gram-negative and facultative anaerobes. Cultures from these patients are usually polymicrobial with the most commonly isolated organisms being: Clostridia, anaerobic Streptococcus, and Bacteroides with synergistic bacteria including aerobes such as E. coli, Klebsiella, Proteus, and Pseudomonas [66, 67].

Patients commonly present with small superficial ulcerations that drain a malodorous reddish brown fluid. Ulcerations are surrounded by varying degrees of skin erythema and necrosis with approximately 25% of patients presenting with subcutaneous emphysema. Affected areas are exquisitely tender to palpation despite the occasional benign appearance of the overlying lesions. A major difference between SNC and NF is that many patients with SNC may have experience some of the above symptoms for 2 weeks or more before seeking medical attention. SNC tends to have a more prolonged and indolent course when compared to the rapid onset and quickly progressing disease process seen in NF [67]. Treatment for these patients however is similar to those with NF, including care in a burn center, cor-

rection of electrolyte and hemodynamic abnormalities, prompt initiation of broad-spectrum antibiotics and wide surgical debridement [65–67]. Because of its slower clinical course, if the SNC patient does show a clinical response with the initiation of antibiotics, then conservative treatment may continue as long as positive clinical progress continues; any signs of worsening disease mandates surgical debridement.

## Purpura fulminans

Purpura Fulminans (PF) is another necrotizing disease of the soft tissue characterized by widespread intravascular thrombosis of the skin with eventual hemorrhagic infarction, septicemia, and disseminated intravascular coagulation (DIC) occurring after acute infections [52, 68]. When associated with adrenal hemorrhage, it is also known as Waterhouse-Friderichsen syndrome [69]. It is believed that PF is initiated through the release of specific endotoxins from inciting bacteria leading to a cascade of septic shock with associated DIC and full thickness skin loss [70]. An additional aspect of the disease pathogenesis is associated with a relative genetic deficiency of Protein C and/or Protein S, leading to vascular thrombosis from an inherent coagulopathy [71–73]. Three types of PF have been identified: inherited (neonatal) PF from abnormalities with Protein C/S, acute infectious PF, and idiopathic PF [52, 74]. The immaturity of the neonatal hepatic system leads to a relative deficiency of Protein C/S as birth, placing them at an increased risk of PF [72, 74].

The onset of this disease commonly occurs after acute bacterial infections and usually leads to full thickness skin loss with the likely need for extremity amputations [75]. Neisseria meningitidis is the causative bacteria most commonly seen in infants and pediatrics while the adults are affected most often by Streptococcus species [69, 76]. There are reports of PF occurring as a result of other infections such has Haemophilus influenzae, varicella, and Legionella pneumonia [77–79].

### Clinical presentation

Patients will often be in the process of recovering from a benign infection when they develop a petechial rash that rapidly progresses to full thickness skin loss. Oftentimes, patients will present with fevers and non-specific flu-like symptoms with development of systemic purpura within 12 to 96 hours of onset of symptoms [79]. Over the course of the next few days the rash will progress to symmetrical, ecchymotic skin lesions involving the lower extremities [74]. Mortality rates are as high as 33–40% in some reports with approximately 90% of patients requiring full thickness skin grafting or amputation at some point during their hospitalization [69, 79]. Once recognized, patients should be transferred to a burn center for definitive care [76, 80, 81].

## Management

Management consists of aggressive fluid resuscitation, supportive care through the use of vasopressors and ventilators, intense wound management, systemic anticoagulation and prompt initiation of broad-spectrum antibiotics. Some studies reported success in disease treatment with administration of activated protein C [82, 83]. The full thickness wounds in patients with PF are similar to those seen in patients with full thickness burn wounds which has led many burn centers to adopt a similar treatment algorithm for patients with NF including serial staged surgical debridement with allografting and full thickness skin grafting once patients have been adequately resuscitated [76, 83–85]. Due to the degree of resuscitative [65–67] volume delivered to these patients on admission, some studies support the implementation of early fasciotomies to increase chances of limb salvage [69, 76]. Due to the extent of skin loss in patients with PF, nutritional optimization is also paramount in these patients to allow for wound healing. These patient's long-term care is similar to that of NF, requiring long-term nutrition, psychosocial, physical and occupational therapy. As many of these patients will be discharged with physical deformities, close follow-up care with a multidisciplinary team is absolutely required.

## Exfoliative diseases of the skin

While exfoliative diseases of the skin are believed to originate from a similar pathologic mechanism, the degree of clinical morbidity and mortality associate with each can vary significantly. In general, these diseases are typically precipitated by a either a specific drug or metabolite or a viral infection leading to a highly variable degree of soft tissue involvement with sloughing of skin at the dermoepidermal junction, which tends to be the hallmark feature of this disease entity [86]. It is believed that this disease process is the result of a hypersensitive, deregulated immune reaction to the inciting drugs due to an inherent inability to detoxify drug-reactive metabolites [87–89].

The two most common exfoliative diseases of the skin encountered are Stevens-Johnson Syndrome (SJS) and Toxic Epidermal Necrolysis (TEN). Both SJS and TENS are severe, acute, potentially life-threatening diseases characterized by extensive epidermal detachment and erosions of the mucous membranes. Inciting factors are innumerable, with viral infections and drugs generally listed as the most common culprits in SJS and TENS, respectively. Nonetheless, prompt referral and transfer to a tertiary burn center is encouraged as the mainstay in treatment.

### Stevens-Johnson syndrome

Stevens-Johnson syndrome (SJS) is an immuno-complex mediated hypersensitivity complex first described in 1922 [90]. Presently, most experts agree that SJS and toxic epidermal necrolysis (TEN) are different manifestations of the same disease. Stevens-Johnson Syndrome (SJS) is a rare condition, with a reported incidence of around 2.6 to 6.1 cases per million people per year. While the majority of cases of Stevens-Johnson syndrome is associated with a hypersensitivity to certain drugs, viral infections and malignancies have also been implicated in the pathogenesis of SJS [91]. Certain infections have been noted to have an increased associated incidence, including herpes simplex virus, influenza, mumps, cat-scratch fever, histoplasmosis, Epstein-Barr virus and mycoplasma pneumoniae [92].

As such, SJS and TEN tend to be considered in the differential diagnosis when presented with a significant desquamating process of the skin and mucous membranes. While minor presentations may occur, significant involvement of oral, nasal, eye, vaginal, urethral, GI, and lower respiratory tract mucous membranes may develop in the course of the illness. Although several classification schemes have been reported, the simplest breakdown depends on the total body surface area involved [90]:

1. Stevens-Johnson syndrome – A "minor form of TEN," with less than 10 % body surface area (BSA) detachment
2. Overlapping Stevens-Johnson syndrome/toxic epidermal necrolysis (SJS/TEN) – Detachment of 10–30 % BSA
3. Toxic epidermal necrolysis – Detachment of more than 30 % BSA

as is the case with TEN, the clinical features typically associated with SJS includes a prodrome of 2–3 days characterized by fever, cough, sore throat, and general malaise before the cutaneous manifestations of SJS become apparent [93]. The acute phase, which is typically associated with the first 8–12 days, is characterized by an acute macular exanthema, with rapidly spreading necrosis of the mucus membranes at first, followed by similar events in the epidermis, e. g. the skin.

Prompt referral to a tertiary burn care center is highly encouraged and has been demonstrated to improve survival in extensive cases of SJS and TENS. Given the degree of overlap in clinical manifestation, SJS is treated in much the same way as TENS. As such, diagnosis and treatment strategies will be discussed in the TENS section.

## Toxic epidermal necrolysis

Ruskin first described a condition similar to TEN in 1948, and in 1956 Lyell reported 4 more patients who had an acute rash followed by skin detachment and mucus membrane involvement [94, 95]. While clinically similar in presentation to staphylococcal scalded skin syndrome (SSSS), i. e. sloughing of epidermal sheets, SSSS and TEN can be differentiated from a histologic perspective, which underlies the importance of the skin biopsy at the time of presentation. In SSSS, there is superficial detachment involving the upper epidermal layers, whereas in TEN there is pan-epidermal necrosis. Recognition of SSSS is as important as treatment considerations are distinct, including the use of antibiotics, rather than viewing antibiotics as causing the disease, as is often the case

for TEN. On the other hand, the histologic difference between Steven-Johnson syndrome (SJS) and TEN is less pronounced. While SJS and TEN are believed to be the same disorder of different severities, with SJS representing an attenuated form of TEN, a significant proportion of SJS cases are not associated with drug ingestion. Despite a similar clinical presentation and course to TEN, the mortality associated with SJS ranges between 1 % and 3 % [96, 97].

The estimated annual incidence of TEN is reported between 0.4 and 1.3 cases per million per year, and can occur in all age groups, including newborns and the elderly [98–100]. Those patients with HIV and AIDS have been found to be at approximately 1000 fold increase of developing TEN when compared to the normal population [101]. Reported mortality varies from 30–50 %, with the primary cause of death being infection and multi-system organ failure [102]. Antibiotics, NSAIDS and analgesics are the most common drugs identified in cases of TEN, with anticonvulsants reported in 18 % of drug induced cases of TEN [88, 103–105].

## Clinical presentation

The clinical features typically associated with TEN include a prodrome of 2–3 days characterized by fever, cough, sore throat, and general malaise before the cutaneous manifestations of TEN become apparent [93]. The acute phase, which is typically associated with the first 8–12 days, is characterized by an acute macular exanthema, with rapidly spreading necrosis of the mucus membranes at first, followed by similar events in the epidermis, e. g. the skin [106]. At the time of skin involvement, Nikolsky sign is universally present – epidermal separation induced by gentle lateral pressure on the skin surface [107]. Mucous membranes, including conjunctival, pharyngeal, tracheal and esophageal, are involved in nearly all reported cases. Typically, the dermis remains undamaged, and dermatologic recovery takes 1 to 3 weeks, depending on the extent of skin detachment (Fig. 6). However, mucosal lesions, including the ocular manifestations of TEN, generally require a longer time to heal [108].

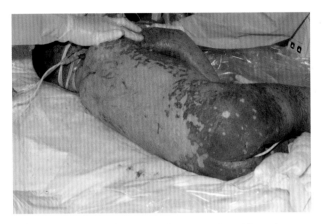

**Fig. 6.** Patient with TENS with characteristic epidermal sloughing at areas of high friction

## Diagnosis

The diagnosis of TEN can often times be made clinically, but differentiating TEN from SJS remains a point of contention. While several proposed diagnostic criteria for SJS and TEN exist, authors do not agree on a universally accepted model. Pathologic examination of perilesional skin can be used to support or exclude a clinical diagnosis of TEN. Characteristic histologic features include extensive keratinocyte death through the apoptotic pathway with separation of the epidermis from the dermis at the dermoepidermal junction. A paucicellular infiltrate, in which macrophages and dendrocytes predominate, has been commonly described. TEN has been characterized immunopathologically by an increased ratio of dermal dendrocytes to dermal lymphocytes, in contrast to the opposite pattern seen in EM where lymphocytes predominate [109].

The mortality associated with TEN ranges from 30–50%, which is significantly higher than episodes of SJS (1–3%). The primary cause of death in TEN is infection and multi-system organ failure. As in burn patients, age and extent of skin detachment are still considered major prognostic factors. However, after controlling for extent of skin detachment, a diagnosis of TEN generally carries a worse prognosis. The SCORTEN (severity-of-illness score for TEN) is a validated model of disease severity which has been shown to accurately predict mortality from TEN based on a seven point checklist [110]. Table 1(a) and (b) demonstrate the seven variables identified

and predicted mortality, respectively. The SCORTEN value is calculated by giving one point to each of the variables present in the first 24h after admission. However, given the lack of consensus on what constitutes a standardized protocol of care, there still remains significant heterogeneity in the treatment of TEN patients [111].

## Treatment

Once the diagnosis of SJS or TEN is suspected, prompt withdrawal of potential causative drug(s) should be the priority, as this particular course of action is one therapeutic technique that has been shown to decrease mortality and improve prognosis [112]. In general, any medication initiated within 3–4 weeks prior to the onset of symptoms should be suspected, and should be strictly avoided, especially in the course of treatment. Principles guiding the care of treatment of SJS and TEN patients are similar to those in extensive thermal burns [113]. The treatment of patients with extensive SJS or TEN is most appropriately provided in intensive care units, or more specifically, burn centers, where staff

**Table 1a.** The SCORTEN scoring system

| SCORTEN | Variables |
|---------|-----------|
| 1. | Extent of Epidermal detachment > 10% |
| 2. | Age > 40 years |
| 3. | Heart rate > 120/min |
| 4. | Bicarbonate > 20 mmol/L |
| 5. | Serum urea nitrogen > 28 mg/dL |
| 6. | Glucose > 252 mg/dL |
| 7. | History of Malignancy |

**Table 1b.** Predicting mortality in TEN based on SCORTEN

| SCORTEN VALUE | PREDICTED MORTALITY RATE (%) |
|---------------|------------------------------|
| 0–1 | 3.2% |
| 2 | 12.1% |
| 3 | 32.4% |
| 4 | 62.2% |
| 5 | 85.5% |
| > 6 | 95% |

is familiar with managing complex epidermal loss and associated complications, i. e. mechanical ventilation, pressor support and wound care [114, 115]. Given the current confusion regarding the pathophysiologic mechanisms responsible for SJS and TENS, it should not be surprising that therapeutic approaches are diverse and relatively ineffective. Presently, there is a lack of consensus on specific treatments for SJS and TEN. As such, patients are treated symptomatically and supportively. Supportive therapies include attention and protection of eroded mucosal surfaces, prevention, early detection and treatment of infection, nutritional support and monitoring of fluid and electrolyte balances.

Given the low incidence of TEN, randomized controlled trials comparing potential therapeutics are rare. Recent therapeutic interventions in TEN are based on the proposed molecular mechanisms involved in the clinical manifestations of TEN, i. e. apoptosis of keratinocytes. As such, the majority of reports in the literature involve single case observations or small, uncontrolled studies. To date, only one prospective, randomized-controlled clinical trial has been reported in the literature [116]. Theoretically, effective treatment strategies should focus on halting keratinocyte apoptosis, either by acting on the keratinocytes directly, or the effectors mediating the process. Table 2 offers a mechanistic overview of reported therapeutic efforts investigated. Needless to say, treatment with corticosteroids remains controversial – early retrospective studies suggested that corticosteroids increased hospital stays and complication rates. As such, corticosteroids are not recommended in the management of either SJS or TEN.

Of particular interest in the treatment of TEN is the use of IVIg. The in-vitro studies of Viard et al. showed that up-regulation of keratinocyte FasL expression is the critical trigger for keratinocyte destruction during TEN[117]. Furthermore, this induced apoptosis could be completely abrogated by the addition of pooled IVIg, which contained naturally occurring anti-FasL antibody. Others speculate that IVIg may also contain products involved in the inhibition of inflammatory cytokines. Following the in-vitro study, the group demonstrated the efficacy in 10 consecutive TEN patients with IVIg doses ranging from 0.2 to 0.75 g/kg/day with marked clinical improvement. Treatment of TEN with IVIg has been reported in several case studies with wide variation in patients and treatment protocols. As a consequence, results have been inconsistent and, at times, conflicting. Several case series support the use of IVIg, suggesting that mortality rates are improved in IVIg treated cohorts [118–121]. Other groups have demonstrated no improvement in outcome [122–124]. Given such conflicting results, it is difficult to draw a conclusion on the efficacy of IVIg in the treatment of TEN. Much of the conflicting results may be attributable to the inconsistency of pooled IVIg lots. Several questions remain unanswered, including what is the optimal neutralizing titer that is necessary to halt the progression, and, more importantly, what is the true target that is affected with pooled IVIg. Well designed prospective studies are needed to address whether IVIg does improve outcome.

**Table 2.** Proposed mechanism and medications attempted in the treatment of TEN

| Proposed mechanism | Medication/Intervention | Level of support |
|---|---|---|
| Inhibition of circulating cytokines, mediators | ▶ Plasmapheresis<br>▶ Anti-TNF antibodies | Case series<br>Case reports |
| Direct Inhibition of keratinocyte apoptosis – Fas/FasL | ▶ IVIg<br>▶ High-dose glucocorticoids | Case series, retrospective reviews<br>Laboratory evidence |
| Inhibition of T-cell activation | ▶ Glucocorticoids<br>▶ Cyclophosphamide<br>▶ Cyclosporin A | Case series, retrospective reviews<br>Case series, retrospective reviews<br>Case series, retrospective reviews |
| Modulation of TNF-α activity | ▶ Thalidomide<br>▶ Pentoxifylline | Prospective, randomized trial<br>Case series, retrospective reviews |

## Conclusion

Necrotizing and exfoliative diseases of the skin are commonly encountered by physicians across multiple medical specialties and remain a diagnostic challenge. When encountered, diagnosis needs to be made as rapidly as possible with swift transfer to burn centers for definitive care. Treatment modalities must be based around a multidisciplinary team approach to patient management. With prompt diagnosis, local wound care, and aggressive nutritional support patients have an increased likelihood of meaningful long-term survival and recovery.

## References

[1] Howell ER, Phillips CM (2007) Cutaneous manifestations of Staphylococcus aureus disease. Skinmed 6(6): 274–279

[2] Bisno AL (1984) Cutaneous infections: microbiologic and epidemiologic considerations. Am J Med 76(5A): 172–179

[3] Chan HL (1983) Bacterial infections of the skin. I: primary and secondary infections. Ann Acad Med Singapore 12(1): 92–97

[4] Connor MP, Gamelli R (2009) Challenges of cellulitis in a lymphedematous extremity: a case report. Cases J 2: 9377

[5] Fontes RA, Jr, Ogilvie CM, Miclau T (2000) Necrotizing soft-tissue infections. J Am Acad Orthop Surg 8(3): 151–158

[6] Bang RL, Gang RK, Sanyal SC, Mokaddas EM, Lari AR (1999) Beta-haemolytic Streptococcus infection in burns. Burns 25(3): 242–246

[7] Stevens DL (2009) Treatments for skin and soft-tissue and surgical site infections due to MDR Gram-positive bacteria. J Infect 59 [Suppl 1]: S32–39

[8] Mueller E, Haim M, Petnehazy T, Acham-Roschitz B, Trop M (2010) An innovative local treatment for staphylococcal scalded skin syndrome. Eur J Clin Microbiol Infect Dis 29(7): 893–897

[9] Satyapal S, Mehta J, Dhurat R, Jerajani H, Vaidya M (2002) Staphylococcal scalded skin syndrome. Indian J Pediatr 69(10): 899–901

[10] Simpson C (2003) The management of staphylococcal scalded skin syndrome in infants. Nurs Times 99(42): 59–61

[11] Elias PM, Fritsch P, Epstein EH (1977) Staphylococcal scalded skin syndrome. Clinical features, pathogenesis, and recent microbiological and biochemical developments. Arch Dermatol 113(2): 207–219

[12] Mirabile R, Weiser M, Barot LR, Brown AS (1986) Staphylococcal scalded-skin syndrome. Plast Reconstr Surg 77(5): 752–756

[13] Patel GK (2004) Treatment of staphylococcal scalded skin syndrome. Exp Rev Anti Infect Ther 2(4): 575–587

[14] Johnston GA (2004) Treatment of bullous impetigo and the staphylococcal scalded skin syndrome in infants. Exp Rev Anti Infect Ther 2(3): 439–446

[15] Patel GK, Finlay AY (2003) Staphylococcal scalded skin syndrome: diagnosis and management. Am J Clin Dermatol 4(3): 165–175

[16] Decleire PY, Blondiaux G, Delaere B, Glupczynski Y (2004) Staphylococcal scalded skin syndrome in an adult. Acta Clin Belg 59(6): 365–368

[17] Oyake S, Oh-i T, Koga M (2001) Staphylococcal scalded skin syndrome in a healthy adult. J Dermatol 28(3): 145–148

[18] Ladhani S (2003) Understanding the mechanism of action of the exfoliative toxins of Staphylococcus aureus. FEMS Immunol Med Microbiol 39(2): 181–189

[19] Hanakawa Y, Schechter NM, Lin C et al (2002) Molecular mechanisms of blister formation in bullous impetigo and staphylococcal scalded skin syndrome. J Clin Invest 110(1): 53–60

[20] Amagai M, Matsuyoshi N, Wang ZH, Andl C, Stanley JR (2000) Toxin in bullous impetigo and staphylococcal scalded-skin syndrome targets desmoglein 1. Nat Med 6(11): 1275–1277

[21] Iwatsuki K, Yamasaki O, Morizane S, Oono T (2006) Staphylococcal cutaneous infections: invasion, evasion and aggression. J Dermatol Sci 42(3): 203–214

[22] Blyth M, Estela C, Young AE (2008) Severe staphylococcal scalded skin syndrome in children. Burns 34(1): 98–103

[23] Hedrick J (2003) Acute bacterial skin infections in pediatric medicine: current issues in presentation and treatment. Paediatr Drugs 5 [Suppl 1]: 35–46

[24] Sharma S, Verma KK (2001) Skin and soft tissue infection. Indian J Pediatr 68 [Suppl 3]: S46–50

[25] Kasperkiewicz M, Schmidt E (2009) Current treatment of autoimmune blistering diseases. Curr Drug Discov Technol 6(4): 270–280

[26] Patricio P, Ferreira C, Gomes MM, Filipe P (2009) Autoimmune bullous dermatoses: a review. Ann N Y Acad Sci 1173: 203–210

[27] Cunha PR, Barraviera SR (2009) Autoimmune bullous dermatoses. An Bras Dermatol 84(2): 111–124

[28] Kabir AK, Kamal M, Choudhury AM (2008) Clinicopathological correlation of blistering diseases of skin. Bangladesh Med Res Counc Bull 34(2): 48–53

[29] Olasz EB, Yancey KB (2008) Bullous pemphigoid and related subepidermal autoimmune blistering diseases. Curr Dir Autoimmun 10: 141–166

[30] Lessey E, Li N, Diaz L, Liu Z (2008) Complement and cutaneous autoimmune blistering diseases. Immunol Res 41(3): 223–232

[31] McCuin JB, Hanlon T, Mutasim DF (2006) Autoimmune bullous diseases: diagnosis and management. Dermatol Nurs 18(1): 20–25

[32] Xu L, Chen M, Peng J et al (1998) Molecular cloning and characterization of a cDNA encoding canine type VII collagen non-collagenous (NC1) domain, the target antigen of autoimmune disease epidermolysis bullosa acquisita (EBA). Biochim Biophys Acta 1408(1): 25–34

[33] Woodley DT, Gammon WR (1989) Epidermolysis bullosa acquista. Immunol Ser 46: 547–563

[34] Puvabanditsin S, Garrow E, Samransamraujkit R, Lopez LA, Lambert WC (1997) Epidermolysis bullosa associated with congenital localized absence of skin, fetal abdominal mass, and pyloric atresia. Pediatr Dermatol 14(5): 359–362

[35] Horvath B, Niedermeier A, Podstawa E et al (2010) IgA autoantibodies in the pemphigoids and linear IgA bullous dermatosis. Exp Dermatol 19(7): 648–653

[36] Kharfi M, Khaled A, Karaa A et al (2010) Linear IgA bullous dermatosis: the more frequent bullous dermatosis of children. Dermatol Online J 16(1): 2

[37] Colombo M, Volpini S, Orini S et al (2008) [Linear IgA bullous dermatosis: the importance of a correct differential diagnosis]. Minerva Pediatr 60(3): 351–353

[38] Akin MA, Gunes T, Akyn L et al (2009) A newborn with bullous pemphigoid associated with linear IgA bullous dermatosis. Acta Dermatovenerol Alp Panonica Adriat 18(2): 66–70

[39] Onodera H, Mihm MC, Jr, Yoshida A, Akasaka T (2005) Drug-induced linear IgA bullous dermatosis. J Dermatol 32(9): 759–764

[40] Khan I, Hughes R, Curran S, Marren P (2009) Drug-associated linear IgA disease mimicking toxic epidermal necrolysis. Clin Exp Dermatol 34(6): 715–717

[41] Navi D, Michael DJ, Fazel N (2006) Drug-induced linear IgA bullous dermatosis. Dermatol Online J 12(5): 12

[42] Knudson RM, Kalaaji AN, Bruce AJ (2010) The management of mucous membrane pemphigoid and pemphigus. Dermatol Ther 23(3): 268–280

[43] Mahoney MG, Wang Z, Rothenberger K et al (1999) Explanations for the clinical and microscopic localization of lesions in pemphigus foliaceus and vulgaris. J Clin Invest 103(4): 461–468

[44] Mazzi G, Raineri A, Zanolli FA et al (2003) Plasmapheresis therapy in pemphigus vulgaris and bullous pemphigoid. Transfus Apher Sci 28(1): 13–18

[45] Bickle K, Roark TR, Hsu S (2002) Autoimmune bullous dermatoses: a review. Am Fam Physician 65(9): 1861–1870

[46] Canoso JJ, Barza M (1993) Soft tissue infections. Rheum Dis Clin North Am 19(2): 293–309

[47] Ryssel H, Germann G, Kloeters O et al (2010) Necrotizing fasciitis of the extremities: 34 cases at a single centre over the past 5 years. Arch Orthop Trauma Surg 130(12): 1515–1522

[48] Patino JF, Castro D (1991) Necrotizing lesions of soft tissues: a review. World J Surg 15(2): 235–239

[49] Light TD, Choi KC, Thomsen TA et al (2010) Long-term outcomes of patients with necrotizing fasciitis. J Burn Care Res 31(1): 93–99

[50] Childers BJ, Potyondy LD, Nachreiner R et al (2002) Necrotizing fasciitis: a fourteen-year retrospective study of 163 consecutive patients. Am Surg 68(2): 109–116

[51] McGee EJ (2005) Necrotizing fasciitis: review of pathophysiology, diagnosis, and treatment. Crit Care Nurs Q 28(1): 80–84

[52] Edlich RF, Winters KL, Woodard CR, Britt LD, Long WB, 3rd (2005) Massive soft tissue infections: necrotizing fasciitis and purpura fulminans. J Long Term Eff Med Implants 15(1): 57–65

[53] Seal DV, Kingston D (1988) Streptococcal necrotizing fasciitis: development of an animal model to study its pathogenesis. Br J Exp Pathol 69(6): 813–831

[54] Wall DB, Klein SR, Black S, de Virgilio C (2000) A simple model to help distinguish necrotizing fasciitis from nonnecrotizing soft tissue infection. J Am Coll Surg 191(3): 227–231

[55] Endorf FW, Klein MB, Mack CD, Jurkovich GJ, Rivara FP (2008) Necrotizing soft-tissue infections: differences in patients treated at burn centers and non-burn centers. J Burn Care Res 29(6): 933–938

[56] Redman DP, Friedman B, Law E, Still JM (2003) Experience with necrotizing fasciitis at a burn care center. South Med J 96(9): 868–870

[57] Barillo DJ, McManus AT, Cancio LC, Sofer A, Goodwin CW (2003) Burn center management of necrotizing fasciitis. J Burn Care Rehabil 24(3): 127–132

[58] Endorf FW, Supple KG, Gamelli RL (2005) The evolving characteristics and care of necrotizing soft-tissue infections. Burns 31(3): 269–273

[59] Faucher LD, Morris SE, Edelman LS, Saffle JR (2001) Burn center management of necrotizing soft-tissue surgical infections in unburned patients. Am J Surg 182(6): 563–569

[60] Steinstraesser L, Sand M, Steinau HU (2009) Giant VAC in a patient with extensive necrotizing fasciitis. Int J Low Extrem Wounds 8(1): 28–30

[61] Hassan Z, Mullins RF, Friedman BC et al (2010) Treating necrotizing fasciitis with or without hyperbaric oxygen therapy. Undersea Hyperb Med 37(2): 115–123

[62] Graves C, Saffle J, Morris S, Stauffer T, Edelman L (2005) Caloric requirements in patients with necrotizing fasciitis. Burns 31(1): 55–59

[63] Saffle JR, Morris SE, Edelman L (2008) Fournier's gangrene: management at a regional burn center. J Burn Care Res 29(1): 196–203

[64] Jeong HJ, Park SC, Seo IY, Rim JS (2005) Prognostic factors in Fournier gangrene. Int J Urol 12(12): 1041–1044

[65] Sada A, Misago N, Okawa T et al (2009) Necrotizing fasciitis and myonecrosis "synergistic necrotizing cellulitis" caused by Bacillus cereus. J Dermatol 36(7): 423–426

[66] Rozmaryn LM (1995) Synergistic necrotizing cellulitis in the hand of a renal dialysis patient: a case report. J Hand Surg Am 20(3): 500–501

[67] Stone HH, Martin JD, Jr (1972) Synergistic necrotizing cellulitis. Ann Surg 175(5): 702–711

[68] Adcock DM, Hicks MJ (1990) Dermatopathology of skin necrosis associated with purpura fulminans. Semin Thromb Hemost 16(4): 283–292

[69] Warner PM, Kagan RJ, Yakuboff KP et al (2003) Current management of purpura fulminans: a multicenter study. J Burn Care Rehabil 24(3): 119–126

[70] Chu DZ, Blaisdell FW (1982) Purpura fulminans. Am J Surg 143(3): 356–362

[71] Chasan PE, Hansbrough JF, Cooper ML (1992) Management of cutaneous manifestations of extensive purpura fulminans in a burn unit. J Burn Care Rehabil 13(4): 410–413

[72] Zenciroglu A, Ipek MS, Aydin M et al (2010) Purpura fulminans in a newborn infant with galactosemia. Eur J Pediatr 169(7): 903–906

[73] Demirel N, Bas AY, Okumus N, Zenciroglu A, Yarali N (2009) Severe purpura fulminans due to coexistence of homozygous protein C deficiency and homozygous methylenetetrahydrofolate reductase mutation. Pediatr Hematol Oncol 26(8): 597–600

[74] Lalitha AV, Aruna D, Prakash A, Nanjunda Swamy HM, Subba Rao SD (2009) Spectrum of purpura fulminans. Indian J Pediatr 76(1): 87–89

[75] Wharton SM, Reid CA (1998) Purpura fulminans localising to a recent burn injury. Burns 24(7): 680–682

[76] Brown DL, Greenhalgh DG, Warden GD (1998) Purpura fulminans: a disease best managed in a burn center. J Burn Care Rehabil 19(2): 119–123

[77] Gast T, Kowal-Vern A, An G, Hanumadass ML (2006) Purpura fulminans in an adult patient with Haemophilus influenzae sepsis: case report and review of the literature. J Burn Care Res 27(1): 102–107

[78] Jordan K, Kristensen K (2010) [Purpura fulminans]. Ugeskr Laeger 172(28): 2064–2065

[79] Kubo K, Chishiro T, Okamoto H, Matsushima S (2009) [Purpura fulminans (symmetric peripheral gangrene): 7-year consecutive case review in Japan]. Kansenshogaku Zasshi 83(6): 639–646

[80] Sheridan RL, Briggs SE, Remensnyder JP et al (1995) The burn unit as a resource for the management of acute nonburn conditions in children. J Burn Care Rehabil 16(1): 62–64

[81] Bichet JC, Mojallal A, Delay E, Ziad S, Foyatier JL (2003) [Surgical management of cutaneous necrosis in the purpura fulminans: report of 2 clinical cases]. Ann Chir Plast Esthet 48(4): 216–221

[82] Minhas KM, Bashir S, Sarwari AR, Parker J (2008) Pneumococcal purpura fulminans successfully treated with activated protein C. South Med J 101(10): 1046–1048

[83] Hassan Z, Mullins RF, Friedman BC et al (2008) Purpura fulminans: a case series managed at a regional burn center. J Burn Care Res 29(2): 411–415

[84] Arevalo JM, Lorente JA, Fonseca R (1998) Surgical treatment of extensive skin necrosis secondary to purpura fulminans in a patient with meningococcal sepsis. Burns 24(3): 272–274

[85] Lowery K, Shirley R, Shelley OP et al (2008) Purpura fulminans skin loss: surgical management protocols at a regional burns centre. J Plast Reconstr Aesthet Surg 61(12): 1520–1523

[86] Dalli RL, Kumar R, Kennedy P et al (2007) Toxic epidermal necrolysis/Stevens-Johnson syndrome: current trends in management. ANZ J Surg 77(8): 671–676

[87] Baby S, Doris S (1999) The Steven Johnson syndrome. A case study. Nurs J India 90(7): 149–150

[88] Wolkenstein P, Charue D, Laurent P et al (1995) Metabolic predisposition to cutaneous adverse drug reactions. Role in toxic epidermal necrolysis caused by sulfonamides and anticonvulsants. Arch Dermatol 131(5): 544–551

[89] Lissia M, Mulas P, Bulla A, Rubino C (2010) Toxic epidermal necrolysis (Lyell's disease). Burns 36(2): 152–163

[90] Gravante G, Delogu D, Marianetti M et al (2007) Toxic epidermal necrolysis and Steven Johnson syndrome: 11-years experience and outcome. Eur Rev Med Pharmacol Sci 11(2): 119–127

[91] Crosby SS, Murray KM, Marvin JA, Heimbach DM, Tartaglione TA (1986) Management of Stevens-Johnson syndrome. Clin Pharm 5(8): 682–689

[92] Auquier-Dunant A, Mockenhaupt M, Naldi L et al (2002) Correlations between clinical patterns and causes of erythema multiforme majus, Stevens-Johnson syndrome, and toxic epidermal necrolysis: results of an international prospective study. Arch Dermatol 138(8): 1019–1024

[93] Dolan P, Flowers F, Araujo O et al (1989) Toxic epidermal necrolysis. J Emerg Med (7): 65–69

[94] Lyell A (1956) Toxic epidermal necrolysis: an eruption resembling scalding of the skin. Br J Dermatol (68): 355–361

[95] Arnold HJ OR, James WD (1990) Contact dermatitis: drug eruptions. In: Andrew's diseases of the skin: Clinical dermatology. WB Saunders, Philadelphia, pp 128–130

[96] Roujeau JC (1997) Stevens-Johnson syndrome and toxic epidermal necrolysis are severity variants of the same disease which differs from erythema multiforme. J Dermatol 24(11): 726–729

[97] Roujeau J, Guillaume J, Fabre J et al (1990) Toxic epidermal necrolysis (Lyell Syndrome): incidence and drug etiology in France, 1981–1985. Arch Dermatol 126: 37–42

[98] Guillaume JC, Roujeau JC, Revuz J, Penso D, Touraine R (1987) The culprit drugs in 87 cases of toxic epidermal necrolysis (Lyell's syndrome). Arch Dermatol 123(9): 1166–1170

[99] Hawk RJ, Storer JS, Daum RS (1985) Toxic epidermal necrolysis in a 6-week-old infant. Pediatr Dermatol 2(3): 197–200

[100] Roujeau JC, Kelly JP, Naldi L et al (1995) Medication use and the risk of Stevens-Johnson syndrome or toxic epidermal necrolysis. N Engl J Med 333(24): 1600–1607

[101] Rzany B, Mockenhaupt M, Stocker U, Hamouda O, Schopf E (1993) Incidence of Stevens-Johnson syndrome and toxic epidermal necrolysis in patients with the acquired immunodeficiency syndrome in Germany. Arch Dermatol 129(8): 1059

[102] Fritsch P, Sidoroff A (2000) Drug-induced Stevens-Johnson syndrom/toxic epidermal necrolysis. Am J Clin Dermatol (1): 349–360

[103] Kaufmann D (1991) Epidemiologic approaches to the study of toxic epidermal necrolysis. J Invest Dermatol (102): 31S-33S

[104] Schopf E, Stuhmer A, Rzany B et al (1991) Toxic epidermal necrolysis and Stevens-Johnson syndrome. An epidemiologic study from West Germany. Arch Dermatol 127(6): 839–842

[105] Shear NH, Spielberg SP, Grant DM, Tang BK, Kalow W (1986) Differences in metabolism of sulfonamides predisposing to idiosyncratic toxicity. Ann Intern Med 105(2): 179–184

[106] Ruiz-Maldonado R (1985) Acute disseminated epidermal necrosis types 1,2 and 3: a study of sixty cases. J Am Acad Dermatol 13: 623–635

[107] Becker D (1998) Toxic epidermal necrolysis. Lancet 351: 1417–1419

[108] Oplatek A, Brown K, Sen S et al (2006) Long-term follow-up of patients treated for toxic epidermal necrolysis. J Burn Care Res 27(1): 26–33

[109] Paquet P, Pierard GE (1997) Erythema multiforme and toxic epidermal necrolysis: a comparative study. Am J Dermatopathol 19(2): 127–132

[110] Bastuji-Garin S, Fouchard N, Bertocchi M et al (2000) SCORTEN: a severity-of-illness score for toxic epidermal necrolysis. J Invest Dermatol 115(2): 149–153

[111] Palmieri TL, Greenhalgh DG, Saffle JR et al (2002) A multicenter review of toxic epidermal necrolysis treated in U. S. burn centers at the end of the twentieth century. J Burn Care Rehabil 23(2): 87–96

[112] Garcia-Doval I, LeCleach L, Bocquet H, Otero XL, Roujeau JC (2000) Toxic epidermal necrolysis and Stevens-Johnson syndrome: does early withdrawal of causative drugs decrease the risk of death? Arch Dermatol 136(3): 323–327

[113] Demling RH, Ellerbe S, Lowe NJ (1978) Burn unit management of toxic epidermal necrolysis. Arch Surg 113(6): 758–759

[114] Herndon DN (1995) Toxic epidermal necrolysis: a systemic and dermatologic disorder best treated with standard treatment protocols in burn intensive care units without the prolonged use of corticosteroids. J Am Coll Surg 180(3): 340–342

[115] Kelemen JJ, 3rd, Cioffi WG, McManus WF, Mason AD, Jr, Pruitt BA, Jr (1995) Burn center care for patients with toxic epidermal necrolysis. J Am Coll Surg 180(3): 273–278

[116] Wolkenstein P, Latarjet J, Roujeau JC et al (1998) Randomised comparison of thalidomide versus placebo in toxic epidermal necrolysis. Lancet 352(9140): 1586–1589

[117] Viard I, Wehrli P, Bullani R et al (1998) Inhibition of toxic epidermal necrolysis by blockade of CD95 with human intravenous immunoglobulin. Science 282(5388): 490–493

[118] Prins C, Kerdel FA, Padilla RS et al (2003) Treatment of toxic epidermal necrolysis with high-dose intravenous immunoglobulins: multicenter retrospective analysis of 48 consecutive cases. Arch Dermatol 139(1): 26–32

[119] Stella M, Cassano P, Bollero D, Clemente A, Giorio G (2001) Toxic epidermal necrolysis treated with intravenous high-dose immunoglobulins: our experience. Dermatology 203(1): 45–49

[120] Trent JT, Kirsner RS, Romanelli P, Kerdel FA (2003) Analysis of intravenous immunoglobulin for the treatment of toxic epidermal necrolysis using SCORTEN: The University of Miami Experience. Arch Dermatol 139(1): 39–43

[121] Tristani-Firouzi P, Petersen MJ, Saffle JR, Morris SE, Zone JJ (2002) Treatment of toxic epidermal necrolysis with intravenous immunoglobulin in children. J Am Acad Dermatol 47(4): 548–552

[122] Bachot N, Revuz J, Roujeau JC (2003) Intravenous immunoglobulin treatment for Stevens-Johnson syndrome and toxic epidermal necrolysis: a prospective noncomparative study showing no benefit on mortality or progression. Arch Dermatol 139(1): 33–36

[123] Brown KM, Silver GM, Halerz M et al (2004) Toxic epidermal necrolysis: does immunoglobulin make a difference? J Burn Care Rehabil 25(1): 81–88

[124] Shortt R, Gomez M, Mittman N, Cartotto R (2004) Intravenous immunoglobulin does not improve outcome in toxic epidermal necrolysis. J Burn Care Rehabil 25(3): 246–255

Correspondence: Richard L. Gamelli, M.D. FACS, Stritch School of Medicine – 420 Loyola University Medical Center 2160 South First Avenue Maywood, IL 60153, USA, E-mail: rgamell@lumc.edu

# Frostbite

Paul Kraincuk[1], Maike Keck[2], David Lumenta[2], Lars-Peter Kamolz[2]

[1]Universitätsklinik für Anästhesie, Allgemeine Intensivmedizin und Schmerztherapie, Vienna, Austria,
[2]Universitätsklinik für Chirurgie, Vienna, Austria

Frostbite (*congelatio* in medical terminology) is the medical condition, where a damage is caused to skin and other tissues due to extreme cold. Frostbite is most likely to happen in body parts farthest from the heart and those with large exposed areas. The initial stages of frostbite are sometimes called "frostnip".

## Classification

Cold injuries can result in a number of distinct conditions including: Frostnip is a superficial cooling of tissues without cellular destruction [1]. Chilblains are superficial ulcers of the skin that occur when a predisposed individual is repeatedly exposed to cold. Frostbite, on the other hand, involves tissue destruction. Hypothermia is a decrease in core body temperature below 35 C. Trench foot or immersion foot is due to repetitive exposure to wet non-freezing temperatures.

### Mechanism

At or below 0 °C (32 °F), blood vessels close to the skin start to constrict. The same response may also be a result of exposure to high winds. This constriction helps to preserve core body temperature. In extreme cold, or when the body is exposed to cold for long periods, this protective strategy can reduce blood flow in some areas of the body to dangerously low levels. This lack of blood leads to the eventual freezing and death of skin tissue in the affected areas. There are four degrees of frostbite. Each of these degrees has varying degrees of pain [2].

### First degree

This is called frostnip and this only affects the surface of the skin, which is frozen. On onset there is itching and pain, and then the skin develops white and yellow patches and becomes numb. The area affected by frostnip usually does not become permanently damaged as only the skin's top layers are affected. Long-term hypersensitivity to both heat and cold can sometimes happen after suffering from frostnip.

### Second degree

If freezing continues, the skin may freeze and harden, but the deep tissues are not affected and remain soft and normal. Second-degree injury usually blisters 1–2 days after becoming frozen. The blisters may become hard and blackened, but usually appear worse than they are. Most of the injuries heal in one month but the area may become permanently sensitive to both heat and cold.

## Third and fourth degrees

If the area freezes further, deep frostbite occurs. The muscles, tendons, blood vessels, and nerves will all freeze. The skin is hard, it feels waxy, and use of the area is lost temporarily, in severe cases permanently. The deep frostbite results in areas of purplish blisters, which turn black and, which are generally blood-filled. Nerve damage in the area can result in a loss of feeling. This extreme frostbite may result in fingers and toes being amputated, if the area becomes infected. If the frostbite has gone on untreated they may fall off. The damage done to the area by the freezing process of the frostbite may take several months to find out and this often delays surgery to remove the dead tissue [3].

### Risk factors

Risk factors for frostbite include using beta-blockers and having conditions such as diabetes and peripheral neuropathy.

### Causes

Factors that contribute to frostbite include extreme cold, inadequate clothing, wet clothes, wind chill, and poor circulation. Tight clothing or boots, cramped positions and fatigue can cause poor circulation. Certain medications, smoking, alcohol use, and diseases that affect the blood vessels like diabetes can do the same. Liquid nitrogen and other cryogenic liquids can cause frostbite to people working in chemical laboratories even under brief exposure. If the weather is very cold and it is windy, wind chill can greatly reduce the time it takes for frostbite to set in. Diabetes can also sometimes lead to frostbite, if diabetics take trips to ice-cold places [4].

### Diagnosis

Plain radiographs, angiography, laser doppler, digital plethysmography, infrared thermography, magnetic resonance imaging, magnetic resonance angiography and triple phase bone scanning can help to predict the severity of frostbite injuries. The most promising studies have used triple phase bone scanning [5] and MRI/MRA [6]. Triple phase bone scanning using 99technetium assesses tissue viability in an effort to allow early debridement of soft tissue and early coverage of ischaemic bony structures [7].

### Treatment

Treatment of frostbite centers on rewarming (and possibly thawing) of the affected tissue. The decision to thaw is based on proximity to a stable, warm environment. If rewarmed tissue ends up refreezing, more damage to tissue will be done. Excessive movement of frostbitten tissue can cause ice crystals that have formed in the tissue to do further damage. Splinting and/or wrapping frostbitten extremities is therefore recommended to prevent such movement. For this reason, rubbing, massaging, shaking, or otherwise applying physical force to frostbitten tissues in an attempt to rewarm them can be harmful [8]. Caution should be taken not to rapidly warm up the affected area until further refreezing is prevented. Warming can be achieved in one of two ways.

### Rewarming

Passive rewarming [9] involves using body heat or ambient room temperature to aid the person's body in rewarming itself. This includes wrapping in blankets or moving to a warmer environment [10]. Active rewarming [9] is the direct addition of heat to a person, usually in addition to the treatments included in passive rewarming. Active rewarming requires more equipment and therefore may be difficult to perform in the prehospital environment [8]. When performed, active rewarming seeks to warm the injured tissues as quickly as possible without burning them. This is desirable as the faster tissue is thawed, the less tissue damage occurs [8]. Active rewarming is usually achieved by immersing the injured tissue in a water-bath that is held between 40–42 °C. Warming of peripheral tissues can increase blood flow from these areas back to the bodies' core. This may produce a degree in the bodies' core temperature and increase the risk of cardiac dysrhythmias [11].

## Surgery

Debridement and or amputation of necrotic tissue are usually delayed. This has led to the adage *"Frozen in January, amputate in July"* [12]. Indications for surgical debridement are unreliable until 2–3 weeks postwarming. Debridement should be deferred until that point unless tissue is causing a life-threatening condition e. g. infection or gangrene [13].

It is difficult to predict at initial presentation what the final demarcation between viable and necrotic tissue will be. Therefor early surgery usually is contraindicated in frostbite, because the nonviable tissue requires time to demarcate. Older series show that debridement prior to 2–3 weeks postwarming significantly increases the amount of viable tissue removed and is harmful to the patient, resulting in an increased amputation rate, mortality, and morbidity.

After a period of watchful waiting commonly accepted indications for surgical debridement include clearly necrotic or nonfunctional tissue. The absence of accurate radiologic assessment of viability has meant that the appropriate level of amputation is not clear until the tissue declares itself. Some authors are now advocating a more aggressive approach with the advent of technetium scintigraphy and advancing role of magnetic resonance imaging [14–17]. Preliminary results suggest that improved imaging may lead to reduction in length of hospital stay and still allow maximum stump length preservation.

The functional outcome of any surgery needs to be considered and ideally, where major limb loss is foreseen, the early involvement of a multidisciplinary rehabilitation team will produce better long term functional results [18].

## Sympathectomy

The role of sympathectomy has yielded mixed results. Sympathectomy performed within the first few hours of injury is said to increase oedema formation and leads to increased tissue destruction. However if performed 24–48h after injury it is thought to decrease tissue loss and to accelerate resolution of oedema. Sympathectomy can also serve as a useful treatment in the late sequelae of frostbite such as hyperhidrosis and pain due to vasospasm [19]. However, since a sympathectomy is irreversible, great caution should be exercised when considering its use in frostbite.

## Vasodilators

Iloprost, a stable metabolite of prostacyclin, is a powerful vasodilator and has been used in the treatment of frostbite with some success [20]. It is used in arterial surgery to mimic the effect of a sympathectomy. Pentoxifyllin is considered to lower pathologically increased levels of fibrinogen yielding some promising results in human trials [21]. Both drugs may protect against damage of the vascular endothelium, improve tissue perfusion and therefore limit tissue damage caused by frostbite. The a-blocker buflomedil has been used to increase peripheral blood flow [22].

## tPA

A small study assessing the effectiveness of tPA in reducing amputation rates in frostbite has recently been reported by Bruen et al. Among the six patients who received tPA within 24h of injury, six of 59 (10%) affected fingers or toes were amputated, compared with 97 of 234 (41%) among those who did not receive tPA. It is postulated that rapid clearance of the microvasculature improves tissue salvage [23].

## Escharotomy and fasciotomy

Escharotomy and fasciotomy have no proven prophylactic role in the management of frostbite. Ischemic injury in frostbite is most often caused by vascular compromise from thrombosis and not by compression from edematous tissue, making decompression unnecessary. Escharotomy or fasciotomy may be indicated in the early phase if compartment syndrome develops [24, 25].

### Prognosis

A number of long-term squeal can occur after frostbite. These include: transient or permanent changes in sensation, electric shocks, increased sweating, cancers, and bone destruction / arthritis in the area affected [26]. Tissue that has recovered from frostbite is more susceptible to further injury and this needs to be kept in mind when advising individuals about a return to environments where they may be at risk.

*Research*

Evidence is insufficient to determine whether or not hyperbaric oxygen therapy as an adjunctive treatment can assist in tissue salvage [26].There have been case reports but few actual research studies to show the effectiveness [27–31]. Medical sympathectomy using intravenous reserpine has also been attempted with limited success [26].

# References

[1] Marx J (2010) Rosen's emergency medicine: concepts and clinical practice, 7th edn. Mosby/Elsevier, Philadelphia, PA, p 1862, ISBN 9 780 323 054 720

[2] Frostbite, eMedicineHealth.com, http://www.emedicinehealth.com/frostbite/article_em.htm, retrieved 4/3/10

[3] Definition of Frostbite, MedicineNet.com, http://www.medterms.com/script/main/art. asp? articlekey=3522, retrieved 4/3/10

[4] Perez E (2006) MD. National Institute of Health. Retrieved May 18, 2006

[5] Bhatnagar A, Sarker BB, Sawroop K et al (2002) Diagnosis, characterisation and evaluation of treatment response of frostbite using pertechnetate scintigraphy: a prospective study. Eur J Nucl Med 29: 170–175

[6] Barker JR, Haws MJ, Brown RE et al (1997) Magnetic resonance imaging of severe frostbite injuries. Ann Plast Surg 38: 275–279

[7] Greenwald D, Cooper B, Gottlieb L (1998) An algorithm for early aggressive treatment of frostbite with limb salvage directed by triple-phase scanning. Plast Reconstr Surg 102: 1069–1074

[8] Mistovich J, Haffen B, Karren K (2004) Prehospital emergency care. Pearson Education, Upsaddle River, NJ, pp 506, ISBN 0–13–049 288–4

[9] Mistovich J, Haffen B, Karren K (2004) Prehospital emergency care. Pearson Education, Upsaddle River, NJ, p 504, ISBN 0–13–049 288–4

[10] Roche-Nagle G, Murphy D, Collins A, Sheehan S (2008) Frostbite: management options. Eur J Emerg Med 15 (3): 173–175, doi:10 1097/MEJ.0b013e3282bf6ed0] PMID 184 609Retrieved 2008–06–30

[11] Marx J (2010) Rosen's emergency medicine: concepts and clinical practice 7th edition. Mosby/Elsevier, Philadelphia, PA, p 1864, ISBN 9 780 323 054 720

[12] Golant A, Nord RM, Paksima N, Posner MA (2008) Cold exposure injuries to the extremities. J Am Acad Orthop Surg 16 (12): 704–715, PMID 19 056 919

[13] McGillion R (2005) Frostbite: case report, practical summary of ED treatment. J Emerg Nurs 31 (5): 500–502, doi:10 1016/j. jen.2005.07.0[02] PMID 16 198 741

[14] Salimi Z (1985) Frostbite: assessment of tissue viability by scintigraphy. Postgrad Med 77: 133–134

[15] Mehta RC, Wilson MA (1989) Frostbite injury: prediction of tissue viability with triple-phase bone scanning. Radiology 170: 511–514

[16] Salimi Z, Wolverson MK, Herbold DR, Vas W (1986) Frostbite: experimental assessment of tissue damage using Tc-99 m pyrophosphate. Radiology 161: 227–231

[17] Barker JR, Haws MJ, Brown RE, Kucan JO, Moore WD (1997) Magnetic resonance imaging of severe frostbite. Ann Plast Surg 38: 275–279

[18] Golant A, Nord RM, Paksima N, Posner MA (2008) Cold exposure injuries to the extremities. J Am Acad Orthop Surg 16 (12): 704–715

[19] Taylor MS(1999) Lumbar epidural sympathectomy for frostbite injuries of the feet. Mil Med 164: 566–567

[20] Cauchy E, Cheguillaume B, Chetaille E (2011) A controlled trial of a prostacyclin and rt-PA in the treatment of severe frostbite. N Engl J Med 364(2): 189–190. PMID: 21226604

[21] Hödl S (2005) Treatment of freezing injury. Wien Med Wochenschr 155 (7–8): 199–203

[22] Cauchy E, Chetaille E, Marchand V et al (2001) Retrospective study of 70 cases of severe frostbite lesions: a proposed new classification scheme. Wild Envir Med 12: 248–255

[23] Bruen KJ, Ballard JR, Morris SE et al (2007) Reduction of the incidence of amputation in frostbite injury with thrombolytic therapy. Arch Surg 142: 546–551

[24] Britt LD, Dascombe WH, Rodriguez A (1991) New horizons in management of hypothermia and frostbite injury. Surg Clin North Am 71: 345–370

[25] McCauley RL, Hing DN, Robson MC, Heggers JP (1983) Frostbite injuries: a rational approach based on the pathophysiology. J Trauma 23: 143–147

[26] Marx J (2010) Rosen's emergency medicine: concepts and clinical practice 7th edition. Mosby/Elsevier, Philadelphia, PA, p 1866, ISBN 9 780 323 054 720

[27] Finderle Z, Cankar K (2002) Delayed treatment of frostbite injury with hyperbaric oxygen therapy: a case report. Aviat Space Environ Med 73 (4): 392–394, PMID 11 952 063

[28] Folio LR, Arkin K, Butler WP (2007) Frostbite in a mountain climber treated with hyperbaric oxygen: case report. Mil Med 172 (5): 560–563, PMID 17 521 112

[29] Gage AA, Ishikawa H, Winter PM (1970)Experimental frostbite. The effect of hyperbaric oxygenation on tissue survival. Cryobiology 7 (1): 1–8] doi:10 1016/0011–2240 (70)90 038–6, PMID 54 750[96] Retrieved 2008–06–30

[30] Weaver LK, Greenway L, Elliot CG (1988) Controlled frostbite injury to mice: outcome of hyperbaric oxygen therapy. J Hyperbaric Med 3 (1): 35–44, Retrieved 2008–06–30

[31] Ay H, Uzun G, Yildiz S, Solmazgul E, Dundar K, Qyrdedi T, Yildirim I, Gumus T (2005) The treatment of deep frostbite of both feet in two patients with hyperbaric oxygen. (abstract). Undersea Hyperb Med 32 (1 [Suppl]), ISSN 1066–29[36] OCLC 269 155[85] Retrieved 2008–06–30

Correspondence: Kraincuk Paul, Ass.-Prof. Dr. med. univ., Universitätsklinik für Anästhesie, Allgemeine Intensivmedizin und Schmerztherapie, Währinger Gürtel 18–20, 1090 Wien, Austria, E-mail: paul.kraincuk@meduniwien.ac.at

# Subject index